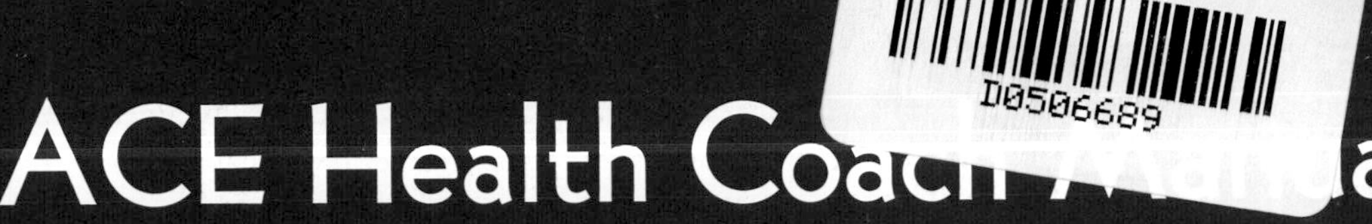

ACE Health Coach Manual

The Ultimate Guide to Wellness, Fitness, & Lifestyle Change

American Council on Exercise®

Editors
Cedric X. Bryant, Ph.D., FACSM
Daniel J. Green
Sabrena Jo, M.S.

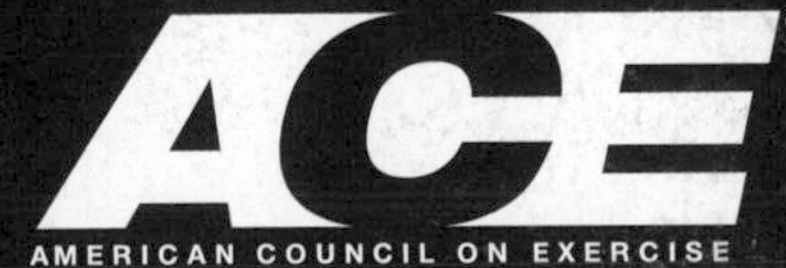

Library of Congress Catalog Card Number: 2012946419

ISBN 978-1-890720-45-2

Printed in the United States of America

D E F G

Distributed by:
American Council on Exercise
4851 Paramount Drive
San Diego, CA 92123
(858) 576-6500
FAX: (858) 576-6464
ACEfitness.org

Project Editor: Daniel J. Green
Technical Editors: Cedric X. Bryant, Ph.D., and Sabrena Jo, M.S.
Art Direction: Karen McGuire
Cover Design: Ian Jensen
Production: Nancy Garcia
Photography: Dennis Covey, Rob Andrew, Eduardo Acorda
Stock photo images: iStock, Thinkstock
Anatomical Illustrations: James Staunton
Index: Kathi Unger
Chapter Models: Lisa Acevedo, Doug Balzarini, Angel Chelik, Linda S. Chemaly, Michael Davis, Patricia A. Davis, Jetta Starr Eveland, Helen Koules, Todd Galati, Nancy Garcia, Robert Garcia, Valerie O'Neill, Michael Marsh, Brittany McCall, Alexandra Morrison, Mike Osuna, Anthony Padilla, Jesse Patton, Gisele Pineda, Pam Wright

Acknowledgments:
Thanks to the entire American Council on Exercise staff for their support and guidance through the process of creating this manual.

NOTICE

The fitness industry is ever-changing. As new research and clinical experience broaden our knowledge, changes in programming and standards are required. The authors and the publisher of this work have checked with sources believed to be reliable in their efforts to provide information that is complete and generally in accord with the standards accepted at the time of publication. However, in view of the possibility of human error or changes in industry standards, neither the authors nor the publisher nor any other party who has been involved in the preparation or publication of this work warrants that the information contained herein is in every respect accurate or complete, and they are not responsible for any errors or omissions or the results obtained from the use of such information. Readers are encouraged to confirm the information contained herein with other sources.

P16-015

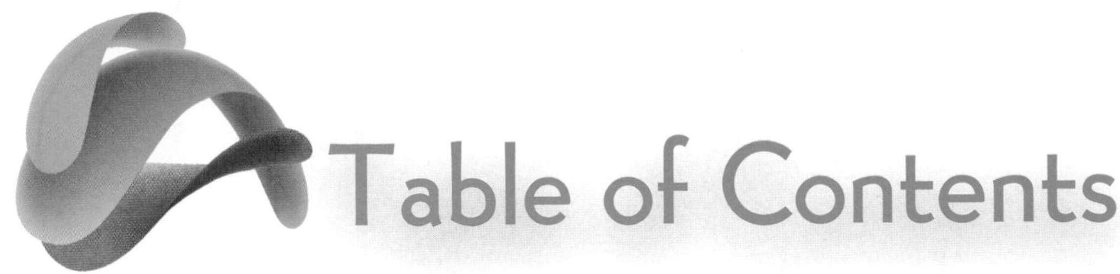

Table of Contents

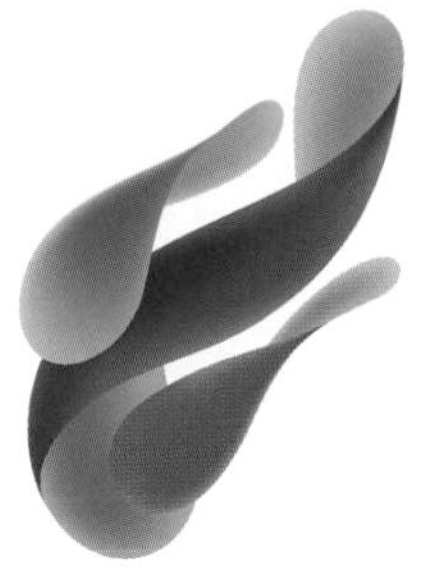

Reviewers

Liz Applegate, Ph.D., is the director of sports nutrition and a faculty member for the Nutrition Department at the University of California, Davis, where she has earned several teaching honors including the 2010 Distinguished Undergraduate Teaching Award. She is the author of several books, including *Nutrition Basics for Better Health and Performance* and *Encyclopedia of Sports and Fitness Nutrition.* She has written more than 300 articles for national magazines and is nutrition editor and columnist for *Runner's World* magazine. She frequently serves as a keynote speaker at industry, athletic, and scientific meetings, and as a consultant to professional athletes.

Mary Bratcher, M.A., is the co-creator of The BioMechanics Method, an educational program that teaches allied health and fitness professionals how to help people alleviate chronic joint and muscle pain through a combination of structural assessment, movement analysis, corrective exercise, and life coaching. She is also an educator, content developer, subject matter expert, committee member, and board member for numerous health and fitness organizations including the American Council on Exercise, PTA Global, PTontheNet, and IDEA Health and Fitness Association.

Mark Jackman, Ph.D., owns Life Signs℠, where for 15 years he has specialized in fitness programs for clients with health conditions or needing weight management. He obtained his doctorate at Duke University, where he did research on occupational stress and health, and has been an upper-level strategic planning manager n the health insurance industry. He is an ACE-certified Personal Trainer, Advanced Health & Fitness Specialist, and Health Coach (formerly Lifestyle & Weight Management Coach), in addition to holding a certification from the American Academy of Health, Fitness, and Rehabilitation Professionals as a Medical Exercise Specialist. He has served on ACE item writing and role delineation panels.

Len Kravitz, Ph.D., is the program coordinator of exercise science and researcher at the University of New Mexico, where he won the "Outstanding Teacher of the Year" award. Dr. Kravitz was honored with the 2009 Canadian Fitness Professional "Specialty Presenter of the Year" award and chosen as the American Council on Exercise 2006 "Fitness Educator of the Year." He also has received the prestigious Canadian Fitness Professional "Lifetime Achievement Award."

Michael R. Mantell, Ph.D., earned his Ph.D. at the University of Pennsylvania and his M.S. at Hahnemann Medical College, where he wrote his thesis on the psychological aspects of obesity. His career includes serving as the Chief Psychologist for Children's Hospital in San Diego and as the founding Chief Psychologist for the San Diego Police Department. Dr. Mantell is a member of the Scientific Advisory Board of the International Council on Active Aging, the Chief Behavior Science Consultant to the Premier Fitness Camp at Omni La Costa, a best-selling author of two books, including the 1988 original *Don't Sweat the Small Stuff, P.S. It's All Small Stuff,* an international behavior science fitness keynote speaker, an advisor to numerous fitness-health organizations, and is featured in many media broadcasts and worldwide fitness publications. He has been featured on Oprah, Good Morning America, the Today Show, and has been a contributor to many major news organizations including Fox and ABC News. Dr. Mantell is a nationally sought after behavioral science coach for business leaders, elite amateur and professional athletes, individuals, and families. He is included in the greatist.com's 2013 list of "The 100 Most Influential People in Health and Fitness."

Christopher R. Mohr, Ph.D., R.D., is the co-owner of Mohr Results, Inc., a nutrition consulting company that works with media outlets and corporations including the Nordic Naturals, SOYJOY, Gatorade, Under Armour, and others. Dr. Mohr is the consulting sports nutritionist for the Cincinnati Bengals. He has authored or co-authored several books, including *The New York Times* bestseller *LL Cool J's Platinum Body* with celebrity LL Cool J. He has written more than 500 articles for consumer publications, such as *Men's Fitness, Weight Watchers, Men's Health,* and *Muscle and Fitness*. Dr. Mohr has bachelor's and master's degrees in nutrition from Penn State University and the University of Massachusetts, respectively. He received his Ph.D. in exercise physiology from the University of Pittsburgh and is also a registered dietitian.

Jack Raglin, Ph.D., FACSM, is a professor and the director of graduate studies of the Department of Kinesiology in the School of Public Health at Indiana University-Bloomington. He is a Fellow in the American Psychological Association, the American College of Sports Medicine, and the American Academy of Kinesiology. Dr. Raglin's research involves integrating the use of psychological and physiological variables to examine various issues in sport and exercise, including overtraining, pre-competition anxiety, performance, and the relationship between exercise and mental health.

Kelly Spivey, Ph.D., has a doctorate in Natural Health and a master's degree in Fitness Management. She has an extensive career in the health and fitness arena, ranging from cardiopulmonary rehabilitation manager to owner/operator of three medically based fitness centers. Dr. Spivey is a Territory Manager for Freemotion Fitness, works with the University of Tampa in the Health Science & Human Performance Department, and serves as a subject matter expert for ACE. She has authored chapters in both the *ACE Personal Trainer Manual* and the *ACE Advanced Health & Fitness Specialist Manual.*

David K. Stotlar, Ed.D., serves as the director of the School of Sport & Exercise Science at the University of Northern Colorado. He teaches on the faculty in the areas of sport management and sport marketing, has had more than 90 articles published in professional journals, and has written more than 50 chapters in various textbooks and books on sport, fitness, and physical education.

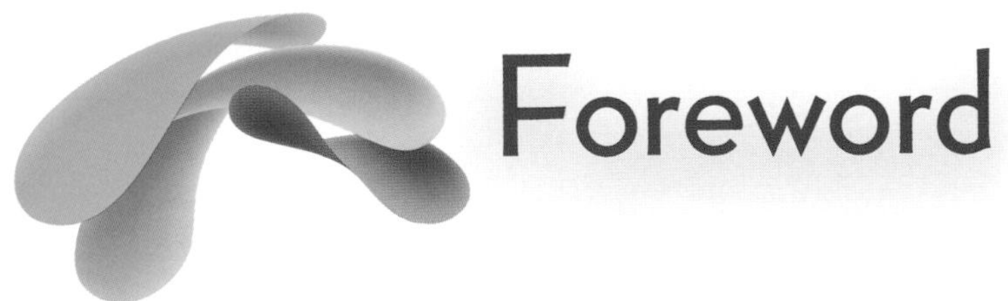

Foreword

The American Council on Exercise is proud to introduce the *ACE Health Coach Manual* and certification, the next evolution in our dedication to educating consumers about the critical need to regularly engage in physical activity. Like ACE-certified Health Coaches, we as an organization seek to inspire, motivate, and encourage Americans to make healthy living an integral part of our society, and this commitment extends beyond physical activity to balanced nutrition, behavioral change, and lifelong weight management. ACE has set for itself the lofty goal of being the centerpiece of the effort to eliminate the obesity epidemic among Americans and around the world. To achieve this goal, ACE has partnered with a number of well-respected organizations, ranging from the International Association of Fire Fighters and AARP to the International Health, Racquet and Sportsclub Association (IHRSA) and even the White House's Joining Forces program. Inherent in this team-building approach is the understanding that no single entity can accomplish such a lofty and important goal alone.

Health coaches are likely to find themselves in a similar situation, albeit on a smaller scale. Health coaches seek to fight the obesity epidemic on a daily basis, from one client to the next. While ACE is forming national and international coalitions to work together on a grand scale, health coaches should form local teams and professional networks that enable them to give each and every client the absolute best chance for success. Out of respect for scope for practice and a desire to facilitate lifelong behavioral change among their clients, the best health coaches form networks of like-minded professionals in their communities. ACE, of course, would like to support you in these efforts, which is why this manual includes chapters on taking "A Team Approach to Health Coaching" and "Helping Clients Establish Self-reliance," the latter of which covers the essential step of enabling clients to experience and maintain success on their own, returning to see members of "their team" as needed.

Much has changed in the fitness industry since 1996—when ACE first introduced the *ACE Lifestyle & Weight Management Consultant Manual* and certification, the precursor to the ACE Health Coach program—but one thing remains constant: it is essential that fitness and allied-health professionals collaboratively find effective ways to reach and motivate the millions of Americans who do not get enough regular physical activity, do not eat healthfully, and have a less-than-optimal quality of life. And while individual health coaches can have a tremendous impact on the lives of their clients, it will take true teamwork to create global change. We are happy that you have chosen to become part of the ACE team, and we are thrilled to become a part of yours.

Scott Goudeseune
President and CEO
American Council on Exercise

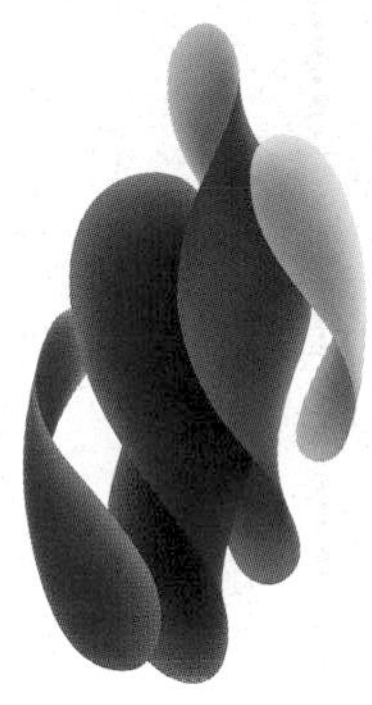

Introduction

As with all manuals from American Council on Exercise, the *ACE Health Coach Manual* offers the most current, complete picture of the instructional techniques and professional responsibilities that ACE-certified Health Coaches need to teach their clients to make meaningful and lasting behavioral changes. This text takes an application-based, interactive approach to presenting this material, which should enable readers to more easily turn theoretical concepts into practical tips. For example, in Chapter 5: Connection Through Communication, the reader will learn about various personality types and how to apply that understanding to improve his or her communication skills. But before moving on to reading subsequent sections, the reader is asked to pause to "Think It Through" by considering a client scenario that brings this concept to life. If, as you work your way through this textbook, you take advantage of these application-based tools, you will not only be more prepared to sit for the certification exam, but also to thrive in real-world situations once you become an ACE-certified fitness professional.

The *ACE Health Coach Manual* is divided into six sections. **Section I: Introduction** kicks off the manual with three chapters that provide a foundational understanding of what it means to be a "coach." Chapter 1 provides an introduction to coaching by briefly outlining many of the concepts and theories that are expanded upon in subsequent chapters, including communication skills, problem-solving models, and interpersonal sensitivity and respect. Chapter 2 is all about teamwork—how to identify appropriate team members as well as techniques for reaching out and making that connection to establish a professional network. Chapter 3 presents several behavioral theory models and explains various determinants of behavior. By understanding and utilizing these concepts, health coaches can maximize clients' adherence and motivation over the long haul.

The two chapters that make up **Section II: Strategies for Effective Communication** teach readers how to make that all-important connection with clients. If a health coach is unable to establish and maintain rapport with his or her clients, all the knowledge in the world about nutritional and exercise science will not make a difference, as clients will not be inspired to continue with the program. From establishing self-efficacy and making sure the physical environment is conducive to lifestyle change to having developed the appropriate listening and questioning skills, it is up to the health coach to maintain an ongoing sense of connection and rapport with each of his or her clients.

Section III: Nutritional and Physiological Sciences begins with an explanation of the basics of nutrition, including the micro- and macronutrients and the processes of digestion and absorption. This is followed by a chapter teaching readers to apply this knowledge through the use of federal dietary recommendations. In addition, this chapter features sections on the importance of nutrition for everyone from elite athletes to children, older adults, and individuals with special considerations, such as diabetes, obesity, and eating disorders. This section continues with an explanation of the physiology of obesity, including the health consequences and etiology of obesity and the effects of genetic and environmental factors. Section III concludes with a discussion of current concepts in weight management. This chapter covers several popular diets, as well as pharmacological agents for weight loss, weight-loss surgery, and a detailed discussion of various eating disorders.

Now that you have gained essential insight into communication techniques, rapport-building, and nutritional science, it is time to begin working with clients. **Section IV: Screening and Assessment** teaches readers how to assess the various elements of a client's health status—physical health, psychological health, exercise readiness, physical fitness, and readiness to change. From body composition to lower-body muscular endurance, the assessments in this section of the manual will enable readers to introduce appropriate lifestyle changes to elicit long-term success.

Once a client has undergone the various assessments and been cleared to exercise, it is time to move on to **Section IV: Program Design and Implementation.** This section, which includes seven chapters, forms the heart of this manual. After explaining the importance of goal-setting and offering tips for doing so effectively, this section offers a thorough discussion of lifestyle modification and behavioral change, which of course lie at the very core of what a health coach does in daily practice. Several tools used in nutritional programming—food diaries, 24-hour recalls, and food-frequency questionnaires among them—are outlined, along with the pros and cons of each. There are two chapters on exercise programming—the first presents general considerations and guidelines and the second delves deeply into the process of categorizing clients along the function–health–fitness–performance continuum of the ACE Integrated Fitness Training® Model and creating an individualized exercise program. The next chapter focuses on helping clients establish self-reliance. This chapter explains the importance of cultivating self-reliance in clients, as this is the only way to ensure long-term weight-management success. Finally, this section concludes with a series of case studies that pull together everything learned thus far in the manual.

The final section—**Section VI: Legal, Professional, and Ethical Responsibilities**—presents such topics as one's status as an employee versus independent contractor, scope of practice, insurance needs, and legal concepts and defenses. It is essential that health coaches not neglect this aspect of the profession.

We are confident that the information presented in this manual will enhance the quality of service provided by health coaches. Ultimately, the true goal—which ACE shares with each of our certified professionals—is to empower people to live their most fit lives. We sincerely hope that this book serves you well in your efforts.

Cedric X. Bryant, Ph.D.
Chief Science Officer

Daniel J. Green
Project Editor

Sabrena Jo, M.S.
Exercise Scientist

SECTION I

INTRODUCTION

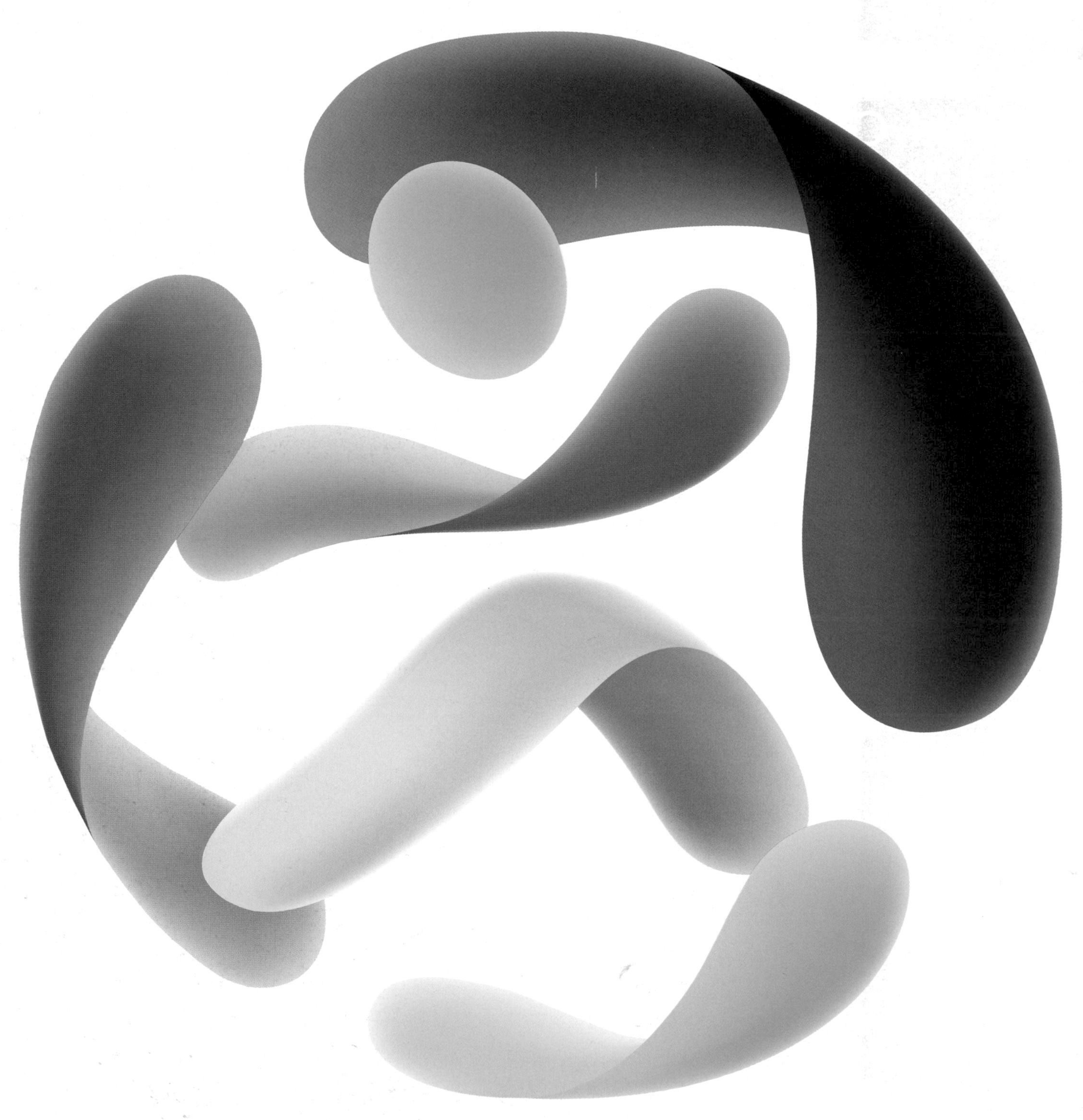

Chapter 1
Introduction to Health Coaching

Chapter 2
A Team Approach to Health Coaching

Chapter 3
Health Behavior Sciences

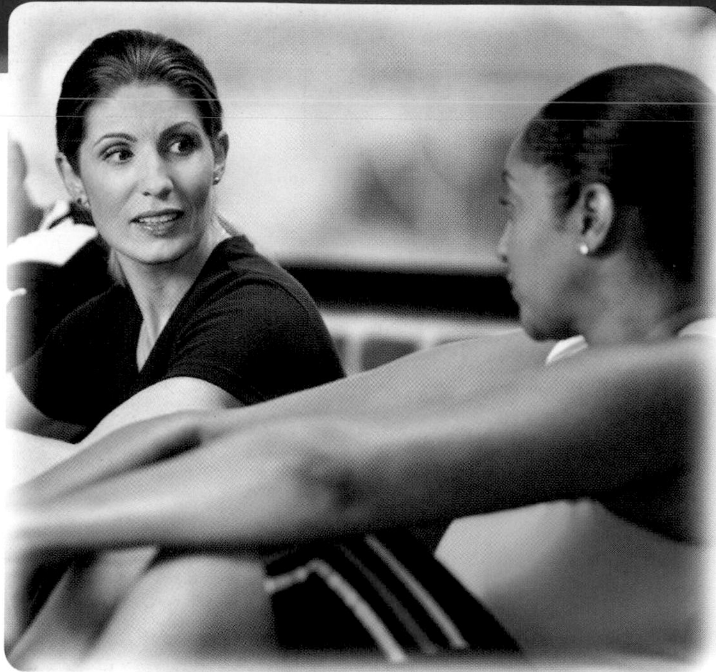

IN THIS CHAPTER:

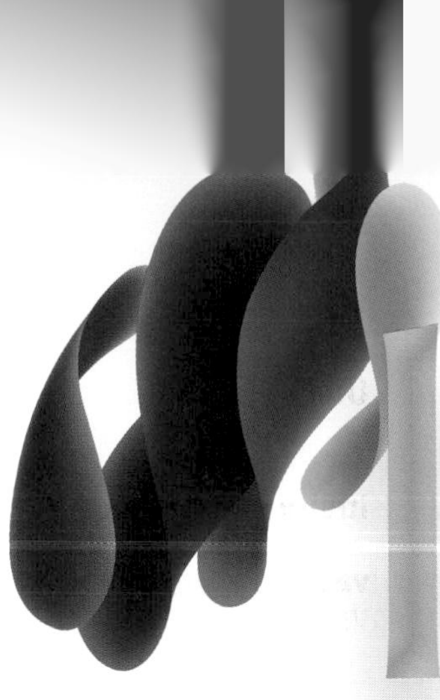

Introduction to Health Coaching

MICHAEL R. MANTELL

Michael R. Mantell, Ph.D., earned his Ph.D. at the University of Pennsylvania and his M.S. at Hahnemann Medical College, where he wrote his thesis on the psychological aspects of obesity. His career includes serving as the Chief Psychologist for Children's Hospital in San Diego and as the founding Chief Psychologist for the San Diego Police Department. Dr. Mantell is a member of the Scientific Advisory Board of the International Council on Active Aging, the Chief Behavior Science Consultant to the Premier Fitness Camp at Omni La Costa, a best-selling author of two books, including the 1988 original Don't Sweat the Small Stuff, P.S. It's All Small Stuff, *an international behavior science fitness keynote speaker, an advisor to numerous fitness-health organizations, and is featured in many media broadcasts and worldwide fitness publications. He has been featured on Oprah, Good Morning America, the Today Show, and has been a contributor to many major news organizations including Fox and ABC News. Dr. Mantell is a nationally sought after behavioral science coach for business leaders, elite amateur and professional athletes, individuals, and families. He is included in the greatist.com's 2013 list of "The 100 Most Influential People in Health and Fitness."*

Non-athletic coaching as a profession has been developing since the early 1990s (Peltier, 2010; Cockerill, 2002; Fournies, 2000). The term "coach," borrowed from sports, has gained expanding acceptance in numerous fields in personal and lifestyle improvement, as well as in business, organizational, and executive performance, and most notably in the fields of health, lifestyle, and wellness coaching. Practicing ACE-certified Health Coaches have always coached their clients through lifestyle changes related to weight management and wellness. Health coaches guide their clients to make weight-related behavioral changes through goal-setting, education, **motivation,** programming, support, appropriate progressions, and referral when necessary.

The present-day health coach is in a unique position to become a well-anchored member of a client's allied health team, bringing a unique understanding of the intertwined emotional, behavioral, physical, nutritional, exercise, and lifestyle factors to clients to help them enhance their well-being and support them as they strive to reach their lifestyle and weight-management goals. In a coaching context, the contemporary health coach will be seen as a health promoter, health educator, and an active partner in unlocking each client's potential to maximize his or her own healthy lifestyle choices.

Grounded in the science of lifestyle and weight management, but also armed with humility, compassion, superior communication skills, **rapport**-building know-how, the ability to elicit motivation, and the capability to increase the capacity to change by fostering positivity, resilience, and **self-efficacy,** the contemporary health coach will be seen by clients as the ultimate partner in facilitating the process of health and lifestyle change, in addition to what has been referred to as the "art of living" (Veenhoven, 2007). The art of living involves four aptitudes related to health improvement:

- *The ability to enjoy:* Health coaches can use "attentiveness" or meditation techniques to encourage the broadening of leisure activities and remove inner barriers that prevent enjoyment.
- *The ability to choose:* Health coaches can help clients understand the options they have, and, through a healthy coaching relationship, assist clients in understanding how those options fit their personality style to assure adherence.
- *The ability to keep developing:* Maslow (1954) described "growth needs," which health coaches can build on by helping clients define and engage in challenging activities, leaving clients with a sense of autonomy, competence, and relatedness to life.
- *The ability to see meaning:* Health coaches can help clients see worth in their lives and value in accomplishing their health-related goals.

Coaching, as described in this manual, is founded in the context of the energetic and imaginative fields of coaching psychology and positive psychology. Focusing on human strengths and well-being, researchers including Peterson (2006), Linley and Harrington (2005), Seligman and Csikszentmihalyi (2000), and Snyder and McCullough (2000) have brought a scientific base to focusing on what brings happiness, fulfillment, and flourishing to life—the elements of lifestyle and health enhancement.

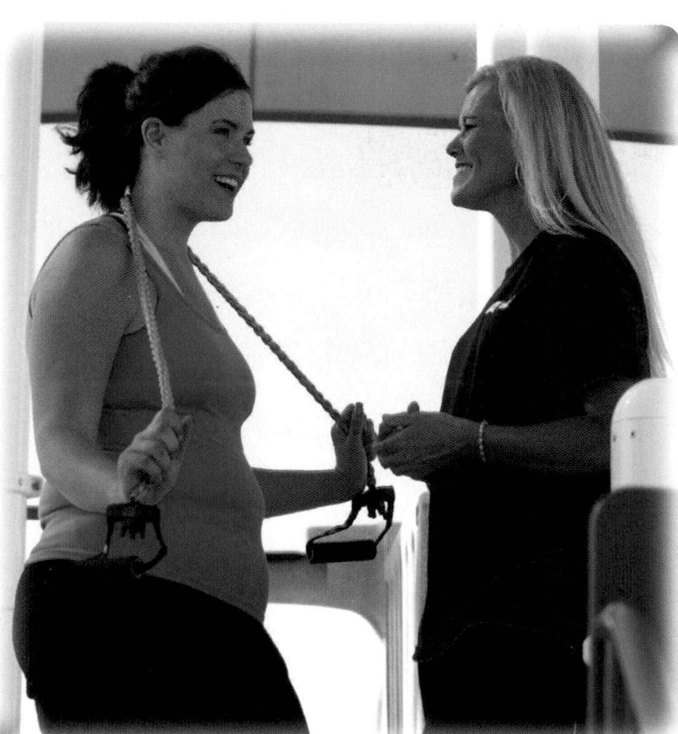

A health coach brings a focus on enhancing, preserving, and maintaining health and preventing illness, and views clients in nonjudgmental terms as *whole beings* who do not need to be repaired, but who may require support and assistance in building on their self-esteem and character strengths. Like the sculptor who "continues to carve to set the angel free," the client-centered health coach has a curious two-way mindset, draws out potential, enables, develops, reflects in a reactive and flexible manner, and is strategy-oriented. The outdated, failed, one-way "expert" model imposes aims and goals, directs, and is tactic-oriented. The health coach, in contrast, helps clients find solutions.

One way of understanding the difference between "coaching" and the "directing" style of leadership is by examining what the client is left thinking after a session. When clients work with a health coach who directs well, for example, they leave thinking, *"My coach is terrific."* When clients work with a true coach, they leave thinking, *"Wow, I'm really good!"*

Good coaches understand that every client is capable of achieving more, and that clients' self-talk—their inner critical voice—is often their only limitation. Coaches understand how to identify those negative, irrational, and erroneous beliefs, and continuously provide full support—not necessarily answers and certainly not criticism. To do so, effective coaches listen more than they talk. Coaches do not give up their "expert" role; they simply understand how to use their expertise in ways that enhance each client's well-being. They make every effort to speak less than clients do, ensure that clients work hard at finding their own answers whenever possible, and offer advice with the client's permission. In addition, coaches rely on nondirective interventions before giving advice, draw on tools to encourage the client's thinking, and are willing to call on others for expertise that they themselves do not have.

This chapter provides an overview of the most contemporary and effective coaching tools available. These concepts are then expanded upon in other chapters. New health coaches will learn about widely used methods to understand and connect with clients, develop an understanding of their own strengths and weaknesses, and be introduced to effective methods to motivate clients—all in the service of building trust and rapport in client relations. This overview will provide the contemporary health coach with a broad glimpse into the most up-to-date approaches to weight management, cognitive coaching, and inter-professional relationships.

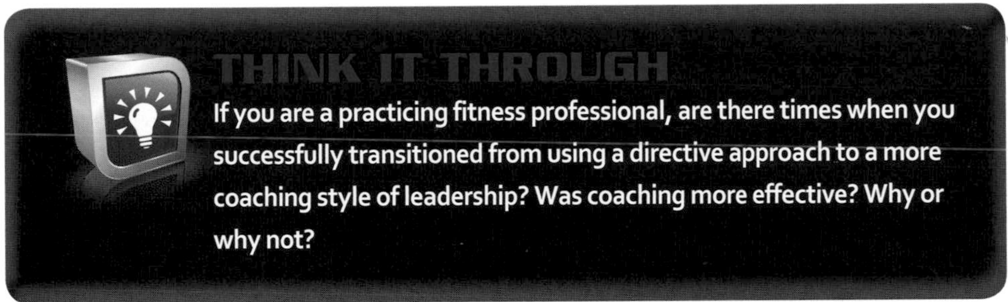

THINK IT THROUGH
If you are a practicing fitness professional, are there times when you successfully transitioned from using a directive approach to a more coaching style of leadership? Was coaching more effective? Why or why not?

Dynamics of the Client–Coach Relationship

Moore et al. (2005) suggest that there is a "relational dynamic between coaches and clients when they enter a zone where they are fully challenged at a high level of skill and awareness." The authors describe this zone, or state, as an "intuitive dance" and a "relational flow" and believe it is necessary to achieve in order to reach a client's goals. Initial structured steps and mechanistic actions transform into a more fluid flow between the health coach and client. The health coach's mastery of related factual knowledge (e.g., exercise, behavioral, and nutritional sciences; screening, assessment, and referral; and program design and implementation) is a necessary ingredient in achieving this relational flow. The client's readiness level is another essential ingredient in arriving at this fluid state. The **emotional intelligence** levels of the health coach and client are also valuable in creating a healthy relationship.

As described by Goleman (1998; 1995), emotional intelligence refers to the ability to recognize one's own feelings, as well as the feelings of others. This is necessary to motivate oneself and manage emotions within the context of the relationship. Emotional intelligence, for both the health coach and client, is based on four competencies within the emotional and interpersonal arena:

- *Self-awareness:* Does the individual have the ability to recognize his or her emotions and understand the effect they have on him or her? Does the individual know his or her own strengths and weaknesses?

- *Self-regulation:* Does the individual have the ability to control impulses, manage emotions, act in resilient ways, and follow through on commitments?
- *Empathy:* Does the individual have social awareness; the ability to understand the emotions, needs, and concerns of others; pick up on these cues; and feel comfortable socially?
- *Social skills:* Does the individual have the ability to manage relationships, communicate clearly, inspire and influence others, work as part of a team, and manage conflict?

Great Coaches—Great People—Great Leaders

- Understand exercise science
- Constantly seek out new information
- Display humility
- Are memorable motivators
- Are compassionate
- Understand each client
- Are exemplary communicators
- Are excellent listeners
- Are personally disciplined
- Are passionate
- Lead by daily example
- Display unrelenting commitment
- Build enduring client relationships for long-term growth

Coaching Roles

- Advisor
- Assessor
- Counselor
- Demonstrator
- Friend
- Facilitator
- Fact finder
- Instructor
- Mentor
- Motivator
- Organizer and planner
- Role model
- Supporter

Personal Awareness—SWOT Analysis

The health coach's attitude affects clients in a variety of ways. The attitude, thoughts, beliefs, and self-talk of an individual determine how that person feels, and in turn how that person will react to a given situation. The behavior of person A then influences the attitude, thoughts, beliefs, and self-talk of person B, which determine how that person will feel and act... and so the circle goes.

Thus, it is important for the health coach to develop a highly refined level of self-awareness. One tool that can help with this process is the **SWOT analysis,** credited to Stanford University's Albert Humphrey (2005), who led the initial work on this method in the 1960s based on work he did with Fortune 500 companies. SWOT analysis stands for strengths, weaknesses, opportunities, and threats.

A basic SWOT analysis is easy to perform. Begin by dividing a piece of paper into four sections and labeling them as depicted in Figure 1-1. The SWOT analysis can be used by a health coach to assess him- or herself, or to analyze a business or opportunity. It is important to be as honest as possible about one's weaknesses, as this exercise will help the health coach turn any perceived weaknesses into new opportunities. For example, if a health coach lists "lack of education" in a specific area of exercise science, this could be viewed as an opportunity to take a continuing education course or workshop to gain the necessary training. When listing threats, the health coach should include anything that might negatively impact either the health coach or the business, from the emergence of a new competitor to a downturn in the general economic climate. The following is a quick rundown of some questions one might ask when conducting a SWOT analysis.

- Strengths
  - ✓ What advantages do I have that others do not?
  - ✓ What do I do better than anyone else?
  - ✓ What values do I believe in that help me succeed?
- Weaknesses
  - ✓ What tasks do I avoid because I do not feel confident doing them?
  - ✓ What will people around me see as my weaknesses?
  - ✓ What personality traits are currently holding me back?
- Opportunities
  - ✓ What technologies can help me move ahead?
  - ✓ What network of strategic contacts do I have or can I create?
  - ✓ What needs in my company or in my industry are not being filled?
- Threats
  - ✓ What obstacles do I face in my work?
  - ✓ What weaknesses could lead to additional threats?
  - ✓ What technologies threaten my work?

The personal SWOT analysis is meant to help the health coach focus on expanding his or her business and personal standing as a health coach.

STRENGTHS	WEAKNESSES
ACE-certified Health Coach B.S. in Kinesiology Excellent one-on-one relationship-building skills	Inadequate business-building know-how Poor social media skills Anxiety about speaking to large audiences
OPPORTUNITIES	**THREATS**
Take a public speaking course Market and emphasize value of personal one-on-one training/coaching Work with a social media and technology coach	Social media applications ("apps") on lifestyle improvement, weight loss, and exercise Attraction to group-fitness/weight-loss programs Economic pressures limit the pool of new clients

Figure 1-1
Sample SWOT analysis

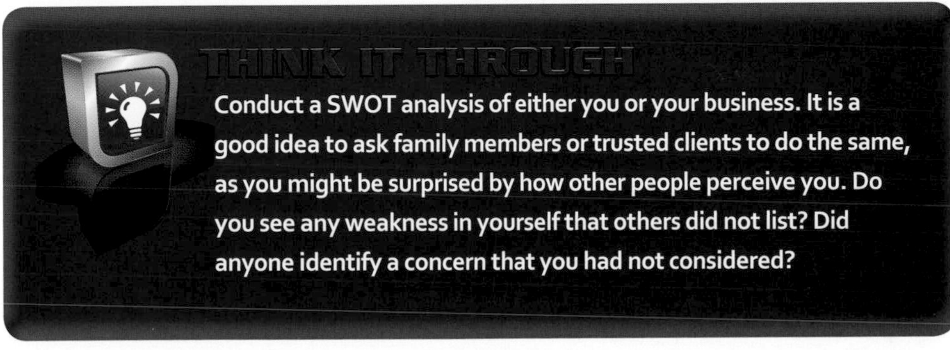

THINK IT THROUGH
Conduct a SWOT analysis of either you or your business. It is a good idea to ask family members or trusted clients to do the same, as you might be surprised by how other people perceive you. Do you see any weakness in yourself that others did not list? Did anyone identify a concern that you had not considered?

The DISC Model of Understanding Personality Types

While self-understanding is essential for the health coach to create healthy interpersonal relationships, the ability to understand the personality styles of clients is invaluable.

The DISC model of understanding personality types will assist the health coach in understanding him- or herself, as well as in rapidly assessing the personality style of his or her clients. This model was developed by Harvard's Dr. William Marston in 1928 and is still widely used today. In the DISC model, there are four personality types: outgoing, reserved, task-oriented, and people-oriented (Figure 1-2) .

Figure 1-2
DISC model of understanding personality types

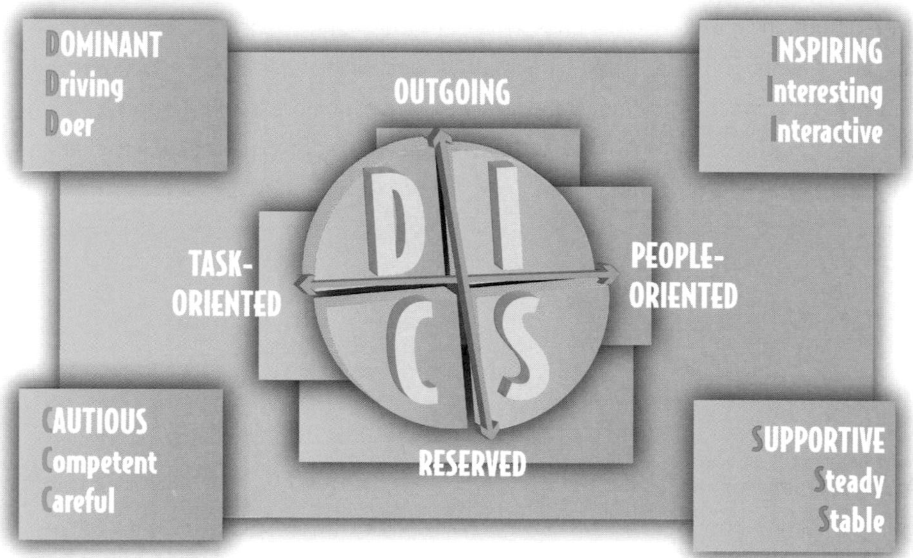

People who talk about what they think or how things are done are often more task-oriented. People who talk in terms of what they feel or how things seem to them are often more people-oriented. An effective health coach will hear these differences and pay careful attention to how he or she handles time and tasks and how he or she speaks and interacts with clients based on their personality styles (see Chapter 5 for more detailed information on the DISC model).

Interpersonal Sensitivity and Respect

Great coaches simply do not pass judgment on their clients. They see the good, the value, the dignity, and the strengths in those with whom they are privileged to work. They can find connection points easily with every client, have the patience to allow clients to advance according their own timetables, and identify with legendary Dallas Cowboys coach Tom Landry's oft-quoted wisdom: "Leadership is getting someone to do what they don't want to do, to achieve what they want to achieve."

Coaches should have a highly refined vision and respect for where clients want to go to achieve their weight, lifestyle, and health goals. They patiently, professionally, and passionately encourage, motivate, enable, and empower their clients to move forward. The health coach should be a solution-oriented, process-respectful, results-oriented, and interpersonally sophisticated enhancer of the client's growth.

An element of respect involves the ability to avoid treating all clients as if they are at the same stage of readiness for change. Health coaches can utilize the **transtheoretical model of behavioral change (TTM)** to carefully assess every client's readiness for change (Prochaska, DiClemente, & Norcross, 1998; Prochaska & DiClemente, 1984) (see Chapter 3).

The health coach understands that people in the **precontemplation** stage have no intent to change at all in the short-term. While individuals in the second stage, the **contemplation** stage, are considering making changes, it is only in the **preparation** stage that the commitment to change genuinely increases and small changes may already be underway. It is easy to want to see clients in the **action** stage, or to rush them to it. When clients arrive at this stage they are engaging in new activities and the coach's support and guidance may be delivered through face-to-face meetings, email, text messages, phone calls, and Skype™ or FaceTime™. Clients who have reached the **maintenance** stage have been engaged in health enhancement, weight management, and lifestyle change for more than six months.

Coaches should note that self-efficacy, or one's perception of his or her ability to change or perform specific behaviors, increases as a person moves through the stages of the TTM (Ounpuu, Woolcott, & Rossi, 1999; Bandura, 1977). Conversely, **habit strength** (Velicer, Rossi, & Prochaska, 1996), or the psychological and physiological factors involved in behaviors the client wants to change, will decrease as one moves through the stages of the TTM.

Listening and Motivational Communication Skills

Active Listening

Active listening is one of the most important skills of an emotionally intelligent coach (see Chapter 5). Not only does it build trust, but it also encourages positive problem-solving in the client. Nonverbal active listening skills involve establishing eye contact, using pauses and silence, knowing how to demonstrate facial expressions that indicate one is present and focused, and appropriate body language that displays interest and attentiveness. Consistent undivided attention is the simplest way to describe what the health coach offers the client when listening.

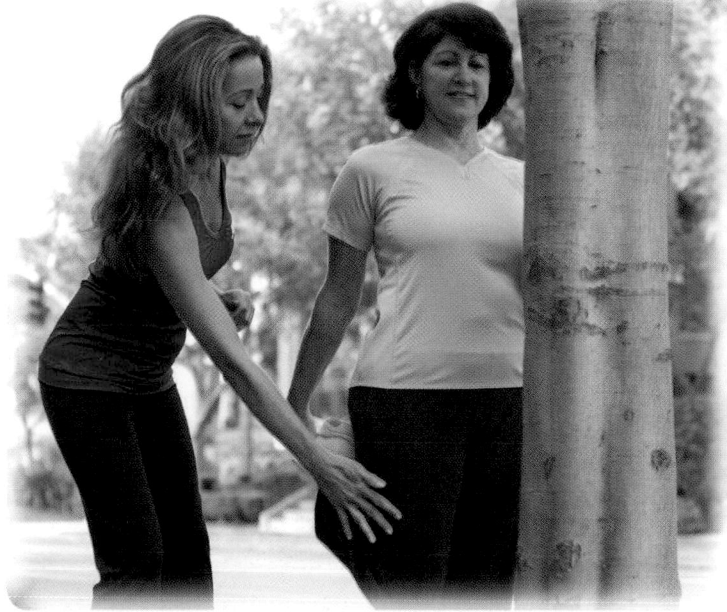

Health coaches can confirm their understanding using the following four-step process:

- Use a confirming statement
- Summarize key facts
- Ask if your understanding is correct
- Clarify misunderstandings

When the health coach "listens" to a client, it is more than just words he or she is listening for. Tone, style, and speed of speech, as well as body language, are all a part of what a good listener focuses on during a conversation. While each of these elements is important, body language is a method of communication that transmits a great deal of information to the health coach who is skilled in "hearing" this type of messaging.

The language of closure to the client literally involves the coach turning away or sitting with arms and legs crossed. The language of openness is demonstrated with open arms, legs and feet pointing toward the client, and relaxed and prolonged eye contact. Leaning forward shows the health coach is interested in what the client has to say. When a person is attentive, the head is tilted slightly forward, while tilting the head slightly to the side demonstrates curiosity. Slow nodding, interest noises ("uh huh"), and even a furrowed brow may demonstrate concentration.

An attentive and engaged health coach looks at the person, avoids any distractions, does not interrupt, nods and smiles to acknowledge points, and emphasizes connecting more than communicating. Maxwell (2010) has identified eight ways to determine when a connection has been made with people, either one-on-one or in a group.

- People give extra effort.
- People say positive things.
- People demonstrate trust.
- People express themselves more readily.
- People feel good about what they are doing.
- People display an emotional connection.
- People are emotionally charged by being together.
- People have growing synergy and their overall effectiveness is greater than the sum of their contributions.

The type of questions the health coach asks may impact external performance. Declarative and interrogative self-statements are related to performance outcome. Declarative self-statements, such as "I will stick to my food plan at the party this evening," are linked to **extrinsic motivation.** On the other hand, interrogative self-statements, such as "Will I stick to my food plan this evening?" encourage **intrinsic motivation,** which is more apparent when clients stick with their plans for their own sake, with no external motivator present.

One of the most well-known basketball coaches of all time, John Wooden, compared extrinsic motivation to the type of enforcement used by a prison guard. The guard can force the chain gang to do what is necessary, but without the guard there the prisoners stop working immediately. Declarative forms of self-talk are like the prison guard. They work for a short while, perhaps to get things moving, but as soon as an "out" is present, the motivation is gone. When the health coach asks open-ended questions, the client is more likely to generate thoughts about accomplishing a goal on his or her own, with no feeling of anything being imposed. The key is for the health coach to ask questions in a way that is less threatening to the autonomy of the client and respects the client's choices. Declarative self-talk and closed-ended questions stifle the conversation. Open-ended questions lead to more questions, planning, and action steps (see Chapter 5 for more information on the various types of questions used during active listening).

Motivational Interviewing

Motivational interviewing is a client-centered approach to assist clients with ambivalence to change (Miller & Rollnick, 2002; Miller, 1983) (see Chapter 5). Motivation can be conceptualized as a state of readiness for change, not a personality trait, and it can fluctuate over time and be influenced for positive change. Motivational interviewing offers the health coach tools with which he or she can facilitate healthy motivation to change by working with the client to explore and resolve ambivalences. As a "fluctuating product of interpersonal interaction," motivation to change, then, is evoked *within* the client, not imposed *on* the client (Rollnick & Miller, 1995). The health coach's task is to expect, anticipate, and recognize ambivalence to change, and help each client examine and resolve his or her ambivalence.

Motivational interviewing is grounded in expressing **empathy** and acceptance of ambivalence. The coach must then sensitively highlight discrepancies between the client's behaviors and goals so the client can make his or her own arguments for change.

Positive Listening

It is important for the health coach to listen without passing judgment or interrupting with advice. The expression of empathy is a critical skill for the health coach to develop. Respect, or the demonstration of an attitude of caring, and assertiveness, or the ability to express feelings openly and directly, are additional skills the health coach needs in healthy communication. However, six negative habits are at the root of poor listening (Lynn, 2002):

- *The faker:* All the outward signs are there: nodding, making eye contact, and giving the occasional "uh-huh." However, the faker is not concentrating on the speaker. His or her mind is elsewhere.
- *The interrupter:* The interrupter does not allow the speaker to finish and does not ask clarifying questions or seek more information from the speaker. He or she is too anxious to speak and shows little concern for the speaker.
- *The intellectual or logical listener:* This person is always trying to interpret what the speaker is saying and why. He or she is judging the speaker's words and trying to place them into a logical box that fits his or her own perceptions. He or she rarely asks about the underlying feeling or emotion attached to a message.
- *The rebuttal maker:* This person only listens long enough to form a rebuttal. The rebuttal maker's point is to use the speaker's words against him or her. At worst, this type of listener is argumentative and wants to prove the speaker wrong. At the very least, this person always wants to make the speaker see the another point of view.

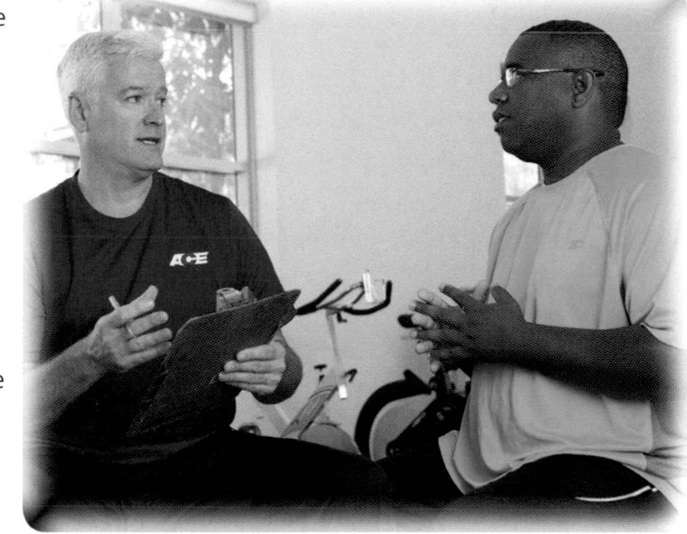

- *The focus thief:* The focus thief uses the speaker's words only as a way to get to his or her message. When the speaker says something, the focus thief steals the focus and then changes to his or her own point of view, opinion, story, or facts. Favorite lines include, "Oh, that's nothing. Here's what happened to me…"
- *The advice giver:* While this habit may be helpful at times, at other times it interferes with good listening because it does not allow the speaker to fully articulate his or her feelings or thoughts. It may prohibit venting, and may belittle the speaker by minimizing his or her concerns with a quick solution. An advice giver does not help the speaker solve his or her own problems.

By being aware of these negative listening habits, the health coach is in a better position to begin correcting any pattern he or she recognizes within him- or herself. It is far better for the health coach to be aware of these patterns before clients become aware of them.

Trust and Rapport-building

In their book, *"The Speed of Trust,"* Stephen M. Covey and Rebecca R. Merrill (2008) note that "trust means confidence." Great coaches understand the need to impart and develop trust. Covey and Merrill describe five "waves of trust":

- Self-trust
- Relationship trust
- Organizational trust
- Market trust
- Societal trust

For the purpose of establishing a quality coaching relationship, it is the relationship trust "wave" that is important to highlight. The health coach must act consistently in ways that are predictable to the client's sense of comfort. Covey and Merrill (2008) identify 13 behaviors that are common to "high-trust" leaders:

- Character-based behaviors
  - ✓ Be honest
  - ✓ Demonstrate respect
  - ✓ Create transparency
  - ✓ Right wrongs
  - ✓ Show loyalty
- Competency-based behaviors
  - ✓ Deliver results
  - ✓ Get better
  - ✓ Confront reality
  - ✓ Clarify expectations
  - ✓ Practice accountability
- Character and competency behaviors
  - ✓ Listen first
  - ✓ Keep commitments
  - ✓ Extend trust

The health coach who commits these rapport-building principles to memory, and who uses them as guiding principles in his or her day-to-day practice, will develop not only a solid group of clients, but also a supportive group of fans.

EXPAND YOUR KNOWLEDGE

The Pillars of Healthy Lifestyle Maintenance

The effective health coach will be of value to his or her clients in a number of areas of healthy lifestyle functioning, within the proper scope of practice. The ACE-certified Health Coach's scope of practice is similar to that of a personal trainer (see Figure 2-1, page 30), but extends beyond the realm of physical fitness to include a focus on other healthy lifestyle factors. The pillars of a healthy lifestyle include:

Physical fitness: This includes the competence to function well in daily activities without injury, resist disease, enjoy leisure time, be healthy, and resiliently cope with emergency events. Cardiorespiratory fitness, body composition, flexibility, muscular endurance, muscular strength, agility, coordination, and reaction speed are all components of physical fitness.

Psychological fitness: The individual has sufficient resilience, energy, and motivation to be able to use his or her intellectual, behavioral, and emotional competencies to meet the demands of everyday life and function in society. This includes the way the individual thinks about him- or herself, his or her life, and others with whom he or she interacts. It also encompasses the way individuals react in response to thoughts and emotions. This area may also encompass spiritual fitness, including positive beliefs and expressions of the deepest parts of the self, an individual's self-awareness, creativity, and the ability to love and be loved.

Nutritional fitness: The individual eats the correct amount of nutrients on a regular schedule to be able to perform at the highest levels, support adaptation, prevent obesity and other diseases, repair the body after damage, fuel bioenergetic needs, and live life in good health.

Interpersonal fitness: The individual has the ability to establish close, meaningful relationships free of conflict—overtly, face-to-face, or even virtually. The ability to fulfill the needs of others and make one's own needs clear are also important elements.

Achievement fitness: Individuals who strive for something that is personally meaningful, regardless of the content, are found to be happier than those who do not strive to achieve. Finding a purpose in life and working ceaselessly toward that purpose encompasses achievement fitness. It requires perseverance, determination, resolution, and diligence—traits that are key elements of healthy living.

Cognitive Coaching

How clients think about their lives and health situations determines how they will feel and act. Many clients will erroneously believe, for example, that "dieting and exercise should be easy." When they are not easy, clients may feel angry, resentful, sad, or depressed. They may believe it is catastrophic that their life situation is not as they *demand* it to be. For the health coach who does not understand the inner self-talk of the client, it would be difficult to comprehend the emotion and behavior being demonstrated. The belief, "dieting and exercise should be easy," is likely a consequence of "must"-type thinking. Ellis (1962) describes what happens when an individual falls into the trap of believing in the three "musts" as follows:

- I *must* do well and win the approval of others for my performances or else I am no good.
- Other people *must* treat me considerately, fairly, and kindly, and in exactly the way I want them to treat me. If they do not, they are no good and they deserve to be condemned and punished.
- I *must* get what I want, when I want it, and I *must not* get what I do not want. It is terrible if I do not get what I want, and I cannot stand it.

It becomes easy to see how these erroneous beliefs can interfere with forward movement in healthy lifestyle and weight-management behaviors.

Albert Ellis (1962), founder of the rational emotive behavioral therapy movement later built on by Aaron Beck (1976) and more recently called "cognitive behavior therapy," describes that how people react to events is determined largely by their view of the events, not the events themselves. Ellis describes this in an A-B-C model, where A is the activating event, B is the beliefs the client has about the event or situation, and C is the emotional and behavioral consequence of the person's beliefs. The health coach moves to D, helping the client dispute, challenge, and question the erroneous beliefs the client holds that lead to disruptive emotions and behaviors.

Ultimately, behavior change rests on the health coach's ability to guide a client to first change his or her thoughts. That is where the all-important "D" step comes in. This is, after all, where the client's real work takes place, in replacing his or her irrational, negative, inaccurate, and illogical thinking with rational, factual thoughts upon which healthy behavioral change can rest.

Typically, the health coach will help the client dispute irrational thinking through a series of questions and methods derived from the work of Burns (1980) and Ellis (1962). One such method, "examine the evidence," involves the health coach helping the client examine the evidence for a belief instead of assuming his or her thought is true. The health coach may help the client dispute his or her belief with questions such as, "What are the facts?" and "What do the facts show?"

The health coach may also help the client think in terms of "shades of gray" as a method to dispute irrational thoughts. Instead of thinking about one's health problems, exercise avoidance, or weight-management challenges in terms of black and white categories, the health coach helps the client evaluate them in shades of gray. Thinking in terms of partial success may help the client feel motivated to continue striving for more progress. Perhaps the client is putting him- or herself down. Instead of continuing on this path, the client can begin to dispute his or her beliefs by talking to him- or herself in the same compassionate way he or she might speak with a close friend or loved one. The health coach may encourage the client to ask, "Would I say such harsh things to a family member or close friend with a similar problem? If I wouldn't, why wouldn't I? What would I say to him or her instead? Can I say those things to myself?"

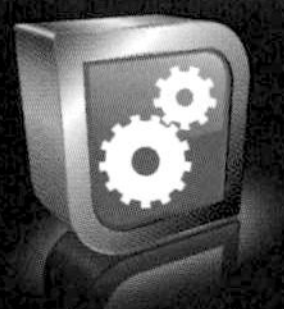

EXPAND YOUR KNOWLEDGE

Cognitive Distortions

A health coach can help a client actively dispute his or her erroneous beliefs by identifying the type of distortions he or she is making from among the following 10 cognitive distortions:

- *All-or-nothing thinking:* Looking at things in black-and-white terms
- *Overgeneralization:* Viewing a negative event as a continual pattern of defeat
- *Mental filter:* Dwelling on the negatives and ignoring the positives
- *Discounting the positives:* Believing that accomplishments or positive qualities are meaningless
- *Jumping to conclusions:* (a) Mind reading—Assuming that people are reacting negatively with no basis in reality; (b) Fortune-telling—Erroneously predicting that things will turn out badly
- *Magnification or minimization:* Blowing negative things out of proportion or diminishing positive things
- *Emotional reasoning:* Reasoning from how one feels: "I feel like a failure, so I must really be one," or "I don't feel I can succeed so I won't try."
- *"Should" statements:* Demanding that oneself or other people "should" or "shouldn't" "must," "ought to," or "have to" be different
- *Labeling:* Calling oneself names. Instead of saying "I made an error," telling oneself "I'm a loser" or "stupid" or "a failure."
- *Personalization and blame:* Blaming oneself or others inappropriately

Source: Burns, D. (1980). *Feeling Good: The New Mood Therapy*. New York: William Morrow.

The goal of cognitive coaching is for the health coach to help clients change their irrational beliefs into rational beliefs. Changing beliefs is the real work of health coaching and is achieved by the health coach sensitively, respectfully, and persistently helping the client recognize irrational beliefs. For example, the health coach might ask, "Why *must* dieting and exercise be easy? Where is it written that it *must* be easy? Just because you want it to be easy, why *must* it be?"

The health coach will find the following questions useful when helping a client reevaluate irrational, erroneous, and inaccurate thinking. The health coach asks the client to self-reflect with these questions:

- What is the evidence for and against thinking that…?
- What would I tell a friend in this same situation who was thinking what I am?
- What is the worst that could realistically happen? How bad would that be?
- Would it really be 100% bad? Would it be the worst thing that could happen?
- It is really true that I must, should, ought to, have to…?
- Are there any other possible explanations besides blaming myself?
- Is there any other conceivable way to look at this positively?

The goal is to help the client move from an *absolutistic demanding*, all-or-nothing approach to health improvement to a *full preference* that things be different, but with the ability to accept it when they are not. This is based on guided discovery, where the health coach asks the client a series of questions in order to bring the client's awareness to his or her thinking.

Regarding weight management, cognitive coaching can be a very useful tool in helping clients identify the unhelpful thoughts that sabotage their healthy behavior, and then respond more effectively. Helping clients develop "rational counter-responses" to their erroneous beliefs is a critical part of coaching.

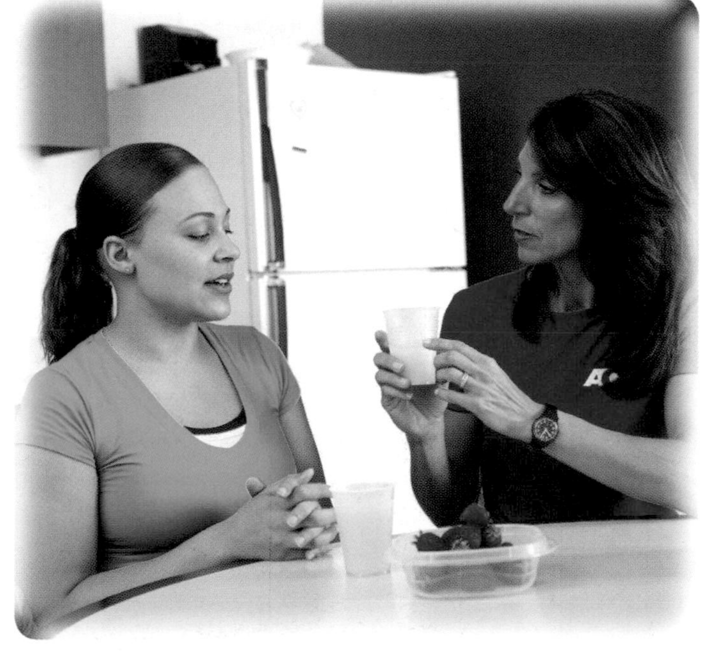

- *"This is awful and horrible…I can't stand it…I have to eat!"* This belief can be countered with "It's not awful. It's just uncomfortable… I'm going to eat in a couple of hours. While I don't like it, I can certainly wait."
- *"Wow, those cupcakes look so good. I need to have one."* The health coach can arm the client with counter-responses such as, "No, I don't need to eat one. I'm having dinner in an hour anyway." "Just because they look good doesn't mean I must eat one." and "Sure they look good, but my desire will go away if I concentrate on something else."
- *"It feels unnatural to make myself eat slowly."* The health coach can help the client develop the more helpful thought, "The more I practice, the more natural it will feel. It doesn't have to feel natural at first. It's an important skill."

Helping clients cognitively distinguish, for example, the difference between hunger and the desire to eat, can be a very valuable coaching goal.

Problem-solving Models

Wasik (1984) proposed a seven-step model of problem-solving for clients to consider, along with questions the health coach can use to facilitate the process (Table 1-1).

Table 1-1

Seven-step Problem-solving Model

Steps	Questions/Actions
Problem identification	What is the concern?
Goal selection	What do I want?
Generation of alternatives	What can I do?
Consideration of consequences	What might happen?
Decision making	What is my decision?
Implementation	Now do it!
Evaluation	Did it work?

Similarly, the GROW model—which stands for "goal, reality, options, and what" offers health coaches an example of a structured approach to behavioral change. It is one of the most established and successful models for personal and professional enhancement in the coaching industry (Whitmore, 2009).

- *Goal:* Questions define the goal as clearly as possible and evoke an emotional response
  - ✓ What do you want to achieve?
  - ✓ What will be different when you achieve it?
  - ✓ What is important about this for you?
- *Reality:* Questions elicit specific details of the situation and context
  - ✓ What is happening now?
  - ✓ Who is involved?
  - ✓ What is the outcome?
  - ✓ What is likely to happen in the future?
- *Options:* Open-ended questions facilitate creative thinking
  - ✓ What could you do?
  - ✓ What ideas can you bring in from past successes?
  - ✓ What have you not tried yet?
- *What/How/When/How:* Focused questions get an agreement to specific actions and criteria for success in **SMART goal** language (specific, measurable, attainable, relevant, and time-bound) (see Chapter 13)
  - ✓ What will you do?
  - ✓ How will you measure whether it was done or not?
  - ✓ When will you do it?
  - ✓ Who do you need to involve?
  - ✓ When should you see results?
  - ✓ Is possible to actually achieve this goal?
  - ✓ Is it a realistic action to move the client to his or her goal?

Neuro-linguistic Programming

"A thought is just a thought," which is commonly heard among neuro-linguistic practitioners, reflects the underlying approach to those who use **neuro-linguistic programming (NLP)** in their mind-body coaching. NLP was created in the early 1970s by Richard Bandler, a computer scientist and Gestalt therapist, and Dr. John Grinder, a linguist and therapist (Bandler & Grinder, 1979). *Neuro* refers to how the mind and body interact, *linguistic* relates to the insights into a person's thinking as expressed through language, and *programming* refers to the study of patterns of thinking and behaving in a client. Similar to cognitive coaching, NLP teaches clients how unhelpful thoughts create obstacles in life. Like cognitive coaching, NLP uses an approach based on careful rapport-building and questions to help the client see through his or her perception of reality. This is called the "meta model" and includes questions that challenge linguistic distortions, clarifies generalizations the client may make, and recovers unrecalled information. NLP questions may be in the form of "What, specifically?" "How, specifically?" "According to whom?" and "How do you know that?"

Coaching for lifestyle and weight management requires empathy, highly advanced emotional intelligence, and outstanding communication skills coupled with a well-anchored bedrock of knowledge about behavior-change methods. Of course, the fundamentals of exercise physiology, weight-management approaches, and ethical considerations are also a part of the successful health coach's education. This combination of expertise allows the health coach to relate to professionals in allied health fields in a way that brings mutual respect and consideration for what is best for clients.

Connecting With Medical Fitness Professionals

For a health coach who has the inclination to network with medical and allied health professionals, particularly those in the growing medical fitness industry, this can represent a significant step in building a practice and career. Creating a list of medical facilities, perhaps those that are focused on fitness and weight-related issues, is the first step. Contacting the physician or community education director is the next step, often with a letter, email, or phone call, requesting an opportunity to meet and chat about health coaching and how it may relate to the physician's or hospital's medical fitness model. Offering to do a free presentation in a class about fitness and obesity may be an excellent way to get one's "foot in the door." Introducing oneself by discussing health coach credentials, explaining the services offered, describing the interest one has in helping patients of the physician or hospital, and expressing the desire to work in concert with the healthcare team, are all part of the initial introduction.

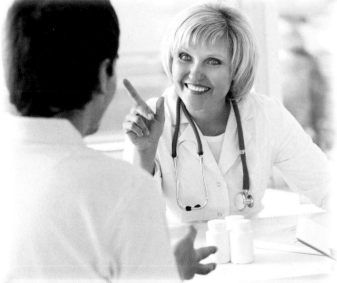

It is important to follow up monthly with a report on those individuals who have been referred by other healthcare professionals. Health coaches should consider providing the physician's offices and appropriate hospital departments with monthly newsletters about the services they offer.

Sending cards, gifts, and other ways of saying "thank you" are critically important.

An introductory letter to successfully network with medical fitness professionals should include a paragraph about each of the following topics:

- The health coach's areas of practice, including up-to-the-minute data about overweight/obesity in America and its related illnesses
- The health coach's credentials, education, and related work
- Some niche or specialized work the health coach does, or the type of service and assessment the health coach will provide
- Request referrals and an opportunity to meet

EXPAND YOUR KNOWLEDGE

Choosing the Right Resources

While the Internet, fitness and health magazines, and the popular media are sources of information many people turn to for guidance when trying to lose weight, the behavioral, exercise, and allied health and medical fields publish peer-reviewed journals that meet well-accepted academic standards. In addition to reading scientific health-, exercise-, and nutrition-related publications, a health coach should become familiar with the following peer-reviewed journals in the areas of coaching and development. Utilizing resources like these expands the health coach's knowledge base and adds credibility to his or her coaching methods.

- *Academy of Management Review*
- *The Annual Review of High Performance*
- *Consulting Psychology Journal: Research and Practice*
- *Coaching: An International Journal of Theory, Research, and Practice*
- *The Journal of Coaching Education*
- *The Coaching Psychologist*
- *Human Resource Development Quarterly*
- *International Coaching Psychology Review*
- *International Journal of Coaching in Organizations*
- *International Journal of Evidence-Based Coaching and Mentoring*
- *International Journal of Mentoring and Coaching*
- *Journal of Change Management*
- *Journal of Educational Research*
- *Journal of Occupational and Organizational Psychology*
- *Journal of Organizational Change Management*
- *International Journal of Training and Development*
- *Training and Management Development Methods*

THINK IT THROUGH

How do you define coaching? Now that you have read this introductory chapter, are there areas of coaching that you had not considered until now? Have you focused on the study of nutrition or exercise science at the expense of developing your communication skills? What can you do to become a more well-rounded fitness professional?

Summary

The future for health and fitness professionals, particularly health coaches, is bright. With over 35% of the American adult population obese, and nearly 17% of children in the same category (Ogden et al., 2012), the health coach is an important member of the allied health continuum. The employment market for fitness workers is expected to jump 29% between 2008 and 2018, according to the U.S. Bureau of Labor Statistics (2010), which notes that, "Increasing numbers of people are spending time and money on fitness and more businesses are recognizing the benefits of health and fitness programs for their employees."

Clients are seeking whole-life fitness coaching, not only to learn how to work out properly, but also how to make important lifestyle changes, especially in the area of weight-related issues. The more well-rounded, connected, and whole-person focused health coach who "empowers" his or her clients will fill this need and surpass other fitness professionals who simply "show." By closely engaging with clients in the full range of healthy lifestyle choice management, the health coach will become a valued and marketable member of the health, fitness, and wellness community. The practice of simply meeting clients at the gym or at a local park for a fitness-training session will fade as the children of baby boomers seek more active availability and input from coaches in order to live more active and happier lives.

References

Bandler, R. & Grinder, G. (1979). *Frogs Into Princes: Neuro Linguistic Programming.* Salt Lake City, Utah: Real People Press.

Bandura, A. (1977). Self-efficacy: Toward a unifying theory of behavioral change. *Psychological Review,* 84, 2, 191–215.

Beck, A.T. (1976) *Cognitive Therapy and the Emotional Disorders.* New York: New American Library.

Burns, D. (1980). *Feeling Good: The New Mood Therapy.* New York: William Morrow.

Cockerill, I. (2002). *Solutions in Sport Psychology.* London: Thomson.

Covey, S.M. & Merrill, R.R. (2008). *The Speed of Trust.* New York: Free Press.

Ellis, A. (1962). *Reason and Emotion in Psychotherapy.* New York: Lyle Stuart Press.

Fournies, F.F. (2000). *Coaching for Improved Work Performance.* New York: McGraw-Hill.

Goleman, D. (1998). *Working with Emotional Intelligence.* New York: Bantam Books.

Goleman, D. (1995). *Emotional Intelligence.* New York: Bantam Books.

Humphrey, A.S. (2005). *SWOT Analysis.* www.businessballs.com/swotanalysisfreetemplate.htm

Linley, P.A. & Harrington, S. (2005). Positive psychology and coaching psychology: Perspectives on integration. *The Coaching Psychologist,* 1 (July), 13–14.

Lynn, A.B. (2002). *The Emotional Intelligence Activity Book.* Amherst, Mass.: HRD Press.

Marston, W.M. (1928). *Emotions of Normal People.* London: K. Paul, Trench, Trubner & Co.

Maslow, A.H. (1954). *Motivation and Personality.* New York: Harper.

Maxwell, J.C. (2010). *Everyone Communicates, Few Connect.* Nashville, Tenn.: Thomas Nelson.

Miller, W.R. (1983). Motivational interviewing with problem drinkers. *Behavioral Psychotherapy,* 11, 147–172.

Miller, W.R. & Rollnick, S. (2002). *Motivational Interviewing* (2nd ed.). New York: The Guilford Press.

Moore, M. et al. (2005). *Relational Flow: A Theoretical Model of the Intuitive Dance of Coaching.* International Coaching Federation: 2005 Coaching Research Proceedings.

Ogden, C.L. et al. (2012). *Prevalence of Obesity in the United States 2009–2010.* NHCS Data Brief, No. 82. Washington, D.C.: Centers for Disease Control and Prevention.

Ounpuu, S., Woolcott, D.M., & Rossi, S.R. (1999). Self-efficacy as an intermediate outcome variable in the transtheoretical model: Validation of a measurement model for applications to dietary fat reduction. *Journal of Nutrition Education,* 31, 1, 16–21.

Peltier, B. (2010). *The Psychology of Executive Coaching: Theory and Application* (3rd ed.). New York: Brunner-Routledge.

Peterson, C. (2006). *A Primer in Positive Psychology.* New York: Oxford University Press.

Prochaska, J.O. & DiClemente, C.C. (1984). Toward a comprehensive model of change. In: Prochaska, J.O. & DiClemente, C.C. (Eds.) *The Transtheoretical Approach: Crossing the Traditional Boundaries of Therapy.* Homewood, Ill.: Dow-Jones.

Prochaska, J.O., DiClemente, C.C., & Norcross, J.C. (1998). Stages of change: Prescriptive guidelines for behavioral medicine. In: Koocher, G.P., Norcross, J.C., & Hill III, S.S. (Eds.) *Psychologists' Desk Reference* (pp. 203–236). Oxford: Oxford University Press.

Rollnick, S.R. & Miller, W.R. (1995). What is motivational interviewing? *Behavioral and Cognitive Psychology,* 23, 325–334.

Seligman, M.E. & Csikszentmihalyi, M. (2000). Positive psychology: An introduction. *American Psychologist,* 55, 1, 5–14.

Snyder, C.R. & McCullough, M.E. (2000). A positive psychology field of dreams: 'If you build it, they will come...' *Journal of Social & Clinical Psychology,* 19, 1, 151–160.

U.S. Bureau of Labor Statistics (2010). *Occupational Outlook Handbook, 2010–11.* Washington, D.C.: Labor Department, Labor Statistics Bureau.

Veenhoven, R. (2007). Subjective measures of wellbeing. In: McGillivray, M. (Ed.) *Human Well-being: Concept and Measurement.* Basingstoke: MacMillan.

Velicer, W.F., Rossi, J.S., & Prochaska, J.O. (1996). A criterion measurement model for health behavior change. *Addictive Behaviors,* 21, 5, 555–584.

Wasik, B. (1984). *Teaching Parents Effective Problem-Solving: A Handbook for Professionals.* Unpublished manuscript. Chapel Hill: University of North Carolina.

Whitmore, Sir J. (2009). *Coaching for Performance* (4th ed.). London: Nicholas Brealey.

Suggested Reading

Arloski, M. (2007). *Wellness Coaching for Lasting Lifestyle Change.* Duluth, Minn.: Whole Person Association.

Botelho, R. (2004). *Motivate Healthy Habits: Stepping Stones to Lasting Change.* Rochester, N.Y.: MHH Publications.

Buckingham, M. & Clifton, D.O. (2001). *Now Discover Your Strengths.* New York: Free Press.

Burns, D.D. (1980). *Feeling Good: The New Mood Therapy.* New York: William Morrow.

Csikszentmihalyi, M. (1990). *Flow: The Psychology of Optimal Experience.* New York: Harper and Row.

Frederickson, B.L. (2003). The value of positive emotions: The emerging science of positive psychology is coming to understand why it's good to feel good. *American Scientist,* 91, 330.

Freudenberger, H.J. (1980). *Burnout: The High Cost of High Achievement.* New York: Bantam Books.

Gavin, J. (2005). *Lifestyle Fitness Coaching.* Champaign, Ill.: Human Kinetics.

Hargrove, R. (2008). *Masterful Coaching* (3rd ed.). San Francisco: Jossey-Bass.

Lyubormirsky, S. (2007). *The How of Happiness: A Scientific Approach to Getting the Life You Want.* New York: Penguin Press HC.

Miller, W. R. & Rollnick, S. (2002). *Motivational Interviewing: Preparing People for Change.* New York: Guilford Press.

Peterson, C. (2006). *A Primer in Positive Psychology.* New York: Oxford University.

Pilzer, P.Z. (2002). *The Wellness Revolution.* Hoboken, N.J.: John Wiley & Sons.

Roizen, M.F. & Oz, M.C. (2006). *You on a Diet: The Owner's Manual for Waist Management.* New York: Free Press.

Seligman, M. (2002) *Authentic Happiness: Using the New Positive Psychology to Realize Your Potential for Lasting Fulfillment.* New York: Free Press.

U.S. Department of Agriculture (2015). *2015-2020 Dietary Guidelines for Americans* (8th ed.). www.health.gov/dietaryguidelines

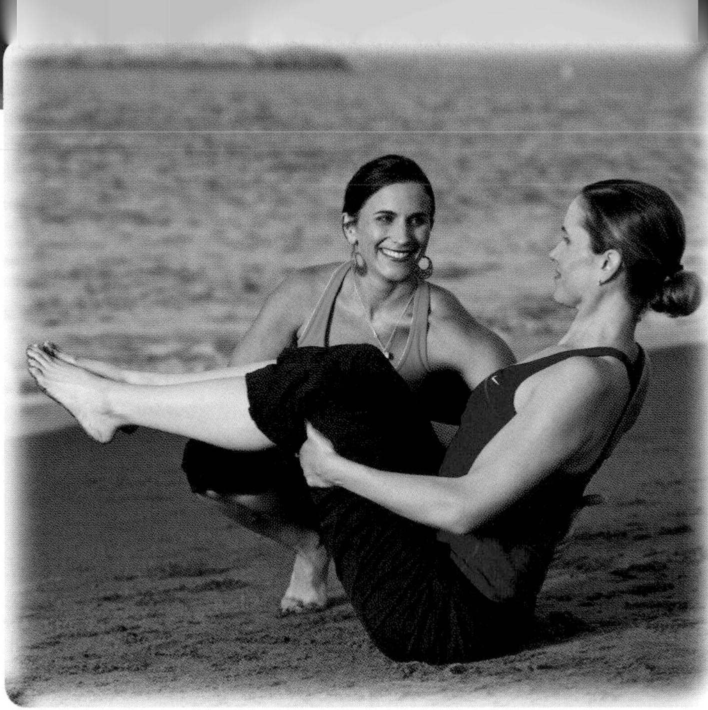

IN THIS CHAPTER:

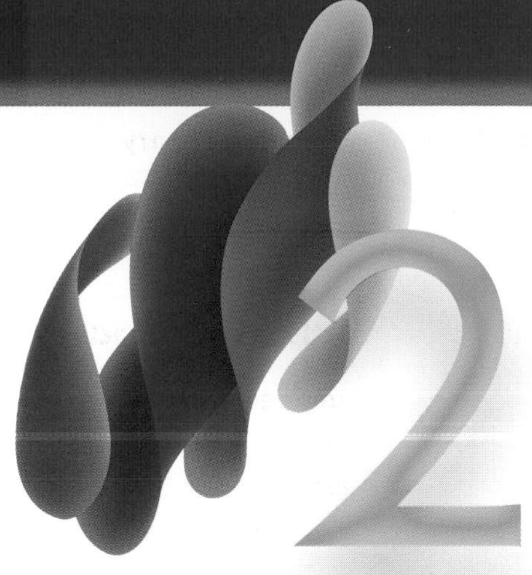

A Team Approach to Health Coaching

NANCEY TREVANIAN TSAI

Nancey Trevanian Tsai, M.D., is assistant professor of neurosurgery at the Medical University of South Carolina and serves on ACE's Board of Directors. She has been an ACE-certified Personal Trainer since 1996 and works with high-performance athletes as well as special populations.

An ACE-certifed Health Coach combines the science of fitness and weight management with the art of coaching and the maintenance of positive change. There are many facets to health coaching, including nutrition education, personal training, time management, and psychology. To achieve long-term behavioral change, all of these aspects will need to be addressed to varying degrees depending upon each client's needs. Just as in sports and business, having a cohesive team approach will increase the odds for sustainable, successful outcomes for both the health coach and the client.

A Brief History of Coaching Theory

A number of theories have arisen in the past 100 years that attempt to describe the process of behavioral modification. These include behaviorism, cognitive development, constructivism, and other derivative and integrative approaches. Having a basic understanding of the clinical research from which current coaching theories arise may help the health coach develop his or her own most effective method in managing client progress toward positive change.

Behaviorism was put forth by Pavlov (1925), who demonstrated that animals can be trained to respond to stimuli in predictable ways. Similarly, Watson (1924) and later Skinner (1953) also applied these principles to humans performing complex activities, termed "operant behavior." Thorndike (1931) used the term "law of effect," stating that actions that were rewarded tended to be repeated, whereas actions that were punished tended to cause the subject to either avoid the behavior or exhibit fear and anxiety when prompted to that action. In essence, behaviorism suggested that external stimuli can induce a change in behavior.

Piaget (1926) spent many years analyzing his children's learning processes to construct his cognitive learning theory, later to be incorporated into constructivism. Chomsky (1959) would critique behaviorism as well, stating that language and learning are intertwined to the extent that if new sentences or word patterns can be created, then new behaviors can also result from new thought correlations. This was to be termed "constructivism," from which much of coaching theory is based and has evolved. Another variation of this is the "learning cycle" put forth by Kolb (1984), suggesting that behaviors are modeled and remodeled based upon reinforcements and new experiences in one's life. The "social learning theory" put forth by Bandura (1986) utilizes behavioral modeling and dynamic interactive techniques to assist those being coached in taking on attributes, values, and behavioral traits of the coach or mentor. This method is, for example, utilized by the military's Special Forces to train its recruits.

Another approach is **neuro-linguistic programming (NLP),** put forth by Bandler and Grinder (1979), which is also largely anchored in cognitive-behavioral psychology. However, it expands this concept by employing techniques such as visualization and hypnosis to augment its effects. When used properly, NLP is reported to improve an individual's self-motivation, which helps to overcome learning blocks. The limitation of NLP is in the lack of clinical evidence for or against its effectiveness.

Most effective coaches today use a combination of these many approaches. A health coach invokes elements of behaviorism with every mention of "goal-setting" and/or "reinforcement." Yet, it seems clear that one's actions are a result of experiences and emotional responses to those experiences, reinforcing the attributes of cognitive development. Furthermore, clients are unique in their responses to the variety of techniques utilized by health coaches, just as each health coach will have a unique ability to execute the theories employed. As such, the traditional practice of coaching teams has evolved to include coaching individuals to optimize the results that can be achieved in the one-on-one setting.

Defining "Lifestyle"

Webster's Dictionary states that lifestyle is "the typical way of life of an individual, group, or culture." It is loosely defined as those attitudes, choices, standards, economic status, and other factors—personal and unique—that constitute the mode of living of a person or group of people. Some personal attributes are more easily altered than others, and each client will have tasks that he or she finds easier or more challenging. Studies have demonstrated that certain demographic variables, such as higher educational achievements and income, are more consistently linked with exercise adherence (Morgan & Morgan, 2005). This is a correlation, and does not specifically infer causation in either direction. However, there are other studies that also suggest, for example, that physicians are more apt to discuss lifestyle choices with patients who are of the higher-income demographic (Taira et al., 1997). When a person decides that a change in lifestyle is needed, he or she must make modifications to support the change toward the desired result. A health coach assists and empowers the individual to make the necessary changes.

Health coaching can be seen as a subset of a larger **scope of practice** involving personal (or "life") coaching. This is a new field with roots in performance psychology that now encompasses executive and leadership training. Rather than simply working through personal problems and/or underlying psychopathology, personal/life coaches work interactively with their clients to effect global changes in career and overall personal satisfaction. Personal/life coaches assess not only a client's fitness and wellness, but also career, financial, and spiritual goals that may be outside the scope of practice for a health coach. However, the strategies employed by life coaches are applicable for effective health coaching.

Client Factors

The **transtheoretical model of behavioral change (TTM)** identifies a number of stages that clients will experience as they progress through their lifestyle modifications (Prochaska & DiClemente, 1984) (see Chapter 3). Typically, a potential client has already moved from the **precontemplation** stage to the **contemplation** stage by the time he or she contacts a health coach. The key to effective coaching is to continuously improve the action process and maintain the results without regressing to old behaviors.

Factors inherent to the client that will move him or her toward, or away from, success include insight into real and perceived barriers. Adapting the transtheoretical model to the health coach client includes developing a relationship through establishment of **rapport** and an intimate trust. By actively listening and asking engaging questions, the health coach can assist the client in identifying patterns of past successes or barriers. By creating awareness to those factors that move a client toward or away from effective actions, the health coach will be able to develop a plan and identify goals that are manageable and have measurable results.

A client's stage of change is determined during an initial assessment. There are many elements to client assessment. Initially, assessments should be made with regard to the client's past efforts to invoke change, his or her current lifestyle and circumstance, the goals he or she would like to achieve, and the timeframe in which to achieve them. A current fitness evaluation can give insight to the client's physical ability, health risks, and body composition. A food diary may give insight into current eating habits and, thus, the level of nutrition education needed. It is worth exploring the barriers to change, such as fear, anxiety, or other emotions that prevent progress. It can be helpful to identify whether a client's belief system and self-talk match his or her intentions. It may be necessary to refer a client to his or her physician to ensure that there are no medical barriers to the changes desired. All of these resources are available, and will help to determine the right combination of coaching tools and personnel for each client.

One of the keys to success when meeting a client for the first time is establishing rapport. It is important to let him or her talk freely about the circumstances that led him or her to seek the expertise of a health coach. There may have been dramatic past experiences, a near-future event (such as a wedding or reunion), or a strong warning from others that led to the decision for lifestyle change. **Active listening** involves being engaged and involved with the information being presented. When a person is being heard actively, he or she may be asked questions that clarify unclear statements. It can be as simple as maintaining good eye contact and displaying empathetic facial expressions. **Empathy** is the quality that allows one who has not personally experienced an emotion to "put themselves in another's shoes." It is different from sympathy, which involves acknowledging a shared emotion from similar experiences. Once the background leading to the individual's decision has been assessed, it is important to clarify goals and establish realistic expectations.

A health coach can let a client know that the lifestyle changes he or she is about to make are not unlike training for a complex sports activity. When an athlete is training for an event or for the next performance goal, objective assessments are made to determine his or her current physical, mental, and emotional status prior to engaging in the activity. Once the current status and goals are identified, barriers to reaching the stated goals are discussed. If a goal has a barrier that is immovable or not negotiable for whatever reason, the goals may need to be reassessed and modified to something more realistic if alternative solutions cannot be established.

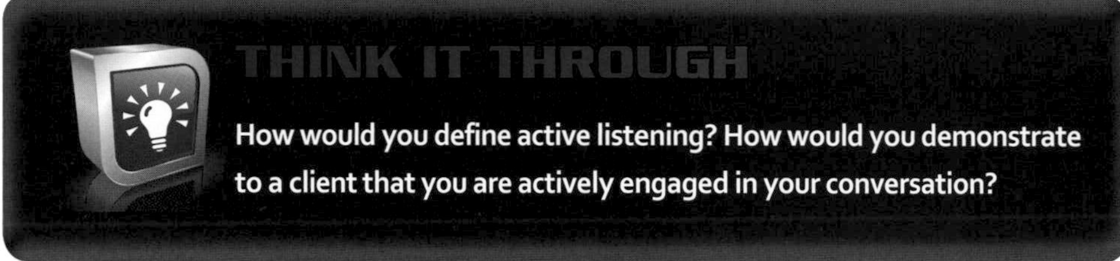
THINK IT THROUGH
How would you define active listening? How would you demonstrate to a client that you are actively engaged in your conversation?

Qualities of an Effective Health Coach

Effective health coaches typically possess a number of specific character traits. Notable traits described by influential writers such as Dale Carnegie (*How to Win Friends and Influence People*), Jim Collins (*Good to Great*), and John Maxwell (*21 Indispensable Qualities of a Leader*) typically include trustworthiness, unconditional acceptance, empathy, loyalty, integrity, and passion. A coach should aspire to be someone in whom the client finds a role model and genuine inspiration. An effective health coach can ideally go further and empower the client to become the leader in his or her own life.

The best coaches will admit that no single person is necessarily effective with everyone. Other factors, such as personality and stylistic differences, come into play when working with a variety of clients. By employing a team strategy, formally or informally, the health coach has access to a greater breadth of experiences in people management. This allows for accelerated service and broader strategies to assist a client in reaching his or her goals. Furthermore, when faced with a situation where those differences prevail despite the best of intentions, a health coach should have the professionalism to suggest that a better "fit" might be had with another coach.

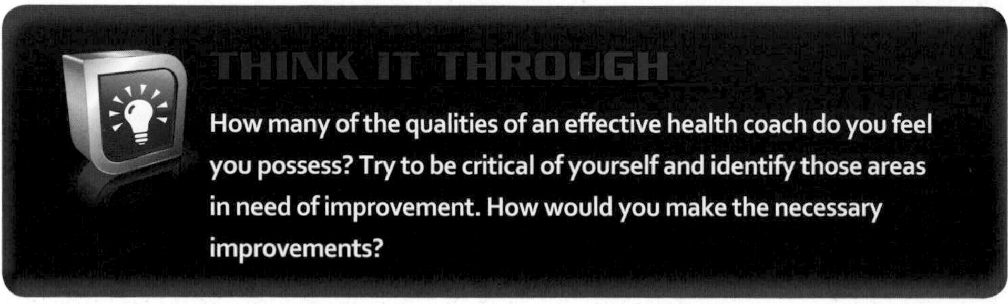

A Team Approach to Coaching

By examining the two extremes of the human physical condition, one can see that a team approach is effective for cultivating change. On the high-performance extreme, at Olympic Training Centers for example, athletes have access to personal trainers, nutritionists, massage therapists, chiropractors, and sport psychologists to assist them as they strive for their goals. There is also a team approach in the healthcare system. On the post-injury and severe illness extreme, physical medicine and rehabilitation hospitals are required to have team meetings each week to discuss the progress of each patient as he or she recovers from devastating medical events such as **stroke,** spinal cord injury, and/or complex surgeries. Between these extremes are individuals who the health coach will assist. Clients will have varying degrees of physical fitness and/or mental advantage or disability, so the strategies employed will need to be adapted for each situation. As such, when working with clients who are seeking to make changes, big or small, utilizing the power of networking and the strength in differences among professionals will improve the odds of success and maintenance of professional boundaries by utilizing synergistic strategies.

The health coach will be able to utilize exercise science, behavioral science, and nutritional science as foundations upon which to build a personalized plan for each client. It is anticipated that an effective health coach will be able to identify which of these areas the client has the most challenge in and address it accordingly. The health coach should have adequate training in these areas to identify the strengths and barriers to change, as well as other specific needs of each client to reach his or her goals. By linking the influences between each foundational science, and calling upon outside specialists for assistance as needed, the client–coach team is able to optimize its odds of success. Additionally, by networking with others who specialize in particular areas that address more difficult or resistant barriers to change, the client–coach team will further optimize the odds for creating safe, sustainable, positive change.

EXPAND YOUR KNOWLEDGE

Understanding the Health Coach's "Intrinsic Team"

Most fitness professionals know that networking and team-building are essential aspects of success, both in terms of individual clients achieving their goals and in the broader sense of having a successful long-term career in the fitness industry. Many health coaches will partner with personal trainers, registered dietitians (R.D.s), psychologists or psychiatrists, and other healthcare professionals, possibly including chiropractors or massage therapists.

While building a quality "extrinsic team" made up of these previously mentioned experts is extremely important, the multifaceted nature of health coaching requires that the health coach form what is sometimes called an "intrinsic team" as well. A health coach has to be an expert in exercise science, nutritional science, and behavioral science, and be able to call upon these various areas of expertise as needed, often multiple times within a single conversation or exercise session. Successful health coaches must seamlessly integrate these various aspects of coaching and the facilitation of long-term behavioral change. Consider a client who, in the middle of an aerobic workout, tells the health coach that he had a serious lapse in his nutrition program since their last session, largely due to being overwhelmed at work and the stresses of being a single father. The health coach must call upon his or her "internal nutrition expert" to help the client get back on track, the "internal behavioral management expert" to assist the client with time and stress management, and the "internal exercise scientist" to maintain the ongoing exercise session. This example clearly demonstrates the unique role of the health coach in the fitness industry—and why the acquisition of this certification represents a great career-development opportunity.

Power in Networking

Any enterprising professional should be involved in social media on one level or another (see pages 43–46). This is a technological extension of an old concept: networking. Every successful business has a board of directors that guides its vision and lends their expertise. Teamwork is recognized as a powerful tool in virtually every civilization in history. *Webster's Dictionary* defines networking as "the exchange of information or services among individuals, groups, or institutions; specifically, the cultivation of productive relationships for employment or business." Fortunately, with the technological advances available today, networking takes little investment and can make a great impact on the success of any business. In fact, a virtual team can be created from the technological tools widely available on the Internet.

Networking occurs both formally and informally. All of the family and friendships one acquires over a lifetime is a network of sorts. Individuals with whom one has a shared past, such as friends from school or neighbors, can be considered part of the informal network. There are no specific confidential or fiduciary duties legally associated with these relationships, and they are typically bound by social etiquette. More formal networks can involve business or legal relationships with individuals or corporate entities. Information exchanged among formal networks can be bound by privacy laws or nondisclosure agreements. Many relationships have elements of both formal and informal networks.

Business relationships are cultivated by an exchange of useful information or services. These can be considered more formal or even legal relationships. As such, they may be subject to contract laws (see Chapter 20). These professional relationships can be a source of guidance or information that is unfamiliar to a health coach, or perhaps serve as a source of new clients. Frequently, the establishment of trust and rapport with potential network members serves as an informal prerequisite to the introduction of other network members or clients.

For each individual, the functionality of physical fitness, optimized nutrition, and adequate stress management work synergistically to promote health and wellness. Being adequately trained in all of these areas will allow each health coach to call upon his or her internal area of expertise (i.e., the intrinsic team) in order to address each challenge appropriately. The health coach must utilize elements from the three foundational elements of health coaching in the effort to create change.

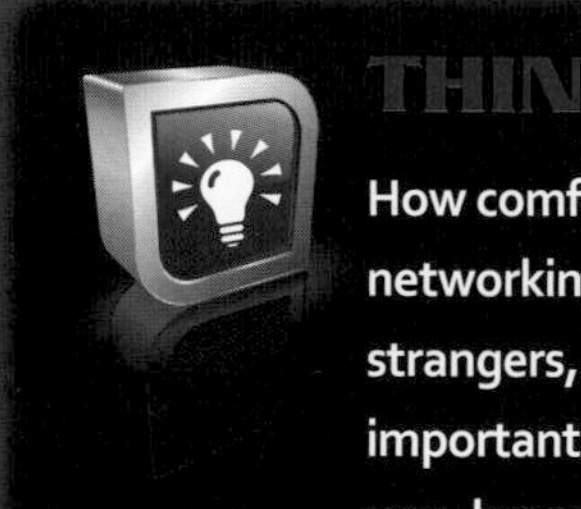

THINK IT THROUGH

How comfortable are you with the notion, and actual process, of networking? Many people struggle when introducing themselves to strangers, actively promoting their services, and making those all-important professional connections. If this is an area of concern for you, how might you address this potential weakness?

Strength in Differences

Just as each client is unique in his or her coaching needs, each coach is also unique in his or her communication style, motivational skills, knowledge base, and technical ability to affect change. The health coach is instructed on the fundamentals of exercise science, nutritional science, and behavioral management in order to utilize an integrative approach to lifestyle management. Knowledge in these three areas can offer different strategies toward successful change. For example, it has been established both in scientific studies and also in popular literature that stress and poor eating habits are frequently correlated. "Emotional eating" is a topic frequently discussed in popular magazine articles. Suggesting, for example, that a client substitute a 10-minute walk for a high-sugar snack is one way to utilize exercise science principles to assist in breaking down a barrier that is not well managed with knowledge in nutritional science and/or behavioral management. The activity has the benefit of both diffusing stress and burning calories instead of consuming them. By focusing on a positive activity, rather than avoiding a negative activity, the client has a better chance of removing the stress–eating barrier. When a client has deep-rooted emotional challenges and is resistant to change, it may be necessary to refer him or her to other team members who have more expertise in addressing these difficult problems.

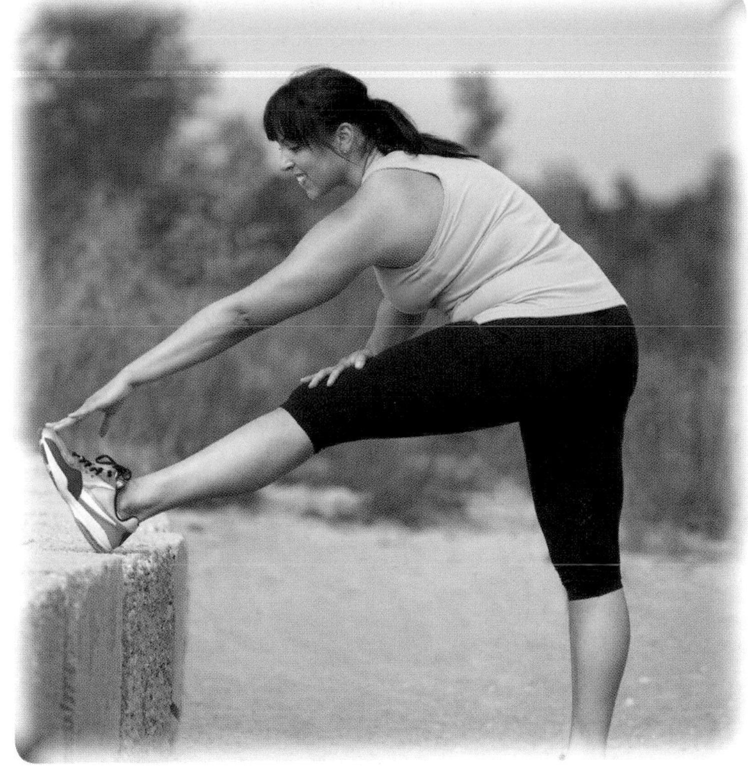

The power in networking stems from the ability of several people to lend their strengths where others might have weaknesses. In medicine, for example, many specialties and subspecialties have developed over the years as physicians have become more well-versed or trained in the understanding of a particular organ or process. As such, it is not uncommon for a patient to see several physicians when admitted into a hospital for care. This team approach to care allows the most effective care plan to be developed for each individual patient, and decreases the burden of knowledge on any one physician.

A small business can utilize the same type of team approach. As small businesses grow, it becomes more cost-effective for owners to work with others who have strengths and interests that will move the organization toward efficient and effective growth. Many of those skills are now automated or programmed to be affordable, but they can lack a personal touch. Doing cost–benefit analyses and having a variety of strategies to communicate with the client will improve the chances of success.

Improving the Odds of Success

Having a team approach allows the best qualities of a health coach to shine, and protects against potential pitfalls when working with challenging clients. One way to do this may be to shift the focus from one foundational science to another to break through barriers. By being able to utilize different strategies from a variety of evidence-based practices, the client–coach team can find an approach that will promote positive and permanent change. It is not uncommon for an individual to state a particular goal (such as weight loss) when he or she really seeks to create change in another part of his or her life (e.g., decrease stress). Another approach may be to call upon network members with more experience with this particular barrier to help develop strategic plans that have proven successful for others in similar situations.

Identifying the Team

The Coach–Client Team

The health coach has changed its designation from "consultant" to "coach" in order to emphasize the collaborative nature of the coach–client relationship. A consultant has a more directive role in relationship to a client, whereas a coach creates the environment to foster change. This team approach allows the health coach to be a co-creator of change by primarily utilizing the client's inherent strengths and assisting as necessary. As a facilitator in the relationship, the health coach can empower the client to learn the skills necessary to analyze and solve the problems identified. In this manner, the coach and client share in the assessment and planning toward new lifestyle behaviors.

The Intrinsic Team

The health coach should have some familiarity with the best practices currently in use for personal training, dietary planning, and behavioral management. These three areas of knowledge represent the basic intrinsic team of resources when coaching clients. There are a number of other professional resources and continuing education that allow the health coach to expand his or her own repertoire of knowledge and tools. The Internet has also made it easy for information exchange. However, not all information is of a high quality. Professional journals have a peer-review process that ensures the validity of the statistical method and soundness of the study design that is reflected in the quality of the studies. Most professions have their own widely accepted journals. Much of the research appropriate to exercise science, nutritional science, and behavioral management can be referenced at www.pubmed.gov. These articles are written with a high level of sophistication and can be difficult to translate into practice by casual readers. Other sources such as the *Cochrane Review* (www.cochrane.org) are written in plain language to assist medical personnel as well as patients when making informed decisions based upon evidence-based, best-practice methods. Even with these resources, there are times when consulting a specialist who gives real-time feedback makes the best use of time for the coach–client team. A diverse network is key to success.

A health coach has the foundational knowledge in exercise science and programming, nutritional science and weight management, and behavioral management needed to reinforce the positive aspects of the changes being made. Although each aspect can be a career in and of itself, it is the successful integration of all three that provides the intrinsic knowledge-based team. Using evidence-based practices will allow the health coach to call upon proven methods to assist the client in moving toward successful lifestyle change.

Exercise Science

Exercise science is the study of the acute responses and chronic adaptations to physical activity. In some colleges, this is a formal area of study in which the students systematically learn from a broad range of topics, including human anatomy, physiology, applied kinesiology, and bioenergetics. There is peer-reviewed literature that provides evidence for programming considerations, as well as an increasing body of research that has identified a positive correlation between regular exercise, disease prevention, and improved cognition and mood. This benefit correlation is maintained throughout all age groups and is integral to a health coach's programming considerations.

Nutritional Science

Nutritional science is the study of the body's physiological and metabolic responses to energy consumption and utilization. Human beings are omnivores, which means they have the ability to consume a wide variety of food substances, including animal and plant materials. Nutritional science has historically placed emphasis on the six major categories of nutrients: carbohydrates, proteins, fats, vitamins, minerals, and water. Researchers are also evaluating the effects of food on physical and psychological **satiety.** Certain amino acids are known to be **neurotransmitter** precursors, which can affect mood. For example, tryptophan is present in large quantities in turkey and is a precursor for serotonin, which partially contributes to the relaxation that follows a typical Thanksgiving dinner. Hydration and **electrolyte** balance during vigorous exercise can affect brain function and performance. When the brain has too few electrolytes, cognition is affected, and the seizure threshold is lowered; too high levels of electrolytes can lead to headaches and irritability. A well-trained health coach ideally should have a grasp of nutritional science beyond the energy-balance principles related to weight loss and weight gain (i.e., calories in vs. calories out).

Behavioral Management

Behavioral management has evolved from informal structures (e.g., etiquette) to a formal specialty that involves an understanding of the determinants of human behavior. Psychology developed as a behavioral science in the 19th century. Widely varying philosophies have pervaded in the study of this discipline. The health coach can utilize strategies that capitalize on a client's optimal sustainable performance conditions and co-create a positive emotional attachment to the new behaviors. The behavioral management area of study is still being developed in terms of proven strategies. Most of the publications are still largely anecdotal. However, most successful practitioners will state that behavioral management relies on the strength of the client–coach relationship, as well as solid communication and negotiation skills.

The Extrinsic Team

It is the rare coach who will possess a high level of competency as well as possess the appropriate professional credentials in fitness, nutrition, and performance psychology. Identifying one's strengths and weaknesses, as well as interests and aversions, will help identify the most suitable client populations. Traditional coaches associated with commercial weight-loss clinics typically possess some fundamental education in nutrition or dietary sciences, but perhaps less so in physical fitness and kinesiology. Sports psychology is a relatively young specialty with few practitioners, but can be an invaluable asset to health coaching. Medical practitioners are useful allies to assess a client whom the health coach may suspect of having underlying conditions that may be barriers to success or warrant further evaluation. Having access to professionals whose knowledge base is complementary can offer more tools to assure success for the client.

Personal Trainer

A personal trainer's scope of practice involves the planning and implementation of exercise programs (Figure 2-1). Currently, none of the 50 states requires a personal trainer to be licensed. Certification is not a legal requirement, but is required for employment in most fitness facilities.

Figure 2-1
The ACE-certified Personal Trainer Scope of Practice

ACE-certified Personal Trainer Scope of Practice

The ACE-certified Personal Trainer is a fitness professional who has met all requirements of the American Council on Exercise to develop and implement fitness programs for individuals who have no apparent physical limitations or special medical needs. The ACE-certified Personal Trainer realizes that personal training is a service industry focused on helping people enhance fitness and modify risk factors for disease to improve health. As members of the allied healthcare continuum with a primary focus on prevention, ACE-certified Personal Trainers have a scope of practice that includes:

- Developing and implementing exercise programs that are safe, effective, and appropriate for individuals who are apparently healthy or have medical clearance to exercise
- Conducting health-history interviews and stratifying risk for cardiovascular disease with clients in order to determine the need for referral and identify contraindications for exercise
- Administering appropriate fitness assessments based on the client's health history, current fitness, lifestyle factors, and goals utilizing research-proven and published protocols
- Assisting clients in setting and achieving realistic fitness goals
- Teaching correct exercise methods and progressions through demonstration, explanation, and proper cueing and spotting techniques
- Empowering individuals to begin and adhere to their exercise programs using guidance, support, motivation, lapse-prevention strategies, and effective feedback
- Designing structured exercise programs for one-on-one and small-group personal training
- Educating clients about fitness- and health-related topics to help them in adopting healthful behaviors that facilitate exercise program success
- Protecting client confidentiality according to the Health Insurance Portability and Accountability Act (HIPAA) and related regional and national laws
- Always acting with professionalism, respect, and integrity
- Recognizing what is within the scope of practice and always referring clients to other healthcare professionals when appropriate
- Being prepared for emergency situations and responding appropriately when they occur

Although personal trainers may have some knowledge of illnesses and injuries, it is not within their scope of practice to make diagnoses or recommend supplements, which can be perceived as providing treatment of medical illnesses. In some states, such as California, to act outside of fitness, or fail to refer to appropriate healthcare professionals, is considered a criminal offense punishable by incarceration. However, this does not prevent some personal trainers from advocating fitness products and nutritional supplements that are sold in the facility where they work.

It is within the scope of practice of the personal trainer to observe and assess the basic **biomechanics** of a client, then plan and implement exercise programs accordingly. In the event that medical concerns are suspected, personal trainers may be required to refer clients to a physician for diagnosis. For example, if a client has reported low-back pain and is noted to have an excessive spinal curvature that cannot be corrected by coaching the client into a more neutral spinal position, the personal trainer should suggest that the client see a physician to have this properly evaluated. Once the treatment options are in place or precautions made known, the exercise program can then resume.

Nutritionist/Registered Dietitian

There are some key differences between a nutritionist and a dietitian. "Nutrition" or "nutritional science" are official programs of study at many colleges. Those who have degrees in nutrition may go on to have careers in other healthcare fields or test to become registered dietitians. The Academy of Nutrition and Dietetics, formerly the American Dietetic Association, has a three-block practice framework for their R.D. members (www.eatright.org):

- Block 1 is foundational knowledge that abides by a code of ethics, possesses science-based knowledge, demonstrates competency established by credentialing exams, acts autonomously, and provides services to individuals or population groups.
- Block 2 involves maintaining the standards of practice that are accepted by the profession at large. This involves implementation of treatment plans for eating disorders as an allied healthcare provider.
- Block 3 involves legal credentialing, organizational privileging, and utilizing best-evidence tools and nationally developed guidelines for practice.

As suggested above, not all nutritionists are registered dietitians, but all R.D.s have education in nutritional science. If a client has an uncontrolled chronic condition (such as diabetes) or a history of diet failures or weight-cycling, a referral to an R.D. may be warranted.

> In January 2012, the American Dietetic Association (ADA) changed its name to the Academy of Nutrition and Dietetics (A.N.D.). Throughout this text, research conducted by the organization prior to this name change is cited to the ADA, while newer studies will be credited to the A.N.D. Refer to www.eatright.org for more information on the reasons behind the name change.

Psychologist/Psychiatrist

Psychology is also a course of study with degrees at the college and graduate school level. There are many subspecialties within psychology designed to assist persons with behavioral or thought disorders. Psychologists cannot prescribe medications, but are often associated with psychiatrists (a medical doctor with post-graduate training in mood, behavior, and thought disorders). One should note that there are clinicians who also engage in counseling, but are not necessarily degreed in psychology. In some states, social workers can function as counselors to the public for psychological services, and there may be little or no licensing requirements. Additionally, pastoral services are frequently used for specific psychological needs, such as grieving. The health coach may need to research the best fit as a team member. A client with a suspected eating disorder should consult with a licensed behavioral specialist.

One subspecialty under psychology that has gained ground in recent years is sports psychology. Mental training methods have been utilized historically, with examples including meditation, guided imagery, and biofeedback. More recent efforts have been made to create a systematic and rigorous program to address the issues that are specific to performance and competition. Most sports psychologists are not exclusive in this practice, as many of them maintain standard clinical clients in order to have a full complement to support their practices.

Healthcare Professionals

Licensed healthcare professionals serve an important role on the health coach team. Evaluation and treatment of a client with multiple risk factors may be necessary prior to engaging in physical activity or over the course of the program (after an injury or protracted illness) in order to diagnose underlying illness or injury that may require medical assistance. For example, a client who has weight gain despite changing eating and exercise habits, who also complains of "bloating" and general lethargy, may have an underlying thyroid condition. Referring to a physician or healthcare practitioner who is able to evaluate and treat this condition may be necessary to remove a barrier to the client's goals. Other clients may have medications that will alter their ability to tolerate increases in their activity levels. For example, timing of insulin injections may interfere with programmed activity. Only a physician is within the legal scope of practice to change prescribed medications.

THINK IT THROUGH

Identify your own areas of focused knowledge as a health coach. Do you excel in the areas of exercise science, nutrition, or behavioral coaching? What types of services do you feel most comfortable providing to your clients? Are there any areas you need to improve upon in terms of continuing education or practical experience?

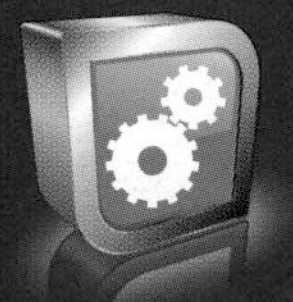

EXPAND YOUR KNOWLEDGE

Understanding the Educational Requirements and Scope of Practice for Each Potential Team Member

Acupuncturist

- L.Ac. (licensed acupuncturist): A license granted by individual state entities, typically to have confirmed national-level certification; able to perform acupuncture and may have complementary medical privileges (e.g., traditional Chinese medicine), and/or lab-ordering privileges depending upon the state licensing laws

Chiropractor

- D.C. (doctor of chiropractic): Post-baccalaureate degree program, typically four years in length; a variety of different chiropractic philosophies and practices exist; do not have prescription writing or surgical privileges; however, depending upon the state, may prescribe and dispense nutritional and herbal supplements

Dietitians

- R.D. (registered dietitian): A baccalaureate-level degree with clinical practicum and national certification testing

Naturopathic Physicians

- N.D. (naturopathic doctor): A four-year, graduate-level naturopathic medical school with all of the same basic sciences as a medical doctor (M.D.), but also studies holistic and nontoxic approaches to therapy with a strong emphasis on disease prevention and optimizing wellness; in addition, the naturopathic physician is required to complete four years of training in clinical nutrition, acupuncture, homeopathic medicine, botanical medicine, psychology, and counseling; licensure is by a state or jurisdiction as a primary care general practice physician; scope of practice varies by state law

Nurses

- L.P.N. (licensed practical nurse): Typically an associate-level degree with clinical practicum
- R.N. (registered nurse), B.S.N. (bachelor of science in nursing): A baccalaureate-level degree with clinical practicum and national certification testing
- M.S.N.: Master of science in nursing
- A.R.N.P. (advanced registered nurse practitioner): Graduate-level degree, typically requiring several years of practical clinical experience; able to prescribe some medications and practice somewhat independently
- Ph.D.: Doctorate in nursing studies; typically a title used in an academic setting

Physicians

- M.D. (doctor of medicine): Typically four years of post-baccalaureate medical school, at least three years of post-graduate training upon completion of the degree; able to prescribe medications and therapies; may have admitting privileges at hospitals
- D.O. (doctor of osteopathy): same academic and clinical training as M.D.s, but also have instruction and practicum in osteopathic manipulation

Behavioral Medicine Practitioners

- Counselor: Baccalaureate- or masters-level degree; some may have social work or other backgrounds with clinical practicum in psychological counseling
- D. Psy. (doctor of psychology): Doctorate level degree in psychology

Physical Therapists

- P.T.A. (physical therapy aide/assistant): Aides are frequently trained on the job, while assistants have an associate-level degree; in some states, the latter is required to have licensure in order to practice
- P.T. (physical therapist): A baccalaureate- or masters-level degree in a physical therapy course of study
- D.P.T. (doctor of physical therapy): A doctorate-level degree with a dissertation defense in physical therapy

Occupational Therapists

- C.O.T.A. (certified occupational therapy aide/assistant): Aides are frequently trained on the job, while assistants have an associate-level degree; in some states, the latter is required to have licensure in order to practice
- O.T. (occupational therapist): Baccalaureate- or masters-level degree in an occupational therapy course of study
- Dr.O.T. (doctor of occupational therapy): A doctorate-level degree with a dissertation defense in occupational therapy

THINK IT THROUGH

How would a health coach network with other professionals help to expand an existing client base? What types of opportunities might exist for collaboration?

Utilizing a Virtual Team

To what extent can technology and/or social media augment a health coach's access to others who have a different scope of practice to improve opportunities in the client–coach team?

Exercise

Draft a referral letter for a client to a qualified health professional. In four sentences or less, communicate how you envision they can get involved and participate in your program.

Communicating With Team Members

When communicating with clients, utilizing the strategies of active listening will ensure that both parties are in relative mutual agreement. For example, a client may state that he or she seems to have a drop in energy in the afternoon, followed by a trip to the coffee shop for a beverage. The client may know intellectually that the coffee drink is adding several hundred calories to his or her total daily intake, but has created a habit over time. These complex behavior patterns typically involve more than just getting a caffeine fix, and may simply be a way to break up the day into another segment before going home. Frequently, the barrier to change will be identified when the client is allowed to talk freely about the circumstances around his or her behavior. Other times, a client may reflect that the barrier may be related to a medication that peaks around mid-day, which may necessitate a discussion with the client's physician. When substitute behaviors require other professionals, being able to communicate the barrier and the end-goals efficiently may result in an integrated solution for the client.

Making Initial Contact

There are many reasons for communicating with extrinsic team members. For some clients, medical clearance may be needed prior to commencing a program involving changes in diet and exercise. This clearance improves the safety margin from which a program may be created. For the health coach, having access to other professionals builds credibility and offers resources for consultation and reference. It also has the potential to build market share for the health coach's services. However, finding and maintaining relationships with other professionals can be a daunting experience for some individuals. It should be a relief to know that most potential team members are more than willing to network services.

When making contact with a physician or other healthcare practitioner, it may be advantageous to start with a physician with whom the health coach is already familiar. Meeting with a client's personal physician is an effective way to gain future referrals. Gain permission from the client to meet his or her physician. The most difficult way to make initial contact is by "cold calling" an office to request an appointment. Once at the appointment, keep the presentation brief and collaborative in nature. Explain the concept of the health coach within a few minutes (no more than three), and describe the importance of having a place to refer patients with medical clearance issues. Providing a written biography that includes education, credentials, and pertinent experience is beneficial, as are referral forms.

Physicians who might be the most open to a team relationship with a health coach include family practice and internal medicine specialists. Many of their patients are generally healthy, with controllable risk factors such as **hypertension, diabetes,** and/or obesity. Members of these populations will benefit most from lifestyle changes. When a health coach collaborates with a primary care provider, the burden of compliance can be shared. Once an effective change has been made in one client, it is likely that the physician will refer other patients to the health coach. There may also be the potential for the physician to refer colleagues, further expanding the team.

EXPAND YOUR KNOWLEDGE

Consultation Notes

The initial contact with a client typically involves gathering useful information. The key to establishing rapport and allowing an opportunity for the client to give the most useful information is the use of active listening. It is recommended that the health coach use an open-ended statement to allow the client to speak freely. Statements such as, "Tell me about yourself," delivered in a private setting, will most likely allow the client to give more complete history of his or her challenges and successes. Allow the client to speak freely, and ask clarifying questions at regular intervals while maintaining good eye contact and mirroring the client's mood and body language. If notes are being taken, write down a few key words rather than transcribing entire sentences. Staying focused and actively engaged with the new client will assist with gathering the most useful and complete history.

Most consultation notes will have elements of the following:

- *Chief complaint:* Identify the challenges that the client is experiencing. It is recommended that dates and circumstances surrounding each of his or her health issues be elicited fully using open-ended, active questioning. Inquire as to specifics regarding the client's eating habits and exercise program. Identify the client's feelings surrounding the challenges and barriers to change, as doing so will offer potential solutions in the planning stage.

Employ the following strategies in active questioning:
- ✓ Explore needs, motivations, desires, skills, and thought processes. Facilitate the client's own thought processes in order to identify solutions and actions.
- ✓ Observe and listen actively to the client's description of his or her life circumstances.
- ✓ Maintain unconditional positive regard for the client. Be supportive and non-judgmental of the client's lifestyle and goals.

- *Past history:* How has the client attempted to work through this challenge in the past? What were successful strategies? What strategies did not work?
- *Current diet/medications/exercise program:* The client may not have analyzed his or her eating, exercise, or behavior styles objectively. The health coach should strive to be unbiased and non-critical to promote honesty.
- *Social history:* Identify the client's environment, support structure, and sources of potential lifestyle stressors.
- *Physical examination:* This involves the assessment of physical abilities, any biomechanical deficiencies or asymmetries, strength/flexibility/endurance factors, and so on. Use objective tests and measurements for future reference. By converting the units from English to metric or vice versa, the emotional attachments to the measurements may be removed. For example, it may be easier for a client to learn that he or she weighs 100 kilograms rather than 220 pounds.
- *Assessment:* List challenges and any correlation with identifiable stressors or barriers.
- *Plan:* Propose strategies to address each item listed under the assessment. Keep the following in mind when partnering with the client on a proposed plan:
  - ✓ Identify realistic goals and objective means of assessing progress.
  - ✓ Develop personal competencies and avoid dependency upon the health coach.
  - ✓ Encourage personal choice to act positively toward each goal.
  - ✓ Work within the framework of the client's competency to achieve change.
  - ✓ Positive emotions assist the individual in making real, lasting change.

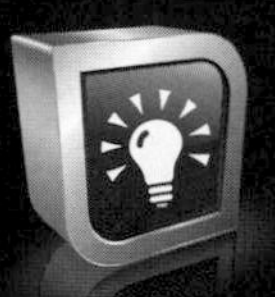

THINK IT THROUGH

Writing a Consultation Note

A 37-year-old female attorney is meeting you for the first time. She states that she gained 65 lb (30 kg) with her second child two years ago, and has kept about 50 lb (23 kg) of the weight since the delivery. She went back to work full-time three months after delivery and carries a full schedule as a family-court attorney. She usually has a cup of coffee with sweetened creamer in the morning, and will pick at the donuts or anything that is left in the break room at around 10:00 a.m. Two days a week she is in court, where she may sit for several hours waiting for her case to be heard. She will frequently grab a fast-food sandwich on her way back to the office, where she sits for several more hours sifting through paperwork and making phone calls. Frequently, she goes to the coffee shop in the afternoon for a large mocha to get a boost of energy.

After work, she commutes about 30 minutes to get home, where she tends to her young children. She reports that they dine out frequently at night, as she and her husband are both too tired to cook. After dinner, she gets the kids ready for bed. Several days a week, she will review her briefs in preparation for the next day and goes through her daily "to do" list. Her weekends are filled with basic household chores, such as laundry, grocery shopping, and organizing the house. She has not exercised regularly since she was in college, and states that just walking up one flight of stairs makes her "winded." Her goals are to lose at least 35 lb (16 kg) and feel less stressed.

Write a sample consultation note for this client.

Updates on Mutual Clients

In general, most professionals create value when they are engaged with client-related activities, even when not face-to-face. As such, time that is spent on client activities that do not involve direct contact with the client, however necessary, becomes administrative time. Most effective team leaders limit the amount of administrative work they must perform personally in order to optimize their schedules. Efficient methods of communicating with other professionals regarding mutual clients have been developed to best serve the client by minimizing the required administrative time.

Recalling specific client information is paramount to team communication. Most professionals will have more clients than they can know in detail. For this reason, there should be some recordkeeping mechanism that allows for recall. When calling or meeting to discuss a mutual client, be ready to give his or her full name, age, gender, and some identifying information (e.g., birth date) to allow the other team member to pull up the documentation of the last visit. Be brief and direct when stating the nature of the discussion, keeping the purpose to two or three sentences at most. Having these details on hand will facilitate the discussion with other team members. Being concise in communications is a positive marker of a professional. It demonstrates that the caller has an appreciation for the value of time for both parties, while keeping the best interest of the mutual client in mind. Using the **SOAP note** format, the vital information about a client can be communicated very efficiently to a healthcare practitioner, typically within one minute. Being able to use this presentation skill with all team members decreases the amount of time performing non-compensated administrative activities, yet effectively harnesses the contributions of each member of the team. Some members of the healthcare team may prefer written updates.

The frequency of contact is somewhat established by those who interface with the particular professional on a regular basis. Typically, team members should expect to receive updates every four to six weeks. More frequent communication may be perceived by the team member as offering too much contact without being able to report on actual change. Communication that takes place less frequently than about every eight weeks runs the risk of being forgotten. For example, pharmaceutical representatives typically make contact with their assigned physicians every four to six weeks to update them on any new research or information that is released by the parent company. Similarly, if a client is also seeing an R.D. or psychologist, four-to-six week intervals are typical, as this allows for measurable change that is used to assess the effectiveness of ongoing programs.

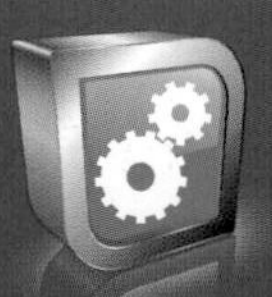

EXPAND YOUR KNOWLEDGE

SOAP Notes

One tool frequently used for healthcare professionals to communicate with each other is the SOAP note—the acronym stands for subjective, objective, assessment, and plan. It is a concise way to summarize a person's condition as it relates to the goal of the visit.

Subjective: This section is used to document a client's feelings or subjective complaints or symptoms. For example, if a client states, "I felt depressed and had two desserts last night," this section documents his or her personal feelings or experiences.

Objective: This section documents actual measurements made by the health coach. The weight or other measurements agreed upon by the client–coach team are recorded in this section. Any noticeable symptoms are also recorded here (e.g., client appeared short of breath today at the usual workload).

Assessment: This section addresses the relatedness of the subjective comments to the objective measures made, and whether any relationship exists between the two. If a clear relationship—either a positive or negative correlation—exists, an action plan can be made to address it as it pertains to the goals of the client. By creating transparent awareness to the relationships between a client's inner state and his or her actions, modifications to the behavior can be made.

Plan: This section outlines the plan agreed upon by the client–coach team to move toward the goals discussed. The plan should have goals that are measurable and attainable on some scale by the next session.

One strategy to create momentum toward success is to have achievable deadlines. Each goal should be broken down into steps that are achievable by the next meeting of the client–coach team. If a step is not achieved fully, the team can then identify the barriers and agree on strategies to overcome them. For example, a client may state that he or she does not have time to exercise. The health coach can work together with the client to identify ways to tie exercise into an existing activity. Simple ways to work in more physical activity include parking farther away from a destination or taking the stairs regularly.

Sample SOAP Note

S: Ms. S. reports that she exercised twice last week. She states that she finds it difficult to stop at the gym, even though it is on her way home from work. She feels that she should get home to make dinner and be with her family each evening, although they frequently go out because she and her husband are too tired to make dinner. The children typically want fast food, but she insists on healthier options. She reports that she feels good when she does go to the gym and seems to have more energy. She seems to require less sleep, but have better quality sleep, when she exercises. She reinforces that she is committed to the idea of regular exercise and better eating, but "life gets in the way."

O: Weight today is 183 lb (83 kg), essentially unchanged from last week.

Food diary: 2,300 kcal per day on average, most of it in the evening within two hours of going to sleep. Pedometer: average 4,500 steps per day, with variance between 3,000 and 8,000 (the latter on the days that she exercises.)

A: Ms. S is a 41-year-old professional woman whose goals are to have more energy and lose 30 lb (14 kg) this year. Her challenges are as follows:

Exercise frequency: goal is to exercise at least 30 minutes, most days of the week. Barriers include getting off work late and her desire to be with family.

Quality and time of food intake: goal is to increase quality and nutrient density of foods eaten, and to distribute the calories more evenly throughout the day. Barriers include established patterns at home and limited availability of quality food.

P: Utilize weekend days to establish new food and exercise patterns to be introduced during the week. We agreed to the following:

She will participate in one, 30-minute outdoor activity with her children near her home, on each of the weekend days, such as walking the neighborhood or the trail at the county park. If she does not go to the gym, she agrees to tell her family that she is walking in the neighborhood for at least 15 minutes when she gets home. She will encourage her family to join her on these walks.

She will cut up fresh fruit and vegetables and place them in snack bags, along with string cheese and small amounts of trail mix, to be taken to work each morning if breakfast is not eaten. She will choose a variety of healthy foods at lunch and eat a soup or salad for dinner.

We will reassess her progress next week.

THINK IT THROUGH

Writing a SOAP Note

You are following up with a client whose goal is to lose 25 lb (11 kg) in time for his high-school reunion. He states that although it was difficult to commit to working out daily, he did feel better after using the stationary cycle for 15 minutes each evening this past week. He states that last week his energy level was higher in the afternoons, even without his usual post-lunch coffee. He continues to crave ice cream after dinner, especially when he sits down in front of the television. His current weight is 215 lb (97.6 kg), down from 218 lb (99.0 kg).

Write a SOAP note for this client.

Effective Networking

There are many business books dedicated to the art of networking. Essentially, networking is about building relationships to strengthen both of the individuals' efforts in pursuing their respective goals. Networking tends to be a collaborative activity, requiring all parties to be both giving and receiving information in similar measure. By contrast, marketing is an activity that seeks to separate one from others in the marketplace. While health coaches can act to promote themselves during the networking process in order to create interest, they can also show interest in others' marketing niches to ensure continuing relationships and collaborations toward common goals. People, in general, like doing business with those they like and trust, regardless of the actual product features. Networking involves utilizing opportunities to build relationships with others who share the health coach's goals.

Co-branding

Co-branding or brand-partnership is when two entities collaborate to create marketing synergy. For example, the makers of Post Raisin Bran® state on its packages that they use "Two scoops of real Sunkist® raisins." Companies market their products together to create brand-recognition value for each of their individual products. The health coach can utilize this strategy when establishing an extrinsic team framework to boost recognition of each individual in the partnership. Co-branding creates synergy by linking the perceived added-value of known entities and their reputations. The potential pitfall to co-branding is when one or more of the partners experience degradation in their image. This can lead to decreased perceived value of the partnership as well.

Strategies for Effective and Efficient Communication

When communicating with members of a coaching team, using accepted templates for progress charting will facilitate discussions about clients. In healthcare, initial consultations and follow-up SOAP notes are widely utilized for the concise summary of an individual's complaint, condition, and proposed changes, in writing or in person. SOAP notes are frequently part of the individual's permanent records within an office or a hospital. Electronic medical records (EMRs) allow other treating physicians to review the records for patients and avoid duplication or the repetition of potential adverse events.

One potential pitfall when communicating with healthcare professionals is using words and vernacular that sound medical, but are inaccurate. In general, healthcare providers are accustomed to plain language used by their patients and prefer to have information delivered simply.

Managing a Client With Medical or Psychological Difficulties

Clients can pose a number of challenges to even the most seasoned health coach. The challenges can be internal to the client and/or external or environmental. Challenges that are internal to the client include battles with **depression, anxiety,** and/or substance abuse. These internal challenges are frequently compounded by problems with fitness motivation, nutritional choices, and base psychological state. For example, someone who is depressed and overweight may have the baseline depression compounded by a poor self-image, which leads to compensatory eating of "comfort foods" that lead to short-term feelings of wellness but add weight over time. This situation then feeds back into the depression because of the feelings of helplessness and a lack of control.

External challenges include family members, such as spouses, who do not share the problems of the client and are not necessarily supportive of the changes. For example, consider a woman who has gained a significant amount of weight after the birth of a child and would like to get to her prenatal fitness state, which may require her spouse to assist with childcare when she is at a workout or agree to a significant change in the types of foods served in the home. Occasionally, a spouse is unwilling or unable to assist, which forms a barrier over which the client may not necessarily have control. These difficulties and barriers should be identified with a focus on developing solutions that are within the client's control whenever possible.

There are a number of barriers to creating a well-balanced activity, nutrition, and psychologically supportive program of change. Occasionally, there are medical reasons for one or more of these challenges, which requires referral to a physician for proper evaluation prior to commencing a program. For example, consider a client who has had increasing difficulty with weight loss, experiences fatigue daily, "retains water," and reports depression. This client may have hypothyroidism, which can only be diagnosed and treated by a physician. A client with diabetes may experience anxiety at the end of a workout because his or her blood **glucose** may be lower than the previous baseline, causing subjective symptoms of malaise that can be rectified with a medication adjustment. Frequently, symptoms that are reproducible (e.g., every time a client exercises he or she feels lightheaded or experiences numbness in both feet) have a medical basis and may warrant a referral back to his or her physician. Once a diagnosis is made, compliance with the treatments suggested should result in positive changes for the client.

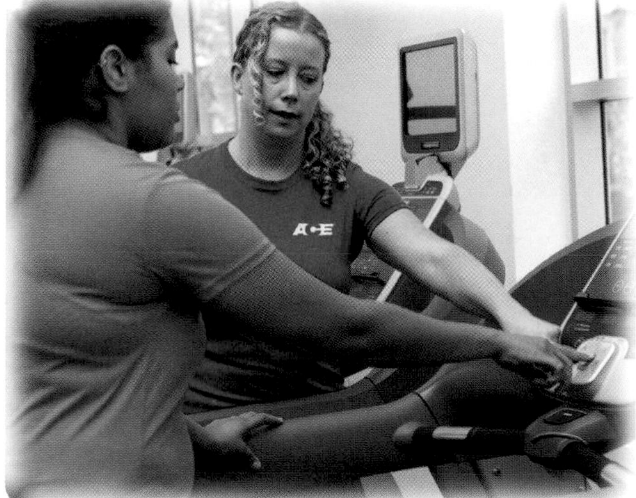

Food allergies are another challenge. True food allergies can be devastating and have serious consequences, including death. True food allergies are usually identified in childhood and include common products such as peanuts, wheat, and eggs. Many people who do not have medical emergencies upon consuming certain products have food sensitivities. Sensitivities to products do not cause anaphylactic reactions, but do produce adverse effects that are predictable. For example, people with lactose intolerance may experience gastrointestinal upset when they eat dairy products. Certain sensitivities to allergenic sources can cause skin and tongue conditions, such as rash or patchy loss of rugae (the rough surface) on the tongue. They are typically self-limiting (i.e., they disappear on their own without any medical intervention), and can be treated symptomatically with oral or topical medications as needed. Of the foods that are generally suggested in a comprehensive lifestyle program, the gluten in whole grains, certain fruits, lean dairy sources, and legumes could be potentially problematic. Fortunately, choice has increased in the typical grocery store as well as in restaurants. A referral to an allergist may be indicated.

Psychological barriers to lifestyle change include depression, anxiety, and/or substance abuse. The challenge may be to identify whether the psychological barrier is primary or secondary. Primary depression or anxiety is typically the result of neurotransmitter imbalance and a genetic and/or psychological predisposition. These conditions can respond dramatically to medications. Secondary depression is due to some other factor manifesting as symptoms. For example, iatrogenic (secondary to medication or other intervention) causes of depression can include medications treating high blood pressure, **epilepsy**, heart arrhythmias, and high **cholesterol.** Alcohol use can also cause symptoms of depression. Reactive depression is an emotional response to situations that are unexpected, such as grieving a death, change in relationship status, or loss of employment. Treatment for primary and reactive depression includes regular exercise, light therapy, psychological support, and medications. Treatment for secondary depression may require a review of the cause and options that will both address the medical condition being treated and decrease the side effects. There is a segment of the population that has higher requirements for sunlight and can suffer from seasonal affective disorder (SAD). One treatment is using UV lights that mimic sunlight. Low-intensity exercise in the early mornings has also demonstrated to be effective in treating SAD, so a client may want to change the time of his or her fitness program to amplify this effect (Peiser, 2009). Seasonal use of antidepressants may also be prescribed for those with particularly severe symptoms.

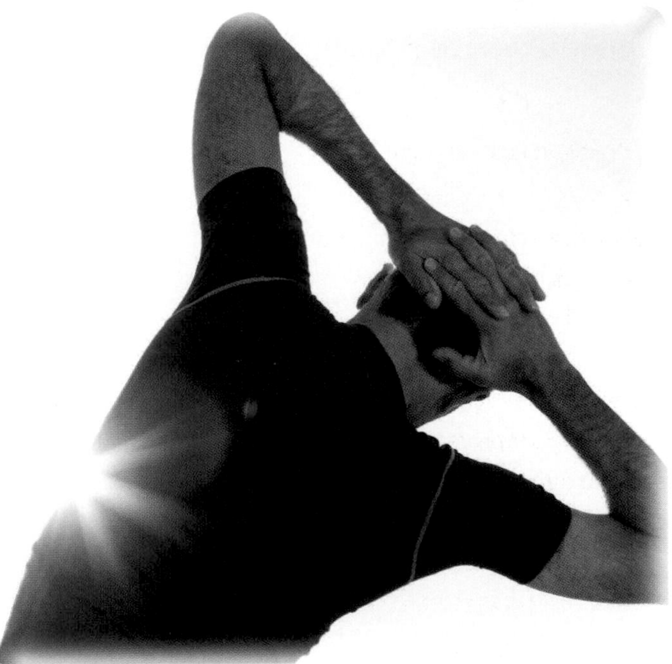

Similar principles exist for anxiety, with some individuals suffering from situational anxiety, such as a fear of public speaking, and others becoming anxious due to past experiences when feeling threatened, such as confronting a hostile spouse or boss. Those who are pathologically anxious can have a panic disorder. Anxiety symptoms may also be related to excessive use of caffeine, amphetamines and their derivatives, and even as a late effect after large amounts of alcohol as the body becomes dehydrated. Treatments for anxiety disorder include psychological counseling, moderate exercise at regular intervals, and medications for more severe symptoms. There are also medications that can cause symptoms that mimic anxiety, such as the use of thyroid replacement drugs, certain antidepressants, and amphetamine-derivatives for attention deficit disorders. Clients with anxiety that is poorly managed may benefit from a referral to either a psychologist or physician to evaluate their risk factors and suggest treatments. Clients with moderate to severe health problems may benefit from a referral to an ACE-certified Advance Health & Fitness Specialist (ACE-AHFS), who will have more training in dealing with specific medical conditions.

Avoiding Pitfalls in Teamwork

Team-splitting Behaviors and Co-treatment

On occasion, a health coach may have clients who exhibit difficult traits. One of those behaviors is termed "splitting." The client say one thing in person, but recount the story completely differently with another team member. Psychologists have deemed people with this type of behavior to have "borderline personality traits." Often, the client may not even be aware that he or she is engaging in the behavior and seem oblivious to the adverse effects it may have on the team. When this occurs, it is important for the health coach to have a meeting with the various team members and discuss perceptions about the behavior and its causes. Once the members agree to a strategy to manage the behavior, arrange a meeting with the client as a team ("co-treatment"), but keep the focus on the positive effects that each member is contributing to the client's progress and ask for feedback and/or concerns that the client may have. After the meeting, if the client uses splitting language during sessions, gently remind him or her of the positive gains mentioned during the meeting and move on to the next task.

Managing a Difficult Client

Some clients will be more challenging than others. Sometimes, the client lacks general sophistication in social etiquette. Others lack effective coping skills. Some clients suffer from psychological problems that stem from anxiety, depression, eating disorders, and/or substance abuse. Access to a counselor, a psychologist, or others who are better equipped to handle difficult conversations may improve the effectiveness of the client–coach relationship.

Most professionals will have at least one or two, if not more, clients who are "high maintenance" or "difficult." The clients may or may not be aware that they simply require more assistance than others in similar situations. Some people seem to thrive on "drama" in their lives because it is familiar to them, and may seem to create drama when there is none simply to maintain a level of consistency in their lives. Not infrequently, this may be where the behavioral management part of the client–coach team will work hardest to break through barriers. The health coach may need to address emotional "baggage" to better assist the client to lose weight. In some cases, simply drawing attention to the issue will effect a change in the behavior. Other times, a referral to a mental health professional may be needed to offer sustainable change. The health coach, as part of the client–coach team, may have triggers that result in limited coping capacity with particular personalities. By knowing the boundaries and barriers of both parties, decisions and behavioral change can be made to optimize the outcome for both team members.

EXPAND YOUR KNOWLEDGE

Personality Disorders and Traits

Frequently referred to as "axis II disorders," personality disorders demonstrate the extremes of poor interpersonal relationship skills. It is important to note that many individuals can exhibit a combination of aspects taken from across the personality trait spectrum. In order to qualify for a diagnosis of a personality disorder, one must exhibit a disproportionate number of behaviors from those listed in the *Diagnostic and Statistical Manual (DSM)* under specific groups. Clinical diagnosis of a personality disorder is limited to the scope of practice of, and should only be made by, a psychiatrist or psychologist. However, being aware of these traits will assist the health coach in understanding the patterns that may underlie some client behaviors. There are three "cluster" references:

- *Cluster A:* Schizoid, schizotypal, and paranoid. These individuals seem odd and eccentric without losing grasp on accepted reality. Not infrequently, these people avoid being in public and prefer to be by themselves.
- *Cluster B:* Narcissistic, histrionic, borderline, and antisocial. These individuals are demanding of attention, dramatic, emotionally unstable, and frequently go through relationships intensely before severing them completely. They have a poor sense of boundaries and have an exaggerated sense of relationships (positive or negative) that hide a fundamental lack of security. Generally speaking, individuals with these traits will offer the most pronounced challenges. These people are drama-magnets.
- *Cluster C:* Dependent, anxious, and obsessive-compulsive. These individuals exhibit anxious and fearful behavior. Coping mechanisms frequently involve dependence upon others or rules and rigid behaviors that offer a sense of security.

Note that some individuals will exhibit strong behaviors without completely meeting the criteria set. Those with subclinical psychopathology are assessed to have "personality disorder traits."

When and How to Discontinue Professional Relationships

It is likely that some professional relationships will need to be discontinued. Sometimes, the end of a contract signals the end of the formal relationship. Other times, the legal or fiduciary relationship has not been completely fulfilled, but the terms of the relationship render the task untenable. It is preferable to sever ties diplomatically, and "agree to disagree."

Most businesses employ an "exit strategy" for dissolving the business or partnership when it ceases to function toward its stated goals. Similar strategies can be built into every client–coach relationship. Stating upfront that if certain landmarks are not achieved within a particular agreed-upon timeframe, the relationship may need to be terminated in order to direct the client toward his or her goals is one way to build in an exit strategy upon initial consultation. Other times, referring to other professionals in order to break through barriers, either as a temporary or permanent arrangement, also moves the client toward positive change. The discontinuation of a professional relationship does not necessarily represent failure, but rather a redirection in order to achieve the desired change.

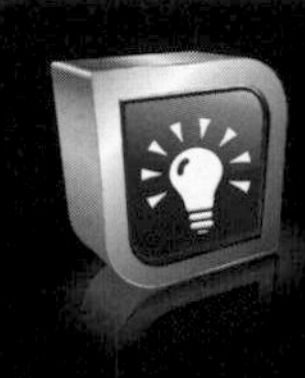

THINK IT THROUGH

What are your plans regarding keeping in touch with past clients? Do you have a policy in place for following up with clients after they have completed their time with you?

Helping a Client Establish His or Her Own Team

At the Olympic Training Center, athletes frequently engage those from other sports to partake in each other's events. Martial arts athletes will learn table tennis, and will teach judo takedowns in return. Since most of the athletes are fairly coordinated and kinesthetically proficient, they are able to compete at a relatively high level of expertise after a short time. In that environment, some athletes are able to cross over to other sports, should they find affinity and desire to compete in a new sport. Many times, their friends are not on their teams, but have skills that are complementary. Archers and marksman have different equipment, but have nearly identical training schedules. Many types of athletes use similar strength-training and mental-management strategies. Nearly all of the athletes engage in mental training with a sports psychologist. It is not uncommon that when specialized athletes take on a new sport recreationally, they become even better at their original sport. In addition to the benefits of cross training, there is a new dimension to their mindset when they engage other high-performance athletes.

Similarly, clients who are able to make changes to their lifestyles should be encouraged to socialize with others who have also transitioned to good habits. It is beneficial to reduce the negative impact of the client's old lifestyle in order to move on toward the new behaviors. Positive emotional bonds reinforce the changes made, and offer clients self-sufficiency in maintaining the change. With social media now a legitimate method of marketing and communication, its power can be utilized to create a virtual team by which both the coach and client can maintain the changes that have been made. Using Twitter, for example, a client can be connected instantly to a whole network of interested parties who can respond to an imminent relapse into a food binge or ask for motivation to proceed with a daily workout. A Facebook post from a branding page can be the morning motivational thought for all of the clients and followers of a business or practice.

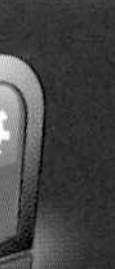

EXPAND YOUR KNOWLEDGE

Virtual Tools for the Health Coach

By Ted Vickey, M.A.

Ted Vickey, M.A., is an entrepreneurial strategist whose clients have included the U.S. Department of Commerce, the Securities and Exchange Commission, Fruit of the Loom, and Osram Sylvania. He is currently a Ph.D. candidate at the National University of Ireland Galway in exercise adherence and technology and is a member of the ACE Board of Directors.

Imagine a health coaching practice where your website ranks on page one of an internet search, where bills are paid, and fees are collected with the touch of a button. In addition, clients' nutrition and physical-activity achievements are wirelessly sent from their mobile phones to your email for tracking. That practice is readily available through the use of technology. There are two types of technology that health coaches should consider as part of their overall coaching practice: business-management tools and connected health tools.

Business-management Tools

Coaching businesses can reap the benefits of various business-management tools, including the creation of a coaching practice website, engagement with clients, professional relationship management, appointment scheduling, accounting, and online credit card processing.

It can be difficult to decide which platform is most suitable for a coaching practice. Which platform allows for easy publishing of a site and can also grow with one's coaching practice? Which platform drives engagement and leads to new clients and/or additional appointments? Which platform has reporting capabilities that can show a return on the initial investment? While the task may seem daunting at first, the reality is that with some trial runs, and even beta-testing with friends and family, creating an online business-management platform may offer tremendous return for very little time investment. No longer must a health coach hire an expensive design company to create a website, although for best results, consulting a website designer is never a bad idea.

Social media and online marketing are increasingly important for health coaches to get a practice noticed and utilized by potential clients on the web. There are a number of good reasons for a coaching practice to participate in and maintain an online presence, including the following:

- Connect and engage with current and potential clients
- Get discovered by people searching for health coaching services
- Create an active and persuasive community around the practice
- Promote content such as webinars, blog articles, or health tips (visit www.ACEfitness.org for free tips you can use in your practice)
- Generate leads for the practice

Health coaches around the world are using Facebook as their primary website, not only to attract new business, but also to remain engaged with former and existing clients. On Facebook, "profiles" are meant for people, while "pages' are meant for businesses. To fully engage and leverage the power of Facebook, be sure to create a page for the coaching practice. Pages are public and are split into different categories, and are therefore searchable. These "branding" pages also allow anyone to become a fan of (or "like") the coaching page without needing administrator approval. Facebook also provides flexible privacy settings to control who sees what parts of your page (*Source:* Hubspot). For additional information about setting up Facebook as your website, conduct an online search for "Facebook for Business."

Health coaches are also using Twitter to stay in touch with clients by sharing short, valuable health-related tips. Twitter is a free service that allows anyone to say anything in 140 characters or less. Twitter allows health coaches to promote particular services directed at a target market; connect with other coaches who share their views; get instant access to relevant, timely opinions; receive a steady stream of ideas, content, links, resources, and tips focused on their area of expertise; and monitor what is being said about the coaching practice (*Source:* Duct Tape Marketing). Twitter is more than promotion; it is also about the sharing of valuable information. For every business/coaching promotion, consider sharing several health tips. For additional information about using Twitter in your coaching practice, search "Twitter for Business."

Another easy-to-use website that can add value to a health coach's practice is LinkedIn (www.linkedin.com). On LinkedIn, health coaches can connect not only with potential clients, but also with other health and wellness professionals in the area, state, and even around the world. Health coaches should be sure to add all relevant information, include a professional picture, request the vanity URL (that can include your name in the URL), and use this resource to connect with other like-minded professionals with a click of the mouse. The LinkedIn help section provides tips to make a profile stand out from the rest. Once a member of LinkedIn, health coaches should join groups and be active by posting questions, providing answers, and engaging with the rest of the group. There are a number of ACE groups on LinkedIn that health coaches can join, all for free.

Other do-it-yourself websites include Tumblr (www.tumblr.com), Pinterest (www.pinterest.com), Instagram (www.instagr.am), and Tout (www.tout.com). Prior to committing to one site, spend some time planning an online strategy. It helps to have a checklist of features that are both user-friendly and useful. Review other professionals who are currently using these tools effectively.

For additional information about business tools for coaching practices, consider searching for these terms: social media, online marketing, online appointment scheduler, online accounting, and credit card processing. Also visit the ACE website (www.ACEfitness.org) for additional resources for building, marketing, and expanding a health coaching practice.

Connected Health Tools

Former Surgeon General C. Evert Koop dreamed of a day where "...cutting-edge technology, especially in communication and information transfer, will enable the greatest advances yet in public health. Eventually, we will have access to health information 24 hours a day, 7 days a week, encouraging personal wellness and prevention, and leading to better informed decisions about health care" (Koop, 1995). That dream is now a reality, as personal trainers, nutritionists, and health coaches are using the power of technology (the Internet, social networking services, and mobile phone applications) as persuasive tools to help clients lead healthier lives.

Specific to the health coaching profession, connected health tools are small, inexpensive client-based mobile applications or websites that eliminate the four walls of a physical building and allow coaching to take place virtually in real time. These tools can transmit health data from the client to the health coach, such as heart rate, physical activity, meal logs, body weight, blood pressure, and sleep habits. This allows the health coach to not only hold clients accountable between appointments, but also allows for real-time immediate feedback and encouragement for daily behaviors. By using connected health technology, health coaches can provide a more personalized experience and potentially reach more individuals with effective health-related advice and information at a very low cost. Griffiths et al. (2006) suggest five reasons for using connected health tools for delivering web-based health, wellness, and fitness interventions:

- Reduced delivery costs
- Convenience to users
- Timeliness
- Reduction of stigma
- Reduction of time-based isolation barriers

Within the healthcare field, interactive technologies can be effectively deployed to take on multiple roles at the same time. For example, a simple online tool can measure calories while at the same time giving a reward upon attainment of a personal goal. This type of self-monitoring is a key ingredient in successful behavioral modification. The power of self-monitoring is not just between client and coach. Research suggests that if several people are connected through the Internet, social support can be leveraged, which has been shown to impact motivation and behavioral change (Chatterjee & Price, 2009). Health coaches should find ways to connect clients with friends, family, or other clients to create an "electronic bond." Accountability emails, online chats, Facebook posts, and Twitter messages can be powerful motivational tools.

Tracking of physical activity is moving away from the paper and pencil of a workout card and more toward digital tracking. Technology allows users to track progress, interact with coaches who can suggest areas for improvement, and self-administer tests and measures. Blood pressure cuffs that connect to the web, body-weight scales that tweet a person's weight, and even sleep-monitoring systems are allowing people to track their personal health data from the comforts of their own homes (www.withings.com). Tracking tools such as BodyMedia (www.bodymedia.com), FitBit (www.fitbit.com), Jawbone UP (www.jawbone.com/up), and Nike Fuel (www.nike.com/fuelband) empower users to collect and share exercise, nutrition, and sleep data. In-depth nutrition apps such as MyNetDiary (www.mynetdiary.com) and Foodzy (www.foodzy.com) are modern, comprehensive diet services that help users track and monitor food intake while displaying a robust nutritional analysis based on personalized guidelines. These tools can be extremely useful for a client who needs that extra motivation to stay the course.

Mobile fitness applications can offer similar tracking options for a fraction of the cost. Apple and Android software provide data collection and motivational tools. The sharing of data within a private group, on Facebook, or on Twitter can provide additional accountability and support for clients. Health information data portals such as Microsoft's Health Vault (www.microsoft.com/en-us/healthvault) and RunKeeper's HealthGraph (www.runkeeper.com) allow for health data to be collected, monitored, and shared not only with the client, but also with other members of the client's healthcare team, including physicians, nutritionists, and personal trainers.

For more information about connected health tools that health coaches can implement in their practice, conduct an online search for mobile fitness applications (or "apps"), personal health-information management, Microsoft Health Vault, and mobile health apps.

THINK IT THROUGH

Design a series of tweets or blog titles focused on simple ways to incorporate more physical activity throughout the day.

Summary

A team approach to affect change and move toward a goal has its foundations in cognitive-behavioral science and can be used synergistically with current evidence-based, best-practice methods in exercise and nutritional sciences. Many professional services, including the healthcare profession, have moved toward a collaborative methodology with the client to promote sustainability of the changes made. Health coaches have the opportunity to work with other members of the allied health team to create lifelong wellness by combining the client's inherent strengths with sound science and effective coaching techniques.

References

Bandler, R. & Grinder, G. (1979). *Frogs Into Princes: Neuro Linguistic Programming.* Salt Lake City, Utah: Real People Press.

Bandura, A. (1986). *Social Foundations of Thought and Action: A Social Cognitive Theory.* Upper Saddle River, N.J.: Prentice-Hall.

Chatterjee, S. & Price, A. (2009). Healthy living with persuasive technologies: Framework, issues, and challenges. *Journal of the American Medical Informatics Association,* 16, 2, 171–178.

Chomsky, N. (1959). *Aspects of the Theory of Syntax.* Boston: MIT Press.

Griffiths, F. et al. (2006). Why are health care interventions delivered over the internet? A systematic review of the published literature. *Journal of Medical Internet Research, 8,* 2, e10.

Kolb, D.A. (1984). *Experiential Learning.* Upper Saddle River, N.J.: Prentice-Hall.

Koop, C.E. (1995). A personal role in health care reform. *American Journal of Public Health,* 85, 6, 759–760. www.pubmedcentral.nih.gov/articlerender.fcgi?artid=1615490&tool=pmcentrez&rendertype=abstract

Morgan S. & Morgan K. (2005). *Health Care State Rankings.* Lawrence, Kans.: Morgan Quitno Press.

Pavlov, I.P. (1925). *Conditional Reflexes.* New York: Dover Publications.

Peiser, B. (2009). Seasonal affective disorder and exercise treatment: A review. *Biological Rhythm Research,* 40, 1, 85–97.

Piaget, J. (1926). *Language and Thought of a Child.* London: Clark University Press.

Prochaska, J.O. & DiClemente, C.C. (1984). *The Transtheoretical Approach: Crossing Traditional Boundaries of Therapy.* Homewood, Ill.: Dow Jones-Irwin.

Skinner, B.F. (1953). *Science and Human Behavior.* New York: Free Press.

Taira, D.A. et al. (1997). The relationship between patient income and physician discussion of health risk behaviors. *Journal of the American Medical Association,* 278, 17, 1412–1417.

Thorndike, E.L. (1931). *Animal Intelligence.* New York: The Macmillan Company.

Watson, J.B. (1924). *Behaviorism.* Chicago: University of Chicago Press.

Suggested Reading

Blackett, T. (1999). *Cobranding: The Science of Alliance.* London: Palgrave MacMillan.

Carnegie, D. (1936). *How to Win Friends and Influence People.* New York: Simon & Schuster.

Collins, J. (2001). *Good to Great.* New York: Harper-Collins.

Frates, E.P. et al. (2011). Coaching for behavioral change in physiatry. *American Journal of Physical Medicine and Rehabilitation,* 90, 12, 1074–1082.

Grossman, R.P. (1997). Co-branding in advertising: Developing effective associations. *Journal of Product & Brand Management,* 6, 3, 191–201.

Grunden, N. (2007). *The Pittsburgh Way to Efficient Healthcare: Improving Patient Care Using Toyota-based Methods.* Pittsburgh, Pa.: Productivity Press.

Guseh, J.S., Brendel, R.W., & Brendel, D.H. (2009). Medical professionalism in the age of online social networking. *Journal of Medical Ethics,* 35, 584–586.

Holmes, T.H. & Rahe, R.H. (1967). The social readjustment rating scale. *Journal of Psychosomatic Research,* 11, 2, 213–218.

Mack, G. (2001). A model for communicating with physicians. *IDEA Personal Trainer,* Sept.

Maxwell J. (2007). *21 Indispensable Qualities of a Leader.* Nashville, Tenn.: Thomas Nelson.

Murchu, I.O., Breslin, J.G., & Decker, S. (2007). Online social and business networking communities. *Proceedings of ECAI 2004 Workshop on Application of Semantic Web Technologies to Web Communities,* 241–267.

Prochaska, J.O., Norcross, J.C., & DiClemente, C.C. (1994). *Changing for Good: A Revolutionary Six-Stage Program for Overcoming Bad Habits and Moving Your Life Positively Forward.* New York: Harper Collins.

Riley, S. (2005). Respecting your boundaries. *IDEA Trainer Success,* Sept.

Selye, H. (1950). Stress and the general adaptation syndrome. *British Medical Journal,* 1, 4667, 1383–1392.

Zimmerman, G.L., Olsen, C.G., & Bosworth, M.F. (2000). A 'stages of change' approach to helping patients change behavior. *American Family Physicians,* 1, 61, 5.

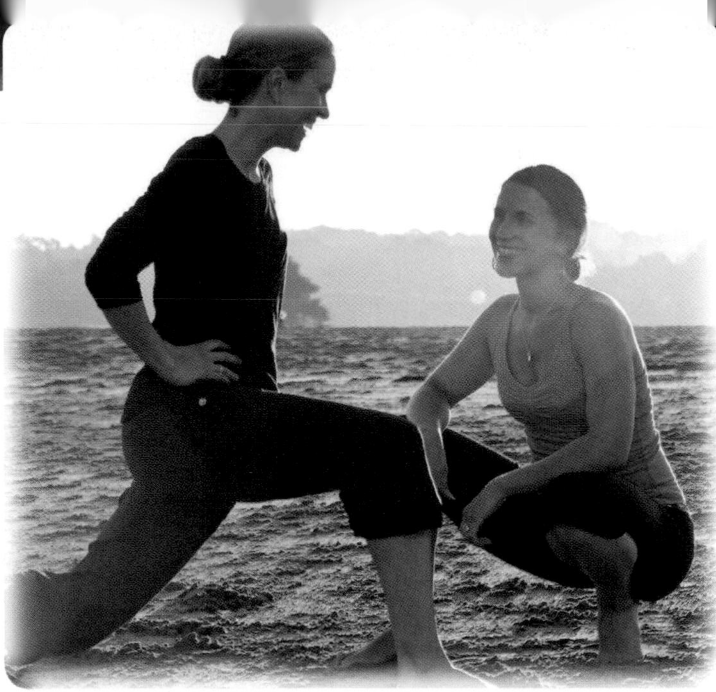

IN THIS CHAPTER:

Tracie Rogers, Ph.D., is a sport and exercise psychology specialist and the director of the MS Human Movement Program at A.T. Still University. She is also the owner of BAR Fitness, located in Phoenix, Arizona. Dr. Rogers teaches, speaks, and writes on psychological constructs related to physical-activity participation and adherence.

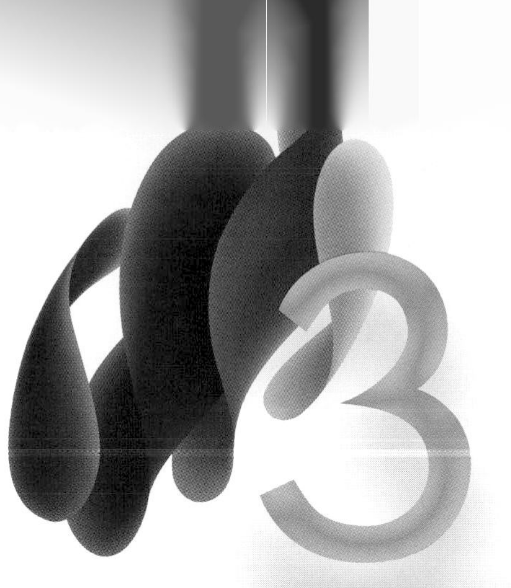

Health Behavior Sciences

TRACIE ROGERS

& MICHAEL R. MANTELL

Michael R. Mantell, Ph.D., earned his Ph.D. at the University of Pennsylvania and his M.S. at Hahnemann Medical College, where he wrote his thesis on the psychological aspects of obesity. His career includes serving as the Chief Psychologist for Children's Hospital in San Diego and as the founding Chief Psychologist for the San Diego Police Department. Dr. Mantell is a member of the Scientific Advisory Board of the International Council on Active Aging, the Chief Behavior Science Consultant to the Premier Fitness Camp at Omni La Costa, a best-selling author of two books, including the 1988 original Don't Sweat the Small Stuff, P.S. It's All Small Stuff, *an international behavior science fitness keynote speaker, an advisor to numerous fitness-health organizations, and is featured in many media broadcasts and worldwide fitness publications. He has been featured on Oprah, Good Morning America, the Today Show, and has been a contributor to many major news organizations including Fox and ABC News. Dr. Mantell is a nationally sought after behavioral science coach for business leaders, elite amateur and professional athletes, individuals, and families. He is included in the greatist.com's 2013 list of "The 100 Most Influential People in Health and Fitness."*

Although the traditional biomedical model that explains diseases from a strictly physiological standpoint led to great advances and understanding in the health and medical community, the approach does not describe the whole picture, and as healthcare costs continue to rise along with the occurrence of lifestyle diseases, it is clear that a more comprehensive approach is needed.

Health psychology emerged in the 1970s as a field of psychology that examines the causes of illnesses and studies ways to promote and maintain health, prevent and treat illnesses, and improve the healthcare system (Sarafino & Smith, 2011). Health psychology took the traditional biomedical model and added the individual to the equation. As a result, it has created a broader picture of the **correlates** of health and illness by examining not only the biological factors, but also the psychological and social factors that affect, and are affected by, a person's health (Engel, 1977). Under a biopsychosocial model, behavioral risk factors, such as smoking, inactivity, alcohol abuse, and excess sugar consumption, have been identified for each of the five leading causes of death.

ACE-certified Health Coaches are in a unique position to greatly impact a client's overall health by decreasing the behavioral risk factors of numerous diseases. Because health coaches are working directly with clients on achieving long-term behavioral change, it is important that they understand the social and psychological factors that influence the adoption and maintenance of health behaviors.

Defining Health and Wellness

The health coach is a change agent above all else, whose primary focus is aiding clients in their quest for healthier living, particularly in the area of weight management and health-related behaviors. The World Health Organization (WHO) defined health in 1946 as "a state of complete physical, mental, and social well-being and not merely the absence of disease or infirmity" (WHO, 1946). Later, in 1986, the WHO said that health is "a resource for everyday life, not the objective of living. Health is a positive concept emphasizing social and personal resources, as well as physical capacities" (WHO, 1986). Physical health is anchored in exercise, proper nutrition and body weight, freedom from substance abuse, and adequate rest. The WHO (1986) defines the other aspect of health, mental health, as "a state of well-being in which the individual realizes his or her own abilities, can cope with the normal stresses of life, can work productively and fruitfully, and is able to make a contribution to his or her community."

Central to understanding health and wellness is recognizing that good health does not mean "being without illness." Rather, health includes wellness—a sense of well-being and having a positive quality of life. Thus, wellness is a positive set of factors related to optimal health, including positive relationships and meaningful work:

- *Emotional:* The ability to express emotions with comfort and in a healthy manner
- *Intellectual:* The ability to learn and use intellectual capabilities to make healthy decisions
- *Social:* The ability to develop satisfying interpersonal relationships
- *Environmental:* The ability to appreciate the external environment and improve environmental conditions
- *Physical:* The ability to achieve a healthy lifestyle in the service of one's own health
- *Spiritual:* The ability to seek meaning and purpose in one's daily life

The Health Coach's Role in Prevention and Risk Reduction

A health coach is a central figure in preventing illness and early death. Encouraging, motivating, and teaching clients to engage in regular physical activity, choose healthy nutrition and eating habits, and properly manage emotional stress, among other lifestyle decisions, all are associated with reduced disease risk and increased wellness. The health coach is particularly focused on **hypokinetic diseases** or conditions, which are associated with too little activity or exercise (*hypo* = too little; *kinetic* = activity). **Cardiovascular disease,** low-back pain, **diabetes,** and **obesity** are examples of hypokinetic diseases.

Health coaches play a large role in coaching for weight management, including providing tools for making decisions that lead to good nutrition and healthful diet habits. These interventions are a significant part of the health coach's important place in preventive healthcare. In this capacity, the health coach can directly reduce and prevent major health risks associated with weight-related conditions, including the following (U.S. Department of Agriculture, 2010):

- Overweight and obesity
- Malnutrition
- Iron-deficiency anemia
- Heart disease
- High blood pressure
- Dyslipidemia (poor lipid profiles)
- Type 2 diabetes
- Osteoporosis
- Oral disease
- Constipation
- Diverticular disease

Medical Fitness

One of the key trends in health and fitness is the development of the field of medical fitness. Integrated health and fitness centers are defining a fast-growing arena in which health coaches will be valued members of the professional team. Clients who are aging, suffering with chronic diseases, in need of physical therapy or post-surgery aftercare, or have a host of multiple risk factors including obesity and a **sedentary** lifestyle, are finding their physicians are often "prescribing" physical activity and health coaching. The goal of medical fitness professionals is aligned with the goals of the health coach and other health and fitness professionals—to improve the health status of clients through coaching, management, and prevention.

The health coach will likely have clients who also have diabetes, obesity, heart disease, hypertension, and other chronic lifestyle-oriented diseases. The medical fitness industry will very likely become a valued source of referrals to those health coaches who have built bridges to this professional community. Showing physicians how the services of a health coach can improve their patient outcomes is invaluable in networking.

Establishing ties with other professionals in this expanding behavioral health science field is advantageous for the health coach. Developing a network of medical fitness centers, hospitals, primary care physicians in local communities, physical therapists, and other health professionals to support mutual growth is an excellent way to begin. The health coach should understand the continuum of care that begins with a primary care physician, moves to a physical therapist, and then moves to a post-rehabilitation or post-medical care specialist. This is where the health coach can enter the system.

Attending local conferences and lectures, taking additional classes, and becoming publicly visible in health-promotion activities in the local community are additional ways for a health coach to connect with medical fitness professionals. This will help the health coach develop a trusting relationship. The health coach needs to demonstrate that he or she is doing something that is valued by the referral network.

Proactively contacting schools, local YMCAs, hospitals, physician's offices, physical therapists, and medical fitness centers is a smart way to enter the healthcare network system. Pamphlets, social media, emails, personal letters, and face-to-face meetings are effective ways to initiate contact (Figure 3-1).

Figure 3-1
Sample email

Dear Dr. ________________________:

I'd like to introduce myself to you for your kind consideration as a referral resource to help your patients in need of weight management, fitness, & health coaching as a part of their overall care. I recently earned my American Council of Exercise certification as a Health Coach, in addition to holding a certification as ________________________________.

My specialty training has prepared me to work with you on behalf of your patients to develop sound, balanced weight-management programs that include nutrition, exercise, and lifestyle change. My training has specifically enabled me to understand the psychological aspects of weight management, the biomechanical and physiological impact of obesity, techniques for lifestyle coaching to facilitate behavior change, the relationship between exercise and nutrition in weight control, and exercise programming and weight-management strategies and progressions.

I'd like to stop by and introduce myself to you and your staff and will give your office a call later this week. Enclosed please find my card and a pamphlet describing the assistance I can offer your patients in supporting the care you provide to them.

Thank you very much.
Mary Smith, ACE-certified Health Coach

Determinants of Behavior

Unfortunately, there is no simple explanation for why some people engage in healthy behaviors and others do not. Additionally, because a person is engaging in one healthy behavior does not mean that he or she is more likely to engage in other healthy behaviors. The complexity of understanding and predicting health behaviors is further complicated with physical activity, as exercise is perceived to take more time and effort than other health behaviors (Turk, Rudy, & Salovey, 1984). However, despite the complex task of successfully promoting activity adoption and maintenance, researchers do have some understanding of factors that influence exercise behavior. There are numerous predictors of health behaviors, including learning, social and individual factors, and motivations and emotions.

Operant Conditioning

It is known that people learn health-related behavior from a variety of sources, including other people and the environment. This is also true of unhealthy behaviors. Health coaches will be more effective at triggering behavioral change if they understand some of the history behind the development of their clients' current behaviors and the keys to learning new behaviors. One way that people learn behavior is through **operant conditioning,** a process by which behavior is influenced by its consequences. Operant conditioning examines the learning process by looking at the relationships between **antecedents,** behaviors, and consequences (Martin & Pear, 2010).

Antecedents

Part of the learning experience is realizing which behaviors have consequences under certain conditions. Antecedents are stimuli that precede a behavior and often signal the likely consequences of the behavior. Antecedents help guide peoples' behavior so that it will most likely lead to positive or desirable consequences. Furthermore, antecedents can be manipulated in the environment to maximize the likelihood of desirable behaviors. This type of influence on behavior is called **stimulus control** and can be a valuable tool in behavior modification (see page 74).

Response Consequences

The most important component of operant conditioning is what happens after a behavior is executed. Different types of consequences lead to different behavioral outcomes, and consequences always involve the presentation, nonoccurrence, or removal of a positive or aversive stimulus. **Positive reinforcement,** or the presentation of a positive stimulus, increases the likelihood that a behavior will reoccur in the future. **Negative reinforcement,** which consists of the removal or avoidance of aversive stimuli following a desirable behavior, (i.e., removing a negative condition in order to strengthen a desired behavior) also increases the likelihood that the behavior will occur again. **Extinction** occurs when a positive stimulus that once followed a behavior is removed, which means that the likelihood of the behavior occurring again is decreased. **Punishment,** which consists of an aversive stimulus following an undesirable behavior, also decreases the likelihood of the behavior occurring again. Despite being effective in decreasing an unwanted behavior, punishment also increases fear and decreases enjoyment.

It is important that health coaches provide appropriate **feedback** and consequences to client behaviors. Health coaches must positively reinforce the things that clients are doing well and must not ignore the things that need improvement. Clients need a clear understanding of the target behaviors, and providing consistent consequences will help decrease program ambiguity (Smith, 2010). Additionally, if clients have clear expectations, they will be more able to succeed by meeting the demands of the program.

APPLY WHAT YOU KNOW

Operant Conditioning

In a lifestyle-modification program, the goal is to increase healthy behaviors in clients' lives. According to the principle of operant conditioning, behaviors are strengthened when they are reinforced. In the health coach context, using reinforcements means that positive or healthy behaviors have consequences that are going to increase the likelihood of the behavior happening again. At the most basic level with a new client, a positive behavior is simply showing up to the gym. If the success of this behavior (which can be a real victory for a new exerciser) is ignored by the health coach, the likelihood of it happening again will decrease. However, if the client is verbally rewarded for showing up and is further rewarded with a positive, pleasant, and supportive workout experience, then the behavior has been positively reinforced and the likelihood of it happening again has been increased. As health coaches, the opportunity to trigger lasting change is always present, and the basic principle of operant conditioning can serve as a good reminder of the influence health coaches have in each and every client encounter.

Habit

As health coaches work to decrease negative health behaviors and increase positive health behaviors, it is important to remember that most behaviors are habits. In other words, over time, behaviors become established in one's life and are executed without much thought or, more importantly, resistance. Health coaches need to be aware of the fact that most health behaviors are habitual because this creates a challenge when working to remove unhealthy behaviors from one's lifestyle. Most people are unable to just stop doing something unhealthy. Instead, clients are more likely to succeed if unhealthy behaviors and habits are replaced with more productive, healthy behaviors. New antecedents and consequences must be implemented to instigate the change of habitual behaviors, and **social support** networks are important for this challenging task.

Social and Individual Factors

Social Support

Social support from family and friends is an important predictor of physical-activity behavior and has been consistently related to activity in both cross-sectional and prospective research designs (Duncan & McAuley, 1993). It is difficult for an individual to maintain a lifestyle-modification program if he or she does not have support at home or at work. When support is broken down into specific types, support from a spouse is shown to be an important and reliable predictor of program **adherence.** Support, or lack thereof, can be presented in many forms, including motivation, confidence, and willingness to also make changes. Health coaches need to be aware of the type of support a client is receiving and should always work to create support within the exercise environment.

The health coach will be also offering a great deal of social support to clients who are seeking weight management and lifestyle change. There are four primary types of social support:

- *Emotional support:* The health coach will provide empathy, concern, acceptance, encouragement, and care (Wills, 1991). The client will typically feel valued when receiving this type of support.
- *Tangible support:* The health coach provides educational services and other concrete and direct methods of assistance. Most clients will easily recognize this instrumental support (Heaney & Israel, 2008).
- *Informational support:* This is problem-solving support that includes advice, guidance, and suggestions, and may involve the use of videos, pamphlets, books, websites, and other sources of information (Krause, 1986).
- *Companionship support:* This involves creating a sense of belonging and a feeling of comfort when attending sessions with others in small groups, as well as discussing comfort-related issues about being in a health club or medical fitness center (Uchino, 2004).

Personality Traits

Personality traits refer to general tendencies that people have in their personality or psychological makeup. Personality traits account for individual differences between people, and are often difficult to define and measure. However, there are some general traits that have been shown to be related to health behaviors. Self-motivation, which is reflective of one's ability to set goals, monitor progress, and self-reinforce, has been shown to have a positive relationship with physical-activity adherence (Dishman, 1982). The more self-motivation that a client brings to the program, the easier it will be for the health coach to implement the program and engage the client, as a self-motivated client is fully prepared to be accountable and active in the program. Additionally, conscientiousness is an important characteristic that represents an individual's tendency to be organized and dutiful, and it has been linked to higher fitness levels and healthy food selection (Bogg & Roberts, 2004). A conscientious client will be aware of program expectations and will work on a regular basis to meet the demands of all aspects of program participation. Additionally, this type of client will be more prepared to make changes in his or her life to fully adopt the lifestyle modifications.

Cognitive Factors

Individuals have a wide variety of knowledge, attitudes, and beliefs about starting and sticking with an exercise program. Modifying the way an individual thinks and feels about exercise has been shown to influence his or her intentions for being active. Health perception, which is a knowledge, attitude, and belief variable, has been linked to adherence, such that those who perceive their health to be poor are unlikely to start or adhere to an activity program. Furthermore, if they do participate, it will likely be at an extremely low intensity and frequency (Dishman & Buckworth, 1997). **Locus of control,** which is a belief in personal control over health outcomes, is another variable in this category, and, in healthy adults, is a consistent predictor of unsupervised exercise activity. Finally, the variable of perceived barriers, such as lack of time, consistently demonstrates a negative relationship with activity-program adherence. The more information and knowledge people have about exercise and healthy eating behaviors, the more likely they will be to succeed in a lifestyle-modification program. Long-term success is ultimately related to one's ability to problem solve and make decisions and program modifications as needed. However, without the knowledge to make accurate judgments and assessments, a person will be unable to successfully self-monitor, which will decrease the likelihood of long-term behavioral change. Additionally, a lack of knowledge about a lifestyle-modification program can add to the problem of unrealistic expectations about the program and an unrealistic assessment regarding the need to change. Health coaches must be proactive in providing continual education to their clients so that they have the necessary cognitive skills to succeed.

It is essential that health coaches be able to explain to clients how internal thoughts—or cognitions—affect behavior. Albert Ellis founded the practice of rational emotive behavior therapy (Ellis, 1994; 1962; Ellis & Harper, 1961), which was later expanded upon by Aaron Beck (1975), and David Burns (1980). This approach is now largely referred to as cognitive behavior therapy or simply coaching. Ellis' model provides the health coach with the understanding and practical approach necessary to harness a client's cognitions in a manner that is directly applicable.

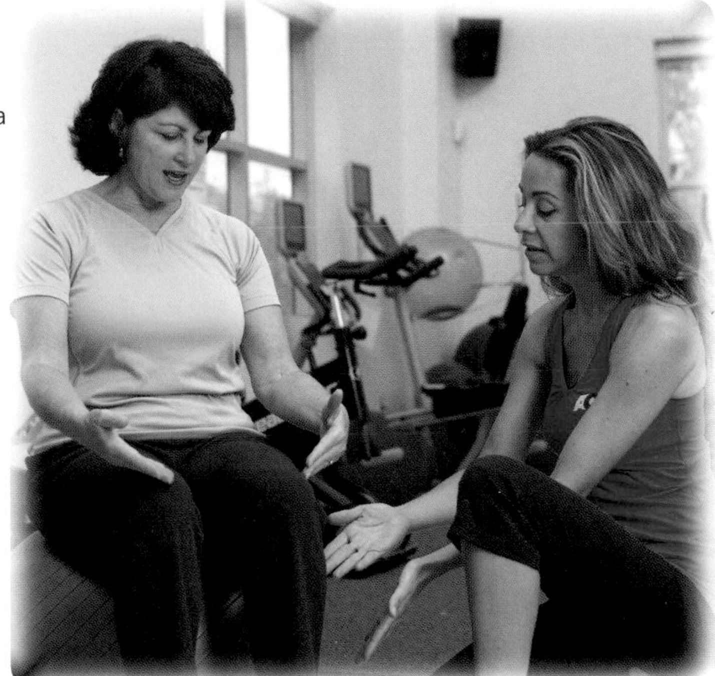

Ellis posits that people's beliefs determine how they feel and behave, not the external events they actually face. First, an external event takes place. The client then has a thought (often irrational, distorted, or inaccurate) about that situation. He or she then has an emotional reaction to the *belief* about the external event, leading to an emotional reaction that causes a response behavior. For example, a client has been contemplating beginning a weight-loss program after his physician suggested that losing weight is necessary for health. The client believes, "I've never had success in the past with losing weight, and I'll never have success in the future. I feel like a failure when it comes to weight loss. I can't stand to feel like a failure—it's intolerable for me." The client feels sad, depressed, and desperate. The client therefore does not move into the planning or action stages of behavioral change.

There are 10 "cognitive irrational distortions," any one of which may lead to anxiety, depression, or anger—all emotions that increase the likelihood that the client will not be successful in adopting a healthy behavior-change plan (Burns, 1980):

- *All-or-nothing thinking:* Look at things in absolute, black-and-white categories
- *Overgeneralization:* Viewing a negative event as a never-ending pattern of defeat
- *Mental filter:* Dwelling on the negatives and ignoring the positives
- *Discounting the positives:* Insisting that accomplishments or positive qualities "don't count"
- *Jumping to conclusions:* (a) Mind reading—assuming that people are reacting negatively when there is no evidence for this belief. (b) Fortune telling—arbitrarily predicting that things will turn out badly

- *Magnification or minimization:* Blowing things way out of proportion or shrinking their importance inappropriately
- *Emotional reasoning:* Reason from how one feels: "I feel like an idiot, so I must really be one," or "I don't feel like doing this, so I'll put it off."
- *"Should" or catastrophe statements:* Criticizing oneself or other people with "shoulds" or "shouldn'ts." "Musts," "oughts," and "have-tos" are similar offenders. "It is horrible, terrible, awful, and catastrophic and it should not be."
- *Labeling:* Identifying with one's shortcomings. Instead of saying "I made a mistake," a client tells him- or herself, "I'm a jerk," "a fool," or "a loser."
- *Personalization and blame:* Blaming oneself for something that the person was not entirely responsible for, or blaming other people and overlooking ways that one's own attitudes and behavior might contribute to a problem.

In the previous example, the client believes, "I've never had success in the past with losing weight, and I'll never have success in the future. I feel like a failure when it comes to weight loss. I can't stand to feel like a failure—it's intolerable for me." This client demonstrates the following cognitive irrational distortions:

- *Jumping to conclusions:* "I'll never have success in the future"
- *Labeling:* "I feel like a failure"
- *Overgeneralization:* "I've never had success in the past with losing weight"
- *Emotional reasoning:* "I can't stand to feel like a failure," implying that if he feels like a failure, then he must be a failure
- *All-or-nothing thinking:* Demonstrated by the "success or failure" approach to weight loss
- *Magnification and a catastrophe statement:* "It's intolerable for me"

The health coach, hearing this type of thinking, needs to help the client change his irrational (inaccurate and erroneous) beliefs into rational beliefs. Before behavioral change can take place, a change of thinking needs to occur.

The health coach may help the client challenge or dispute his or her irrational thoughts about himself, exercise, weight loss, or any health-behavior plan and replace these thoughts with accurate and motivating thoughts using methods adapted from Burns (1980), such as the following:

- *Examine the evidence:* Instead of assuming that the client's irrational thought is true, help the client examine the evidence for it. Ask, "What are the facts? What do they show?"
- *Experimental technique:* Help the client create an experiment to test the validity of his or her irrational thought, in much the same way that a scientist would test a theory. Ask, "How could you test this thought to find out if it's really valid?"
- *Socratic method:* Ask several questions that will lead to the inconsistencies in irrational thoughts. For example, the health coach may encourage the client to ask him- or herself, "When I say that I'm a failure, do I mean that I fail at some things some of the time, or all things all of the time?" If the client says, "some things some of the time," the health coach can point out that this is true of all human beings. If the client says, "all things all of the time," the health coach can point out that this is not true of anyone, since no one fails at everything.

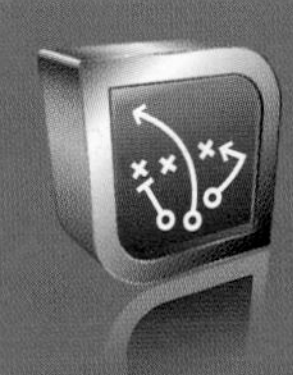

APPLY WHAT YOU KNOW

Replacing Irrational Thoughts

The health coach may also help the client replace irrational cognitions with healthier, more productive and factual thinking by helping the client answer questions such as the following:

- What is the evidence for and against this thought?
- What would I tell a friend in this same situation (as opposed to what I tell myself)?
- What is the worst that could realistically happen? How bad would that be?
- It is really true that I must, should, ought to, have to…?
- Are there any other possible responses besides blaming myself?
- Is there any conceivable way to look at this positively?
- Is thinking this way helping the situation, myself, or others, or only making it worse?
- How have I tolerated these situations in the past?

Motivation and Emotion

Health coaches will be most successful in implementing lifestyle-modification programs when they realize that each and every client is unique and brings his or her own qualities to the program. Motivational and emotional factors, including desires, preferences, and stress, all can potentially impact the success of a program. It is up to the health coach to understand these individual variables and work to customize each program to meet client needs.

Behavioral Theory Models

Each client will present new challenges and require the health coach to develop unique techniques to achieve program adoption and maintenance. Because adopting a healthy lifestyle is complex, numerous models have been developed to explain the factors affecting health behaviors. One important factor in any lifestyle-modification program is the client's readiness to make a change. This individual readiness for change is the focus of a well-accepted theory examining health behaviors called the **transtheoretical model of behavioral change (TTM)** (Prochaska & DiClemente, 1984). It is important that health coaches understand this theory and are able to apply it at various stages of a client's weight-management program.

Transtheoretical Model of Behavioral Change

The TTM is one of the most often referenced models of intentional behavioral change in the health arena (Prochaska & Velicer, 1997). It is a complex, complete, and comprehensive approach to coaching clients who want to make healthier lifestyle choices regarding weight, stress, exercise, and other health coach areas of practice. The health coach who develops skill in using the TTM will be well equipped to help clients with health-related lifestyle choices that result in increased quality of life and reduced risk of morbidity and mortality.

The core components of the TTM model include stages of change, processes of change, **decisional balance, self-efficacy,** and situational temptations to **relapse.** These cognitive and performance-based elements help the health coach properly focus on the decision-making abilities of the individual.

Stages of Change

The first component of the TTM consists of five stages of behavioral change.

- **Precontemplation:** People in this stage are sedentary, and are not even considering an activity program. These people do not see activity as relevant in their lives, and may even discount the importance or practicality of being physically active. The main goal of the health coach is to encourage the client to start thinking about change. Encouragement, personalizing healthy lifestyle information, expressing concern about specific symptoms, and asking the client what he or she sees as advantages to change, are all appropriate techniques at this stage. Essentially, the health coach provides information and helps the client analyze personal risk. Media resources, referrals to other health professionals, and personalized handouts are examples of what the health coach can offer to clients at this stage. Validating the client's lack of readiness, ensuring the client understands the decision is entirely his or hers, and encouraging exploration, not action, are additional key methods to help the client move to the contemplation stage. *The client may say, "I won't."*
- **Contemplation:** People in this stage are still sedentary. However, they are starting to consider the importance of activity and have begun to identify the implications of being inactive. Nevertheless, they are still not prepared to commit to making a change. The health coach should encourage the client to review the pros and cons of healthy behavioral change. Asking the client to list benefits and obstacles to change is an excellent technique at this stage. Ask the client how he or she would overcome the barriers listed. Say to the client, "I've found that some of my clients find this technique to be helpful and I believe you might as well." This is the stage to help the client review the personal pros and cons of the contemplated lifestyle change. Keep in mind that interest and thinking about change does not represent a readiness to change. *The client says, "I might."*
- **Preparation:** People in this stage perform some physical activity, as they are mentally and physically preparing to adopt an activity program. Activity during the preparation stage may be a sporadic walk, or even a visit to the gym, but it is still inconsistent. People in the preparation stage are ready to adopt and live an active lifestyle. At this stage, the health coach encourages the client to create a plan for making healthy lifestyle changes and overcoming challenges. The client is looking for specifics in creating his or her plan. Suggestions for investigating weight-loss programs, health clubs, planning how a diet and/or exercise program can fit into his or her lifestyle and schedule, and identifying friends with whom the client may share the lifestyle change are examples of what the health coach can provide at this stage. *The client says, "I will."*
- **Action:** During this stage, people are engaging in regular physical activity, but have been doing so for less than six months. The assistance of the health coach is most important in this stage. Specific goals help the client see progress. The health coach needs to be as encouraging as possible, ensure social support, focus on long-term advantages, and continue offering support when obstacles appear. The health coach assists the client in putting his or her plan into action by offering support and encouragement, celebrating any and all success, and continuing to review solutions to any difficulties that arise. The coach provides information and references for further study, including access to Smartphone "apps" (see page 72). The key is to provide the client with useful information on how to

anticipate and overcome obstacles that reduce motivation and interfere with adherence. Goal-setting—using **SMART goals**—is particularly useful during the action stage (see Chapter 13). *The client says, "I am now."*

- **Maintenance:** This stage is marked by regular physical-activity participation for longer than six months. This is essentially a continuation of the action stage. Preventing relapse is key here. Staying focused on the risks of slipping backward is most important to the client. Internal rewards will help the client cope with any temptation to revert to old behaviors. The health coach helps the client maintain the changed behavior with continued encouragement and by exploring how the client might handle temptations to find reinforcement in unhealthy behaviors and face relapse. The health coach monitors and supports the new behaviors. Planning ahead for situations that tempt and undermine self-efficacy is helpful at this stage. *The client says, "I am."*

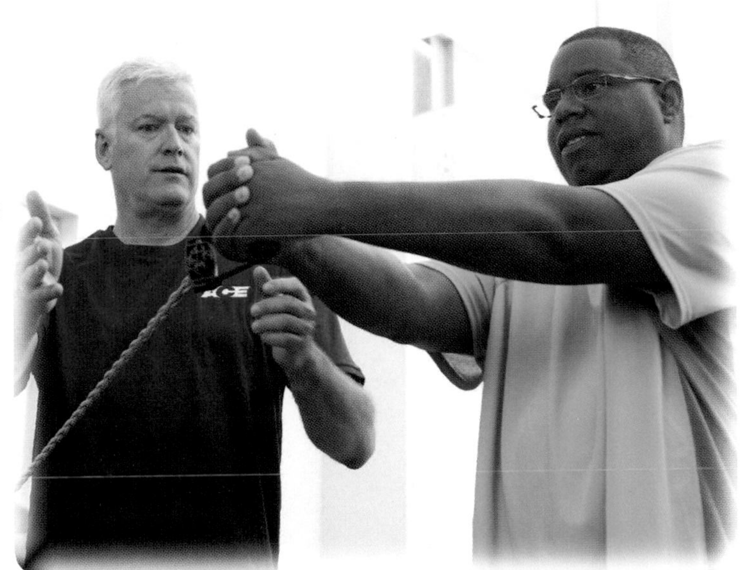

The most important point to remember is that behavioral change is an incremental, spiral, nonlinear process, not a single event. Clients in all stages sometimes find it difficult to maintain their new behaviors and can relapse, often to the precontemplation stage. Ask a client, "On a scale of 1 to 10, how ready do you believe you are to make this change or adopt this healthy behavior?" Answers below 4 suggest that the client is at the precontemplation stage. Keep in mind that this model explains how clients modify their own behaviors.

Processes of Change

The second component of the TTM consists of the processes of change that are used to pass from one stage to the next. Each transition has a unique set of processes and is based on specific individual decisions and mental states, such as individual readiness and motivation. The most effective change strategies are stage-specific interventions that target the natural processes people use as they move from one stage to the next (Table 3-1). The first step is to identify the current stage of each client. If someone is in a fitness facility or has called a fitness facility, he or she is likely not a precontemplator. By listening to the types of questions being asked and to the types of hesitations an individual has, the health coach should be able to identify the current stage of change and choose an appropriate intervention. The general goal of any intervention should be to advance the individual to the next stage of change.

Self-efficacy

The third component of the TTM is self-efficacy, which, in the lifestyle-modification context, is the belief in one's capabilities to be physically active and to maintain healthy nutrition (Bandura, 1986; 1977). Self-efficacy is an important component of lifestyle modification because it is strongly related to program adoption and maintenance. A circular relationship exists between self-efficacy and behavioral change, such that a person's self-efficacy is related to whether he or she will participate in activity, and a person's participation in activity influences his or her self-efficacy level. Therefore, self-efficacy acts as both a determinant and

Table 3-1

The Stages of Behavioral Change

Stage	Traits	Goals	Strategies
Precontemplation	Unaware or under-aware of the problem, or believe that it cannot be solved (e.g., latent pain)	Increase awareness of the risks of inactivity, and of the benefits of activity Focus on addressing something relevant to them Have them start thinking about change	Validate lack of readiness to change and clarify that this decision is theirs Encourage reevaluation of current behavior and self-exploration, while not taking action Explain and personalize the inherent risks Utilize general sources, including media, Internet, and brochures to increase awareness
Contemplation	Aware of the problem and weighing the benefits versus risks of change Have little understanding of how to go about changing	Inform them of available options Provide cues to action and some basic structured direction	Validate lack of readiness to change and clarify that this decision is theirs Encourage evaluation of the pros and cons of making change Identify and promote new, positive outcome expectations and boost self-confidence Offer invitations to become more active (e.g., free trials)
Preparation	Seeking opportunities to participate in activity (combine intent and behavior with activity)	Structured, regular programming with frequent positive feedback and reinforcements on their progress	Verify that the individual has the underlying skills for behavior change and encourage small steps toward building self-efficacy Identify and assist with problem-solving obstacles Help the client identify social support and establish goals
Action	Desire for opportunities to maintain activities Changing beliefs and attitudes High risk for lapses or returns to undesirable behavior	Establish exercise as a habit through motivation and adherence to the desired behavior	Behavior-modification strategies Focus on restructuring cues and social support toward building long-term change Increase awareness to inevitable lapses and bolster self-efficacy in coping with lapses Reiterate long-term benefits of adherence Require continual feedback on progress
Maintenance	Empowered, but desire a means to maintain adherence Good capability to deal with lapses	Maintain support systems Maintain interest and avoid boredom or burnout	Reevaluate strategies currently in effect Plan for contingencies with support systems, although this may no longer be needed Reinforce the need for a transition from external to internal rewards Plan for potential lapses Encourage program variety
Lapse	Encounter lapses that they are unable to overcome	Return to action	Identify reasons for lapse Identify current stage of change to progress once again toward action Maintain existing systems and relationships and offer appropriate support

an outcome of behavioral change. Additionally, there is a reliable relationship between a person's self-efficacy for activity and his or her stage of behavioral change, such that precontemplators and contemplators have significantly lower levels of self-efficacy than people in the action and maintenance stages. This relationship makes intuitive sense, as those in the precontemplation and contemplation stages are not exercising, which may be reflective of the belief that they do not have the ability to be active, while those in the action and maintenance stages are engaged in a regular activity program, and thus demonstrating a belief in the ability to be active. It is important to note that the most important and powerful predictor of self-efficacy is past performance experience. Therefore, an individual who has had past success in adopting and maintaining a physical-activity program will be more efficacious in his or her ability to be active in the future.

The documented relationship between stage of change and self-efficacy also implies that if self-efficacy is improved, the client may be helped in progressing through the stages. This is especially important for the people in the contemplation and preparation stages, as they are thinking about being active, or want to be active, and are working toward the point where they can be active regularly. By helping such individuals increase their self-efficacy, the health coach may be able to move them through to the action stage more quickly.

Two aspects of self-efficacy, temptation and situational confidence, are inversely related to one another throughout the stages of change (i.e., when confidence is high, temptations have a weaker appeal; when confidence is low, temptations can become overwhelming). Positive shifts in a client's decisional balance and self-efficacy—especially in overcoming temptations—are particularly useful to the health coach in determining whether a client is moving forward in the stages of change.

APPLY WHAT YOU KNOW

Building Confidence

Most new lifestyle-modification clients will start the program with very low self-efficacy for exercise ability and program success. As a health coach, what are you doing to combat this issue from the very start of the program? Because past performance experience is the most important source of self-efficacy information, each early experience should be focused on creating success and building confidence. A big mistake many fitness professionals make is to schedule an entire session of assessments. Put yourself in the client's place: How do assessments make you feel? When you are out of shape and overweight, what is the result of the assessments? Your goal should be to make each new client leave the first session feeling good and looking forward to being part of the program. Figure out what assessments are absolutely critical and only conduct those tests. Put thought into how you do the assessments as well. Do not make them feel like a test, and in some instances, do not even let the client know you are collecting assessment information. Instead, collect the information you need from simple assessments that are worked into an introductory workout session. Think about the consequences of the things you do and make changes to build self-efficacy, enjoyment, success, and adherence.

Decisional Balance

The final of the four components of the TTM is decisional balance, which refers to the numbers of pros and cons an individual perceives regarding adopting and/or maintaining an activity program (Janis & Mann, 1979). When making any decision, people naturally weigh the pros and cons of each choice. The same is true for exercise. The decision to be physically active has to be "worth it" to an individual and health coaches must remember that this is a difficult and complex decision for people to make. Precontemplators and contemplators perceive more cons (e.g., sweating, sore muscles, time, finances, and boredom) related to being regularly active than pros. As a fitness professional and active person, it might be hard to understand that these cons would prevent someone from engaging in exercise, but it is important to remember that the perceived cons do not have to be logical or realistic to prevent an individual from being active. As people progress through the stages of change, the balance of pros and cons shifts, so that people in the action and maintenance stages perceive more pros than cons. The active behavior of people in these later stages reflects this change in decisional balance.

The natural change in decisional balance that occurs as people progress through the stages of change implies that influencing their perceptions about being active may help in encouraging them to start an activity program. When working on shifting people's decisional balance, health coaches must use the appropriate processes of change related to moving from one stage to the next. For example, when working with a precontemplator or contemplator, a health coach should emphasize the wide variety and general overall benefits of being physically active and avoid arguing about the cons the client perceives about exercise. Often, the cons perceived by non-exercisers are a result of misinformation and a lack of experience. Additionally, it is important to discuss both short- and long-term benefits. A health coach does not want to merely emphasize the long-term weight-loss benefits of an activity program, but also the more immediate benefits, including increased energy, improved mood, and enhanced mastery.

It is important to note that relapse can occur at any stage of the TTM, including during the maintenance stage. Any change that may occur in an individual's life, such as moving, starting school, a job change, or suffering an injury, can trigger a relapse into irregular activity or even no activity. The commitment of long-term exercisers should not be taken for granted, as this behavior can change and relapse can occur on any given day.

THINK IT THROUGH

A 42 -year-old client indicates that she currently engages in physical activity for about 30 minutes a day, a couple of days each week, by walking with her friends in the morning. Her friends are content with this walking schedule, but she states that she is looking to make activity a more regular part of her life and wants to challenge herself to be fit, strong, and healthy, but is not sure what to do next. She has not worked out in a gym in about 10 years, and is really motivated to start, but she is intimidated by jumping into a group class because she thinks everyone will look at her. In addition, she does not know how to use any equipment to work out on her own. She also wants to start making healthy food choices for her and her family. Based on this basic information, the health coach concludes that this client is in the preparation stage, has high self-motivation, and wants to be challenged.

What is the next step for getting this client started on a program? What are your thoughts about her support system and how will you address this in her program? Is she seeking to learn or to just be told what to do? How will this impact your program choices? What type of goals would you work with her to set? How prepared is she to make and adhere to a lifestyle-modification program?

Additional Theories

In addition to examining how readiness to change influences health behavior, researchers have been interested in people's beliefs about their health and how these beliefs influence the adoption or non-adoption of health behaviors.

Health Belief Model

The **health belief model** predicts that people will engage in a health behavior (i.e., exercise and/or healthy eating) based on the perceived threat they feel regarding a health problem, as well as the pros and cons of adopting that behavior (Becker, 1974). Perceived threat, which is defined as the degree to which a person feels threatened or worried by the prospect of a particular health problem, is influenced by several factors:

- The perceived seriousness of the health problem, or the feelings one has about the seriousness of contracting an illness or leaving it untreated. People take the severity of the potential consequences of the problem into consideration, and the more serious the consequences are perceived to be, the more likely people are to engage in a health behavior.
- The perceived susceptibility to the health problem is based on a person's subjective appraisal of the likelihood of developing the problem. People have a higher perceived threat and an increased likelihood to engage in a health behavior when they believe that they are vulnerable to a health problem.
- Cues to actions, or events, either bodily, such as physical symptoms, or environmental, such as health-promotion information, motivate people to make a change. The more people are reminded about a potential health problem, the more likely they are to take action and engage in a health behavior.

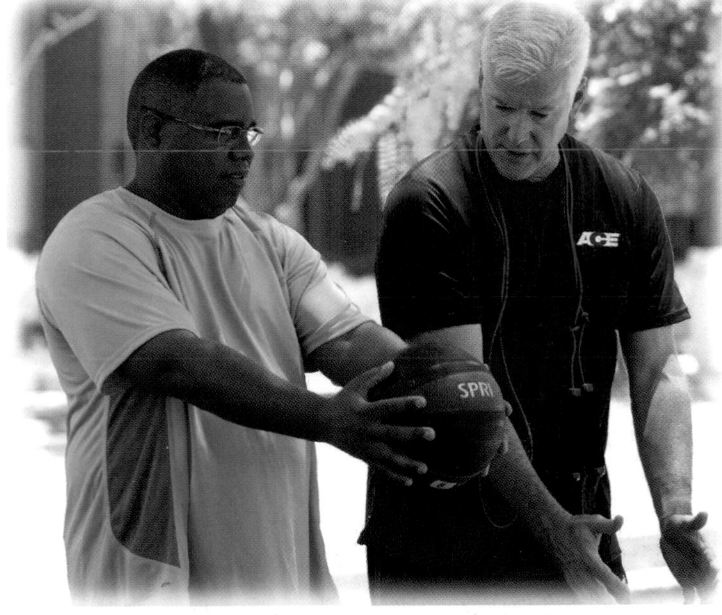

The pros and cons of engaging in a health behavior are examined by the health belief model in terms of perceived benefits and perceived barriers of the health behavior. In other words, the client will assess the benefits, such as getting healthier and looking better, along with the barriers, such as financial cost and time, of making a lifestyle modification. According to the health belief model, if individuals perceive more barriers than benefits regarding a health behavior, they will be unlikely to make a behavioral change.

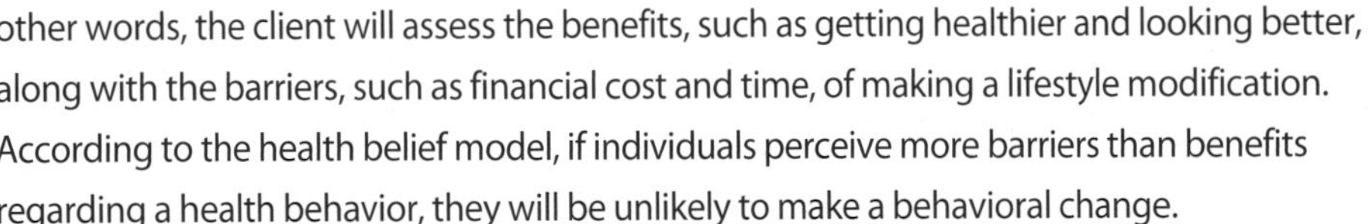

However, if the perceived benefits outweigh the perceived barriers and the perceived threat of illness is high, people are likely to take preventative action, thus engaging in exercise and healthy nutrition behaviors. Health coaches should understand the perceptions their clients have regarding illness and a healthy lifestyle, including their perceived benefits and barriers to program participation. If individuals perceive little threat of developing an illness related to their lifestyle choices, the modification program is going to be difficult to implement without making the seriousness of the illness more apparent and making the individual feel more susceptible to developing the condition. Health coaches should continuously use appropriate cues to action by introducing health information along with educating the client about physical symptoms.

Self-efficacy

Self-efficacy is an important concept to understand when studying exercise and health behavior. As previously mentioned, self-efficacy is the belief in one's own capabilities to successfully complete a task. Self-efficacy beliefs are thought to influence thought patterns, affective responses, and action. Additionally, self-efficacy is positively related to motivation (Bandura, 1986). In the lifestyle-modification context, self-efficacy focuses on exercise behavior and healthy nutrition behaviors. What is the client's belief about his or her ability to be active, be fit, eat healthy, and adhere to a program? This is important information to gather from all clients, as their self-efficacy levels will influence their program success. Furthermore, it is essential to understand how people develop self-efficacy. There are six sources of self-efficacy information:

- Past performance experience is the most influential source of self-efficacy information. What is the client's past experience with being physically active? This information is going to strongly influence his or her current self-efficacy level.
- Vicarious experience can come from observing or learning about someone else's success. For a client who is starting a new lifestyle-modification program, observing someone else who is already successfully doing so, especially if the person is perceived to be similar to the client, can increase the client's self-efficacy.

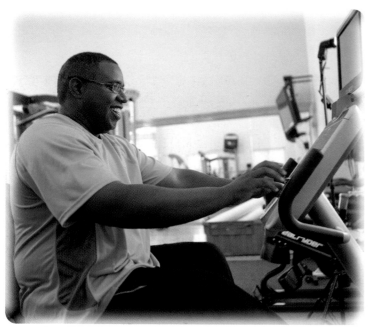

- Verbal persuasion typically comes in the form of feedback (teaching) or motivational (encouraging) statements. These statements are most likely to influence self-efficacy if they come from a credible and knowledgeable source.
- A client's appraisal of his or her own physiological state as it relates to program participation can lead to perceptions of arousal, pain, or fatigue. These appraisals cause people to make judgments about their ability to successfully participate. This can be as simple as a perception of an elevated heart rate or even sweating being viewed as a negative physiological state. For an individual who has been sedentary, physical activity will most certainly trigger "new" physiological responses, and no matter how typical these responses are to exercise (or even how positively they are often viewed by regular exercisers), if they are perceived negatively, the feelings of not being able to do it will compound and self-efficacy will decrease. It is important to monitor and educate clients on the physiological responses that normally occur during physical activity and to create positive interpretations of them.
- The appraisal of one's emotional state or mood related to program participation can lead to positive and negative perceptions. Negative mood states, such as fear, anxiety, anger, and frustration, are related to lowered levels of both self-efficacy and participation.
- Imaginal experiences that a client has regarding program participation (positive or negative) will influence his or her actual self-efficacy levels. People preparing to start,

or even just thinking about starting, a new exercise program have very likely imagined themselves working out. Often, these imagined experiences are not positive, as they are created with the doubt and fear that many new exercisers feel. Such negative visualizations or thoughts further decrease self-efficacy levels and highlight the importance of creating immediate positive experiences for people to use in future thoughts and dreams.

It is always important to assess and understand clients' self-efficacy levels, because self-efficacy is related to ultimate success in a program. Self-efficacy influences three important participation variables:

- *Task choice:* Individuals with high self-efficacy are more likely to choose challenging tasks, as compared to individuals with low self-efficacy, who are more likely to choose very easy, non-challenging tasks.
- *Effort:* Individuals with high self-efficacy are more likely to display maximal effort when engaged in a lifestyle-modification program.
- *Persistence:* Individuals with high self-efficacy are more likely to overcome obstacles and challenges and stick with a program. Those with low self-efficacy are more likely to drop out as soon as a challenge arises.

Based on what researchers know about the construct of self-efficacy, health coaches should be aware of clients' efficacy levels for program participation and attempt to understand why clients feel the way they do. This is best achieved through quality communication, observation, and continued interaction.

EXPAND YOUR KNOWLEDGE

Other Behavioral Change Theories

There are additional theories of behavioral change of which a health coach should be aware. While these are not as commonly used in the fitness industry as the TTM and health belief model, there are elements of each theory that a health coach might find useful.

The Theory of Reasoned Action (TRA)/Planned Behavior

This theory is used to understand and predict the determinants of health-related behaviors. It states that the intention to perform a healthy behavior is related to the actual performance of that behavior. It assumes that behavior is due largely to rational decision-making. Subjective norms, or what an individual believes others think about his or her ability or decision to perform a behavior, along with personal attitudes and self-efficacy, form an individual's intentions. In the TRA model, the decision to engage in a healthy behavior is determined by these factors (Montaño, Kasprzyk, & Taplin, 2008; Ajzen & Fishbein, 1980).

Social Cognitive Theory (Social Learning Theory)

The uniqueness of this theory is that it extends beyond individual factors and includes environmental and social factors in health behavior. It suggests that behavior can be explained by understanding the interaction between the individual (cognitions), his or her environment, and his or her behavior. Change in one element will impact the other two. This model emphasizes the thoughts of an individual and how those thoughts impact behavior (Bandura, 1986).

Promoting Health Behavior Change

To maximize behavioral change and adherence, behavior-modification programs must build knowledge about living an active and healthy lifestyle in each client a health coach encounters. Client education is a key component of every step of the lifestyle-modification process and health coaches should avoid making assumptions about what clients and potential clients already, or should already, know. Information needs to be provided in a straightforward, basic, non-threatening, and consistent manner. Some people may not want to hear about the science of exercise and nutrition, but instead are seeking basic information and strategies that can be directly applied to their lives. An effective approach for these individuals is to explain to them how to do it in a real-world, one-step-at-a-time approach. If a client wants more information, he or she will typically ask. One potential mistake made by fitness professionals is providing too much information too soon in a much too complicated way. The education health coaches provide to their clients must serve the purpose of triggering change and teaching people what they need to do and how to do it one step at a time.

Communication

All client–health coach relationships should start with formal and informal conversations in which the health coach learns about the client's past activity experiences, activity abilities and preferences, and activity-related hesitations. This information will help health coaches start to identify potential and actual barriers and challenges to adopting and maintaining an activity and healthy nutrition program. The more health coaches learn about their clients at the start of a program, the more likely it is that they will be able to customize the program to meet each client's needs and maximize adherence.

Additionally, health coaches should learn about each client's social-support network at the start of the program and should continue to be aware of this information throughout the duration of the program. Does the rest of the family participate in physical activity? Do family members and friends support the client in starting a lifestyle-modification program? Does the client have a work environment that supports and encourages an active lifestyle? This information will present itself over time, but it is important to start gathering as much information as possible during initial interactions with a client.

Health coaches should also make an attempt to identify their clients' attitudes, opinions, and feelings about physical activity. If health coaches deal with individuals who have not engaged in regular activity in the recent past, they might be dealing with clients who have misconceptions about being active. Through education, positive experiences, and rapport-building, health coaches can start building self-efficacy and replacing illogical exercise perceptions with ones that represent a more realistic interpretation of successfully living a physically active life.

Finally, health coaches need to provide education in effective goal-setting techniques and self-monitoring strategies. They must empower clients to take their activity experiences into their own hands and give them the knowledge and self-efficacy to succeed.

If health coaches keep these guidelines in mind for all lifestyle-modification programs, they will be off to a good start in creating effective programs for their clients. It is critically important to remember that interventions do not end when program participation begins. For behavioral interventions to be effective, these program components need to continue through the duration of program participation. These interventions need to become part of the regular activity program and health coaches need to continue to communicate, assess, and educate to maximize the likelihood of long-term adherence and successful behavioral change. Additionally, the best behavioral interventions are multifaceted, meaning that they include a variety of intervention techniques. Health coaches must not get overly focused on one facet, but instead incorporate a variety of strategies for optimal success. Interventions must also be systematic and complete, meaning that health coaches cannot neglect the behavior-change aspect as they get caught up in the physical components of the program.

Avoid Making Assumptions

Many of the frustrations that health coaches encounter are a result of miscommunications or misunderstandings, and these can often be linked back to health coaches thinking that their clients should already know how to do something with which they are in fact unfamiliar. Whether it is about food choices or quantity, effort level and intensity of exercise, calories consumed or burned, sleep habits, or ways to incorporate activity throughout the day, educating clients is arguably the most important service health coaches provide.

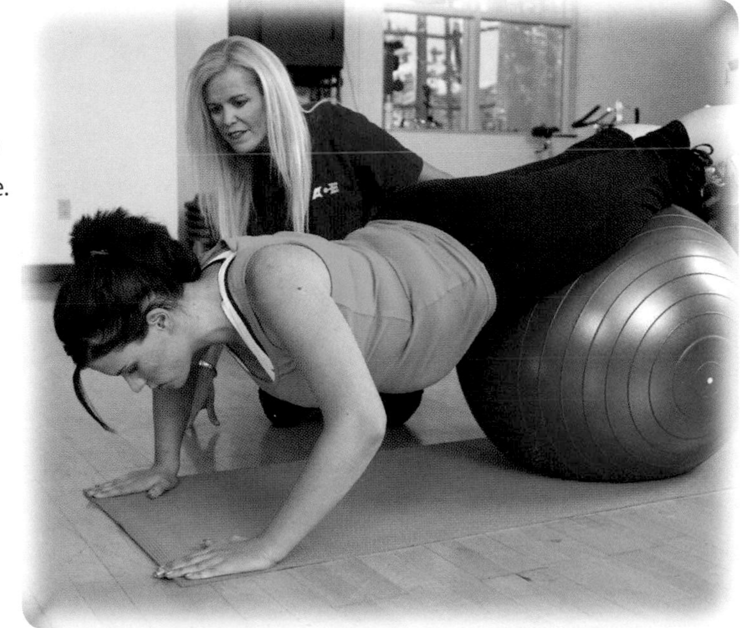

Health coaches may find that clients are often happy to simply follow a program that has been developed for them. However, this type of approach is not teaching the client the *why* of the program components, nor does it address the unique personality type of each client. Instead, health coaches should incorporate education and teaching into each encounter with clients and provide explanations and education about the various program components, empowering the client with choices, knowledge, and autonomy as much as possible. Additionally, a health coach should strive to understand the different personality types of his or her clients. The DISC model (see Chapter 5) will help the health coach interact most effectively to promote success in behavioral change. Some clients will want to be directed on what to do and others will want help to come to their own conclusions.

The personal beliefs health coaches have, the assumptions they make about themselves and others, and the way they think things should be, may directly affect how they will relate with clients. Therefore, it is essential for a health coach to understand his or own cognitive distortions.

Perceptions and interpretations interfere with an individual's ability to perceive and think accurately. Identifying hidden fears, desires, biases, and judgments about oneself and others is a critical part of understanding the obstacles in rational thinking and the ability to connect with others.

For example, if a health coach holds negative beliefs about "people who do not try hard," this will color how he or she interacts with some clients. Biased, long-term, automatic responses to people interfere with healthy relationships. These basic assumptions and attitudes will become manifest in the relationship with the client.

The health coach needs to understand his or her own beliefs and emotions and recognize their impact on how he or she deals with clients, makes decisions with them, plans for them, and motivates them. A health coach who understands his or her own strengths and weaknesses is in a much more secure place in relating appropriately with clients. A sound sense of self-worth, independent of how well a client does in response to the health coach's coaching, is important. This understanding helps keep disruptive emotions and impulses in check.

- What does the health coach believe clients *should, ought to, must,* and *have to* do?
- What does the health coach believe is truly *terrible, awful, horrible,* or *catastrophic* in the client's behavior?
- Is the health coach aware of any negative *labels* he or she uses for clients?
- Is the health coach aware of any projections, or "*fortune telling*" about the client's expected performance?
- Is the health coach *generalizing* about the client's behavior?

These questions can assist the health coach in teaching clients to control their thoughts in ways that move them to healthy decision-making, unencumbered by inaccurate or irrational thoughts.

APPLY WHAT YOU KNOW

Defining Success

Have you ever thought about the definition of a successful lifestyle-modification program? Is it one that is scientifically sound, or maybe that helped a client reach his or her goals? While these are key components of all programs, it is important to look at the bigger picture. Consider this definition: *A successful program is one that the client sticks with over time.* In other words, it is important for all fitness professionals to step back from the inner workings of program design and remind themselves that the ultimate goal is simply behavioral change. Health coaches should be celebrating the small victories and creating activity experiences that people *want* as part of their lives.

Relapse Prevention

Once a client has successfully adopted a lifestyle-modification program, the health coach should start implementing strategies for relapse prevention (see Chapter 14). Relapse from regular physical-activity participation is a common occurrence, and health coaches must educate their clients about potential relapse and prepare them with coping strategies to deal with adherence challenges. Because the vast majority of people face program barriers, such as time, finances, prioritizing, scheduling, support issues, or a dislike of, or dissatisfaction with, the program, it is important to develop strategies before adherence problems arise. Ultimately, the program has to be valued by the client for long-term adherence to occur.

EXPAND YOUR KNOWLEDGE

Relapse

Client relapse from program adherence is an inevitable part of the work of a health coach. Health coaches must always remember that the lifestyle-modification program is only one part of the client's life, and priorities can shift at any moment so that a client is required to put time and energy into other areas. Whether it is illness, travel, work, or family, there are countless life variables that can interfere with a structured program. Health coaches can help prepare clients to deal with relapse. The first step of this is the education that should be an integral part of the program from day one. If the health coach has been educating a client on *how* to make changes in his or her life, instead of just telling the client what to do, he or she will be better prepared to maintain certain program components during stressful, busy, or difficult times. Another key to dealing with relapse is support. Even if the health coach's contact with the client has decreased, letting the client know that the health coach understands his or her needs and is there to answer any questions or help in any way is critically important. Because relapse is often related to factors out of the client's control, being a constant and predictable source of support will be appreciated and will increase the likelihood of program re-adoption.

It can be frustrating to work with a client who exhibits a lack of commitment to his or her lifestyle-modification program. However, in the real world, this frustration will not help a health coach change people's lives. Being a supportive educator who understands not only that circumstances and priorities change, but also that adhering to a lifestyle-modification program is a difficult challenge that will have many ups and downs, is a key to being a successful health coach and building a successful business.

Building Support

An important strategy for relapse prevention is to help increase and maintain social support for living a healthy lifestyle. Health coaches must be creative in developing support systems at home. Get the family involved to some degree in the program so they can understand the commitment the client has made to lifestyle modification. A more direct way that health coaches can increase support is by creating support systems within the exercise or activity environment. This can be done in many ways, but the key is to utilize opportunities for group involvement and social interaction and make clients feel as though they belong in the program. The goal should be for all clients to feel as though they belong to, and are part of, something special and unique.

EXPAND YOUR KNOWLEDGE

Community- and School-based Programs

While most of the work that health coaches do is with clients in a one-on-one or small-group setting, the current and future needs of society call for qualified health coaches to develop, promote, and run successful community- and school-based programs. Historically, most community campaigns have been educational in nature, with the goal being spreading the word about a particular aspect of healthy living, such as the benefits of being physically active, the risks of cardiovascular diseases, or the dangers associated with smoking. Health coaches can make an important community impact by switching up this traditional, mass media approach, and instead focusing on a specific group or target population. Using the existing energy and camaraderie of a school, workplace, or community center can be a huge benefit to program support and compliance. The group should set goals, provide insight into program preferences and expectations, and have opportunities to execute the program together. Communication with the group should be done creatively and in multiple formats. Depending on the population, social media may be an effective tool to bring the group together to share a message, provide support, and keep everyone updated. A large group-based program should offer multiple opportunities for program participation, as well as regular opportunities to discuss program participation (e.g., challenges, successes, and modifications).

An example of a potentially effective school-based intervention would be working with one school for an entire school year. The school could adopt "Being Healthy and Fit" as the motto for the year. The goal would be to increase physical-activity levels and improve dietary habits for students, faculty, and staff. The program should include educational sessions with topics that range from basic background information to specific strategies for implementation. Unique opportunities could be created for faculty and staff, as well as for students to work together in subgroups. The faculty could be brought in as educators in the program and provide tips for healthy living. Basic assessments of groups and individuals could be performed at various points throughout the year and success measured and appropriate incentives offered. Contests could be created between and within the different groups in the school, as well. The options are endless, and although the work in this type of program is extensive, it is the type of work that needs to be done to make a difference, provide education, and change habits. Additionally, this same type of program could be implemented in any workplace environment. The immediate benefit of this type of programming, if properly implemented, is that there is an instant support network of people working toward common goals. With this comes a common understanding of the struggles and challenges associated with a lifestyle-modification program and also a team with whom to celebrate everyone's victories.

Assertiveness

Another strategy that can be used to help prevent program relapse is encouraging clients to be assertive. Assertiveness is an important trait for achieving success and is defined as the honest and straightforward expression of one's thoughts, feelings, and beliefs. Typically, when individuals are not assertive, it is because they lack self-confidence or they feel vulnerable. The more assertive clients are regarding their progress, concerns, accomplishments, and struggles, the more likely they are to speak up and let others know what they need. They will be more willing and able to problem-solve and find solutions that will help them achieve long-term success.

Self-regulation

The more effective that clients become at self-regulating their behaviors, schedules, time, and priorities, the more likely they will be to adhere to the program. Health coaches cannot try to regulate clients' behavior for them or to control and script their every move. Instead, health coaches must teach clients to self-monitor and to make behavior changes that will optimize their success. Teaching self-regulation strategies will provide clients with control over their own lives and provide the confidence they need to succeed. Once clients perceive control over their behavioral outcomes and believe they can do it, they are more able to deal with barriers and challenges as they arise. While this seems like a straightforward concept, fitness professionals often have a difficult time giving up control and teaching clients to take over.

Self-monitoring refers to the practice of clients keeping track of information regarding their own activity participation. This information should include their successes and difficulties in adhering to their lifestyle-modification program. Self-monitoring provides clients with a wealth of information about situations, people, and events that are barriers to adherence. This technique requires a great amount of client commitment and interest in becoming regularly active, but can be very effective in identifying barriers and developing strategies for long-term adherence.

Paying attention to one's own nutrition, weight, level of exercise intensity, and daily physical-activity behavior is among the most useful methods of identifying necessary changes, setting realistic goals, and improving controllable fitness lifestyle behaviors. Simply monitoring one's behavior is a very powerful stand-alone intervention. However, even among those most highly motivated clients, adequate self-monitoring is a hard-to-reach goal without proper support.

The value of self-monitoring is clear. Everyone enjoys actually seeing progress on a scale or self-monitoring tool. In addition, clients can quickly recognize a lapse in progress as an immediate reminder that progress is not "all or nothing." Self-monitoring will lead to more rapid self-correcting behaviors. The more visual the data, the more likely it will have inspirational value and engage the client.

Self-monitoring requires a great deal of forethought, attentiveness, and sustained motivation—the very skills that so many clients lack as they move through the stages of readiness. The health coach can make use of a wide range of tools and technological applications that will help clients self-monitor more easily and effectively than if left completely on their own.

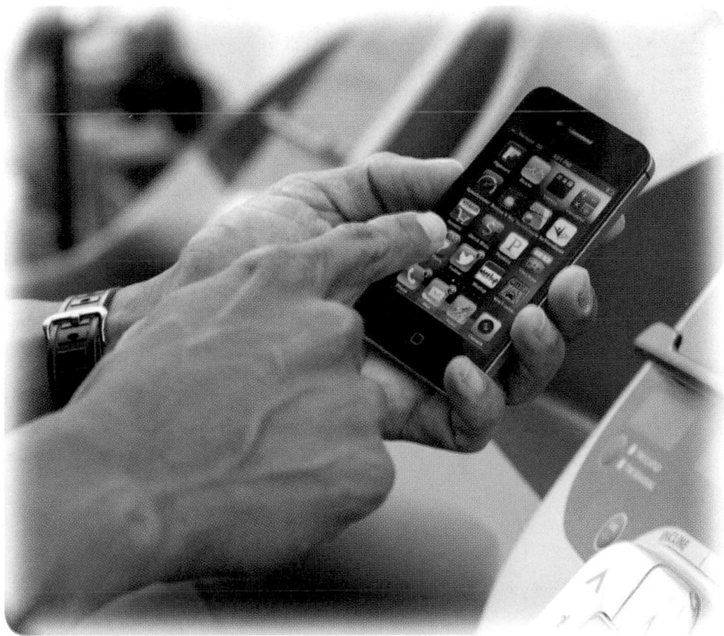

The list on page 72 is meant only to highlight the types of tools and "apps" that are available. There are literally thousands of old and new technologies available on which clients can rely. There are text messaging programs, mobile reminders, biomonitoring, biofeedback, actigraphs, accelerometers, and GPS programs developed daily for Smartphones, tablets, and computers that address smoking cessation, weight monitoring, activity levels, heart rate, mealtime planning, sleep cycles, self-talk, exercise programs, and alcohol intake monitoring.

The health coach may present self-monitoring as a valuable method of helping the client achieve the goals he or she has established and identified as necessary for lifestyle improvement. The health coach will first identify the client's comfort, interest, and accessibility to help choose technology-based tools or paper-and-pencil worksheets. This is, like all coaching, a collaborative method. The health coach does not urge the client to choose one tool over another, but may spend a session, or part of a session, reviewing different tools and apps with the client. The client needs to choose his or her own set of self-monitoring tools so as to "own" them and not let the actual tool or app become an area of resistance.

As with all such interventions, the health coach should use open-ended questions to understand the client's thoughts and feelings, obstacles and barriers, and past successes and challenges with self-monitoring. The health coach may assess the client's stage of readiness to adopt self-monitoring and use motivational interviewing to assist the client in seeing the value of putting a self-monitoring program to use.

Once the client adopts a self-monitoring toolkit, the health coach would be wise to follow up in the first day or two to see how the client is coming along using this approach. The health coach should be available for questions, reflecting on the success or struggle the client may experience. If the app can send information to the health coach, have the client do so regularly, and always send a return text or email commenting on the progress in motivational ways. If it is a paper-and-pencil worksheet, be sure to review the document in every session. A paper-and-pencil self-monitoring worksheet may include keeping track of body weight, aerobic activity, strength and balance activities, eating patterns, and food diaries.

Health coaches can visit the following websites to learn more about technology-based self-monitoring tools:

- www.quantifiedself.com
- http://dttac.org/diabetesprevention/pdfs/Online_Self-Monitoring_Resources.pdf

The following is a list of Smartphone apps that health coaches can use with their clients:

- Weight Watchers Barcode Scanner US
- Weight Watchers Mobile
- Calorie Counter & Diet Tracker by MyFitnessPal
- Pedometer Free
- Nike+GPS
- Garmin Fit
- Sleep Cycle Alarm Clock
- My Daily Journal

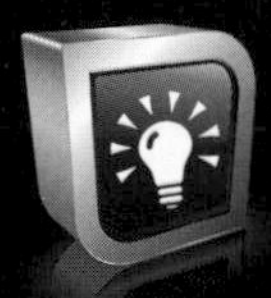

THINK IT THROUGH

If you are sick or on vacation, are your clients able to safely complete a workout? Would they know what to do? Do a little test. During your next workout with a veteran client, ask if he or she can identify the exercises by name, or if he or she knows the purpose of the exercises. How effective are you at educating your clients? Total dependence on a health coach does not benefit the client in the long run. Make sure you are not only telling your clients what to do, but teaching them to be able to do it themselves. Health coaches should teach skills, build confidence, create independence, and work together with clients to make lasting lifestyle changes. What can you do to improve your clients' ability to maintain their programs on their own if necessary?

High-risk Situations

Identifying high-risk situations will make health coaches more prepared to deal with program barriers and program relapse. Vacations, schedule changes, injuries, and holidays are some common situations in which many people relapse. Health coaches must be prepared for these events as they arrive and talk to their clients about the challenges of remaining physically active through these times. Also, identify clients who appear to be most at risk for program relapse.

Those who have poor time-management skills, a lack of social support, or busy schedules are prime examples of people who will likely relapse. Health coaches should provide extra education, support, and guidance for these people as they adopt their programs and deal with barriers in sticking to the programs. Additionally, health coaches must be observant of their clients' emotional states by watching for signs of being overwhelmed and worn out. Health coaches will be better able to help their clients maintain behavioral plans if they take the time to teach them additional coping skills, including time management and prioritizing, work with them on developing a plan for adherence, and remain supportive, understanding, and empathetic.

Adherence and Motivation

Behavioral Modification

Motivating clients to successfully stick with their lifestyle-modification programs can be one of the biggest challenges a health coach will face. In order to succeed at this task, health coaches must teach clients behavior-modification strategies, which are tools to help in the adoption and maintenance of activity programs. Whether clients are just beginning the program or have been participating for a long time, behavior-modification strategies are helpful and important tools for motivation and adherence. Just like turning on the television when getting home from work can become a habit in a person's life, being physically active and participating in activity throughout the day is also a habit. When health coaches help people find time in their schedules for regular activity, they often simultaneously help them identify undesirable behaviors or habits they can eventually replace with physical activity and healthy eating.

When tested in research, behavior-modification programs and tools have been shown to be consistently successful in helping people be regularly physically active. Behavior-modification methods change behavior by using the principles of operant and classical conditioning to help people learn to be more active (Dishman, 1991). There are numerous behavior-modification strategies, two of which are discussed in this section.

Written Agreements

Written agreements can be useful tools for helping people stick with their activity programs because they help to build accountability. A written agreement can either be between the health coach and the client or between the client and him- or herself. A written agreement should clearly specify what is expected of the client but should also be straightforward and simple. One reason that agreements are successful is that they decrease ambiguity and clarify behaviors, commitments, and attitudes that the client expects of him- or herself and that the health coach expects of the client. Written agreements are going to be less successful if the client does not take an active role in creating the contract or if they are too complex. Telling people what to do and what is expected of them is never as helpful for behavior change as people setting their own expectations. Within a written agreement, the health coach should also be specific in clarifying his or her own role in the activity program, along with the client's role. The health coach and the client should both sign the agreement and hold each other accountable for the expected behaviors. Be flexible with the written agreement, and if circumstances or goals change, revise the agreement so that it is always applicable to the activity program.

Stimulus Control

Stimulus control is an important modification and motivational strategy that involves altering the environment to encourage healthy behaviors and make following the modification program as easy as possible. Stimulus control is related to operant conditioning, as it refers to manipulating the stimuli in the environment to trigger the behavior of exercise or healthy eating. Stimulus-control strategies that health coaches can recommend to their clients include the following:

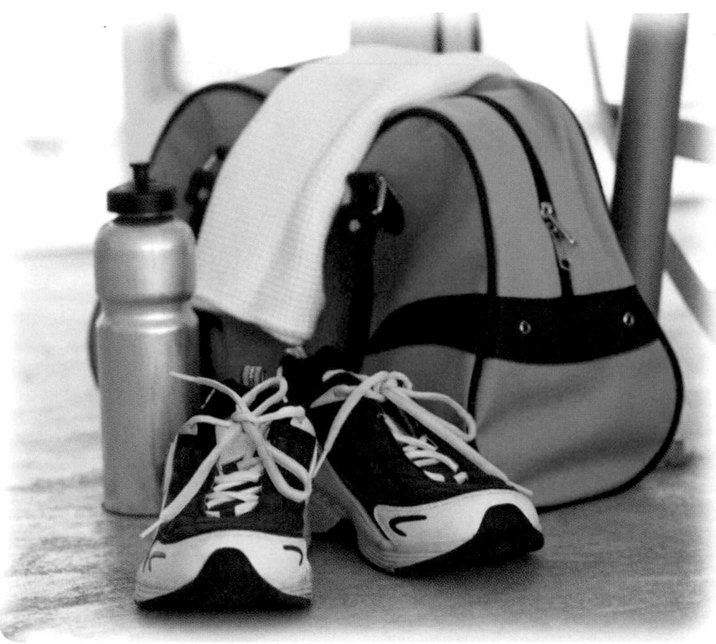

- Having workout clothes, socks, and shoes ready for early-morning workouts
- Keeping a gym bag in the car with all necessary workout items
- Posting signs on pantry and refrigerator doors listing the foods they should be eating
- Making a grocery list and staying away from purchasing non-listed items (if it is not in the house, it will not be eaten)
- Carrying or wearing comfortable shoes at work so that clients can take the stairs instead of the elevator
- Being part of a group or club that engages in physical activity together (such as a running, walking, or hiking group)

Another effective stimulus-control technique is to socialize with other people who live healthy lifestyles. By associating with people who have similar goals and interests, clients will create support systems for behavioral change. Another effective strategy is to join a fitness facility located in the direct path between home and work, and then scheduling workout times that concur with the times a person typically drives by the facility. If health coaches start hearing of excuses from a client about why he or she is missing workouts or is unable to adhere, it may be a cue that a stimulus-control strategy is needed. Health coaches should always strive to make their clients' lifestyle-modification programs as convenient as possible in their everyday lives.

Shaping

Shaping occurs when reinforcements are used to gradually achieve a target behavior. This process begins with the performance of a basic skill that the client is currently capable of doing. The skill demands are then gradually raised and reinforcement is given as more is accomplished. This process of continually increasing the demands at an appropriate rate and providing positive reinforcement leads to the execution of the desired behavior and serves as a powerful behavioral control technique. Part of the reason that shaping is so effective is that it starts with having the client execute a task at an appropriate skill level (Smith, 2010). It is important to remember that each client is going to have his or her own starting point and that health coaches will be most effective when they identify this level and design their programs from that starting point. Expecting too much from clients initially can lead to dropout, as they may feel overwhelmed and incapable.

APPLY WHAT YOU KNOW

Increasing the Enjoyment Factor

What is it about a program that keeps a client coming back? Sometimes even the most comprehensive and carefully designed programs do not lead to program adherence. What is missing? Maybe it is time to look at the situation from a different perspective. What experience is the program creating in the client's life? The biggest competition of fitness professionals is not other facilities, trainers, or coaches. The real competition is the couch, family time, TV, friends, work, and so on. The program a health coach creates has to have value enough in the client's life for it take priority over other demands in order for long-term adherence to happen. How do the program, the facility, and the people involved make the client feel? Is the program *fun?* Do the clients enjoy the experience of being involved in the program? If health coaches take some time to create an environment where people want to be, they will attract and retain more clients.

Cognitive Behavioral Techniques

In addition to behavior-modification strategies, cognitive behavioral techniques are also effective at promoting program adherence. Cognitive techniques alter behavior by changing how people feel and think. By using cognitive techniques, people are able to first identify and then change problematic beliefs that prevent them from making desired changes. Cognitive techniques can be used independently as intervention tools for behavioral change, or in conjunction with other behavior-modification strategies (Dishman, 1991).

Goal-setting

Goal-setting is an effective and easy-to-use cognitive behavioral technique (see Chapter 13). However, for goal-setting to be optimally effective, it needs to be a regular part of the activity program. A common mistake made with goal-setting is creating program goals with a client and then filing these goals away never to look at them again. This type of goal-setting is not going to maximally benefit program adherence. Instead, clients need to be continually aware of their goals. Proper goals should be SMART goals, meaning that they should be specific, measurable, attainable, relevant, and time-bound. It is the health coach's role to educate clients about these guidelines and help them create appropriate goals. It is important to avoid setting too many goals. Keeping the number of goals manageable and attainable prevents the health coach from overwhelming the client. Also, health coaches should avoid setting negative goals. If a client wants to set a goal to not miss any workouts, the health coach can reword the goal to be positive: "Attend every scheduled workout session." When negative goals are set, it makes clients think about the behavior they want to avoid, when they should really be thinking about the behavior they want to achieve. Also, it is essential that the health coach and client set both short- and long-term goals, as well as outcome goals and performance goals. Health coaches want their clients to achieve success in each workout. The most important thing that health coaches can do to make goal-setting an effective behavior-change technique is to attend to the goals on a regular basis. Health coaches must adjust goals as needed and use them as tools to direct attention and effort, and to promote persistence.

Feedback

Feedback is a powerful technique that involves both the health coach and the client. When most fitness professionals think of feedback, they think of providing reinforcement and encouragement to their clients. This is known as **extrinsic feedback,** and is critically important for initial program adoption. However, the type of feedback most important for long-term program adherence is **intrinsic feedback,** which is provided by the clients themselves. To encourage the development of intrinsic feedback for clients, health coaches must taper off the amount of extrinsic feedback they provide and work with the client to replace the extrinsic feedback with more self-assessment. If health coaches continue to reinforce every good behavior their clients engage in, the clients will never need to provide self-feedback and will never learn to monitor their own behavior. Health coaches must give clients the opportunity to provide their own reinforcement, encouragement, error correction, and, in some instances, punishment. By providing excessive amounts of extrinsic feedback, health coaches may cripple their clients' ability to achieve long-term adherence and independence.

The Importance of Ongoing Communication

Understanding a theory of behavioral change is not the same as being able to apply it when working with real clients. The most important skill that health coaches can have in terms of the application of any theoretical concept is communication. Effective communication techniques will allow health coaches to gather necessary information to determine the best course of action for program design and implementation. Client–health coach communication is an ongoing process and no single event, intervention, or conversation is going to change the stage of behavior (see Chapter 5 for more details on client–health coach communication). Instead, the relationship must be viewed as a journey in which each interaction and intervention is a steppingstone to increased self-efficacy, program enjoyment, and long-term adherence.

Summary

Trying to predict health behavior is complex and requires the examination of numerous correlates. Understanding the theoretical models is important to create a foundation of knowledge about health behavior and behavioral change. However, it is also critical that health and fitness professionals are aware of, and continuously evaluate, the numerous psychological and social factors that influence health. Furthermore, the success of a lifestyle-modification program will be related to the health coach's ability to implement ongoing behavior-modification strategies and continual relapse-prevention techniques. Understanding how difficult making a lifestyle change can be will give the health coach a better ability to create a program that inspires lasting behavioral change.

References

Ajzen I. & Fishbein, M. (1980). *Understanding Attitudes and Predicting Social Behavior.* Englewood Cliffs, N.J.: Prentice-Hall.

Bandura, A. (1986). *Social Foundations of Thought and Action: A Social Cognitive Theory*. Englewood Cliffs, N.J.: Prentice-Hall.

Bandura, A. (1977). Self-efficacy: Toward a unifying theory of behavioral change. *Psychological Review,* 84, 191–215.

Beck, A.T. (1975). *Cognitive Therapy and the Emotional Disorders*. Madison, Conn.: International Universities Press.

Becker, M.H. (1974). The health belief model and personal health behavior. *Health Education Monographs,* 2, 324–473.

Bogg, T. & Roberts, B.W. (2004). Conscientiousness and health-related behaviors: A meta-analysis of the leading contributors to mortality. *Psychological Bulletin*, 130, 887–919.

Burns, D. (1980). *Feeling Good: The New Mood Therapy*. New York: William Morrow.

Dishman, R.K. (1991). Increasing and maintaining exercise and physical activity. *Behavior Therapy,* 22, 345–378.

Dishman, R.K. (1982). Compliance/adherence in health-related exercise. *Health Psychology,* 1, 237–267.

Dishman, R.K. & Buckworth, J. (1997). Adherence to physical activity. In: Morgan, W.P. (Ed.). *Physical Activity & Mental Health* (pp. 63–80). Washington, D.C.: Taylor & Francis.

Duncan, T.E. & McAuley, E. (1993). Social support and efficacy cognitions in exercise adherence: A latent growth curve analysis. *Journal of Behavioral Medicine,* 16, 199–218.

Ellis, A. (1994). The sport of avoiding sports and exercise: A rational emotive behavior therapy perspective. *The Sports Psychologist*, 8, 248–261.

Ellis, A. (1962). *Reason and Emotion in Psychotherapy.* New York: Lyle Spencer.

Ellis, A. & Harper, R.A. (1961). *A Guide to Rational Living*. Oxford, England: Prentice-Hall.

Engel, G.L. (1977). The need for a new medical model: A challenge for biomedicine. *Science,* 196, 129–136.

Heaney, C.A. & Israel, B.A. (2008). Social networks and social support. In Glanz, K., Rimer, B.K., & Viswanath, K. (Eds.) *Health Behavior and Health Education: Theory, Research, and Practice* (4th ed.). San Francisco, Calif.: Jossey-Bass.

Janis, I.L. & Mann, L. (1979). *Decision Making.* New York: Macmillan.

Krause, N. (1986). Social support, stress, and well-being. *Journal of Gerontology,* 41, 4, 512–519.

Martin, G. & Pear, J. (2010). *Behavior Modification: What It Is and How to Do It* (9th ed.). Englewood Cliffs, N.J.: Prentice-Hall.

Montaño, D.E., Kasprzyk, D., & Taplin, S.H. (2008). The theory of reasoned action and theory of planned behavior. In: Glantz, K., Lewis, F.M., & Rimer, B.K. (Eds.) *Health Behavior and Health Education: Theory, Research, and Practice* (4th ed.). San Francisco, Calif.: Jossey-Bass.

Prochaska, J.O. & DiClemente, C.C. (1984). *The Transtheoretical Approach: Crossing Traditional Boundaries of Therapy.* Homewood, Ill.: Dow Jones/Irwin.

Prochaska, J.O. & Velicer, W.F. (1997). The transtheoretical model of health behavior change. *American Journal of Health Promotion,* 12, 38–48.

Sarafino, E.P. & Smith, T.W. (2011). *Health Psychology: Biopsychosocial Interactions* (7th ed.). New York: John Wiley & Sons.

Smith, R.E. (2010). A positive approach to coaching effectiveness and performance enhancement. In: Williams, J.M. (Ed.). *Applied Sport Psychology: Personal Growth to Peak Performance.* New York: McGraw-Hill.

Turk, D.C., Rudy, T.E., & Salovey, P. (1984). Health protection: Attitudes and behaviors of LPNs, teachers, and college students. *Health Psychology,* 3, 189–210.

Uchino, B. (2004). *Social Support and Physical Health: Understanding the Health Consequences of Relationships*. New Haven, Conn.: Yale University Press.

U.S. Department of Agriculture (2015). *2015-2020*

Dietary Guidelines for Americans (8th ed.). www.health.gov/dietaryguidelines

Wills, T.A. (1991). Social support and interpersonal relationships. *Prosocial Behavior, Review of Personality and Social Psychology,* 12, 265–289.

World Health Organization (1986). *Ottawa Charter for Health Promotion.* First International Conference on Health Promotion, Ottawa, Canada.

World Health Organization (1946). Preamble to the Constitution of the World Health Organization as adopted by the International Health Conference, New York, 19–22 June 1946; signed on 22 July 1946 by the representatives of 61 States (Official Records of the World Health Organization, no. 2, p. 100) and entered into force on 7 April 1948.

Suggested Reading

Bandura, A. (2001). Social cognitive theory: An agentive perspective. *Annual Review of Psychology,* 52, 1–26.

Bandura A. (1997) Self-efficacy: Toward a unifying theory of behavior change. *Psychological Review,* 184, 191–215.

Dishman, R.K. (1994). *Advances in Exercise Adherence*. Champaign, Ill.: Human Kinetics.

Dishman, R.K. (1990). Determinants of participation in physical activity. In: Bouchard, C. et al. (Eds.). *Exercise, Fitness, and Health* (pp. 75–102). Champaign, Ill.: Human Kinetics.

Dishman, R.K. & Buckworth, J. (1996). Increasing physical activity: A quantitative synthesis. *Medicine & Science in Sports & Exercise,* 28, 706–719.

Dishman, R.K. & Sallis, J. (1994). Determinants and interventions for physical activity and exercise. In: Bouchard, C. et al. (Eds.). *Exercise, Fitness, and Health*. Champaign, Ill.: Human Kinetics.

Janz, N.K. & Becker, M.H. (1984) The health belief model: A decade later. *Health Education Quarterly,* 11, 1–47.

McAuley, E., Pena, M.M., & Jerome, G.J. (2001). Self-efficacy as a determinant and an outcome of exercise. In: Roberts, G.C. (Ed.). *Advances in Motivation in Sport and Exercise.* Champaign, Ill.: Human Kinetics.

Morgan, C.F. et al. (2003). Personal, social, and environmental correlates of physical activity in a bi-ethnic sample of adolescents. *Pediatric Exercise Science,* 15, 288–301.

U.S. Department of Health and Human Services (2012). *Healthy People 2020.* Washington, D.C.: U.S. Government Printing Office.

SECTION II

COMMUNICATION STRATEGIES FOR EFFECTIVE COACHING

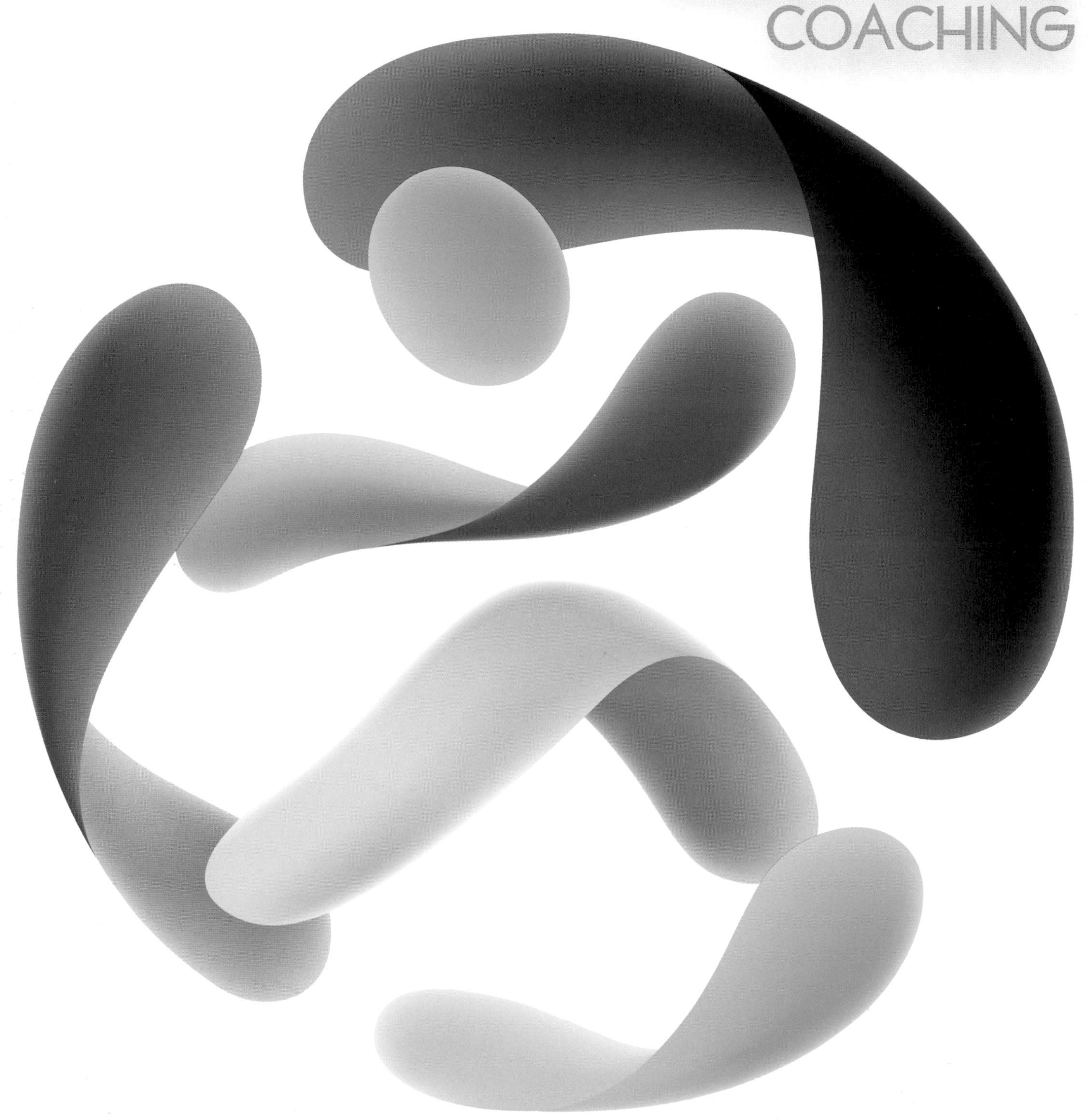

Chapter 4
Building Rapport

Chapter 5
Connection Through Communication

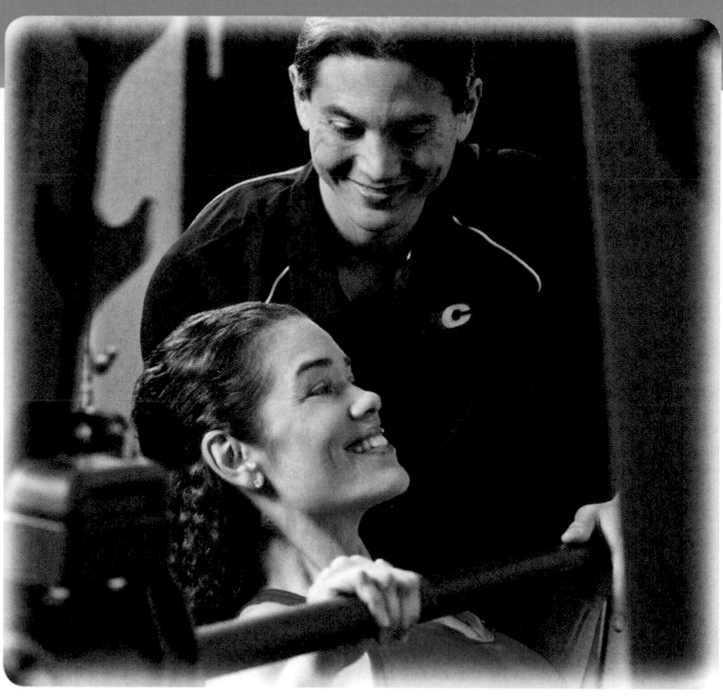

IN THIS CHAPTER:

Understanding the Individual
- *Self-efficacy*
- *Past Experience*
- *Expectations*

Communication Skills
- *Listening*
- *Empathy*

Environment
- *Physical Environment*
- *Psychological Environment*

Defining Program Success
- *Program Goals*
- *Adherence*

Summary

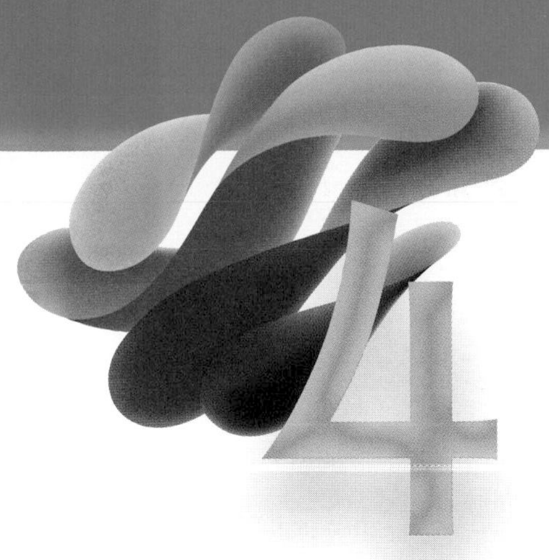

Building Rapport

TRACIE ROGERS

Tracie Rogers, Ph.D., is a sport and exercise psychology specialist and the director of the MS Human Movement Program at A.T. Still University. She is also the owner of BAR Fitness, located in Phoenix, Arizona. Dr. Rogers teaches, speaks, and writes on psychological constructs related to physical-activity participation and adherence.

Conscientious and diligent fitness professionals spend countless hours each year taking continuing education courses, earning new certifications, reading research, and working to develop evidence-based, safe, and effective lifestyle-modification programs.

This type of commitment to knowledge and understanding of the principles of exercise and program design is critically important in building and maintaining a solid reputation for one's business and for the greater community of fitness professionals. However, the vast majority of fitness professionals are initially drawn to this industry because of the unique opportunities that they have to help change lives. The truth is that no program, no matter how perfectly designed, can change someone's life without the backing of trust and understanding. In other words, ACE-certified Health Coaches will not succeed if they are unable to establish trusting relationships with their clients, regardless of how great the program design.

Most new clients starting a lifestyle-modification program are dealing with feelings of stress, apprehension, and insecurity, and it is the job of the health coach to acknowledge and address these emotions and perceptions by establishing quality **rapport** with the client from the start. In fact, health coaches are in a position to truly empower clients to succeed because of the opportunity to build a relationship and work together throughout the duration of the program. Lifestyle-modification programs typically involve regular sessions and direct interaction with the health coach, which provides the health coach with the time and opportunity to build a relationship that will improve client experience, **adherence,** and success.

Understanding the Individual

Rapport can be defined as a relationship of trust and mutual understanding, and health coaches must be very quick to establish such a relationship after meeting a new or potential client. A negative initial interaction can be very difficult to overcome, so health coaches must be prepared and open-minded during each and every interaction. Additionally, health coaches must act with intent to build rapport. This means that each conversation and interaction requires focused thought and purpose, always with the clients' needs in mind.

Many individuals are intimidated by the idea of a fitness professional and fitness environment, and health coaches must be aware of such preconceptions and work to break those barriers. Most fitness professionals not only look fit, but are very passionate about their knowledge and are almost too eager to immediately share that knowledge with anyone who will listen. It is not beneficial or appropriate for a health coach to tell a client everything he or she knows and the science behind it. Such information sharing can be overwhelming and intimidating and is about the health coach, not the client. Regardless of the intention of the health coach, this behavior results in a very self-centered conversation, and this defeats the purpose of the work being done. There will be a time for the health coach to demonstrate how much he or she knows through quality program execution, but if the interactions are focused on the health coach and his or her knowledge from the start, walls will be put up and no rapport will be established. The primary focus of the health coach should always be on the client, and building rapport is about listening, learning, and patience. In other words, the process of effectively building rapport requires the health coach to be selfless and out of the spotlight.

The goal in establishing rapport is to build a relationship that is based on a foundation of trust and credibility (Orlick, 2008). This chapter highlights the importance of health coaches gaining an understanding of the individual's needs, fears, and apprehensions and discusses techniques that health coaches can use to gain this understanding. The more that a health coach can learn about a client, the more effective he or she will be in executing a successful program.

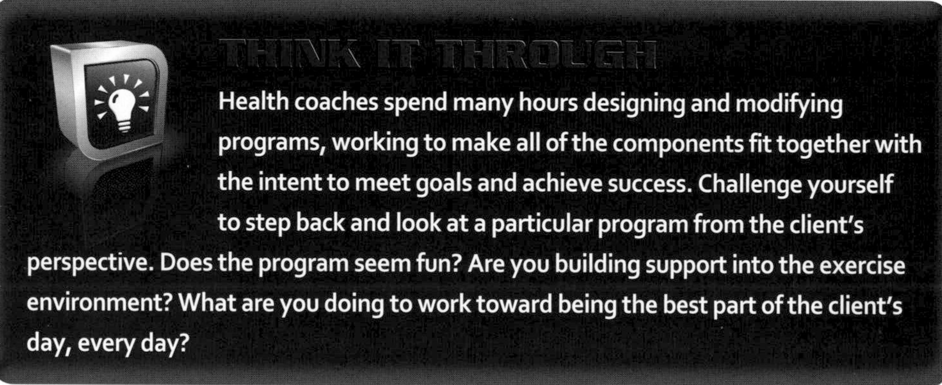

THINK IT THROUGH
Health coaches spend many hours designing and modifying programs, working to make all of the components fit together with the intent to meet goals and achieve success. Challenge yourself to step back and look at a particular program from the client's perspective. Does the program seem fun? Are you building support into the exercise environment? What are you doing to work toward being the best part of the client's day, every day?

Self-efficacy

Self-efficacy, for a health coach's purpose, refers to an individual's belief in his or her ability to successfully engage in and/or complete a lifestyle-modification program. It may also relate to one's belief in his or her ability to actually achieve success and reach desired goals (Bandura, 1986). Health coaches should be able to quickly gauge a client's self-efficacy level from the very beginning and throughout the duration of the program. If self-efficacy is low, and the program is not designed or modified to help increase self-efficacy, the individual will grow more discouraged and will likely drop out. Self-efficacy is a dynamic construct, meaning that it can change from day to day. The goal, of course, is to constantly work to increase each client's belief in his or her ability to succeed, and health coaches should be thinking about this goal during each conversation and workout.

A client's self-efficacy can significantly influence the dynamic of a conversation and the building of rapport. An individual with low self-efficacy is likely feeling doubt related to everything from his or her physical ability to engage in the program to the willpower needed to stick with the program (Bandura, 2004). This type of low self-efficacy will make it more difficult to get the individual to share and communicate information about his or her needs and goals, and if the health coach is unable to clearly identify the client's needs, establishing rapport will be a challenge. Even more important is that if the health coach does not identify the low self-efficacy levels and continues on with program design and implementation without attention to the self-doubt and fear, the client will not develop trust, will continue to build walls, have a negative perception of program participation, and likely drop out. If low self-efficacy is not identified and addressed early in a program, the client will feel threatened with each program challenge and will experience elevated levels of physiological and psychological strain associated with program participation (Bandura, Reese, & Adams, 1982). This stress response will lead to program withdrawal as a coping mechanism, especially if the client does not have rapport and trust with the health coach.

Health coaches should not invest too much time trying to identify exact levels of self-efficacy at the very beginning of the relationship with a new client, but instead should identify key thoughts and behaviors that indicate self-efficacy levels, including fear, excuses, and body language. Chances are that most new clients have some fear and self-doubt related to program participation and success. Therefore, health coaches should approach each program with the goal to build efficacy from the very start. The initial interactions and training sessions should be designed to create low-stress, successful experiences that make clients feel good about their ability to successfully engage in the program. These initial positive experiences will build trust, which will increase rapport in the client–health coach relationship. As the program continues, it is important for health coaches to remain cued into the changing efficacy levels of clients. Health coaches must be able to identify signs of doubt, frustration, fear, or stress related to specific program components or general program participation. When these signs of low self-efficacy emerge, it is important to make modifications that generate success, create support, and provide positive feedback and encouragement. The easiest way for a health coach to do this is to modify each program component to include something the client enjoys and can master. Whether it is changing a workout for the day or week to include the client's favorite exercises in order to generate success and enjoyment, or modifying a nutrition plan back to something that the client has previously mastered, there are times in a lifestyle-modification program when going back to the basics and creating success and enjoyment is necessary. This may also include increasing the amount of positive feedback and encouragement that is provided, and, even if it sometimes seems unnecessary, the client needs to know that the health coach believes that he or she can stick with the program and succeed, especially when efficacy levels are low. These suggestions may appear to be moving the client in the wrong direction, but being aware of when such steps and changes are needed will increase program success, adherence, and enjoyment in the long run.

Past Experience

Most people have some past experience with attempting to be healthy, stay active, or lose weight. No matter what the previous experience entailed, or how much the health coach may disagree with the previous methods used, it is likely, especially in this context, that each previous experience failed. Therefore, it is important for health coaches to show compassion for the client's previous efforts and to work toward understanding the factors related to the unsuccessful attempts. This is best done by being nonjudgmental regarding previous lifestyle choices and modification attempts. Discounting previous effort or choices will create barriers and decrease trust. Instead, it is important to continue to listen and try to understand, as previous failed attempts at making lifestyle changes indicate that the client may be bringing emotional baggage, unreasonable expectations, and low self-efficacy. Taking the time to learn about support systems, expectations, barriers, and preferences as they relate to previous programs can be a valuable tool for future program design and also for establishing trust. It is important in these conversations that the health coach focuses on the client in the present and on the health coach's belief in the client's ability to succeed (Dishman, 1994). Additionally, the health coach should use information about previous experiences as an opportunity to learn about preferences, barriers, and attitudes related to lifestyle-modification programs. The client might bring negative emotions and opinions (e.g., "I can't do that") based on the past experiences, and health coaches have to be prepared to highlight small victories. In other words, health coaches should create a program that is going to provide the client with a path for success.

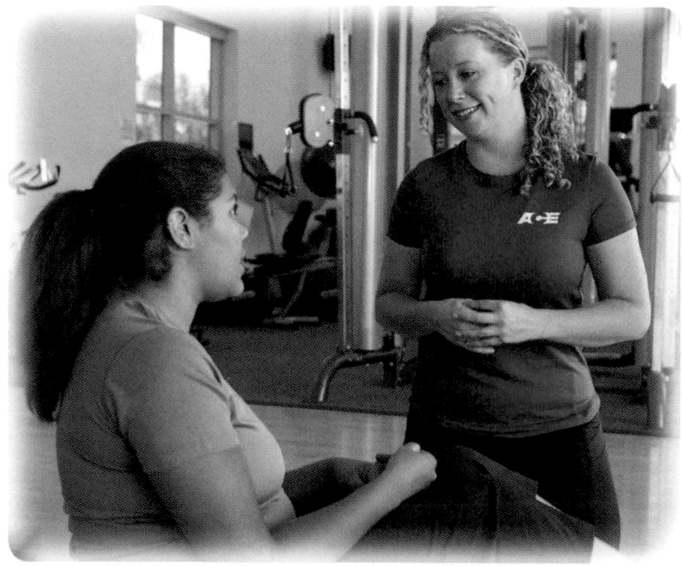

Expectations

Every client will bring his or her own expectations and goals for program participation. It is critical that the health coach knows and understands client expectations from the very beginning of program participation. It is common for initial program expectations to be unrealistic, and it is up to the health coach to work with the client to modify the expectations while building trust and rapport by establishing quality communication, focusing on the client, and understanding client needs. The health coach must also be careful to not get caught up in focusing on only program outcomes or guaranteeing results. This type of outcome-focused conversation does not help build rapport or establish a quality foundation for a long-term relationship.

Discussions about program expectations should focus on the roles of the client and health coach in the program. It is important to understand how the client views the role of the health coach, as well as his or her own role in the program (Eys et al., 2010). It is not uncommon for clients to put the responsibility of program success on the health coach, removing personal responsibility from the equation, which protects them from being at fault when something fails. While health coaches understand that the success is ultimately up to the dedication and commitment of the client, the client–health coach relationship should be viewed as a team, and it is important to create a foundation of realistic expectations verbally, or through a written contract, about the roles and responsibilities of everyone involved (Eys et al., 2010). It can also be beneficial to include the perceived roles of family and other support systems, so that clients know from the start the importance of getting everyone on board.

Additionally, health coaches and clients should discuss their expectations of what the program will entail, and this should include perceived and actual expected daily activities and commitments (both client and health coach) and the required behaviors to fulfill the expectations. The more clarity and consistent information related to the role of the client and the health coach that is established from the start of the relationship, the stronger the foundation will be for successful program execution and satisfaction (Beauchamp et al., 2002).

THINK IT THROUGH

Create a chart that maps out how you envision your responsibilities and the client's responsibilities over the course of a six-month lifestyle-modification program. Think critically about your role and consider how you might explain the chart to a new client who feels that keeping him on track and reaching his goals is your responsibility.

Communication Skills

The success of any relationship is based on the quality of the communication that exists in the relationship. Communication can be a difficult skill to learn and, because it is a dynamic and complex construct, it requires constant practice and attention to maintain effectiveness. Nevertheless, being able to effectively express one's thoughts, feelings, and needs, while also understanding the thoughts, feelings, and needs of others, is crucial for long-term success and for building rapport. Specifically, communication can influence attitudes, motivation, expectations, emotions, and behavior (Yukelson, 2010), which are all key components of a successful lifestyle-modification program.

Health coaches face some unique challenges in communicating with clients, especially at the start, because of the emotions and apprehensions that a client can bring to the conversation. A new client is often skeptical and may be looking for any excuse to abandon the program, so health coaches must be careful to not put up any barriers and instead focus on making the client feel comfortable. One way to connect with an individual and build rapport is to match or mirror his or her verbal and nonverbal behaviors, the goal of which is to be in sync with the client on numerous factors, including voice volume, speed of talking, and body language. For example, if the client is speaking very softly, it is helpful for the health coach to also lower his or her voice to match the volume of the client. This technique will help make the client feel comfortable, secure, and understood, and by matching the client's behavior, the health coach is reassuring the client that he or she is in good hands while also validating the client's feelings. Body language, gestures, facial expressions, and body positioning are all critical nonverbal components of a quality interaction (Mehrabian, 1981). See Chapter 5 for a more in-depth discussion of communication techniques.

It is also important for health coaches to be aware of their own natural communication tendencies and style. Because a key role of health coaches is to provide education to their clients, it is very easy and natural to constantly act as the teacher, provide answers and information, and make corrections. While the role of the educator will have an important place throughout the program, it is not appropriate or beneficial for it to be prominent during initial interactions. Therefore, health coaches should take the time to pay attention to their natural or "automatic" tendencies during conversations and work on communication with a focus on the client.

Listening

The most important thing health coaches can do to improve the quality of their communication with clients is to practice being better and more engaged listeners. **Active listening** is about being involved in the information being presented and asking questions to clarify points and express compassion (see Chapter 5 for more information on active listening). Active listening is the highest level of listening behavior and demonstrates a caring attitude and a true desire to understand what the client has to say (Rosenfeld & Wilder, 1990; Pietsch, 1974). Health coaches should demonstrate listening skills and focus on the conversation through verbal and nonverbal cues. It is important to appear engaged in the conversation by not taking extensive notes or getting distracted by other external cues (e.g., phones, emails, and clutter). Anything that moves the focus from what is being said will be picked up on by the client and perceived as disinterest. Additionally, health coaches should be prepared to ask questions, clarify points, and offer encouragement and understanding. These are components of reflective listening and demonstrate attention and care about what is being said (Yukelson, 2010).

Listening is a skill that is always easier said than done, especially for health coaches. This is because health coaches frequently find themselves in situations in which they really do have the answer or some good information to share. However, as mentioned previously, there will be time for sharing and demonstrating knowledge, but that knowledge will not be received if the client does not first feel secure and comfortable. Health coaches must practice listening, asking questions, and allowing the client to be heard. This validation of feelings and experiences is critically important in creating a foundation of trust and establishing rapport.

Empathy

Empathy is a learned skilled that is demonstrated by showing concern and genuine interest. It truly is an understanding of what the other person is feeling and experiencing and it demonstrates an attitude of caring and concern (Egan, 2010). Health coaches can show empathy by being an active part of the conversation, summarizing what they heard in their own words, and following up with detailed questions (see Chapter 5). This process not only demonstrates that they care about the clients' feelings and experiences, but that they also understand their clients' situations and needs. As mentioned above, being empathetic in communication takes practice and a focused effort. Health coaches should pay attention to this during conversations with clients and should always work to improve their ability to be actively engaged and invested in what the client is saying.

It is important that health coaches acknowledge that the lifestyle-modification journey can be difficult and long—lifelong in most cases. The process of living a healthy lifestyle should never be dismissed as simple or easy, because clients are viewing it as a major change requiring a serious commitment. Instead, health coaches must be empathetic and express understanding related to the feelings of the client. If health coaches fail to take the time to be empathetic of the clients' emotions associated with starting a new lifestyle-modification program, frustration and misunderstanding will eventually take over, damaging rapport and creating a barrier to program success.

Environment

Physical Environment

The majority of client–health coach interactions take place in some type of fitness environment. Whether it is a large gym, a private studio, or a workout space located in a medical/healthcare office, health coaches often do not have control over all aspects of the space in which they work. However, is important that health coaches take control of some elements of the physical environment. For example, the consultation and exercise spaces should be clean and organized. Health coaches should be mindful of clients' first impressions when they walk in the door, as this impression will influence client expectations and the quality of communication during initial interactions. Does it feel warm and inviting, or is it intimidating and unwelcoming? What does the music sound like? How are the employees dressed? What does it smell like? Is it a mess? Did anyone greet the client? Is it a place where people want to hang out? On a monthly basis, health coaches should walk into the facility with the viewpoint of a client and observe the environment using all five senses. Small changes can make a big difference in relation to first impressions and the overall feeling of the facility, and this can influence the trust and security felt in the client–health coach relationship.

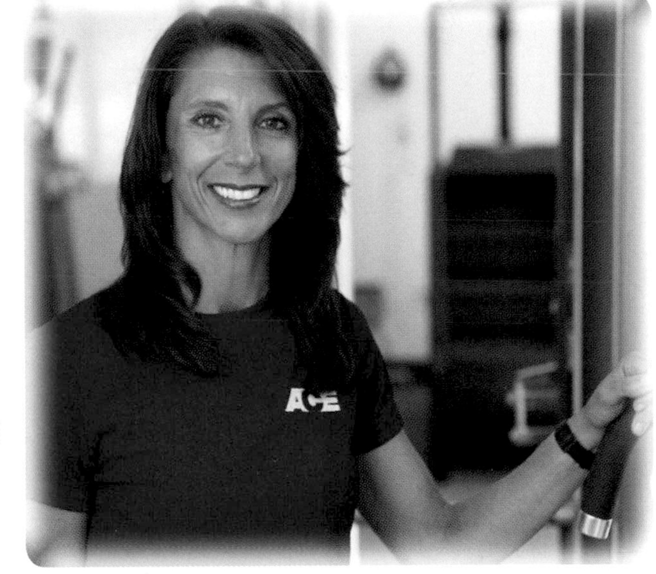

In addition to the physical environment, health coaches should be aware of the way they look and the message this sends. The first element of the client interaction involves the way the health coach dresses and physically presents him- or herself. Health coaches should always be dressed and groomed to look professional and should not look (or smell) like they just finished a workout or be showing off their physiques. Health coaches should also be aware of their body language during the first encounter with a new (or potential) client. When making first impressions, health coaches need to appear cordial, friendly, welcoming, and unintimidating. This is best done through welcoming body language, courteous greetings, smiling, and eye contact. From the very start, clients should have the impression that they are the focus and that their needs are the priority. All health coaches should take the time to evaluate their personal appearance and general demeanor and should be aware of how it may make others feel.

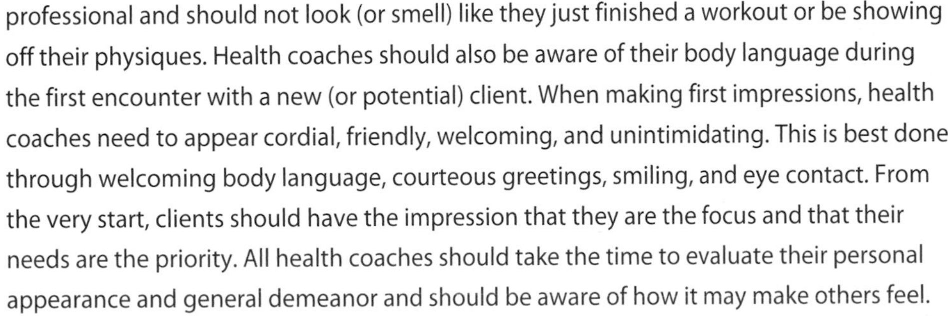

Psychological Environment

Arguably more important than the physical environment is the psychological environment of the facility and the program. This is related to the customer-service experience of the lifestyle-modification program. Health coaches often put a tremendous amount of thought and care into all aspects of program design, but then forget about the client experience. Without a positive experience with the program, long-term success will be difficult to attain. Every client should feel appreciated and be regularly thanked for being part of the program. Health coaches should always remember that clients are customers, and even though they may be seen numerous times each week, the experience of the program should be worth their time and money every single day. Clients should be treated with friendliness and respect in each interaction, and health coaches must work to avoid creating the perception that they are doing their clients a favor. This perception, as terrible as it may seem, can happen very easily and without intent. Therefore, health coaches must remind themselves each day to be thankful and appreciative of the opportunity to be a part of their clients' lives.

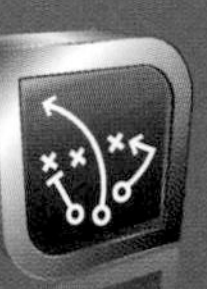

APPLY WHAT YOU KNOW

Simple Things Health Coaches Can Do to Make Their Clients Feel Valued and Appreciated

- Be sure clients are greeted every time they enter and exit the facility.
- Send handwritten thank you notes after the first meeting and periodically throughout program participation.
- Be aware of the things clients are sharing about their lives. It is important that health coaches make clients feel like they care and are paying attention.
- Celebrate clients' successes with them, no matter how small or large.
- Say thank you.

Defining Program Success

The success of a lifestyle-modification program is often measured very objectively through pounds and inches lost and changes in health factors, including **blood pressure, cholesterol,** and **diabetes.** It is fairly straightforward to set goals related to such outcomes and to measure program progress by evaluating these variables. For a health coach, these changes indicate that the program is effective and that goals are being met, and these outcomes should be celebrated. However, it is important for health coaches to realize that other, less outcome-related variables, such as support, enjoyment, and satisfaction may be the true measures of long-term success and adherence.

Program Goals

Every lifestyle-modification program should start with some sort of goal-setting process, and depending on the individual, his or her needs, and the situation, these goals may be very specific and organized or more general and broad. It is critically important for the health coach to be part of the goal-setting process and for both the client and the health coach to be on board in the plan to achieve the goals. Without discounting the importance of setting quality goals in every program, health coaches must be careful to not let the goals take over the purpose of the program. The program must always be about the client, not just about outcomes or his or her goals. Life happens, circumstances and needs change, and if the focus is not on the client, but only on the desired outcome, the relationship will suffer and the client will likely drop out. The point is to not let goals dictate the relationship, as this will make the health coach appear out of touch with the client and his or her real needs. Such a perception will significantly damage trust and rapport. Goals and the goal-setting process should help build an understanding of program components and client expectations and should aid in program design. The goals should then be a dynamic construct that become part of the program, not the focus of the program. The focus should instead be on the client experience during all parts of the program.

For health coaches, the main goals are to change lives, increase activity levels, and improve dietary habits, and these victories should be celebrated as they happen. The best gift a health coach can give is to create an experience that teaches someone to enjoy living a healthy lifestyle. Therefore, it is not always about the outcome goals, but also about the big picture, and if not used properly, a strict goal-setting plan can ultimately hurt the relationship. Health coaches should teach (and practice) flexibility and fun, and focus on the daily *process,* instead of on daily *progress.* Refer to Chapter 13 for information on how a realistic approach to goal-setting can have a tremendous impact on a client's lifelong commitment to health and well-being.

THINK IT THROUGH

After two months of consistent participation in your program, one of your clients tells you that she is very disappointed and is considering dropping out. She has not met her initial goal of losing 20 or more pounds during this timeframe and has decided that she "is just not meant to lose the weight." How would you respond? What other measures of success can be introduced?

APPLY WHAT YOU KNOW

Goal-setting and Rapport

The process and importance of goal-setting as part of a lifestyle-modification program is well documented in most fitness programming literature. The problem with goal-setting is not a lack of understanding about how to do it, but a reluctance to actually systematically implement it. Most fitness professionals view goal-setting as an opportunity to gather key information needed for program design and to measure program progress. While this is a key benefit of goal-setting, the process of goal-setting can be a tremendous opportunity to gain a better understanding of client expectations, desires, and even doubts. Health coaches should use goal-setting as an additional opportunity to create conversation, listen, and build rapport. When clients start talking about their goals, they are typically providing great insight into what they need and want out of the lifestyle-modification program. Additionally, setting goals can and should happen naturally through open conversation about the client's needs and expectations. Health coaches should then maintain these conversations throughout the program in order to effectively reassess client needs and make adjustments to the goals and overall program as necessary.

Adherence

While the qualifications, reputation, and experience of the health coach may bring clients through the door, the rapport built and experiences created are going to keep them there. Even a perfectly designed, scientifically sound program that leads to results is not enough to keep people coming back for more. The program must be a positive experience in the clients' lives and they must perceive value in the time spent with the health coach and making lifestyle changes. The program must be something they enjoy. The time commitment must be worth making over the long-term.

Rapport is an important determinant of adherence to an exercise program. Rapport is not something established in the first consultation and then ignored as the focus shifts to program execution. Instead, the health coach should continuously focus on developing and maintaining trust and rapport through each interaction. Health coaches should be in tune with how the client is feeling about the program factors (progress, components, and demands) that relate to how the program is fitting into his or her life.

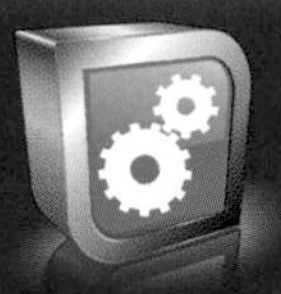

EXPAND YOUR KNOWLEDGE

Rapport: The Foundation of the Every Stage of the ACE Integrated Fitness Training Model

The greatest impact a health coach can have on a client's life is to help that person change his or her habits and establish a positive relationship with exercise. For this reason, rapport is the foundation of the ACE Integrated Fitness Training® (ACE IFT®) Model (see Chapters 16 and 17). Exercise programming has traditionally had a primary focus on helping clients make physiological changes, placing early emphasis on fitness assessments for program design and tracking progress. However, to the out-of-shape client, a complete battery of initial assessments can be detrimental to early program success by reinforcing his or her negative self-image and beliefs that he or she is hopelessly out of shape or overweight. The most important initial adaptations come from helping a client modify behavior to establish a habit of regular exercise. A health coach can have an immediate impact on a client's health by first creating a positive exercise experience that can lead to exercise adherence, and then gradually progressing the training plan by applying program-design strategies that produce results.

Successful health coaches provide integrated training solutions to clients by helping them have positive experiences with exercise. Applying strategies for fitness-related behavioral change and exercise adherence, along with implementing comprehensive exercise programs that help clients reach their unique fitness and wellness goals are two primary functions of health coaches who want to help clients achieve meaningful results.

Even with some initial apprehension, it is common for new clients to be excited about starting a new program. It is a new challenge, they have high hopes for success, and they often feel proud of themselves for making the initial commitment. However, as the program progresses, the real work begins, and the excitement of the newness wears off. For some, the work will be harder than expected and will create a psychological barrier and decrease self-efficacy. For others, the hard work will be viewed as part of the process and a challenge to overcome. Health coaches need to be sure they have time to talk to their clients about how they are feeling about the program and not assume that every client is on track. During these ongoing conversations, health coaches should find out what program components are liked and disliked, what part of the program is the most difficult to stick with, what the challenges are in integrating the program into their lives, if the clients are feeling supported, and if they are having fun. This information seems straightforward, but many health coaches fail to allot the specific time needed to gather it, and this can not only decrease rapport, but also negatively influence adherence.

It is important to remember that clients are much more likely to maintain program participation if the program is something they value in their lives and that they truly enjoy. Health coaches need to take the time to think about these concepts, not only in the lives of their clients, but also in their own lives. Self-reflection and understanding can be a valuable tool in establishing relationships and relating to the struggles clients face and the commitments that clients are working so hard to make.

APPLY WHAT YOU KNOW

Ask Yourself: "What role does exercise play in my life?"

This simple question can provide a lot of insight in how you design programs and view client commitment, so use yourself as an example. It is likely that you are busy and work long hours, as most fitness professionals do. You may have a spouse and children and make an effort every day to balance the work, home, and personal aspects of your life. Without a plan, it is probably easy for exercise to be squeezed out of your schedule, even though you spend hours each day in a gym. However, because it is a priority for you to be active, you have found time in your schedule to make it happen. Maybe that means that you work out early in the morning before your day starts, or that you get your workout in during lunch, or even late at night. You probably do an activity or workout that you enjoy and you likely also bring variety to what you do on a weekly basis. The point is that whether it is a class at the gym, a strength-training program, or a run on the quiet streets before the sun comes up, you know that you have to get your workout in before, between, or after the crazy parts of your day. Ask yourself: What does this workout time *really* mean to you? Is it the *only* time in your day that is dedicated to you? No phone calls, emails, questions to answer, homework, dinner to cook, kids to bathe, classes to teach, toys to pick up, or dishes to wash. Do you look forward to the time for yourself as much as you do the actual workout and the benefits of the workout? Whatever it means, it is powerful because it works! Sure, there are times you could spend an hour or two catching up on paperwork, but then you would miss the opportunity to do something for yourself. In return, your behavior is setting an example of being committed to an active lifestyle for your friends, family, and children.

Your challenge is to answer these questions for yourself. What does your daily exercise routine mean to you, and what role does being active and fit play in your life? This task will help reinforce the importance and power of the work you do and will help you understand the role you play in your clients' lives. It will also help you see the bigger picture beyond weight loss, sets and repetitions, and diet logs. A lifestyle-modification program is about so much more than a scientifically sound program or losing weight. It is about providing a positive experience and outlet for people to feel empowered and to succeed. It is about changing lives and this is as rewarding as it gets!

Summary

Taking the time to establish a relationship with each client is an important part of what health coaches do on a daily basis. Working through a lifestyle-modification program without a foundation of mutual trust, respect, and rapport will lead to frustration, misunderstanding, and ultimately failure. Health coaches are in a unique position to influence change and to empower others with the knowledge and skills to take control of their own health, and they should not lose sight of this bigger picture and purpose as they work through program design and implementation details. Maintaining the client–health coach relationship should always be the first priority, because with a quality relationship, the program components will be easier to implement, the program will be more fun, and the likelihood of success and long-term adherence will be increased.

Clients squeeze fitness into their free time, so the health coach's biggest competition is often the couch; time with children, family, and friends; and so on. The health coach's job is to create an experience that makes the program a priority for people when they have so many choices of how to spend their free time and money. Some clients may never love the actual exercise that is being performed, but the goal should be for them to love the experience of participating in the exercise. Before focusing solely on clients achieving their goals, health coaches should focus on helping them connect with others, build friendships, and enjoy the time dedicated to themselves. The building of rapport is an essential element of creating this type of environment.

References

Bandura, A. (2004). Self-efficacy. In Craighead, W.E. & Nemeroff, C.B. (Eds.) *The Concise Corsini Encyclopedia of Psychology and Behavioral Science* (3rd ed.). pp. 860–862. Hoboken, N.J.: Wiley.

Bandura, A. (1986). *Social Foundations of Thought and Action: A Social Cognitive Theory.* Englewood Cliffs, N.J.: Prentice-Hall.

Bandura, A., Reese, L., & Adams, N.W. (1982). Microanalysis of action and fear arousal as a function of differential levels of perceived self-efficacy. *Journal of Personality and Social Psychology,* 43, 5–21.

Beauchamp, M.R. et al. (2002). Role ambiguity, role efficacy, and role performance: Multidimensional and mediational relationships within interdependent sport teams. *Group Dynamics: Theory, Research, and Practice,* 6, 3, 229–242.

Dishman, R.K. (Ed.). (1994). *Advances in Exercise Adherence.* Champaign, Ill.: Human Kinetics.

Egan, G. (2010). *The Skilled Helper: A Problem Management and Opportunity Development Approach to Helping* (9th ed.). Pacific Grove, Calif.: Brooks/Cole.

Eys, M.A. et al. (2010). The sport team as an effective group. In: Williams, J.M. (Ed.). *Applied Sport Psychology: Personal Growth to Peak Performance.* New York: McGraw-Hill.

Mehrabian, A. (1981). *Silent Messages: Implicit Communication of Emotions and Attitudes* (2nd ed.). Belmont, Calif.: Wadsworth.

Orlick, T. (2008). *In Pursuit of Excellence* (4th ed.). Champaign, Ill.: Human Kinetics.

Pietsch, W.V. (1974). *Human Being: How to Have a Creative Relationship Instead of a Power Struggle.* New York: New American Library.

Rosenfeld, L. & Wilder, L. (1990). Communication fundamentals: Active listening. *Sport Psychology Training Bulletin,* 1, 5, 1–8.

Yukelson, D.P. (2010). Communicating effectively. In: Williams, J.M. (Ed.). *Applied Sport Psychology: Personal Growth to Peak Performance.* New York: McGraw-Hill.

Suggested Reading

Dreeke, R. (2011). *It's Not All About "Me".* Self-published.

Marcus, B.H. & Forsyth, L. H. (2009). *Motivating People to Be Physically Active* (2nd ed.). Champaign, Ill.: Human Kinetics.

Raines, C. & Ewing, L. (2006). *The Art of Connecting.* New York: AMACOM.

Sarafino, E.P. & Smith, T.W. (2011). *Health Psychology: Biopsychosocial Interactions* (7th ed.). New York: John Wiley & Sons.

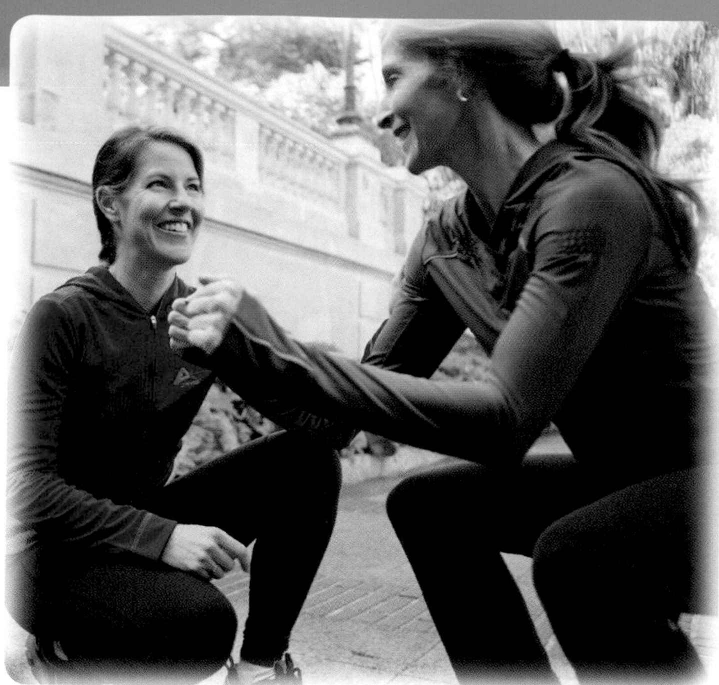

IN THIS CHAPTER:

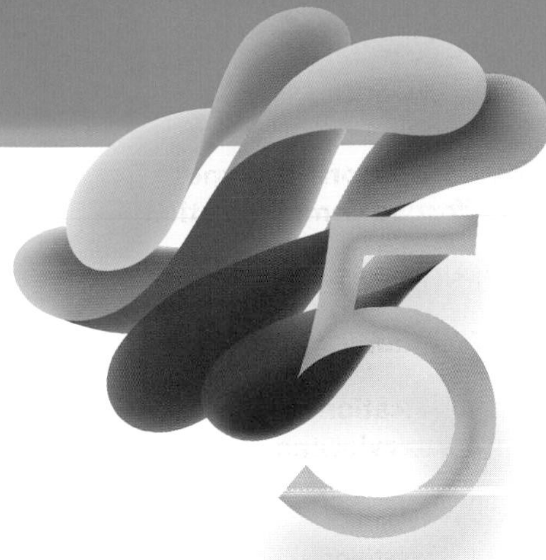

Connection Through Communication

MICHAEL R. MANTELL

Michael R. Mantell, Ph.D., earned his Ph.D. at the University of Pennsylvania and his M.S. at Hahnemann Medical College, where he wrote his thesis on the psychological aspects of obesity. His career includes serving as the Chief Psychologist for Children's Hospital in San Diego and as the founding Chief Psychologist for the San Diego Police Department. Dr. Mantell is a member of the Scientific Advisory Board of the International Council on Active Aging, the Chief Behavior Science Consultant to the Premier Fitness Camp at Omni La Costa, a best-selling author of two books, including the 1988 original Don't Sweat the Small Stuff, P.S. It's All Small Stuff, *an international behavior science fitness keynote speaker, an advisor to numerous fitness-health organizations, and is featured in many media broadcasts and worldwide fitness publications. He has been featured on Oprah, Good Morning America, the Today Show, and has been a contributor to many major news organizations including Fox and ABC News. Dr. Mantell is a nationally sought after behavioral science coach for business leaders, elite amateur and professional athletes, individuals, and families. He is included in the greatist.com's 2013 list of "The 100 Most Influential People in Health and Fitness."*

It is impossible to not communicate. Verbally, nonverbally, in writing, and text messaging—one cannot avoid communicating. The interpersonal experience of communicating is deeply embedded in human behavior. There is in reality, or in virtual reality, no place where communication does not take place. Even turning one's back and walking out of the door communicates something.

Harold Dwight Lasswell is considered to be among the leading social and political scientists of the twentieth century. He investigated social structures, political phenomena, interviewing techniques, and statistical measurement, among other areas of relevance to communication theory. His work in interpersonal communication has application for the ACE-certified Health Coach. When trying to understand the act of transmitting information, signs, or symbols from one person to another over distances in space and time, it is helpful to use Lasswell's maxim: "*Who* says *what* in *which channel* to *whom* with *what effect*?" (Lasswell, 1953) (Figure 5-1). While Lasswell applied this model to societal communication, it can readily be applied to one-on-one communication, the single purpose of which is to connect with another person. The model is an easy one to grasp, and it fits all types of communication a health coach and client will have.

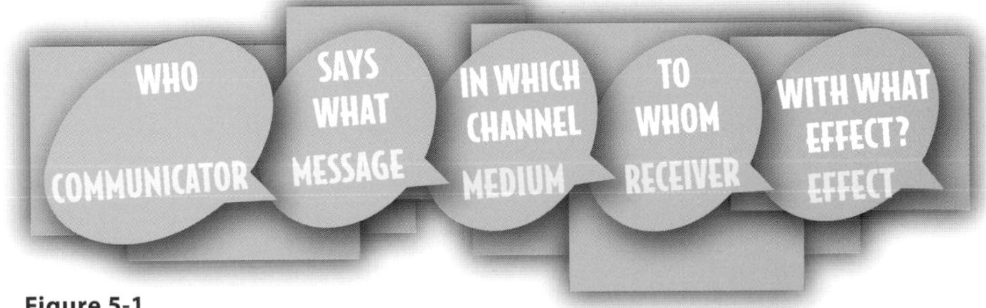
WHO
COMMUNICATOR
SAYS WHAT
MESSAGE
IN WHICH CHANNEL
MEDIUM
TO WHOM
RECEIVER
WITH WHAT EFFECT?
EFFECT

Figure 5-1
Lasswell's model of communication

Drawing on areas of research including sociology, psychology, biology, anthropology, political science, economics, linguistics, semiotics (the study of signs, symbols, and signification), rhetoric (the study of persuasion), engineering, mathematics, gender and sexuality studies, and computer science, scholars who study communication do not consistently agree on one conceptualization of communication. Yet, somehow people seem to intuitively know when they are communicating well and when they are not. The skills taught in this chapter will move the health coach from communicating intuitively, unwittingly, and perhaps "unconsciously" to a mindful, strategic, and purposeful level of communicating with clients, while delivering multiple experiences through a holistic lens, thereby creating dedicated clients who will lead healthier, more fulfilled lives.

The health coach of tomorrow will be called on to connect in deep and meaningful ways with clients' values and needs to help them achieve their behavioral- and lifestyle-modification goals. The ability to do so is solidly anchored in the ability of the health coach to communicate thoroughly and completely, on every level, with his or her increasingly health-conscious clients. The health coach's attempts to reveal a client's aspirations, build a client's self-efficacy, and produce extraordinary results rests on superior connections and **rapport**—both of which are built on communication skills.

The clients of tomorrow will seek more personalized and permanent connections with their health coaches to achieve effective weight management, improved health, and increased quality of life, as well as to find deeper meaning in their lives. As the boundaries become blurred between fitness and coaching, effective communication skills will serve as the vital rapport-building connection between health coaches and their clients.

The ACE Integrated Fitness Training® (ACE IFT®) Model builds upon rapport, or connection, between coach and client (see Chapter 16). Without a strong, genuine, trusting connection, it is unlikely that the relationship between a health coach and a client will be as effective or as lasting. To develop this foundational element in communication requires the health coach to develop superior self-knowledge, trust-building skills, and communication know-how.

John Maxwell (2010) defines connection as, "The ability to identify with people and relate to them in a way that increases your influence with them." Covey and Merrill (2008) observe that trust, like connection, is foundational in a relationship. Trust means the client will have confidence in the relationship and in the education the health coach offers. Specifically, Covey and Merrill (2008) describe self-trust and relationship trust as being two elements that are important to building a trusting connection.

Self-trust, or credibility, is built on the following elements (adapted from Covey & Merrill, 2008):

- *Capabilities*
  - ✓ Talents
  - ✓ Knowledge
  - ✓ Attitudes
  - ✓ Style
  - ✓ Skills
- *Results*
  - ✓ Take responsibility for results
  - ✓ Finish strong
  - ✓ Expect to succeed
- *Integrity*
  - ✓ Make and keep commitments to oneself
  - ✓ Stand for something
  - ✓ Be open
- *Intent*
  - ✓ A clear motive
  - ✓ A sound agenda
  - ✓ Consistent behavior

Relationship trust is built on the following elements (adapted from Covey & Merrill, 2008):

- *Character-based behaviors*
  - ✓ Be honest
  - ✓ Demonstrate respect
  - ✓ Create transparency
  - ✓ Right wrongs
  - ✓ Show loyalty
- *Competency-based behaviors*
  - ✓ Deliver results
  - ✓ Get better
  - ✓ Confront reality
  - ✓ Clarify expectations
  - ✓ Practice accountability
- *Character and competence behaviors*
  - ✓ Listen first
  - ✓ Keep commitments
  - ✓ Extend trust

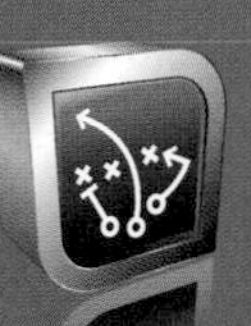

APPLY WHAT YOU KNOW

Coach Connection Checklist

The health coach should ask him- or herself the following questions regarding each and every client:

- Did I do my best?
- Did I answer my client's questions effectively?
- Did I understand and relate to my client?
- Did I add value to the conversation with my client?
- Did we develop a specific plan?
- Did I make a difference in my client's life?

Adapted from Maxwell, J.C. (2010). Everyone Communicates, Few Connect. *Nashville, Tenn.: Thomas Nelson.*

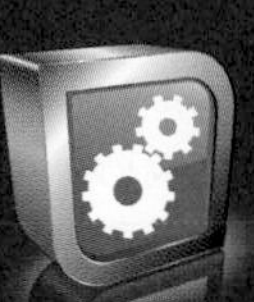

EXPAND YOUR KNOWLEDGE

Components of Connecting With Clients

- *Visual connection:* The health coach is always well groomed, dresses appropriately, smiles, maintains a receptive body stance, and moves with confidence.
- *Intellectual connection:* The health coach knows his or her subject matter and demonstrates confidence in the use of language, avoiding language that is hesitant, doubt-filled, or unclear.
- *Attitude connection:* The health coach maintains an open, friendly, visible positivity in approaching the client. The health coach should always say "hello" first.
- *Verbal connection:* The health coach uses positive, memorable language and examples, and is always aware of his or her tone, timing, inflexion, and pace.

Adapted from Maxwell, J.C. (2010). Everyone Communicates, Few Connect. *Nashville, Tenn.: Thomas Nelson.*

Understanding Personality Types Promotes Effective Communication

It is important to begin communication efforts by knowing the language of the client. It is also important to consider the following questions when structuring communication in a coaching relationship (Crookes, 1991):

- Why does the health coach want to communicate?
- With whom is the health coach communicating?
- Where and when can the message best be sent?
- What is it that needs to be communicated?
- How will the health coach best communicate this information?

As briefly described in Chapter 1, Marston (1928) developed the widely used DISC method of assessing personality types (Figure 5-2). Understanding this model is helpful in creating strategically purposeful communication with clients, since it will assist the health coach in understanding his or her own style of communication as well as that of the client.

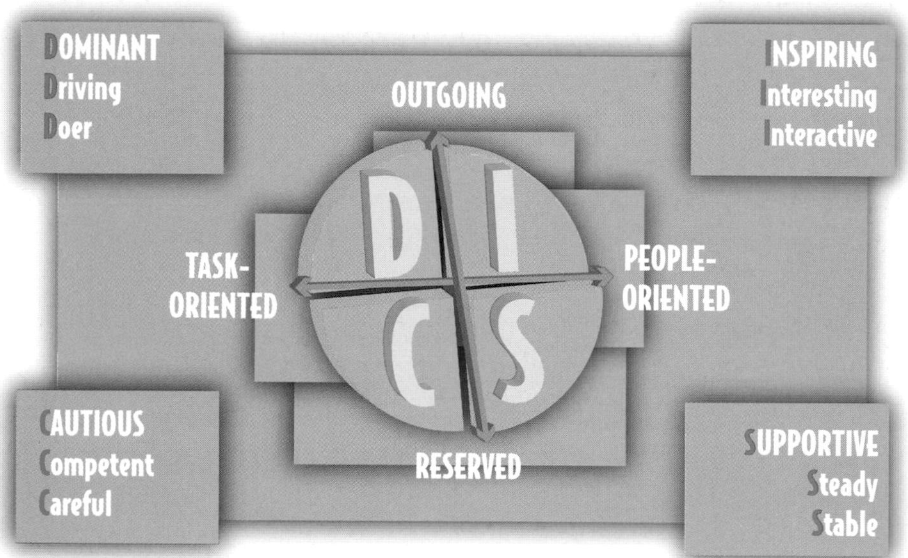

Figure 5-2
DISC model of understanding personality types

Communication involves (1) planning to communicate, (2) creating a carefully constructed message (encoding), (3) choosing the best channel through which to send that message, (4) interpreting a message (decoding), and (5) offering feedback. These steps are influenced by a person's experiences, inner thoughts, expectations, hopes, dreams, values, needs, and personalities. That is where the DISC model, with its four personality types, is valuable. Rapidly distinguishing these four quadrants allows the health coach to see clients as fitting into one area or another.

- **D** = Dominant personality types are fast-paced, direct, outgoing, and task-oriented. These are the "get it done now," results-oriented people. They prefer to be treated with respect and demand to see results quickly. They want to know the "what" of a situation. It is best, when coaching these clients, to maintain eye contact; stay engaged; offer confident, assertive, direct, and to-the-point communication; and avoid withdrawing. These individuals thrive on control, choice, and challenge, and prefer assertive interaction. If the health coach does not have a dominant personality, these clients may appear aggressive and unappreciative, and the health coach may erroneously feel that the client simply does not like him or her. If a dominant client is not challenging the health coach, it may mean that he or she is not interested in what is being said, rather than disapproving. Get to the point quickly with D-type individuals, provide options, show respect, focus on the outcome, and be nonverbally assertive with continuous eye contact and tone of voice. Health coaches who appear organized and who avoid chitchat will work well with D-type clients.

- **I** = Inspiring personality types are also outgoing, but are more people-oriented than D-types, and likely a bit more like many health coaches. These clients are fast speakers, movers, and decision-makers. They want to have fun and will appear to connect easily. These are the folks who enjoy the health coach's admiration, approval, and recognition. These individuals enjoy interacting and socializing, and place value on what others think of them. Health coaches can think in terms of I-types wanting to know the "who" involved in a situation. The health coach will need to gently keep these clients focused, demonstrate approval and positive feedback, stay engaged through verbal and nonverbal methods, and ask clients how they feel about matters discussed. Health coaches working with I-type clients should show enthusiasm, share stories and personal experiences, appear friendly, and inquire about the client's family and friends. Technical details will derail the effectiveness of communication with these clients.
- **S** = Supportive personality types are reserved and people-oriented, focus on relationships, and enjoy helping others. They speak slowly and softly. S-type individuals are not interested in data, tasks, or facts. They avoid confrontations and are not comfortable with quick decisions. These clients are best communicated with in ways that leave them feeling secure, assured, and appreciated. They want to see the health coach's gentle confidence and are willing to have the health coach make the final, carefully thought-out, decision. These types are curious about the "how" of a situation. Health coaches should ensure that feelings are considered fairly when trying to connect with these individuals. Show these clients care by using gentle hand gestures and voice tones, asking indirect questions, and progressing slowly. Steer clear of pushing the S-type person into decisions and avoid a loud, pushy approach in any interaction.
- **C** = Cautious personality types are reserved, task-oriented people who want data and facts, and prefer less emotion. Focusing on feelings will not work with these clients. They want quality information that is correct and accurate. They speak in a monotone voice—slowly, deliberately, and purposefully. Health coaches are encouraged to bring data, website information, research articles, and other supporting information to these clients. Physically, they prefer space and distance. Because they show little emotion, it may be easy to misconstrue their intent. Health coaches should provide them with quality answers and valued results, and demonstrate excellence in every aspect of the relationship. C-type clients value trustworthiness and integrity, they may appear skeptical, and they want to know the "why" of a situation. Recommendations for communicating with C-type clients are to talk slowly, use third-party support for recommendations, discuss thoughts (not feelings), and always provide logic. Also, be careful not to avoid the client's technical questions.

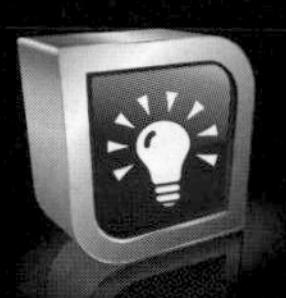

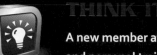

THINK IT THROUGH

A new member at the gym where you work as a health coach and personal trainer approaches you for some help with her weight-loss program. She is very soft-spoken and, after meeting with you to discuss her various options, seems very hesitant to make a decision about how to proceed. Instead, she asks how the different programs would work and if you could give your opinion on what would be the best option for her. Where does this client fit within the DISC model? How would you approach working with this client?

Beyond using the DISC model in understanding the client and one's own personality style, and determining how to deliver coaching in a successful, positively impactful manner, another framework may also be useful in coaching. Developed by John Heron (2001; 1989), there are two basic categories for the health coach to consider when planning an intervention—authoritative and facilitative—each of which has three elements.

If the health coach is moving in an authoritative manner, he or she is offering information, providing a challenge, or making specific suggestions as to what the client should be doing. The authoritative approach consists of the following interventions:

- *Prescriptive:* The health coach offers advice, guidance, and information, and offers direct suggestions for what clients can do to help themselves facilitate desired outcomes. A coach should never tell a client what to do, even when acting from an "authoritative approach."
- *Informative:* The health coach offers his or her own experiences and point of view. When explaining the principles of what to do, the goal is to help the client develop a deeper understanding of why the health coach is directing the client in one direction or another.
- *Confronting:* The health coach mirrors, or reflects, what the client has said, offers his or her own thoughts about what the client has said in a very direct way, tells the client what he or she thinks are the obstacles that lie ahead, and offers ideas for the client to follow to avoid those stumbling blocks.

In contrast to the authoritative approach, if the health coach is moving in a facilitative manner, he or she is helping the client find his or her own solutions or decisions. The facilitative approach consists of the following interventions:

- *Cathartic:* The health coach helps the client express emotions, fears, or thoughts that he or she has not previously confronted. In terms of weight management, this may be especially helpful when having a discussion focusing on the client's self-image and body-image. The health coach will be called on to be empathetic, non-judgmental, and an exceptionally good listener.
- *Catalytic:* The health coach will ask questions to encourage new thinking, generate new solutions, and create new options. The health coach will follow with **active listening,** mirroring, validating, and empathizing.
- *Supportive:* The health coach builds the confidence of the client through focus on empowerment, confidence, and the client's own strengths and accomplishments. The health coach offers praise, support, commitment, and admiration.

THINK IT THROUGH

Can you think of situations in which the authoritative approach would be the best option for a health coach? In what scenarios might the facilitative approach be a wiser choice?

Regardless of the personality style and the type of intervention the health coach decides upon, communication must be (Crookes, 1991):

- *Clear:* The message must be simple and coherent.
- *Concise:* Stick to the message and avoid being long-winded.
- *Correct:* Correct information fits the client and is free of any errors.
- *Complete:* The client will have everything he or she needs to be fully informed to take action.
- *Courteous:* Communication should be friendly, open, honest, non-threatening, and free of any hidden insults or conflict.
- *Constructive:* Always be positive, free of negativity or any critical qualities, and focused on what can go right.

Making a Positive First Impression

The first meeting of the health coach and the client is memorable and noteworthy. The client will not forget it and will form lasting impressions of the health coach in the initial moments of the first meeting, whether by phone, email, website introduction, or in person.

In Chapter 1, the concept of different types (or waves) of trust was introduced. Covey and Merrill (2008) describe the first "wave of trust" as "self-trust," and this type of trust must be evident to the client from the very first meeting. This "wave of trust" consists of the integrity, intent, and capabilities of the health coach.

The integrity factor of the health coach is foundational. The client will see how the health coach makes commitments and keeps those commitments, what the health coach stands for, and how open and transparent he or she is. The client will also readily see the motive, agenda, and behavior of the health coach, encompassing what Covey and Merrill (2008) refer to as intent. This involves how the health coach demonstrates care for the client, goal-setting, and whether the behavior of the health coach backs up his or her words.

The talents, attitudes, skills, knowledge, and style of the health coach—that is, the overall capabilities of the health coach—become important only if the client knows and feels that he or she cares. Specifically, in the first meeting, it is important for the health coach to communicate care by simply being on time and presenting him- or herself in a professionally attired, well-groomed manner. Meeting in a health club may mean "gym attire," while meeting elsewhere may require "business casual" or "formal business" attire. The health coach must bear in mind that not all clients will see gym attire as necessarily appropriate if their first meeting is not in the gym. The key is to be appropriate for the situation. Attire, like anything else, speaks volumes about the health coach's level of professionalism.

During the first meeting, the client will consider the health coach's facial expressions, body language, small talk, attentiveness, and courtesy when "reading" the health coach. Introducing oneself with a firm handshake also conveys confidence and professionalism.

Nonverbal Communication

Mehrabian (1971) noted that when communicating a message, 7% of the message is comprised of spoken words, 38% is related to the tone of voice, and a whopping 55% consists of body language. In other words, nonverbal language makes up more than 90% of the message communicated.

Scientific research on nonverbal or body language began in 1872 with Charles Darwin. Darwin demonstrated that the chief expressions displayed by man are the same throughout the world. He recorded weeping, blushing, anger, sulking, and contempt, and looked at the sneer, the pout, and the frown. Darwin's book, *The Expression of Emotion in Man and Animals,* was the first to use photography to demonstrate scientific findings on nonverbal language (Darwin, 1872). The health coach may not need to refer to a text written in the late 1800s to understand how to read and use body language, but perusing Darwin's book is illustrative of the universal nature of nonverbal language.

Notably, researchers Ambady and Gray (2002) found that body language is trusted over any other element of communication, particularly verbal content. Body language includes how the health coach and client position their bodies, how close they are to each other, facial expressions, eye contact/movement, their individual levels of physical contact, how each holds objects, breathing, perspiration, tone of voice, and posture.

There are six generally accepted and genetically based human facial expressions recognized worldwide:

- Happiness
- Disgust
- Fear
- Sadness
- Surprise
- Anger

The health coach will recognize that, without confirmation from a number of indicators, reading one element of body language and assuming with certainty that it means anything, is likely misleading. Context, sufficient evidence, culture, ethnicity, age, gender, and faking and deception, among other indicators, are all necessary to consider. Several consistent signals are needed to arrive at an accurate conclusion. Common body language indicators include the following:

- *Crossed arms:* The client is closed and not listening; this is a defensive posture
- *Light touch on the arm:* An attention getter when done professionally and appropriately
- *Nose rub:* May imply deception
- *Use of a barrier (purse, equipment in the gym):* Personal space is being invaded
- *Hand under the chin:* Decision time has arrived
- *Feet pointed toward the door:* Client is ready to leave
- *Eyes generally looking right/up:* Guessing, fabricating, or lying
- *Eyes generally looking left/up:* Recalling, retrieving facts, or truthfulness
- *Tight-lipped smile:* Secrecy or withholding of feelings
- *Biting lip:* Tension
- *Head tilted to one side:* Non-threatening, submissive, and thoughtful
- *Palms up/open:* Truthfulness and honesty
- *Cracking knuckles:* Comforting habit and attention-seeking
- *Seating that is approximately 45 degrees from each other:* Normal, comfortable, and cooperative arrangement for the health coach and client

The health coach may use a mirroring technique when creating rapport with a client to build **empathy,** understanding, and trust. Doing so with matching body language establishes unconscious feelings of connection.

All body movements should be relaxed, natural, and comfortable. Body posture that is similarly reflective of comfort and ease, and is natural, communicates an openness that will be perceived by the client. Positioning the shoulders back with the head in line with a neutral spine (not dropping forward), and sitting facing the client without invading the client's space, typically communicate safety. The health coach should ensure that body posture conveys enthusiasm and is stress-free. Similarly, the tone of the health coach's voice should include normal variations in inflection, demonstrate energetic enthusiasm, and avoid monotony.

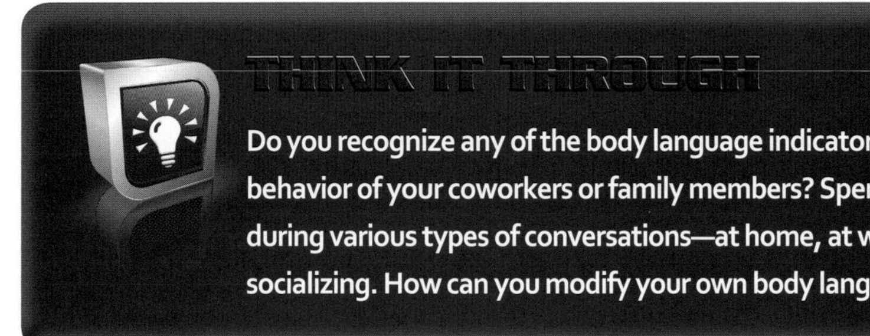

THINK IT THROUGH

Do you recognize any of the body language indicators in your own behavior or the behavior of your coworkers or family members? Spend a few days really paying attention during various types of conversations—at home, at work, and even when out shopping or socializing. How can you modify your own body language to better serve your clientele?

Verbal Communication and Motivational Interviewing

There is evidence that client-centered approaches to healthcare consultations—which are promoted by the health coach approach to coaching—may have better outcomes than traditional advice-giving (Britt, Hudson, & Blampied, 2004). **Motivational interviewing** in a client-centered way helps clients overcome ambivalence to change (Miller & Rollnick, 2002; Miller, 1983). Miller and Rollnick (2002) note that "motivation should not be thought of as a personality problem. Rather, motivation is a state of readiness to change, which may fluctuate from one time or situation to another. This state is one that can be influenced."

The health coach, when communicating with clients who may not be in a state of readiness to change, may find motivational interviewing a useful communication tool in influencing clients for positive change. As a "fluctuating product of interpersonal interaction," motivation to change, then, is evoked within the client, not imposed on the client (Rollnick & Miller, 1995). The health coach's task is to expect, anticipate, and recognize ambivalence to change, and then help the client examine and resolve his or her ambivalence.

There are five core principles of motivational interviewing of which a health coach should be aware (Miller & Rollnick, 2002):

- Express empathy
- Develop awareness of negative consequences
- Roll with resistance
- Support self-efficacy
- Avoid argumentation

The motivational interview model should be thought of as behavioral change with the specific purpose of evoking and strengthening personal motivation for change. In conjunction with the **stages-of-change model,** the collaborative nature of the interaction is particularly clear. Clients always make their own changes.

As the client and health coach move toward a particular goal, the health coach will sometimes observe ambivalence in the client about behavioral change. The task of the coach is to help the client resolve his or her ambivalence in the direction of positive change, though at times this may require the health coach to actually create ambivalence for the client in order to move forward. The health coach elicits and strengthens the client's "change talk" in a non-confrontational manner, through elaborating, affirming, reflecting, and summarizing, all active listening tools. In fact, if the conversation is not specifically about change in a collaborative manner that respects the autonomy of the client, it is not motivational. The health coach communicates in a way that evokes the client's best thinking, personal motivation, and commitment to the goals established. Engaging, guiding, and evoking are the watchwords of motivational interviewing.

The motivational interviewing model readily works with Prochaska and DiClemente's stages-of-change model (Prochaska, DiClemente, & Norcross, 1998; Prochaska & DiClemente, 1984) (see Chapter 3). Below are the steps of the model and the related actions the health coach will engage in when adhering to motivational interviewing methods (Ockene, 1997; Simkin-Silverman & Wing, 1997).

- **Precontemplation**
  - ✓ Validate the client's position
  - ✓ Clarify the client's decision
  - ✓ Encourage the client to reevaluate, not act on, his or her current position
  - ✓ Discuss and personalize the risk of not taking action
  - ✓ Raise the client's awareness of the need for change
  - ✓ Raise doubt
  - ✓ Increase perceptions of the risks of not engaging in more healthful behaviors
- **Contemplation**
  - ✓ Validate the client's lack of readiness
  - ✓ Clarify the decision the client is making
  - ✓ Encourage the client to evaluate the costs and benefits of lifestyle or behavioral change
  - ✓ Help the client identify new positive outcome expectations
  - ✓ Increase the client's desire for change by exploring his or her ambivalences and discrepancies and not taking sides on the client's positions
- **Preparation**
  - ✓ Identify obstacles and assist with problem-solving
  - ✓ Identify with the client's social-support systems
  - ✓ Confirm the client's skills for behavioral change while encouraging the client to take small steps
  - ✓ Assist the client in creating strategies for change and exploring a plan for overcoming obstacles
- **Action**
  - ✓ Focus on the client's social-support system
  - ✓ Bolster the client's **self-efficacy**
  - ✓ Focus on long-term benefits
  - ✓ Support the progression of change at this stage by encouraging "right-sized" steps and exploring with the client how the process is working

- **Maintenance**
  - ✓ Help the client plan for continued support
  - ✓ Reinforce intrinsic motivation
  - ✓ Discuss how the client will cope with relapse
  - ✓ Focus on maintaining the changes the client has made
- **Relapse**
  - ✓ Assist the client by evaluating triggers for relapse, reassessing motivation, and identifying barriers to further relapse
  - ✓ Help the client plan stronger coping methods
  - ✓ Focus on what has been learned

By understanding the client's frame of reference through reflective and active listening, expressing nonjudgmental acceptance and affirmation, reinforcing the client's self-motivational statements, monitoring the client's readiness to change, and ensuring that resistance is not generated by advancing ahead of the client's stage of change, the health coach can develop a successful framework for communicating in a way that leads the client to achieve his or her behavior- and lifestyle-modification goals.

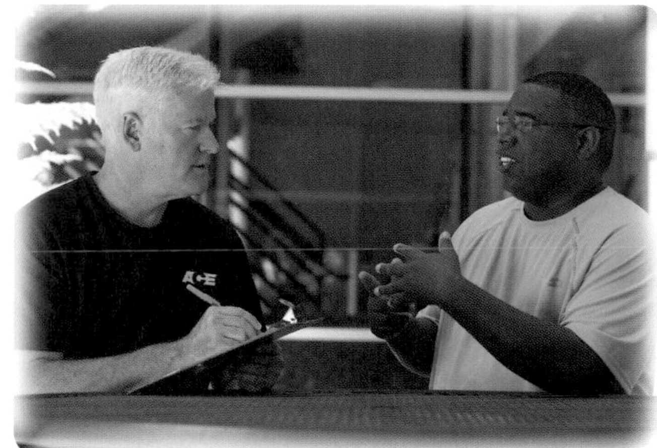

The health coach can attempt to help the client gain awareness of the potential issues that brought him or her to the health coach, the consequences he or she experiences or will experience during the program, and the risks he or she faces if no change is made—as well as the benefits of changing. The client's solution and goals are set by the client with the assistance of the health coach. A health coach's understanding of the client's personality style based on the DISC model can help both the health coach and the client in the goal-setting process (see Chapter 13).

The essential steps of motivational interviewing include:

- Empathizing with the client and using active listening skills to demonstrate understanding of the client's perspective
- Helping the client by identifying where his or her unhealthy lifestyle conflicts with his or her desire to live a healthier life
- Avoiding resistance by using empathy, not confrontation
- Supporting the client's self-efficacy by focusing on confidence-building and looking at what can be accomplished

Specifically, the health coach begins by encouraging the client to talk about a typical day. "Let's discuss your typical day. What happens and how do you feel? How do your weight-management concerns enter the picture?"

Next, the health coach communicates the value of the client setting the agenda for the coaching session. The health coach should encourage the client to communicate specific concerns and personal problem areas such as weight management, **diabetes,** physical activity, and smoking. The health coach can summarize these problems and concerns and identify what the client sees happening with no change. "How have things changed for you because of your weight? What do you believe will happen if you continue as you are now? If things were to improve, what needs to be different? What do you believe are the costs of changing and the benefits of changing?" By answering these questions, the client will better understand the pros and cons of his or her current behavior.

The discussion about **decisional balance** takes place with the client leading the way (see Chapter 3). When the health coach understands the client's readiness to make some changes, asking "Where does that leave you now?" leads to a discussion of solutions and goals. This example is very client-centered, with the health coach leading with motivation-oriented questions. This semidirective communication style, particularly in coaching for lifestyle change, is used to establish rapport, elicit change in a positive client-centered way, and draw commitment language from the client (Amrhein et al., 2003). More information about motivational interviewing is available at www.motivationalinterviewing.org.

Questioning Skills

The heart of effective communication is listening; the foundation is made up of good questions. Health coaches need to understand how to ask five types of questions:

- Open-ended questions
- Closed-ended questions
- Funnel questions
- Probing questions
- Leading questions

These types of questions form the structure of listening and provide an invaluable method for mining for data about the inner life of a client.

Open-ended Questions

Open-ended questions begin with the words "what," why," and "how." However, asking "why" is sometimes the start of an aimless discussion, leading to the all-too-common response, "I don't know." "What" and "how" are much more dynamic and useful. Effective options include:

- "Describe that for me."
- "Tell me more."
- "How would you like things to be different?"
- "How can I help you?"
- "What are the positive things and what are the negative things about your situation?"

These open-ended stems allow the health coach to actively listen. These techniques are useful when the health coach wants to open a conversation, learn more detail, understand a client's views, or keep a conversation going.

Closed-ended Questions

Closed-ended questions elicit "yes" or "no" answers or simple factual responses and provide little room for continuing to pursue dialogue—unless the health coach skillfully turns to an open-ended question. Closed-ended questions come in handy when the health coach simply is checking on a factual point, confirming understanding, or coming to a decision. Closed-ended questions typically end conversations.

Consider the difference between the following exchanges, the first of which begins with a closed-ended question and the second of which begins with an open-ended question:

- *"Did you have any delayed-onset muscle soreness after your workout?"*
  "No."
- *"How did you feel after your last workout?"*
  "It was fine except for my quads—wow! They were really talking to me. I appreciated you calling and leaving a message to see how I was doing."
  "No problem on the call. Sorry I missed you. So what did you do for your soreness?"

Funnel Questions

The use of funnel questions involves beginning with closed-ended questions and slowly moving into more detailed types of open-ended questions. This technique is useful when the health coach wants to learn more detail about a client's specific concern. It also helps pique the attention of the client and build the client's confidence and comfort to delve into areas of a personal concern.

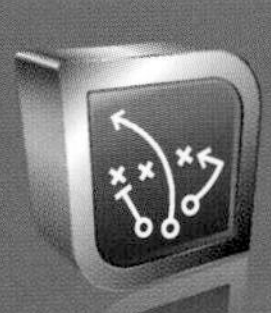

APPLY WHAT YOU KNOW

Funnel Questions

Start with closed-ended questions and then drill down by asking more open-ended questions:

- **Were you able to stick to your eating plan this week?**
- **What was the most difficult obstacle for you in sticking to your plan?**
- **What foods were the most difficult to avoid?**
- **What steps did you take to overcome the urge to eat at the party?**
- **What thoughts did you have as rational responses to your urges to eat?**
- **What else could you have done to avoid eating the foods you wanted to avoid?**
- **How did you feel after you left the party?**
- **Why did you feel that way?**
- **Tell me more about your feelings...**

Probing Questions

Probing questions, which sometimes begin with "who," "what," "where," "when," or "why," coupled with the word "exactly," assist the health coach in ensuring that all of the elements of a problem are fully described. This is particularly useful with highly resistant clients. "Could you tell me more?" "Could you give me an example?" "Why exactly was that?" "Could you expand?" "What exactly do you mean?"

Leading Questions

Finally, leading questions, or semidirective questions, as seen in motivational interviewing, encourage the client to move toward goals and embrace suggestions the health coach may believe are worthwhile for the client to pursue. "Beginning an activity program that includes daily walks sounds like a good idea, *doesn't it?*"

Coaching is about expanding people's capacity to create their desired future. It is not about *telling* people what to do, but instead asking them to examine the thinking behind what they are doing so it is consistent with their goals. Coaching is about being present, asking questions, and listening (Hargrove, 1999).

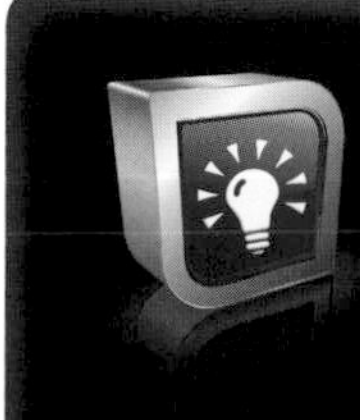

THINK IT THROUGH

Ask family members, friends, or trusted clients to help you role-play the first meeting with a new client. Experiment with various types of questions and observe how the conversation varies depending on the choices you make.

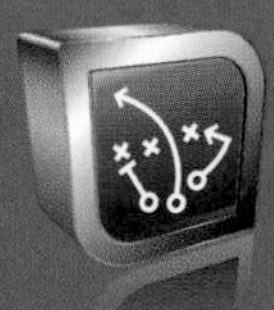

APPLY WHAT YOU KNOW

The OARS Model

The health coach may borrow the OARS model from motivational interviewing in many areas of facilitative communication with clients:

- *O = Ask open-ended questions:* The goal is for the client to open up and share his or her thoughts/feelings—"What do you believe are some good reasons to begin this weight-loss and exercise program?"
- *A = Affirm the client's thinking:* Validate the client's desires, needs, and thinking—"It makes sense that you would feel the way you do, given that ____."
- *R = Listen reflectively:* Demonstrate to the client that the health coach hears and comprehends what the client says by rephrasing or mirroring what the client says—"Let's see if I get what you are saying: __________________________."
- *S = Summarize*: The health coach briefly restates what the client says and means—"So in summary, I hear you say __________________________."

Active Listening Skills

Active listening is a method of listening and responding with special focus on the speaker with one goal—to improve understanding. Communication skills depend on encoding and decoding messages accurately. Listening is required for both elements of this transmission.

Among the many skills involved in communicating, the one primary skill, the skill that makes all the difference, is grounded in the notion that it is not about talking, it is about listening. Specifically, it is about *active listening.*

Active listening means that the health coach accurately understands, interprets, and values what the client says. This requires concentration, eye contact, receptivity, the ability to restate the message, questioning for clarity, empathy, complete objectivity free of personal bias, not interrupting, and strategic pauses.

The Talmudic saying, "We don't see or hear things as they are, but rather as we are," applies. Personal bias, distractions, thinking about other things, and planning what will be said next all interfere with objective comprehending, retaining the information, and responding appropriately. Instead of active listening, there may be passive *not* listening or pseudo-listening.

One model of active listening simply requires the health coach to "mirror" what he or she has heard as accurately as possibly, free of editorializing, adding to, or subtracting from what was said (Hendrix, 2008). Asking if what was heard and "mirrored" was accurate and complete gives the speaker the opportunity to correct the health coach's understanding and adds to the recognition that the client is being heard properly. Summarizing what was heard and again asking the client if the summary was 100% accurate gives the client the sense of being connected and listened to. It also gives the health coach the structure to stay focused.

The next step requires the health coach to demonstrate understanding by telling the client that, given what the health coach understands about the client, what the client is saying makes perfect sense.

Finally, the health coach is encouraged to demonstrate empathy by communicating what he or she imagines the client is feeling. An accuracy check is always useful.

Consider the following example, which depicts the three steps of active listening (Hendrix, 2008):

- *Mirroring:* "I want to see if I get what you are saying. You are saying ______________. Is that correct? Is there anything that I am missing?"
- *Validating:* "It is reasonable you would say this, given that you ______________."
- *Empathy:* "I imagine you might be feeling ______________. Is that a fair assumption?"

The key elements of active listening, verbally or nonverbally, include paying careful attention, demonstrating visually that the health coach is listening, providing feedback, avoiding judgment, and responding appropriately. Asking questions at an appropriate time and using nonverbal body language appropriately to demonstrate listening and positive encouragement are essential.

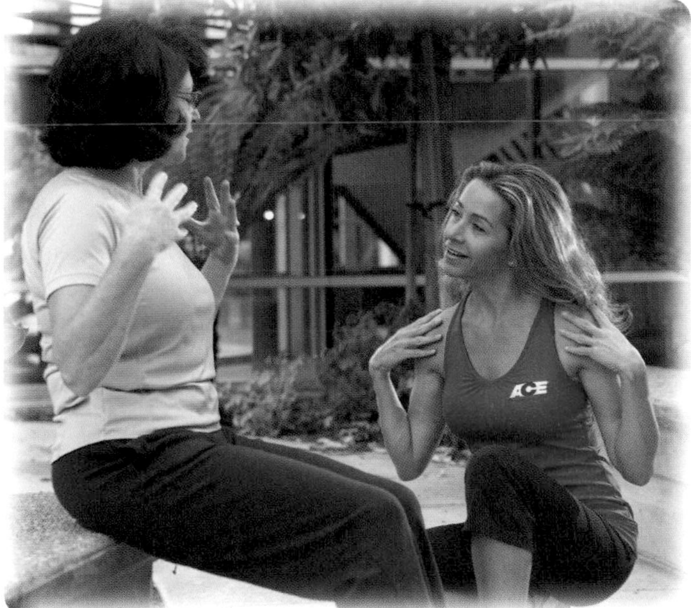

Verbal listening skills include:

- *Paraphrasing:* The health coach is able to repeat words back to the client in a way that demonstrates a general and accurate understanding of what the client said. "Let me repeat back to you what I think you just said, so that I can be sure I understood correctly." This lets the client know that the health coach is trying to understand.
- *Clarifying:* A method of expounding and refining understanding, checking to be sure that what was said was understood. "Please correct me if I am wrong. I understood you to say…"
- *Reflecting:* The health coach attempts to empathize, or reflect, the feeling the client expresses. "It sounds to me like you feel...." Reflective listening involves the words the speaker uses, the words the listener hears, what the listener thinks the speaker means, and what the speaker actually means. This is a key to motivational interviewing, and comprises much of the work the health coach will do in terms of active listening.
- *Explaining:* This involves offering an interpretation of what the health coach heard. "I wonder if you considered…" Similar to "validating" in active listening, this collaborative, non-directive step focuses on opening the client's mind to another possibility based on what the coach believes makes sense given the client's current thoughts and goals.
- *Linking:* The health coach keeps the client's thoughts connected with a simple, "… and then" or "please continue."

- *Summarizing:* The health coach synthesizes what he or she heard the client say in a sentence or two. "So it seems, just to summarize, that you are making three important points. One…" This prevents the health coach from falling into "selective perception," where the listener is expecting the speaker to react in a certain way. Including a question in the summary is also effective. "What might be some other options for you besides the three you mentioned?"
- *Encouraging:* The health coach, during all forms of communication, should always offer supportive comments such as "good point," "well said," or a simple "uh-huh."

Nonverbal listening skills include:

- *Facial expressions:* Health coaches should be alert, face the client, avoid looking around, and nod appropriately. Friendliness, warmth, and happiness may easily be expressed through facial expressions.
- *Body language*: Health coaches should sit facing the client, or at a 45-degree angle, with an open posture while leaning forward.
- *Eye contact:* It is important to maintain eye contact with the client while the client is speaking.
- *Personal space:* Health coaches should avoid being too close or too far away from the client, and watch for signals of discomfort such as the client rocking, swinging the legs, tapping the toes or fingers, or trying to find a more comfortable position or location.
- *Silence:* Maintaining silence, and not interrupting, reflects that the health coach is actively listening.

Finally, to be sure that one has been clearly understood, it may be valuable to ask the client some variation of the following question: "So that I can make sure I communicated clearly, would you please tell me what you heard me say?"

Here are some key points to remember when trying to connect with a client (Raines & Ewing, 2006):

- A health coach can communicate with anyone if he or she uses the right approach.
- Even if the health coach does not believe he or she can find a point of agreement, it is important to keep trying. A connection will eventually be made.
- Although the health coach should plan a strategy, he or she should not make a final decision about what to say until after listening to the other person.
- The health coach should mirror the other person's vocal variations or nonverbal behavior to establish rapport.
- To find out if someone is receiving the message correctly, the health coach should heed verbal and nonverbal cues and ask questions.
- The health coach should examine how his or her entrenched beliefs and reactions may be impeding communication with others.
- The health coach must not assume that people are similar just because they share superficial characteristics, such as age, ethnicity, or religious background.
- It is important to be curious and maintain an open mind. A health coach can learn new things from anyone.
- The health coach should acknowledge differences. Diversity in a group can be a positive connector.
- Curiosity should be based on deep respect.
- The better the health coach knows him- or herself, the better he or she will be able to appreciate others' viewpoints.

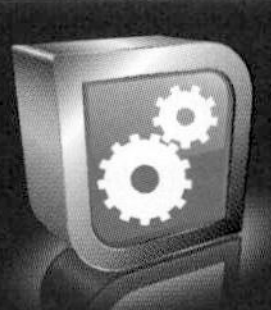

EXPAND YOUR KNOWLEDGE

Developing Active Listening Skills

Health coaches who want to further develop their active listening skills should consider an action plan that consists of:

- *Identifying areas that need improvement:* Health coaches should consider their verbal and nonverbal communication skills, as well as the potential obstacles that may prevent them from being effective communicators. Health coaches can ask people they trust and consider online assessments:
  - www.optimalthinking.com/quiz-communication-skills.php
  - www.managementhelp.org/communicationsskills/index.htm.
- *Measuring these improvements in specific ways:* After identifying specific areas that need improvement, health coaches can create a SMART goal chart to monitor progress (see Chapter 13). Specific, measureable, attainable, relevant, and time-bound goals are the best way to monitor progress. If receptive body language is a problem area, a SMART goal might be, "I will sit in an open position, monitoring my unfolded arms in my lap, in every conversation I have today. I will ask for feedback from two people I trust each day."
- *Taking active steps to achieve these improvements:* Coaching, self-monitoring, requesting feedback, observing oneself daily, reflecting back at the end of a day upon conversations and connections, and utilizing audio and video recording of coaching sessions are all methods to move forward in achieving success in communication skills.

Barriers to Effective Communication

Cultural Bias

An effective health coach acknowledges culture as a predominant force in communication. Connecting and rapport-building require the health coach to reflect and respect the attitudes and values of each client. Race, ethnicity, language, nationality, religion, age, gender, and sexual orientation are all important dimensions in understanding how to best design a message. The concept of **cultural competence** refers to the ability of the health coach to respond respectfully to people of all cultures, languages, classes, races, ethnic backgrounds, religions, and other diversity factors that affirm the value and worth of all people. The health coach must be able to recognize when he or she does not have the cultural competence to sensitively and effectively communicate with a client.

Perception is affected by the way people select, organize, and evaluate stimuli. It is not likely that people of different national groups, with different cultural backgrounds, will see the world in a similar way. People's interests, cultural backgrounds, and values act as filters that distort, block, or even create what they choose to see and hear. People often perceive what they expect to perceive based on what they have been trained to see according to their cultural background (Adler, 2008). This can challenge communication and jeopardize the ability to create a healthy connection with others.

An example of how bias plays a role in effective communication can be seen in the following example. Read this sentence and simply count the number of times the letter "f" appears:

> FINISHED FILES ARE THE RESULT OF YEARS OF SCIENTIFIC STUDY
> COMBINED WITH THE EXPERIENCE OF YEARS.

Most non-native English speakers see all six. Many native English speakers see only three. Why? The word "of" is not "important" in understanding the sentence, and so most native English speakers skip over it. And once skipped, it is as if the words do not exist even when the reader looks for them. Also, the word "of" sounds like it has a "v" in it, so native English speakers do not "hear" the "f" when reading the sentence. In contrast, non-native English speakers deem every word important in understanding and are more careful readers.

This is an example of cultural bias impeding communication. Imagine when it comes to the complex interplay of exercise, food, facial expressions, eye-contact patterns, gestures, diet, and values. Until these biases are understood and accounted for, building a connection may be a very difficult experience.

Communication Errors

Health coaches who demonstrate a lack of credibility by overpromising or overstating facts and not being forthright cause serious damage to the connection-building process. Lacking clarity, warmth, and effective listening skills are common communication mistakes that unskilled communicators make. Similarly, being disrespectful to clients, having an annoying voice or tone, acting in a critical or harsh manner, patronizing, parenting, or using inappropriate humor will also injure the relationship that is the foundation to any positive assistance the health coach can offer a client.

Ordering/directing, warning/threatening, giving too much advice, preaching or moralizing, telling clients what they should do, judging, withdrawing, distracting, and constantly bringing discussions back to one's self are additional trouble spots in communication.

Dealing With Dissatisfied Clients

There are times when, regardless of how talented a health coach may be in the area of communicating, a client will find a reason to be dissatisfied. The prepared health coach understands this as a challenge to overcome, not a reason to simply turn his or her back and focus on the next client. Nearly every relationship can be repaired.

The health coach must understand that he or she is primarily in the service business. This requires a change of focus from coaching to serving. This mindset allows the health coach to immediately shift into the client's perspective when the client expresses dissatisfaction. The health coach should act in a nondefensive, open, and accepting manner. Active listening is critical at this point to ensure that the client believes he or she is being heard and valued. The health coach may begin by inviting the client to review what happened and assuring the client by saying, "I'd like to understand this situation from your vantage point." While the client is reviewing what he or she experienced, the health coach should not interrupt, solve the problem, or jump to any conclusions. Instead, the health coach must simply listen attentively.

Reflective listening will be useful—after the client finishes speaking. The health coach can begin by repeating what was heard: "So I can be sure I understand your concerns, what I heard you say is…." Validating the client's concerns is also essential: "I can understand why you'd feel that way given…."

The third step, after listening carefully as the client shares his or her experience and then validating the client's concern, is to respond with empathy. The health coach should demonstrate an understanding of what the client feels: "I can imagine you are feeling…."

The health coach then needs to find a solution, typically by asking the client what he or she would like to have happen, if it is not apparent. The health coach should immediately take proper action and work to resolve the situation if possible. It is always worthwhile to follow up in a day or two with a phone call, email, text message, or a quick face-to-face meeting to be sure the situation is repaired. When writing to clients, be sure to avoid misspelled words, overt grammatical errors, and incomplete sentences.

THINK IT THROUGH

Sally, a long-time client of yours, surprises you by expressing some serious reservations about continuing her program. It is clear that she has reached a plateau in terms of her weight loss, but she refuses to accept your explanation for why this may have occurred. Instead, Sally counters that it is your responsibility as her health coach to make sure that she stays on track and continues losing weight. How would you handle this situation so that you can retain Sally as a client and help her get back on track with her program?

The Value of Follow-up

The effective communicator uses all channels of communication to build a connection. Providing clients with the health coach's direct phone number, email address, and other means of communication is highly encouraged. Following up significant interactions with a text message, email, or phone message is an effective relationship-building tool.

This is what communication is really all about. Being "available, affable, and able" are the three A's of a high level of practice for the health coach. Creating a clear understanding for clients regarding one's availability as a health coach is the most important aspect of creating a healthy and beneficial client–health coach relationship.

Additionally, when writing welcome letters, correspondence with medical and other allied health professionals, or instructions to clients, it is always important for the health coach to use a friendly and professional tone. At the same time, when following up with a client after a session, checking in to see how a client is doing with a food plan, or offering a quick reminder about the next appointment, health coaches should keep in mind that clients are typically accustomed to communicating in short, informal text or email messages. It is important for health coaches to continue with a professional tone, but not in a way that may be construed as long-winded or off-putting.

Summary

Connecting with clients is the foundation of a successful client–health coach relationship. Given that 7% of a message is the content, 38% is the tone of voice delivering the message, and 55% of the communication is body language (Mehrabian, 1971), it is clear that the "what" of the message is less important than "how" the health coach delivers it.

Trust-building, creating positive first impressions, developing excellent verbal and nonverbal communication skills (including active listening and questioning proficiencies), and understanding and effectively communicating with the different personality types form the foundation by which the health coach will better connect with the clients he or she is serving. In addition, the health coach must develop the ability to overcome barriers to communicating for the purpose of affecting positive change and helping clients live healthier, happier lives.

References

Adler, N.J. (2008). *International Dimensions of Organizational Behavior* (5th ed.). Mason, Ohio: Thomson Southwestern.

Ambady, N. & Gray, H.M. (2002). On being sad and mistaken: Mood effects on the accuracy of think-slice judgments. *Journal of Personality and Social Psychology*, 83, 4, 947–961.

Amrhein, P.C. et al. (2003). Client commitment language during motivational interviewing predicts drug use outcomes. *Journal of Consulting and Clinical Psychology*, 71, 5, 862–878.

Britt, E., Hudson, S.M., & Blampied, N.M. (2004). Motivational interviewing in health settings: A review. *Patient Education and Counseling*, 53, 147–155.

Covey, S.M. & Merrill, R.R. (2008). *The Speed of Trust*. New York: Simon and Schuster.

Crookes (1991). Complan column. *Athletics Coach*, 25, 3, 13.

Darwin, C. (1872). *The Expression of Emotion in Man and Animals*. London: John Murray.

Hargrove, R. (1999). *Masterful Coaching Fieldbook*. San Francisco: Jossey-Bass/Pfeiffer.

Hendrix, H. (2008). *Getting the Love You Want*. New York: Henry Holt.

Heron, J. (2001). *Helping the Client* (5th ed.). London: Sage Publications.

Heron, J. (1989). *Six-Category Intervention Analysis* (3rd ed.). Surrey, England: Human Potential Resource Group, University of Surrey.

Lasswell, H.D. (1953). The structure and function of communication in society. In: Bryson, L. (Ed.) *The Communication of Ideas*. New York: Harper & Co.

Marston, W.M. (1928). *Emotions of Normal People*. London: K. Paul, Trench, Trubner & Co.

Maxwell, J.C. (2010). *Everyone Communicates, Few Connect*. Nashville, Tenn.: Thomas Nelson.

Mehrabian, A. (1971). *Silent Messages*. Belmont, Calif.: Wadsworth.

Miller, W.R. (1983). Motivational interviewing with problem drinkers. *Behavioral Psychotherapy*, 11, 147–172.

Miller, W.R. & Rollnick, S. (2002). *Motivational Interviewing: Preparing People for Change Behavior* (2nd ed.). New York: Guilford Press.

Ockene, J.K. et al. (1997). Provider training for the patient-centered program for the development of smoking intervention skills. *Archives of Internal Medicine*, 157, 2334–2341.

Prochaska, J.O. & DiClemente, C.C. (1984). Toward a comprehensive model of change. In: Prochaska, J.O. & DiClemente C.C. (Eds.) *The Transtheoretical Approach: Crossing the Traditional Boundaries of Therapy*. Homewood, Ill.: Dow-Jones.

Prochaska, J.O., DiClemente, C.C., & Norcross, J.C. (1998). Stages of change: Prescriptive guidelines for behavioral medicine. In Koocher, G.P., Norcross, J.C., & Hill, S.S. (Eds.) *Psychologists' Desk Reference*. Oxford: Oxford University Press.

Raines, C. & Ewing, L. (2006). *The Art of Connecting*. New York: AMACOM.

Rollnick, S.R. & Miller, W.R. (1995). What is motivational interviewing? *Behavioral and Cognitive Psychology*, 23, 325–334.

Simkin-Silverman L. & Wing R. (1997). Management of obesity in primary care. *Obesity Research*, 5, 603–612

Suggested Reading

Covey, S.M. & Merrill, R.R. (2008). *The Speed of Trust*. New York: Simon and Schuster, Inc.

Goulston, M. (2010). *Just Listen: Discover the Secret to Getting Through to Absolutely Anyone*. New York: American Management Association.

Hartland, D. & Tosh, C. (2001). *Guide to Body Language*. London: Caxton Publishing.

Lowndes, L. (2003). *How to Talk to Anyone*. New York: McGraw-Hill.

Maxwell, J.C. (2010). *Everyone Communicates, Few Connect*. Nashville, Tenn.: Thomas Nelson.

Miller, W.R. & Rollnick, S. (2002). *Motivational Interviewing: Preparing People for Change Behavior* (2nd ed.). New York: Guilford Press.

Patterson, K. et al. (2011). *Crucial Conversations*. New York: McGraw-Hill.

Walker, K. et al. (2002). *Communication Basics, LEADS Curriculum Notebook, Unit II, Module 2-1*. Manhattan, Kans.: Kansas State University.

SECTION III

NUTRITIONAL AND PHYSIOLOGICAL SCIENCES

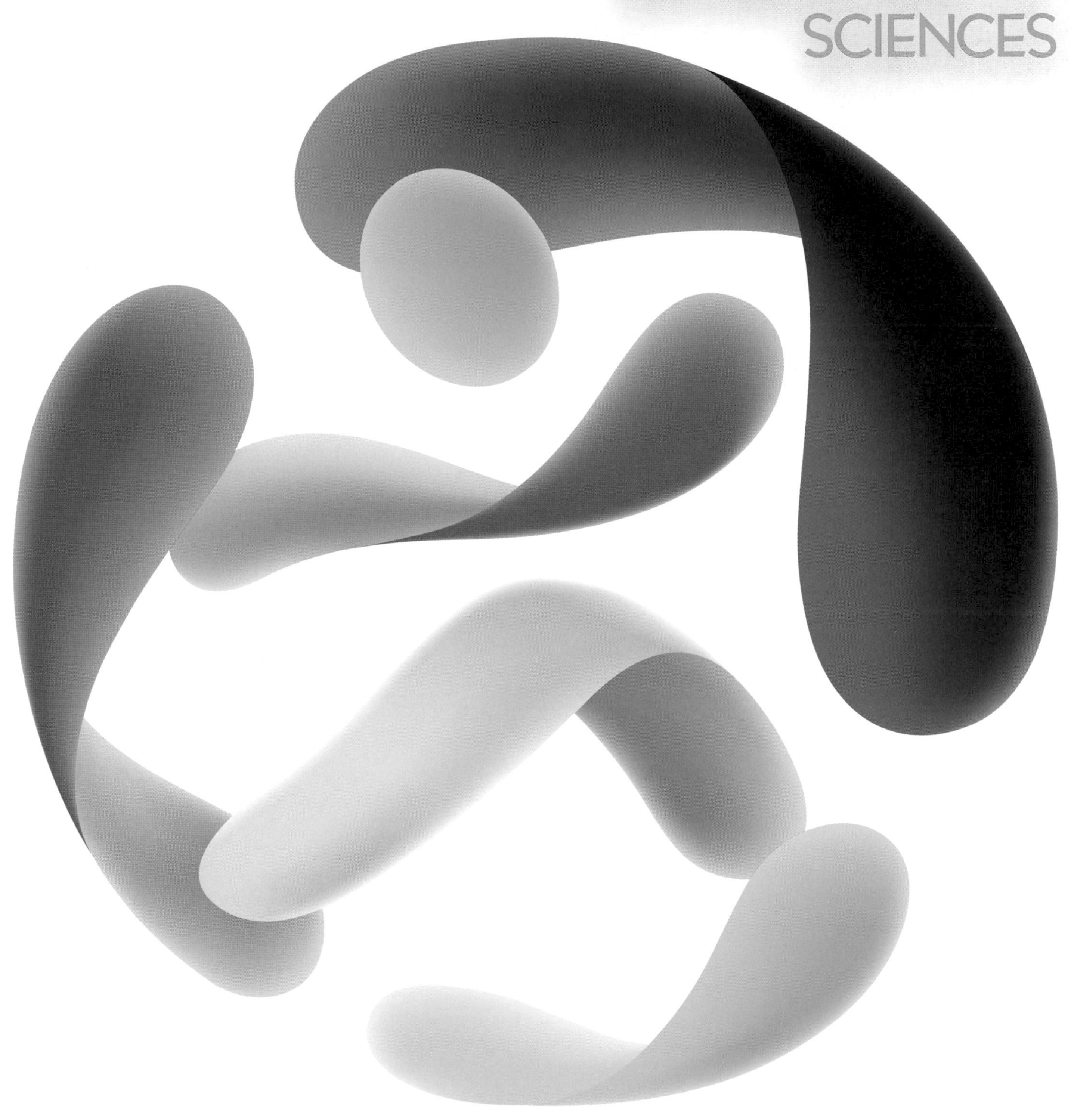

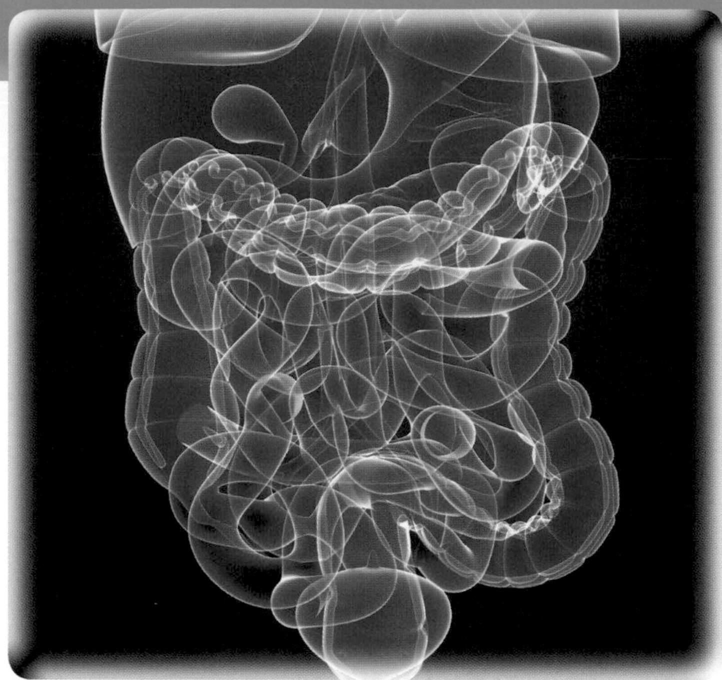

IN THIS CHAPTER:

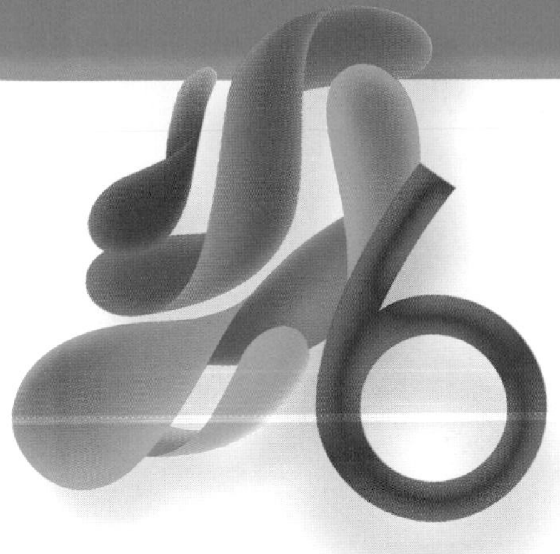

Basic Nutrition and Digestion

NATALIE DIGATE MUTH

Natalie Digate Muth, M.D., M.P.H., R.D., is a pediatrician, registered dietitian, Board-Certified Specialist in Sports Dietetics (CSSD), and Senior Consultant - Nutrition for the American Council on Exercise (ACE). She is also an ACE-certified Personal Trainer and Group Fitness Instructor, an American College of Sports Medicine Health and Fitness Instructor, and a National Strength and Conditioning Association Certified Strength and Conditioning Specialist. She is author of more than 50 articles, books, and book chapters, including the books "Eat Your Vegetables!" and Other Mistakes Parents Make: Redefining How to Raise Healthy Eaters *(Healthy Learning, 2012) and the upcoming textbook* Sports Nutrition for Allied Health Professionals *(F.A. Davis, in press).*

Most clients know that eating a healthful diet is good for their bodies. What they may not understand is why certain foods are considered healthier than others or how different food groups work differently in the body, such as how **protein** helps build muscle or why **carbohydrate** is the best energy source for endurance training.

An understanding of basic nutrition, **digestion,** and **absorption** will help ACE-certified Health Coaches better explain nutrition recommendations and suggestions; provide clear answers to clients' questions; and have a broader knowledge base when they attend educational conferences, read about scientific findings in relevant articles, and communicate with their colleagues. From a discussion of the processes of **nutrient** digestion and absorption to **macronutrient** and **micronutrient** structure and function, this chapter provides a foundation of knowledge in nutritional science, an exciting scientific field that encompasses biology, chemistry, biochemistry, physiology, and psychology.

From a carbohydrate-rich and nutrient-packed citrus fruit to a protein-dense, fat-laden, and iron-loaded cut of steak, every food and beverage that a person eats or drinks gets broken down into its component parts—macronutrients (carbohydrate, protein, and **fat**), micronutrients (**vitamins** and **minerals**), and water. These nutrients enable the body to carry out numerous and complex functions, such as providing energy to fuel activity, strength to muscles and other tissues, and protection of vital organs. Every nutrient serves an essential role in the body, which is why it is so important to consume a nutrient-rich and varied diet.

Macronutrients

The macronutrients, which by definition are needed by the body in large amounts, include carbohydrate, protein, and fat. Through the digestive process, the macronutrients are broken down into their basic building blocks of **monosaccharides, amino acids,** and **fatty acids.** They are then absorbed by the body and delivered to the cells to support the body's many vital functions.

Carbohydrate

Carbohydrates not only are the body's preferred source of immediate energy—and, in fact, the only energy source for the brain and red blood cells—carbohydrates also store energy, and in the case of fiber, may help improve digestive health and **cholesterol** levels.

Structure

Carbohydrates are built from subunits of monosaccharides, sugar compounds made up of carbon with water attached (as the name implies: "hydrated carbon," or carbohydrate).

Monosaccharides and Disaccharides

Three monosaccharides found in nature can be absorbed and utilized by humans—**glucose, fructose,** and **galactose.** Glucose is the predominant sugar in nature and the basic building block of most other carbohydrates (Figure 6-1). Fructose, or fruit sugar, is the sweetest of the monosaccharides and is found in varying levels in different types of fruits. Galactose is most often found linked with glucose to form **lactose,** which is a **disaccharide** and the principal sugar found in milk. Monosaccharides are rarely found free in nature. Instead, they are usually found joined together as disaccharides, **oligosaccharides,** or **polysaccharides.** Irrespective of the type of carbohydrate, each contains 4 calories per gram. In addition to lactose, other disaccharides include **maltose,** which consists of two glucose molecules bound together, and **sucrose** (table sugar or granulated sugar), which is formed by combining glucose and fructose. Most caloric sweeteners are disaccharides. Raw sugar, granulated sugar, brown sugar, powdered sugar, and turbinado sugar (Sugar in the Raw®) are all sucrose. Honey is a natural form of sucrose that is made from plant nectar and harvested by honeybees, which secrete an **enzyme** that hydrolyzes sucrose to glucose and fructose. Thus, honey is a mixture of fructose, glucose, and a bit of sucrose dissolved in water. Corn sweeteners, such as the high-fructose corn syrup commonly found in sodas, baked goods, and some canned products, are a liquid combination of primarily glucose with much smaller amounts of maltose. Sorbitol, which is used in many diet products, is produced from glucose and found naturally in some berries and fruits. It is absorbed by the body at a slower rate than sugar, which may be beneficial for those attempting to control their blood sugar.

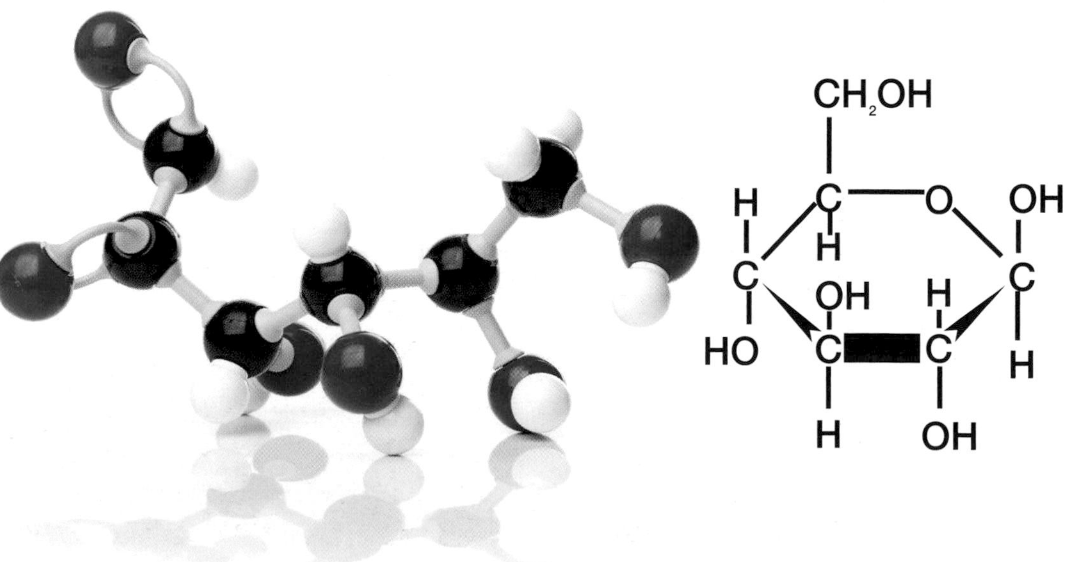

Figure 6-1
Glucose, which is also known as dextrose or grape sugar, has as its molecular formula $C_6H_{12}O_6$.

Note: Carbon is represented by the black balls, oxygen by the red balls, and hydrogen by the white balls.

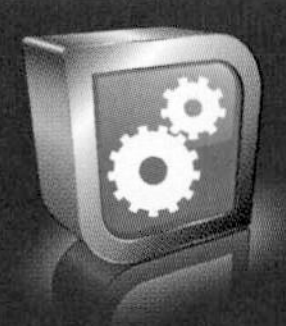

EXPAND YOUR KNOWLEDGE

Does High-fructose Corn Syrup Really Make You Fat?

Corn syrup can be enzymatically converted to change some of its glucose to fructose, yielding high-fructose corn syrup (HFCS). HFCS first made its debut in the American food supply around 1970, when it accounted for about 0.5% of total sweetener use. It is produced when corn syrup undergoes processing to convert glucose to fructose. By the mid-2000s, almost half of all sweetened foods were sweetened with HFCS. HFCS makes up a large proportion of added sweeteners in beverages and processed and packaged foods, including many canned foods, cereals, baked goods, desserts, flavored and sweetened dairy products, candy, and fast food. Two forms of HFCS are used in the U.S. food supply: HFCS-55, which is found mostly in carbonated beverages and is 55% fructose, 41% glucose, and 4% glucose polymers, and HFCS-42, which is found mostly in processed foods and contains slightly less fructose (42% fructose, 53% glucose, and 5% glucose polymers) (Duffey & Popkin, 2008). Food manufacturers prefer fructose to pure sugar (which is comprised of the sugar sucrose) because it is cheaper, which is in large part due to corn subsidies and other government policies aimed to increase corn production that have led to corn prices that are actually less than the cost of production. In addition, high tariffs on imported sugar cane make sweetening with all-natural sugar costly to food manufacturers.

After the publication of several animal studies and human studies of marginal quality that showed that HFCS may contribute to obesity, **insulin resistance,** and **diabetes,** as well as decreased feelings of fullness after consumption, health advocates and the media became alarmed that HFCS may contribute to negative health outcomes, including the surge in obesity. Subsequent large-scale human studies have not shown an increased risk of overweight, obesity, or metabolic disorders like diabetes when HFCS is consumed in reasonable amounts (Rizkalla, 2010). However, the number of long-term high-quality controlled studies is limited. Of course, this is not to say that clients can eat all the HFCS they want without risk of ill consequences. Rather, HFCS probably does not increase health risk *more than* sugar or other sweeteners. That said, the typical American still consumes about 13% of daily calories from added sugars [U.S. Department of Agriculture (USDA), 2015], which is approximately 270 extra **empty calories** per day that provide minimal nutritional value. In total, the typical American eats about 20 pounds (9 kg) worth of added sugar over the course of a year.

Anyone trying to lose or control his or her weight or curb the risk of insulin resistance or diabetes should aim to minimize consumption of HFCS as well as other added sugars, including sucrose (table sugar) and other caloric sweeteners. As clients carefully scan ingredient lists, they will soon find that it does not matter whether they eat foods and drinks with pure sugar, HFCS, or any of the other many added sugars—trying to cut added sugars in the diet is a major challenge. This is part of the reason why large-scale policies to reduce the added sugars—including HFCS—in the food supply are necessary to help Americans reduce excess caloric intake and achieve and maintain a healthy weight.

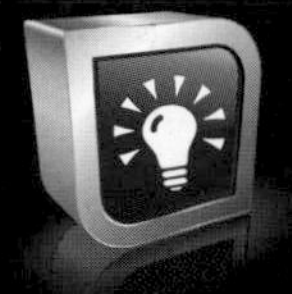

THINK IT THROUGH

During your initial meeting, a new client, Jen, a 20-year-old college student, tells you that she is surprised that she has not lost weight in recent months because she stopped eating foods with high-fructose corn syrup and replaced them with snacks with other sweeteners. How would you respond to this statement, and what advice would you give Jen to facilitate better weight management in the future?

Artificial and Plant-based High-intensity Sweeteners

Noncaloric sweeteners—which are calorie-free because the body cannot metabolize them—are also used to add sweetness to foods and beverages. Aspartame, also known as Equal® in packaged sweeteners and NutraSweet® in foods and beverages; Acesulfame K, which is called Sunett® in cooking products and Sweet One® as a tabletop sweetener; saccharin; sucralose (Splenda®); and neotame all are approved for use in the United States. While early studies found that certain sweeteners may cause bladder cancer in laboratory rats, subsequent studies have found no association in humans. Sugar extracted from the stevia plant is now a widely available natural alternative to artificial sweeteners.

Whether noncaloric sweeteners actually contribute to weight loss is a source of debate and controversy. While, in theory, the decreased caloric intake resulting from the use of a noncaloric sweetener instead of a high-calorie sugar should result in fewer calories consumed and therefore weight loss, some studies have shown the opposite effect. Ultimately, research into the effects of noncaloric sweeteners on appetite, energy balance, and weight control is ongoing with mixed results (Mattes & Popkin, 2009).

EXPAND YOUR KNOWLEDGE

In Stores Now: Stevia—The All-natural Plant-based Sweetener

Once limited to the health-food market as an unapproved herb, the plant-derived sweetener known as stevia is now widely available and rapidly replacing artificial sweeteners in consumer products. Thirty times sweeter than sugar and with no effect on blood sugar and minimal aftertaste, stevia is predicted to reach sales of about $700 million in the next few years, according to the agribusiness finance giant Rabobank (2009).

Stevia's history goes back to ancient times. Grown naturally in tropical climates, stevia is an herb in the Chrysanthemum family that grows wild as a small shrub in Paraguay and Brazil, though it can easily be cultivated elsewhere. Paraguayans have used stevia as a food sweetener for centuries, while other countries including Brazil, Korea, Japan, China, and much of South America also have a shorter, though still long-standing, record of stevia use. There are more than 100 species of stevia plant, but one stands out for its excellent properties as a sweetener—*Stevia rebaudiana*, which contains the compound rebaudioside A, the sweetest-flavored component of the stevia leaf. Rebaudioside A chemically acts very similar to sugar in onset, intensity, and duration of sweetness and is free of aftertaste. Most stevia-containing products contain mostly extracted Rebaudioside A with some proportion of stevioside, which is a white crystalline compound present in stevia that tastes 100 to 300 times sweeter than table sugar (Kobylewski & Eckhert, 2008).

Though widely available throughout the world, in 1991 stevia was banned in the U.S. due to early studies that suggested the sweetener may cause cancer. A follow-up study refuted the initial findings and in 1995 the U.S. Food and Drug Administration (FDA) allowed stevia to be imported and sold as a food supplement, but not as a sweetener (FDA, 1995). Several companies argued to the FDA that stevia should be categorized similarly to its artificial sweetener cousins as "Generally Recognized as Safe" (GRAS). Substances that are considered GRAS have been determined to be safe through expert consensus, scientific review, or widespread use without negative complications. They are exempt from the rigorous approval process required for food additives. In December 2008, the FDA declared stevia GRAS and allowed its use in mainstream U.S. food production (Goyal, Samsher, & Goyal, 2010). It has taken food manufacturers a few years to develop the right stevia-containing recipes, but stevia is now present in a number of foods and beverages in the U.S., such as Gatorade's® G2, VitaminWater® Zero, SoBe® Lifewater Zero, Crystal Light®, and Sprite® Green. Around the world it has been used in soft drinks, chewing gums, wines, yogurts, candies, and many other products. Stevia powder can also be used for cooking and baking (in markedly decreased amounts compared to table sugar due to its high sweetness potency).

Stevia is marketed under the trade names of Truvia® (Coca-Cola® and agricultural giant Cargill®), PureVia® (Pepsi-Cola® and Whole Earth Sweetener Company®), and SweetLeaf® (Wisdom Natural Brands®). While it is known by three different names, the sweetener is essentially the same product, though the different versions contain slightly different proportions of rebaudioside A and stevioside. Both Coke and Pepsi intend to use stevia as a soft-drink sweetener in the U.S., but have not yet unveiled their stevia-version Coca-Cola or Pepsi (although they have trialed it with a few of their less popular products such as Coke's Sprite Green).

Though stevia is likely as safe as artificial sweeteners, few long-term studies have been done to document its health effects in humans. A review conducted by toxicologists at UCLA that was commissioned by nutrition advocate Center for Science in the Public Interest raised concerns that stevia could contribute to cancer (Kobylewski & Eckhert, 2008). The authors noted that in some test tube and animal studies, stevioside (but not rebaudioside A) caused genetic mutations, chromosome damage, and **deoxyribonucleic acid (DNA)** breakage. These changes presumably could contribute to malignancy, though no one has actually studied if these compounds cause cancer in animal models. Notably, initial concerns that stevia may reduce fertility or worsen diabetes seem to have been put to rest after a few good studies showed no negative outcomes. In fact, one study of human subjects showed that treatment with stevia may improve glucose tolerance. Another found that stevia may induce the pancreas to release insulin, thus potentially serving as a treatment for type 2 diabetes (these studies are reviewed in Goyal, Samsher, & Goyal, 2010). After artificial sweeteners were banned in Japan more than 40 years ago, the Japanese began to sweeten their foods with stevia. Since then, they have conducted more than 40,000 clinical trials on stevia and concluded that it is safe for human consumption. Still, there is a general lack of long-term studies on stevia's use and effects.

All in all, stevia's sweet taste and all-natural origins make it a popular sugar substitute. With little long-term outcome data available on the plant extract, it is possible that stevia in large quantities could have harmful effects. However, it seems safe to say that when consumed in reasonable amounts, stevia may be a good natural plant-based sugar substitute.

Oligo- and Polysaccharides

An oligosaccharide is a chain of approximately three to 10 simple sugars. **Fructooligosaccharides,** which are oligosaccharides that are mostly indigestible, may help relieve constipation, improve **triglyceride** levels, and decrease production of foul-smelling digestive by-products.

A long chain of sugar molecules is referred to as a polysaccharide. **Glycogen,** an animal carbohydrate found in meat products and seafood, and **starch,** a plant carbohydrate found in grains and vegetables, are the only polysaccharides that humans can fully digest. Both are long chains of glucose and are referred to as **complex carbohydrates** (versus **simple carbohydrates,** which are short chains of sugar). Historically, much debate has centered around whether consumption of simple or complex carbohydrates is better for athletic performance. The role of a particular carbohydrate in athletic performance may be better determined by its **glycemic index (GI)** than its structure. GI ranks carbohydrates based on their blood glucose response: High-GI foods break down rapidly, causing a large glucose spike, while low-GI foods are digested more slowly and cause a smaller glucose increase. The glycemic index is described and evaluated in more detail in Chapters 7 and 9.

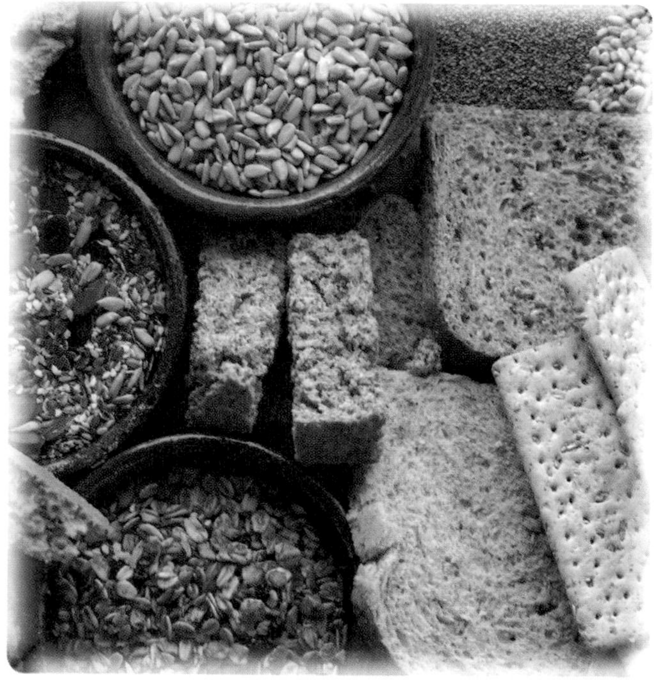

Animals store excess carbohydrates as glycogen in the liver and in muscle. Although glycogen can be found in animal products, most glycogen stores are depleted before meat enters the food supply. Plants store carbohydrates as starch granules. Edible plants make two types of starch: amylase (a small, linear molecule) and the more prevalent amylopectin (a larger, highly branched molecule). Because starches are longer than disaccharides and oligosaccharides, they take longer to digest. Still, humans are able to easily break down and digest starches with specific self-produced enzymes. However, the rest of the plant, which is formed largely of the carbohydrate cellulose and other fibers such as hemicellulose, lignin, gums, and pectin, is indigestible. This fiber passes through the human body undigested, as humans do not produce the necessary enzymes to break the sugar bonds, though some fiber does undergo fermentation in the **large intestines,** thereby providing a small amount of energy for normal gut bacterial growth. While other carbohydrates contain 4 calories per gram, fiber probably contributes about 1.5 to 2.5 calories per gram [Institute of Medicine (IOM), 2005].

Fiber is classified as **dietary fiber** and **functional fiber.** Dietary fiber is that fiber obtained naturally from plant foods, while functional fiber is obtained in the diet from isolated fibers added to food products. Together they comprise "total fiber." **High-viscosity fibers** (typically those that used to be referred to as **soluble fiber**) include gums (found in foods like oats, legumes, guar, and barley), pectin (found in foods like apples, citrus fruits, strawberries, and carrots), and psyllium seeds. These fibers slow **gastric emptying,** or the passage of food from the stomach into the intestines. Consequently, they help to increase feelings of fullness. Also, the delayed gastric emptying slows the release of sugar into the bloodstream. The slow and steady release of sugar into the bloodstream, rather than a rapid surge, helps to avert an insulin spike. High levels of insulin are associated with weight gain (and, for many, insulin resistance as a consequence of weight gain) and increased risk of **cardiovascular disease.** By binding bile acids in the small intestines, fiber also interferes with the absorption of fat and cholesterol and the recirculation of cholesterol in the liver. Once bound to fiber, the unabsorbed cholesterol can then be excreted in feces.

Low-viscosity fibers (previously referred to as **insoluble fibers**) such as cellulose (found in whole-wheat flour, bran, and vegetables), hemicellulose (found in whole grains and bran), and lignin (found in mature vegetables, wheat, and fruit with edible seeds like strawberries and kiwi) play an important role in increasing fecal bulk and provide a laxative effect. Clearly, fiber serves many important and beneficial roles in the human body. Still, most people get nowhere near the recommended 14 grams/1,000 calories per day (approximately 25 to 35 grams per day for most adults; children over two years old should eat their age plus 5 grams per day) (IOM, 2005). With increased consumption of fruits, vegetables, legumes, and whole grains, most Americans could easily achieve this fiber goal.

Metabolism and Storage

Glucose is the body's preferred energy source. Blood glucose gets delivered to working cells, where it is broken down to carbon dioxide and water, releasing **adenosine triphosphate (ATP)**, the body's usable energy source.

Carbohydrates consumed in the diet that are not immediately used for energy are stored in the liver and muscle as glycogen. Approximately 90 grams of glycogen is stored in the liver, which translates to approximately 360 calories. A minimum of 150 grams of glycogen is stored in muscle, which translates to approximately 600 calories, though this amount can be increased up to fivefold with physical training (Mahan, Escott-Stump, & Raymond, 2011). **Carbohydrate loading** also increases glycogen stores (see Chapter 7). Because glycogen contains many water molecules, it is large and bulky and therefore unsuitable for long-term energy storage. Thus, if a person continues to consume more carbohydrates than the body can use or store, the body will convert the sugar into fat for long-term storage.

Protein

Proteins form the major structural component of muscle, as well as that of brain, nervous system, blood, skin, and hair. This macronutrient serves as the transport mechanism for iron, vitamins, minerals, fats, and oxygen within the body, and is a key to acid-base and fluid balance. Proteins form enzymes that speed up chemical reactions and create **antibodies** that the body uses to fight infection. In situations of energy deprivation, the body can break down proteins for energy, yielding 4 calories per gram of protein.

Structure

Proteins are built from amino acids, which are carbohydrates with an attached nitrogen-containing amino group and, in some cases, sulfur. Proteins form when amino acids are joined together through **peptide bonds.** The completed protein is a linear chain of amino acids. These structures fold, creating a unique three-dimensional polypeptide. Individual polypeptides may remain free-standing or bind together to form a larger complex. Figure 6-2 illustrates the peptide bond and folding protein.

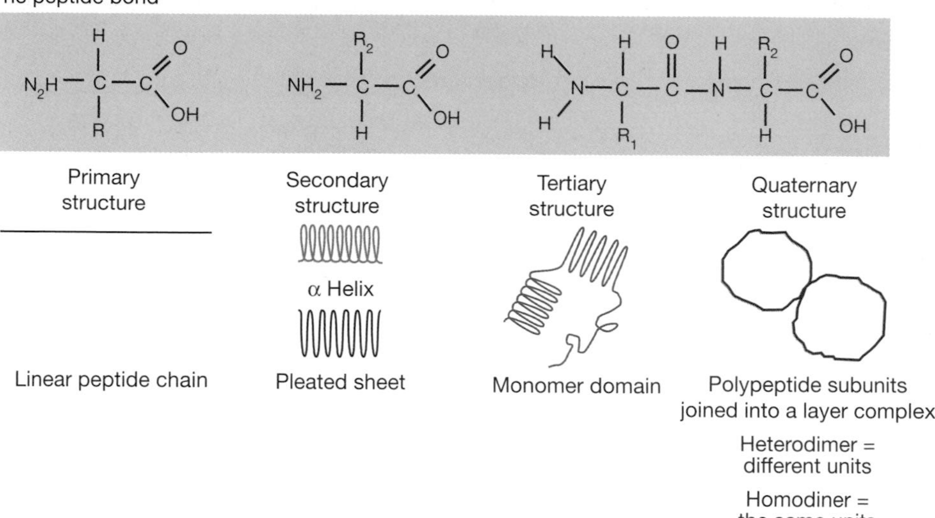

Figure 6-2
The peptide bond and folding protein

Reprinted with permission from Mahan, L.K., Escott-Stump, S., & Raymond, J.L. (2011). *Krause's Food and the Nutrition Care Process* (13th ed.). Philadelphia: W.B. Saunders Company.

The body can produce most of the amino acids that make up proteins, but there are eight to 10 **essential amino acids** that, by definition, are amino acids that cannot be made by the body and must be consumed in the diet. The others are called **nonessential amino acids** because they can be made by the body. A specific food's protein quality is determined by assessing its essential amino-acid composition, digestibility, and **bioavailability,** which is the degree to which an amino acid can be used by the body. Generally, animal products contain all of the essential amino acids in amounts proportional to need (called **complete proteins**), whereas plant foods do not and are called **incomplete proteins.** Notable exceptions are soy and quinoa, which are examples of plant-based complete proteins (low in one or more essential amino acids). Thus, soy and quinoa are better sources of quality protein than other plants. However, vegetarian clients can boost protein quality and get all the essential amino acids they need by combining complementary incomplete plant proteins. Excellent combinations include grains-legumes (e.g., rice/beans) and legumes-seeds (e.g., falafel) (Figure 6-3).

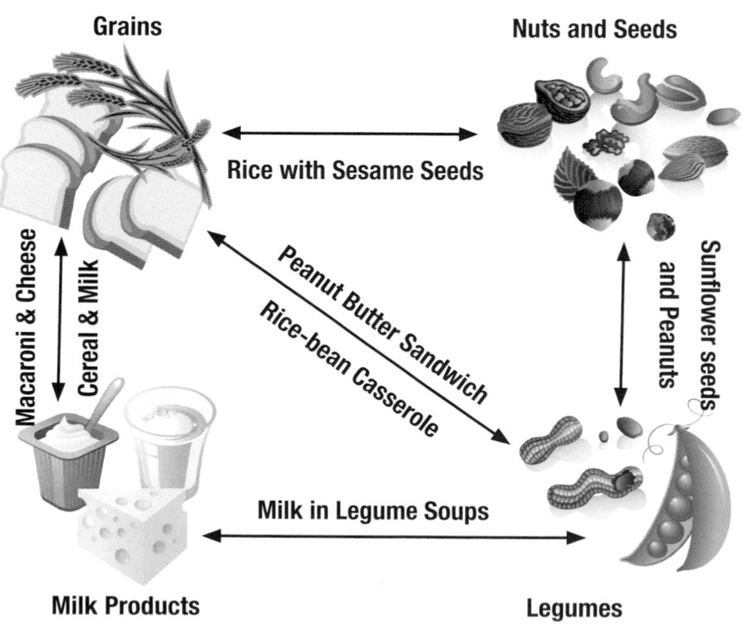

Figure 6-3
Protein complementarity chart

Adapted with permission from Lappé, F.M. (1992). *Diet for a Small Planet.* New York: Ballantine Books.

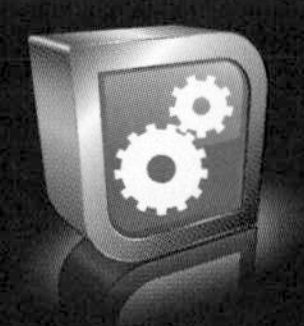

EXPAND YOUR KNOWLEDGE

How Many Essential Amino Acids Are There?

ACE texts, as well as many other reference texts and articles, often state that there are eight to 10 essential amino acids. But what exactly does that mean? It seems that it should be easy to determine whether an amino acid is essential (i.e., not produced by the body) or nonessential (i.e., produced by the body). So, why the range?

Eight amino acids are essential for everyone: valine, leucine, isoleucine, methionine, phenylalanine, threonine, tryptophan, and lysine. Historically, the amino acid histidine was thought to only be essential to infants and children. However, a culmination of studies seems to suggest that it is also essential for adults. The amino acid cysteine is nonessential for most people, but the body is unable to produce it in the elderly, infants, and some individuals with certain chronic diseases, making cysteine an essential amino acid for these special populations.

Metabolism and Storage

The body's need for dietary proteins results from the constant breakdown and regeneration of the body's cells. The immediate supplier of amino acids for cell regeneration comes from the cell's free amino acid pool, which is made of dietary amino acids and the recycled amino acids from cell turnover. Because amino acid recycling is inherently inefficient, dietary amino acid intake is necessary to replace losses.

Unlike carbohydrate and fat, the body does not store protein. The continuous recycling of amino acids through the removal and addition of nitrogen allows the body to carefully regulate protein balance. Protein balance is measured in terms of **nitrogen balance,** which is a measure of nitrogen consumed (from dietary intake protein) and nitrogen excreted (from protein breakdown). In a healthy body, the amount of protein taken in is exactly matched by the amount of protein lost in feces, urine, and sweat. The muscle tissues undergo continual breakdown and resynthesis, with a fraction of muscle protein destroyed and an equal fraction rebuilt daily using amino acids from the amino acid pool. Negative nitrogen balance, in which the body breaks down more protein than it can create **(catabolism),** occurs during times of high stress such as with severe infections and trauma. Positive nitrogen balance, in which the body produces more protein than it breaks down (**anabolism),** occurs in times of growth such as childhood, pregnancy, recovery from illness, and in response to resistance training when overloading the muscles promotes protein synthesis. Importantly, just because an athlete consumes a high-protein diet does not necessarily mean that he or she will be in positive nitrogen balance and experience muscle growth. For example, an endurance athlete who consumes a high-protein, low-carbohydrate diet (and thus has minimal glycogen stores) will rely heavily on muscle protein for fuel; as a result, he will experience decreased athletic performance and worsened muscular strength and endurance.

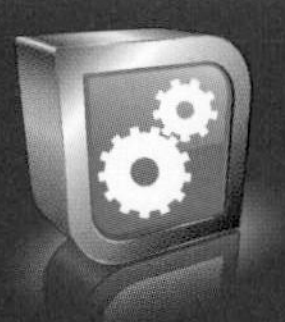

EXPAND YOUR KNOWLEDGE

Myth: You Cannot Eat Too Much Protein

Myth: As far as weight is concerned, you cannot eat too much protein. Anything beyond what your body needs will get excreted in urine.

Logic: Because the body has little capacity to store proteins, it makes sense that anything consumed beyond what the body immediately needs will be excreted in the urine (similar to water-soluble vitamins).

The science: It is true that the body has limited ability to store protein. It is also true that a portion of the protein does get excreted in the urine (the nitrogen group that shows up in urine as urea). However, the other portion of the protein (the carbon group) is readily converted to glucose or fat, depending on the body's current needs. Ultimately, protein consumed beyond what the body needs has the same fate as excess carbohydrate or fat—conversion into stored fat.

THINK IT THROUGH

Your new client, Ashley, has just graduated college and would like your help with staying physically active since she will no longer be playing on her collegiate volleyball team. She informs you that her next fitness-related goal is to run a marathon within the next six months. In your initial interview, you discover that Ashley eats a low-carbohydrate, high-protein diet because she believes it helps her burn more body fat and helps her better manage her weight versus eating a diet with more carbohydrates. What would you say to Ashley to help educate her about the role of carbohydrates in the diets of endurance athletes, such as marathon runners?

Fat

The most energy-dense of the macronutrients, fat provides 9 calories per gram, as compared to both carbohydrate and protein, which provide 4 calories per gram. Because of this high caloric value, foods that are high in fat should be consumed in moderation if weight control is the goal, but they should not be avoided altogether. Mono- and **polyunsaturated fats** are heart-healthy and excellent sources of essential nutrients (though still calorie-dense).

Fats serve many critical functions in the body, including insulation, cell structure, nerve transmission, vitamin absorption, and hormone production. But some fats—notably

saturated fats and **trans fats**—also lead to clogging of the arteries, increased risk for heart disease, and myriad other health problems. Consumption of these fats should be avoided or strictly limited.

Structure

To understand how various fats function in the body, first consider their structures (Figure 6-4). All fats are made up of hydrogen, carbon, and oxygen, and all fats are insoluble in water. Beyond that, they are a very **heterogeneous** group of molecules.

Fatty acids, which are usually found linked to other molecules in nature, are long hydrocarbon chains with an even number of carbons and varying degrees of saturation with hydrogen. Saturated fatty acids contain no double bonds between carbon atoms, are typically solid at room temperature, and are very stable. Foods high in saturated fat include red meat, full-fat dairy products, and tropical oils such as coconut and palm oils. Saturated fat indirectly increases levels of **low-density lipoprotein (LDL),** which is referred to as the "bad" cholesterol because of its tendency to promote arterial plaque formation.

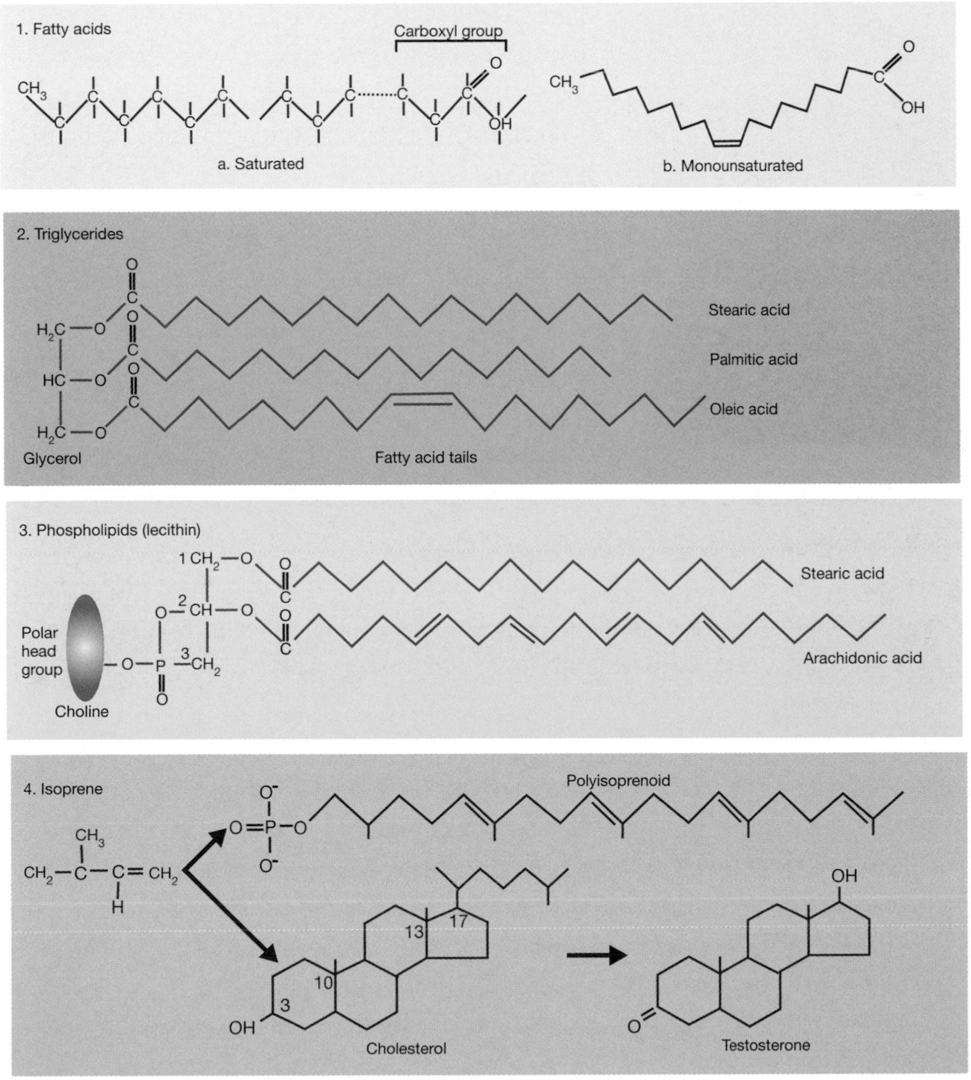

Figure 6-4
Structures of physiologically important fats and lipids

Reprinted with permission from Mahan, L.K., Escott-Stump, S., & Raymond, J.L. (2011). *Krause's Food and the Nutrition Care Process* (13th ed.). Philadelphia: W.B. Saunders Company.

Unsaturated fatty acids contain one or more double bonds between carbon atoms, are typically liquid at room temperature, and are fairly unstable, which makes them susceptible to oxidative damage and a shortened shelf life. **Monounsaturated fats** contain one double bond between two carbons and may increase levels of **high-density lipoprotein (HDL),** which is known as the "good cholesterol" for its association with lowering plaque build-up within the arteries. Common sources include olive, canola, and peanut oils. Polyunsaturated fat contains a double bond between two or more sets of carbons. Sources include corn, safflower, and soybean oils, and cold-water fish (e.g., tuna, salmon, mackerel, and cod).

Essential fatty acids are a type of polyunsaturated fat that must be obtained from the diet. Unlike other fats, the body cannot produce **omega-3 (linolenic acid)** or **omega-6 (linoleic acid) fatty acids**. Omega-3 fatty acids come in three forms: alpha-linolenic acid (ALA), eicosapentaenoic acid (EPA), and docosahexanoic acid (DHA). ALA is the type of omega-3 fatty acid found in plants. It can be converted to EPA and DHA in the body, but the research supporting the benefits of ALA is much less compelling than that for EPA and especially DHA. EPA and DHA omega-3 fatty acids are naturally found in egg yolk (amounts vary depending on the chicken feed), as well as in cold-water fish and shellfish (e.g., crab, shrimp, and oyster). Overall, omega-3s reduce blood clotting, dilate blood vessels, and reduce inflammation. They are important for eye and brain development (and are especially important for a growing fetus in the late stages of pregnancy); act to reduce cholesterol and triglyceride levels; and may help to preserve brain function and reduce the risk of mental illness and attention deficit hyperactivity disorder (ADHD), though more research is needed to confirm these mental health benefits. Notably, most Americans tend not to get enough omega-3 fatty acids. Though natural food sources are best, people who do not meet this recommendation may benefit from supplementation or from the consumption of fortified foods. In fact, the American Heart Association (AHA) recommends that, under the care of a physician, individuals with elevated triglycerides take a 2 to 4 gram EPA+DHA supplement (Miller et al., 2011).

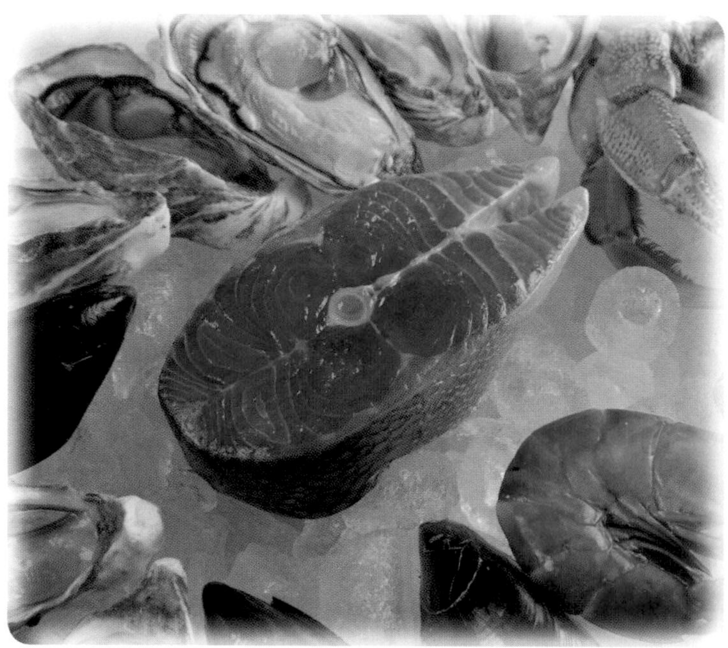

While there is no established **Dietary Reference Intake (DRI)** for the optimal amount of EPA+DHA intake for the general population, the Institute of Medicine (IOM) has established an **Adequate Intake (AI)** for ALA, the precursor to EPA+DHA. The IOM considers 1.1 grams per day of ALA to be the minimal amount necessary for normal growth and neural development. The IOM suggests that 10% of the needed ALA could come from EPA or DHA, which suggests a daily intake of about 100 mg per day (IOM, 2005). Some expert panels have recommended much higher intakes of 250 to 500 mg per day due to the significant health benefits attributed to these fatty acids, and the low risk of complications such as bleeding, even at this higher range (Harris, 2010). Of note, while many products claim to be fortified with omega-3s, it is important for consumers to read the label. If the omega-3s are mostly ALA, they are unlikely to be optimally converted to EPA and DHA and likely have fewer of the health benefits.

Omega-6, which is generally consumed in abundance in the American diet, is an essential fatty acid found in flaxseed, canola, and soybean oils, as well as green leafy vegetables. Unlike omega-3s, which reduce inflammation, omega-6 fatty acids have been shown to contribute to inflammation and blood clotting. The balancing act between omega-6 and omega-3 is essential for maintaining normal circulation and other biological processes. In the past, scientists had hypothesized that reducing consumption of omega-6 fatty acids and increasing consumption of omega-3 fatty acids may lower chronic disease risk, but more recent research has shown that maintaining a high consumption of both omega-3 and omega-6 fatty acids has cardiovascular health benefits (Harris, 2010). The AHA recommends that Americans consume 5 to 10% of calories as omega-6 polyunsaturated fatty acids—that is about 12 g/day for women and 17 g/day for men (Harris et al., 2009).

In nature, most fatty acids are found as part of triglycerides, which are formed by joining three fatty acids to a glycerol (carbon and hydrogen structure) backbone. Triglycerides are the chemical form in which most fat exists in food as well as in the body.

Trans fat, listed as "partially hydrogenated" oil on a food ingredient list, results from a manufacturing process that makes unsaturated fat solid at room temperature with a goal of increasing its stability and thereby prolonging its shelf life. The process involves breaking the double bond of the unsaturated fat and adding a hydrogen molecule. The product is a heart-damaging fat that increases LDL cholesterol even more than saturated fat. Legislation requiring food manufacturers to include the amount of trans fat on the nutrition label if it is more than 0.5 grams per serving has resulted in many processed foods that were once high in trans fat, such as chips, crackers, cakes, peanut butter, and margarine, to be made "trans-fat free." Health coaches should advise their clients to read the label's ingredients list for "hydrogenated" or "partially hydrogenated" oil to determine if a food contains trans fat. If so, the food should be avoided.

Phospholipids such as lecithin and sphingomyelin are structurally similar to triglycerides, but the glycerol backbone is modified, so that the molecule is water-soluble at one end and water-insoluble at the other end. Phospholipids play a critical role in maintaining cell-membrane structure and function. Lecithin is also a major component of HDL, which serves to remove cholesterol from cell membranes. Common food sources of lecithin include liver, egg yolks, soybeans, peanuts, legumes, spinach, wheat germ, and animal products.

Cholesterol, a fat-like, waxy, rigid four-ring steroid structure, plays an important role in cell-membrane function. It also helps to make bile acids (which are important for fat absorption), metabolize fat-soluble vitamins (A, D, E, and K), and make vitamin D and some steroid hormones, such as **estrogen** and **testosterone.** Saturated fat, once it is converted to cholesterol in the liver, is the main dietary cause of **hypercholesterolemia** (i.e., high blood levels of cholesterol), though high levels of cholesterol are also found in animal products such as egg yolks, meat, poultry, fish, and dairy products.

Too much cholesterol in the bloodstream causes a variety of health problems. For cholesterol to be transported from the liver to the body's cells (in the case of endogenously produced cholesterol), or from the small intestine to the liver and adipose tissue (in the case of exogenously consumed cholesterol), it must be transported through the bloodstream. Because cholesterol is fat-soluble, it needs a water-soluble carrier protein to transport it. When the cholesterol combines with this protein en route to the body's cells, it becomes an LDL, which when oxidized can attach to inner linings or walls of arteries, where it forms a plaque and may ultimately cause **atherosclerosis.** HDLs remove excess cholesterol from the arteries and carry it back to the liver, where it is excreted.

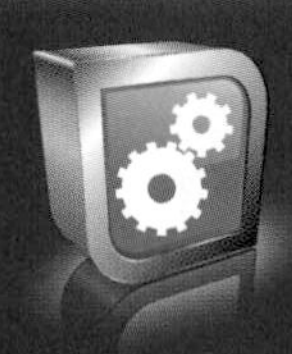

EXPAND YOUR KNOWLEDGE

Are Eggs Good or Bad?

Because of the always growing body of research, nutrition recommendations sometimes change. While this can be extremely frustrating for clients and the general public, it highlights the importance of health professionals, including health coaches, staying on top of the latest research and findings.

Historically, one of the most controversial foods has been the egg. Is it healthy or not? It used to be that eggs were well-known for their potential health-damaging effects, given their high cholesterol content (there are 213 mg of cholesterol in one egg yolk. Then eggs were applauded for their high protein content and, more recently, for the notable amount of heart-healthy DHA omega-3 fatty acid in egg yolk (about 50 mg and eight times that in DHA-enriched eggs). At about 15 cents each, eggs contain a load of nutrients at a very cheap price. But are they safe and healthy to eat?

A single egg has 70 calories, 6 grams of protein including all of the essential amino acids, 13 vitamins and minerals, and DHA omega-3 fatty acids. Few other foods could boast such a high nutritional density (Figure 6-5).

Nutrition Facts	
1 Serving Per Container	
Serving Size	**1 egg (50g)**
Amount Per Serving **Calories**	**70**
	% Daily Value*
Total Fat 3g	**7%**
Saturated Fat 1.5g	**8%**
Trans Fat 0g	
Cholesterol 215mg	**71%**
Sodium 65mg	**3%**
Total Carbohydrate Less than 1g	**0%**
Protein 6g	**10%**
Vitamin A	6%
Vitamin C	0%
Calcium	2%
Iron	4%
Not a significant source of Dietary Fiber or Sugars.	

Figure 6-5
Egg nutrition label

On the other hand, eggs also contain a high amount of cholesterol. While dietary cholesterol is not very closely associated with elevated cholesterol levels in the body (that has more to do with saturated fat intake). In fact, the *2015-2020 Dietary Guidelines for Americans* removed cholesterol as a nutrient to limit, while still noting that most foods high in cholesterol also tend to be high in saturated fat (with eggs as a notable exception). In addition to their cholesterol amounts, eggs also are a possible source of foodborne illness. Salmonella infection may be prevented most of the time with good food-handling techniques, including special care when preparing eggs to make sure they are fully cooked. That said, eggs pose a potential health risk, especially for the elderly and immune-suppressed people.

Ultimately, whether or not clients choose to include eggs in their daily diets will depend on taste preferences and their conclusions regarding the risks versus the benefits, but there is no doubt that eggs are an inexpensive source of a variety of nutrients.

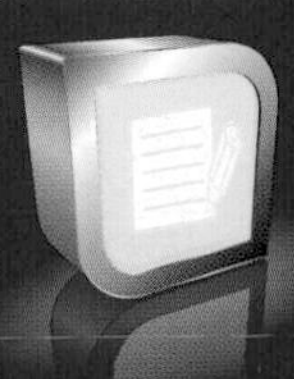

DO THE MATH

Analyzing the Nutrition Label (Figure 6-5)

1. If a client eats three eggs for breakfast, how many calories from saturated fat will he or she eat?
2. What percentage of total calories from an egg come from saturated fat?
3. How many calories from protein are contained in a single egg?

Answers:

1. 1.5 grams saturated fat x 9 calories per gram x 3 eggs = 40.5 calories
2. 1.5 grams saturated fat x 9 calories per gram = 13.5 calories from saturated fat per egg. 13.5 calories saturated fat/70 total calories per egg = 19% of calories from saturated fat.
3. 6 grams of protein x 4 calories/gram of protein = 24 calories from protein

Metabolism and Storage

Fat consumed in the diet beyond what is immediately needed as an energy source is stored primarily as an energy reserve in adipose tissue, though it can also be used to replenish intramuscular triglyceride stores or remain in the bloodstream as free-floating fatty acids. Assuming 15% body fat, the average 176-pound (80-kg) young adult man stores about 26.4 lb (12 kg) of body fat. That translates to about 108,000 calories of fat (12,000 grams x 9 calories/gram). Most of this fat can be mobilized to provide energy to fuel exercise. Beyond serving as an energy source, fat also plays an essential role in thermal insulation, protection and cushioning for vital organs, and as a transport medium for **fat-soluble vitamins.**

Essentials of Digestion and Absorption

In addition to the oxygen that enters the body through the lungs and is efficiently transported to the body's cells, the cells also need a constant supply of nutrients to provide energy and carry out basic metabolic functions. These nutrients can either come from storage (such as glycogen, stored fat, stored fat-soluble vitamins, or calcium stored in bones) or from breakdown of food through the **digestive system** (Figure 6-6). Some nutrients such as proteins and water-soluble vitamins are not effectively stored in the body and must be regularly obtained from foods to prevent deficiency.

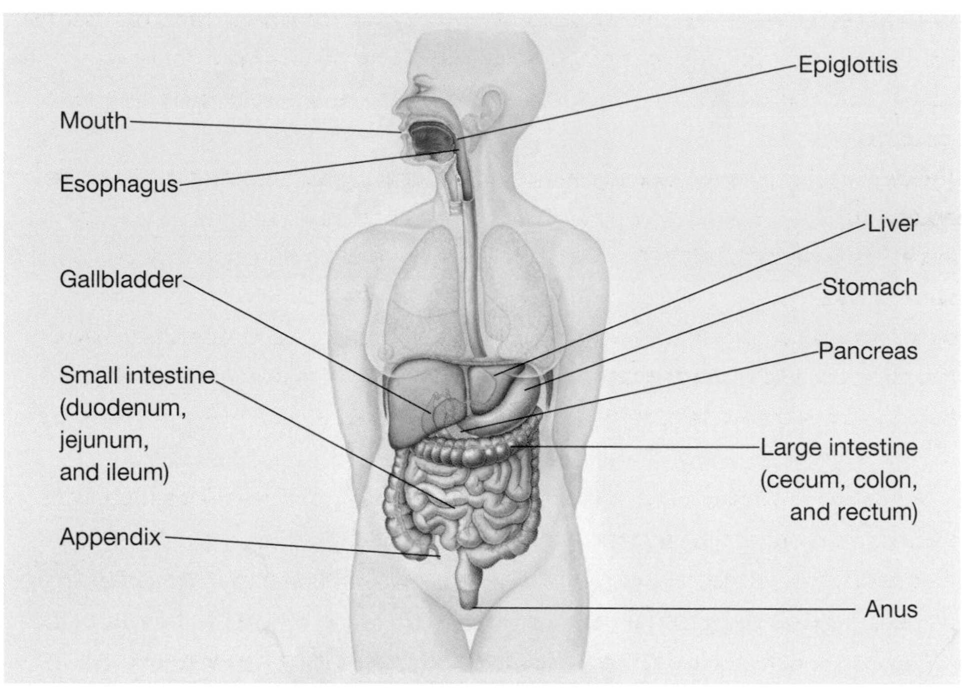

Figure 6-6
The digestive system

The Digestive Pathway

The body has a remarkable ability to transform a food into its individual nutrients through the process of digestion. To understand this process, one can trace the digestive path of a half-cup serving of cottage cheese—a food that contains carbohydrate, protein, and fat as well as other micronutrients.

From the simple thought of eating to the sights and smell of food or drink, the body readies the digestive system. Through activation of the **parasympathetic nervous system,** which is the part of the **autonomic nervous system** responsible for digestion, as soon as a liquid touches the tongue, salivary enzymes get ready to break it down to its individual nutrients. If the substance is a food instead of a drink, chewing the food also helps to activate the salivary enzymes. Digestion of the carbohydrate components of the cottage cheese begins in the saliva with release of the salivary enzyme *a*-amylase, which cleaves (i.e., breaks down) large polysaccharides into oligosaccharides and disaccharides. Chewing the cottage cheese breaks it down even more so that the salivary enzymes can come in contact with more of the surface area of the food.

With swallowing, the cottage cheese passes down the throat and into the **esophagus.** Muscles in the esophagus push the food through into the stomach in a wavelike motion called **peristalsis.** From here, each of the different macronutrient components of the cottage cheese is broken down differently.

Carbohydrate Digestion and Absorption

Partially digested carbohydrates (remember the salivary enzymes in the mouth begin the process of carbohydrate digestion) pass untouched through the stomach into the **small intestine.** The small intestine is the site of the majority of food digestion and absorption. With some help from pancreatic digestive juices and bile produced in the liver and stored in the **gallbladder,** the majority of food digestion occurs in the **duodenum,** the approximately 1-foot-long first portion of the small intestines. From there, the food, now called **chyme,** passes to the second and third portions of the small intestines, the **jejunum** and **ileum.** Together comprising about 20 feet of convoluted intestine, the jejunum and ileum are where the majority of food absorption occurs.

In the small intestines, **lactase** digests milk sugar, which is found in the cottage cheese, into its component parts—the monosaccharides glucose and galactose. (**Lactose intolerance** results from a deficiency in the enzyme lactase. This inability to break down lactose causes symptoms like cramps, bloating, diarrhea, and flatulence.) Other carbohydrates are broken down by various other pancreatic enzymes, including maltase, *a*-dextrinase, sucrase, and trehalase into monosaccharides. The monosaccharides are then absorbed through the intestinal **brush border,** a membrane ideal for absorbing large amounts of nutrients due to its numerous tiny finger-like projections known as **villi.**

Nutrients cross the brush border in different ways depending on how well they dissolve in water (solubility), their size, and their relative concentration. Once sugars are absorbed into the bloodstream, they get fast-tracked directly to the liver (known as **portal circulation**) for processing and distribution of nutrients to the rest of the body. While the liver takes up much of the glucose from the bloodstream as well as most all of the fructose and galactose, the remaining glucose is taken up by the body's cells under the influence of insulin.

Protein Digestion and Absorption

The goal of protein digestion is to break dietary protein down into individual amino acids that can be absorbed and later used by the body. Each protein has a unique three-dimensional structure determined by its amino-acid composition. In order for a protein to be digested, it must first lose its unique shape (a process called **denaturation**).

Protein digestion begins in the stomach. As soon as the body anticipates eating (whether from external cues like seeing or smelling food or internal cues like thinking of food), the stomach releases the hormone **gastrin.** The gastrin stimulates the stomach to release hydrochloric acid. The resulting rapid acidification of the stomach denatures proteins and triggers the activation of the enzyme **pepsin.** Pepsin breaks the peptide bonds between amino acids to shorten long protein complexes into shorter polypeptide chains. The stomach mixes and churns the food and releases the mixture in small quantities to the small intestine over the course of one to four hours. The pancreas then releases enzymes into the small intestine, which activate **trypsin**, an enzyme responsible for further breaking down proteins into single amino acids or amino acids joined in twos (dipeptides) or threes (tripeptides). The dipeptides and tripeptides are absorbed into the intestinal epithelial cells, cleaved into single amino acids, and passed to the bloodstream. Once absorbed into the bloodstream, the amino acids are transported to the liver.

For an amino acid to be of any use to the body, the liver first removes the amino acid nitrogen group through **deamination.** The nitrogen forms urea, which is then excreted in urine. Alternatively, in some cases the nitrogen can be transferred from one compound to another through **transamination.** For example, if the body has an inadequate supply of carbohydrate or fat to fuel exercise, muscle protein is catabolized for energy, providing up to 10% of the total energy for exercise (Brooks, 1987).

Fat Digestion and Absorption

Lipid digestion begins in the mouth with the release of **lingual lipase,** which cleaves short-

and medium-chain fatty acids. The **gastric lipase** released from the stomach further digests these fats. The mixing and churning of the **bolus** of food in the small intestines helps to break long-chain lipids into droplets to increase their surface area for digestion by pancreatic enzymes.

The presence of fat in the small intestines triggers the release of the hormone cholecystokinin (CCK). This hormone stimulates the release of **gastric inhibitory peptide** and **secretin,** which decrease gut movement and slow digestion. This explains why high-fat meals increase feelings of fullness compared with lower fat meals. In the small intestine, bile acids **emulsify** the lipids, further increasing surface area so that pancreatic lipases can break the lipids into fatty acids, cholesterol, and lysolecithin. Products of lipid digestion and fat-soluble vitamins are carried by **micelles** to the absorptive surface of the intestinal cells, where they diffuse across the luminal membrane and are converted back into triglycerides, cholesterol, and phospholipids. While medium-chain triglycerides can pass directly into the portal circulation, the long-chain triglycerides join an apoprotein to form a **chylomicron.** These fats and fat-soluble vitamins are transferred into the **lymphatic system** and passed to the bloodstream through the thoracic duct, a large lymphatic vein that drains into the heart. The fatty acids contained within chylomicrons floating in the bloodstream can be delivered to working cells where the enzyme **lipoprotein lipase** cleaves off the fatty acid. These fatty acids can be used in the metabolic process of fatty-acid oxidation to produce energy. Any fatty acids not immediately needed by the cells pass to the liver, where they are repackaged and shuttled to the adipose tissue, where they are stored as fat.

Getting Rid of Waste

After the macronutrients and micronutrients have been digested and absorbed, all of the waste and indigestibles left over in the small intestine (such as fiber) are passed through the ileocecal valve to the 5-foot-long large intestine, where a few minerals and a significant amount of water are reabsorbed into blood. As more water gets reabsorbed, the waste passing through the large intestine gets harder until it is finally excreted as solid waste through the rectum and anus. Food can stay in the large intestine from hours to days. Total transit time from mouth to anus usually takes anywhere from 18 to 72 hours. Therefore, what is considered to be a "normal" frequency of bowel movements can range from three times daily to once every three days or more (Figure 6-7).

Micronutrients

Micronutrients, by definition, are only needed in small amounts in the body. The World Health Organization (WHO) refers to these nutrients as the "magic wands" that enable the body to produce enzymes, hormones, and other substances that are essential for proper growth and development (WHO, 2010). When the body is deprived of micronutrients, the consequences are severe. But when the micronutrients are consumed in just the right amounts, they lead to optimal health and function.

Vitamins

Vitamins are organic (carbon-containing), non-caloric micronutrients that are essential for normal physiological function. Vitamins must be consumed in the diet, with only three exceptions: vitamin K and biotin, which can be produced by normal intestinal flora (bacteria that

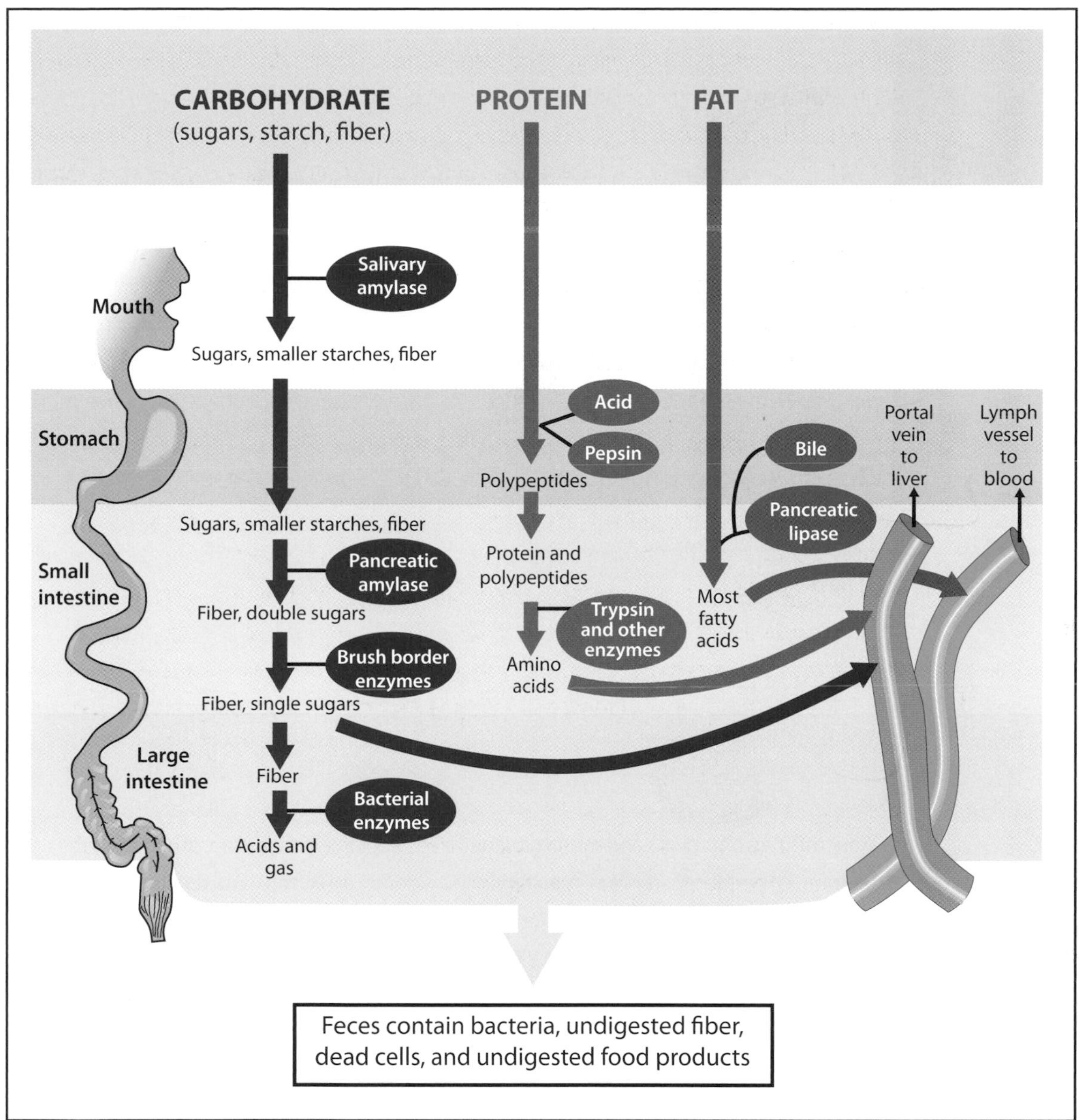

Figure 6-7
Summary of macronutrient digestion and absorption

Source: Adapted from McArdle, W.D., Katch, F.I., & Katch, V.L. (2008). *Sports and Exercise Nutrition* (3rd ed.). Philadelphia: Lippincott Williams & Wilkins.

live in the intestines and are critical for normal gastrointestinal function), and vitamin D, which can be self-produced with sun exposure. No "perfect" food contains all the vitamins in just the right amount. Instead, a variety of nutrient-dense foods must be consumed to ensure adequate vitamin intakes. Many foods (such as breads and cereals) are enriched or fortified with some nutrients to cut the risk of vitamin deficiency. Some foods contain inactive vitamins, which are called **provitamins.** The human body contains enzymes to convert these inactive vitamins into active vitamins.

Humans need 13 different vitamins, which are divided into two categories: water-soluble vitamins (the B vitamins and vitamin C) and fat-soluble vitamins (vitamins A, D, E, and K). Choline—called a "quasi-vitamin" because it can be produced in the body, but also provides additional benefits through consumption of foods—plays a crucial role in **neurotransmitter** and platelet functions; may help prevent Alzheimer's (McDaniel, Maier, & Einstein, 2003) and fatty liver disease (Fischer et al., 2010); and is essential for normal fetal brain development (Zeisel &

Table 6-1				
Vitamin Facts				
Vitamin	RDA/AI*		Best Sources	Functions
	Men†	Women†		
A (carotene)	**900 µg**	**700 µg**	Yellow or orange fruits and vegetables, green leafy vegetables, fortified oatmeal, liver, dairy products	Formation and maintenance of skin, hair, and mucous membranes; helps people see in dim light; bone and tooth growth
B1 (thiamin)	**1.2 mg**	**1.1 mg**	Fortified cereals and oatmeals, meats, rice and pasta, whole grains, liver	Helps the body release energy from carbohydrates during metabolism; growth and muscle tone
B2 (riboflavin)	**1.3 mg**	**1.1 mg**	Whole grains, green leafy vegetables, organ meats, milk, eggs	Helps the body release energy from protein, fat, and carbohydrates during metabolism
B6 (pyridoxine)	**1.3 mg**	**1.3 mg**	Fish, poultry, lean meats, bananas, prunes, dried beans, whole grains, avocados	Helps build body tissue and aids in metabolism of protein
B12 (cobalamin)	**2.4 µg**	**2.4 µg**	Meats, milk products, seafood	Aids cell development, functioning of the nervous system, and the metabolism of protein and fat
Biotin	30 µg	30 µg	Cereal/grain products, yeast, legumes, liver	Involved in metabolism of protein, fats, and carbohydrates
Choline	550 mg	425 mg	Milk, liver, eggs, peanuts	A precursor of acetylcholine; essential for liver function
Folate (folacin, folic acid)	**400 µg**	**400 µg**‡	Green leafy vegetables, organ meats, dried peas, beans, lentils	Aids in genetic material development; involved in red blood cell production
Niacin	**16 mg**	**14 mg**	Meat, poultry, fish, enriched cereals, peanuts, potatoes, dairy products, eggs	Involved in carbohydrate, protein, and fat metabolism
Pantothenic acid	5 mg	5 mg	Lean meats, whole grains, legumes, vegetables, fruits	Helps release energy from fats and vegetables
C (ascorbic acid)	**90 mg**	**75 mg**	Citrus fruits, berries, and vegetables—especially peppers	Essential for structure of bones, cartilage, muscle, and blood vessels; helps maintain capillaries and gums and aids in absorption of iron
D	15 µg	15 µg	Fortified milk, sunlight, fish, eggs, butter, fortified margarine	Aids in bone and tooth formation; helps maintain heart action and nervous system function
E	**15 mg**	**15 mg**	Fortified and multigrain cereals, nuts, wheat germ, vegetable oils, green leafy vegetables	Protects blood cells, body tissue, and essential fatty acids from destruction in the body
K	120 µg	90 µg	Green leafy vegetables, fruit, dairy, grain products	Essential for blood-clotting functions

* Recommended Dietary Allowances are presented in bold type; Adequate Intakes are presented in non-bolded type.

† RDAs and AIs given are for men aged 31–50 and nonpregnant, nonbreastfeeding women aged 31–50; mg = milligrams; µg = micrograms

‡ This is the amount women of childbearing age should obtain from supplements or fortified foods.

Niculescu, 2006). Table 6-1 includes the vitamin DRIs.

Water-soluble Vitamins

Thiamin (vitamin B1), riboflavin (vitamin B2), niacin (vitamin B3), pantothenic acid (vitamin B5), pyroxidine (vitamin B6), biotin (vitamin B 7), folate (vitamin B9), cobalamin (vitamin B12), and vitamin C are referred to as the water-soluble vitamins. Their solubility in water (which gives them similar absorption and distribution in the body) and their role as **cofactors** of enzymes involved in metabolism (i.e., without them, the enzyme will not work) are common traits. With the exception of vitamins B6 and B12, water-soluble vitamins cannot be stored in the body and are readily excreted in urine. This decreases the risk of toxicity from overconsumption and makes their regular intake a necessity.

Certain B vitamins—thiamin, riboflavin, niacin, and pantothenic acid—are cofactors in energy metabolism. In other words, these vitamins are necessary to unlock the energy in food.

Thiamin

Thiamin is essential for carbohydrate metabolism. It also is thought to play a nonmetabolic role in nerve function. Signs of thiamin deficiency include decreased appetite, weight loss, and cardiac and neurologic irregularities that progress to beriberi—a constellation of symptoms that includes mental confusion, muscular wasting, swelling, decreased sensation in the feet and hands, a fast heart rate, and an enlarged heart. Thiamin deficiency is rare in the U.S. because of supplementation in rice and cereal products. Deficiency occasionally manifests in alcoholics, who are often malnourished and have impaired thiamin absorption.

Riboflavin

Riboflavin assists in carbohydrate, amino-acid, and lipid metabolism. It also helps with **antioxidant** protection through its role in reduction-oxidation (redox) reactions. Consumption of meat, dairy products, and green leafy vegetables helps prevent riboflavin deficiency, which causes eye problems, including sensitivity to light, excessive tearing, burning and itching, and loss of vision, as well as soreness and burning of the mouth, tongue, and lips.

Niacin

Niacin acts as a cofactor for more than 200 enzymes involved in carbohydrate, amino-acid, and fatty-acid metabolism. Lean meats, poultry, fish, peanuts, and yeast contain ample amounts of niacin. Muscular weakness, anorexia, indigestion, and skin abnormalities are early signs of niacin deficiency and can cause the disease pellagra, which is characterized by the "three Ds": dermatitis (eczema), dementia, and diarrhea.

Pantothenic Acid

Pantothenic acid, which is present in all plant and animal tissues, forms an integral component of coenzyme A and acyl-carrier protein. These proteins are essential for metabolism of fatty acids, amino acids, and carbohydrates, as well as for normal protein function. Because this vitamin is ubiquitous, deficiency is rare.

Vitamin B6

Vitamin B6 (pyridoxine) plays an important role in many bodily functions, including protein metabolism, red blood cell production, **glycogenolysis** (in which glycogen is broken down to glucose), conversion of the protein tryptophan to niacin, neurotransmitter formation, and immune-system function. Meats, whole-grain products, vegetables, and nuts contain high concentrations of vitamin B6, though bioavailability of the nutrient is highest in animal products. Deficiency leads to decreased neurologic and dermatologic function and weakened immunity.

Folate

Folate (vitamin B9; also known as folic acid in its supplement form) is named for its abundance in plant foliage (like green leafy vegetables). Folate plays a crucial role in the production of DNA, formation of red and white blood cells, formation of neurotransmitters, and metabolism of amino acids. Deficiency is relatively common, as folate is easily lost during cooking and food preparation, and also because most people do not eat enough green leafy vegetables. Folate deficiency early in pregnancy can be devastating for a developing fetus and can lead to neural tube defects such as spina bifida. For this reason, all women of childbearing age are advised to take a daily folic acid supplement. Deficiency also causes megaloblastic anemia, skins lesions, and poor growth. Notably, excessive consumption of folate can mask a vitamin B12 deficiency.

Vitamin B12

Vitamin B12 (cobalamin) is important for the normal function of cells of the gastrointestinal tract, bone marrow, and nervous tissue. The richest sources of vitamin B12 include clams and oysters, milk, eggs, cheese, muscle meats, fish, liver, and kidney. Long-time **vegans** are at risk for deficiency, as are the elderly, who tend to have a decreased ability to absorb the nutrient. Deficiency leads to megaloblastic anemia and neurologic dysfunction, in which neurons become demyelinated (i.e., the nerves cannot effectively transmit electrical impulses). This causes numbness, tingling, and burning of the feet, as well as stiffness and generalized weakness of the legs.

Biotin

Biotin (vitamin B7) is the ultimate "helper vitamin." Typically bound to protein, it carries around a carboxyl (-COOH) group, which it lends to any of four different enzymes that are important in various metabolic functions. Ultimately, biotin plays an important role in the metabolic functions of pantothenic acid, folic acid, and vitamin B12. The most important sources of biotin include milk, liver, egg yolk, and a few vegetables (e.g., mushrooms and cauliflower). Deficiency is uncommon.

Vitamin C

Vitamin C plays an important role as an antioxidant. Deficiency can result in scurvy (a disease that can cause dark purplish spots on the skin and spongy or bleeding gums). Vitamin C is also necessary in the production of collagen, a fibrous protein that is an essential component of skin, bone, teeth, ligaments, and other connective structures. Vitamin C improves iron absorption, promotes resistance to infection, and helps with steroid, neurotransmitter, and hormone production. Citrus fruits and green leafy vegetables are excellent sources of vitamin C. Signs of deficiency include impaired wound healing, swelling, bleeding, and weakness in bones, cartilage, teeth, and connective tissues.

Fat-soluble Vitamins

Vitamins A, D, E, and K are the fat-soluble vitamins and are often found in fat-containing foods. They are stored in the liver or adipose tissue until needed, and therefore are closely associated with fat. If fat absorption is impaired, so is fat-soluble-vitamin absorption. Unlike water-soluble vitamins, fat-soluble vitamins can be stored in the body for extended periods of time and eventually are excreted in feces. This storage capacity increases the risk of toxicity from overconsumption, but also decreases the risk of deficiency.

Vitamin A

Vitamin A and its provitamin beta-carotene are important for vision, growth, and development; the development and maintenance of epithelial tissue, including bones and teeth; immune function; and reproduction. Animal products, including liver, milk, and eggs, are rich in preformed vitamin A. Dark green leafy vegetables and yellow-orange vegetables and fruit contain lots of provitamin A carotenoids. (A good rule of thumb: The deeper the color, the higher the level of carotenoids.) Deficiency of vitamin A is the most common cause of blindness in the developing world. It begins with night blindness and progresses to poor growth and increased susceptibility to infection. Excess consumption, which overwhelms the capacity of the liver to store the vitamin (generally resulting from supplement misuse), leads to dryness and cracking of the skin and mucous membranes, headache, nausea, vomiting, and liver disease. Intake of more than 20,000 international units (IU) of vitamin A in pregnant women is associated with fetal malformations; pregnant women are therefore advised to limit intake to less than 10,000 IU per day.

Vitamin D

Vitamin D is essential for calcium and phosphorus absorption and homeostasis. Vitamin D is referred to as the "sunshine vitamin," because small amounts of sunlight exposure (about 10 to 15 minutes twice a week) induce the body to make sufficient vitamin D from cholesterol. Fish liver oils provide an abundance of vitamin D. Smaller amounts are found in butter cream, egg yolk, and liver. Typically, Americans get the majority of their vitamin D intake from fortified milk. Regardless of the source, adequate vitamin D intake is critical. Without it, adults can develop **osteomalacia,** a condition in which the bones become weak and susceptible to pseudofractures, leading to muscular weakness and bone tenderness. This increases the risk of fracture, in particular of the wrist and pelvis. Low vitamin D intake may also play a role in the development of **osteoporosis** in postmenopausal women. Without vitamin D, children whose bones have not yet fully developed will experience impaired mineralization, which can lead to rickets and bowing of the legs. Too much vitamin D causes elevated calcium and phosphorus levels and may lead to headache, nausea, and eventually calcification of the kidney, heart, lungs, and the tympanic membrane of the ear (i.e., the eardrum), leading to deafness.

Vitamin E

Vitamin E, which is also known as alpha-tocopherol, plays a fundamental role in the metabolism of all cells. It may help protect against conditions related to oxidative stress, including aging, air pollution, arthritis, cancer, cardiovascular disease, cataracts, diabetes, and infection, though research remains contradictory and inconclusive. (A more detailed discussion of the role of antioxidants is presented on page 149.) Vitamin E is only synthesized by plants. The richest sources of vitamin E are polyunsaturated plant oils, wheat germ, whole grains, green leafy vegetables, nuts, and seeds. Vitamin E is easily destroyed by heat and oxygen. Therefore, its richest source, oils, should be stored in a cool, dark location. Vitamin E deficiency is rare in humans and tends to only occur in cases of fat malabsorption and transport problems. Toxicity is uncommon, though when present may decrease the absorption of other fat-soluble vitamins, impair bone mineralization, and lead to prolonged clotting times. This is especially relevant for individuals on anticlotting medication, such as warfarin (Coumadin).

Vitamin K

Vitamin K, which is produced by bacteria in the colon and present in large amounts in green leafy vegetables (especially broccoli, cabbage, turnip greens, and dark lettuce), is important for blood clotting and maintenance of strong bones. Due to vitamin K's critical role in blood clotting, individuals on blood-thinning medications that interfere with vitamin K absorption—such as heparin or warfarin (Coumadin)—need to carefully adjust their vitamin K intake through diet under the supervision of a physician. Insufficient vitamin K intake can lead to hemorrhage, and potentially fatal anemia. Fortunately, vitamin K deficiency is rare, and usually only found in association with lipid malabsorption, destruction of intestinal flora (often due to chronic antibiotic therapy), and liver disease. Newborns are at risk for vitamin K deficiency, as the vitamin does not cross the **placenta** and is negligible in breast milk. For this reason, newborn infants routinely receive a vitamin K shot after birth to prevent (or slow) a rare problem of bleeding into the brain weeks after birth. Toxicity of vitamin K only occurs with excessive intake of the synthetic or supplemental form, which is called menadione. At doses of about 1,000 times the **Recommended Dietary Allowance (RDA),** vitamin K can cause severe jaundice in infants and hemolytic anemia.

Minerals

With roles ranging from regulating enzyme activity and maintaining acid–base balance to assisting with strength and growth, minerals are critical for human life. Unlike vitamins, many minerals are found in the body as well as in food. The body's ability to use the minerals is dependent upon their bioavailability. Nearly all minerals, with the exception of iron, are absorbed in their free form—that is, in their ionic state unbound to organic molecules. When a mineral is bound to other molecules, mineral absorption is impaired, thus decreasing the mineral's bioavailability. Typically, minerals with high bioavailability (>40% absorption) include sodium, potassium, chloride, iodine, and fluoride. Minerals with low bioavailability (1 to 10% absorption) include iron, zinc, chromium, and manganese (bioavailability is 20 to 30% for heme iron). All other minerals, including calcium and magnesium, are of medium bioavailability (30 to 40% absorption).

An important consideration when consuming minerals, and particularly when taking mineral supplements, is the possibility of mineral–mineral interactions. Minerals can interfere with the absorption of other minerals. For example, zinc absorption may be decreased through iron supplementation. Similarly, zinc excesses can decrease copper absorption. Too much calcium limits the absorption of manganese, zinc, and iron. When a mineral is not absorbed properly, a deficiency may develop.

Minerals are typically categorized as macrominerals (major elements) and microminerals (trace elements). Macrominerals include calcium, phosphorus, magnesium, sulfur, sodium, chloride, and potassium. Microminerals include iron, iodine, selenium, zinc, and various other

Table 6-2

Mineral Facts

Mineral	RDA/AI*		Best Sources	Functions
	Men†	Women†		
Calcium	1,000 mg	1,000 mg	Milk and milk products	Strong bones, teeth, muscle tissue; regulates heart beat, muscle action, and nerve function; blood clotting
Chromium	35 µg	25 µg	Corn oil, clams, whole-grain cereals, brewer's yeast	Glucose metabolism (energy); increases effectiveness of insulin
Copper	**900 µg**	**900 µg**	Oysters, nuts, organ meats, legumes	Formation of red blood cells; bone growth and health; works with vitamin C to form elastin
Fluoride	4 mg	3 mg	Fluorinated water, teas, marine fish	Stimulates bone formation; inhibits or even reverses dental caries
Iodine	**150 µg**	**150 µg**	Seafood, iodized salt	Component of hormone thyroxine, which controls metabolism
Iron	**8 mg**	**18 mg**	Meats, especially organ meats, legumes	Hemoglobin formation; improves blood quality; increases resistance to stress and disease
Magnesium	**420 mg**	**320 mg**	Nuts, green vegetables, whole grains	Acid/base balance; important in metabolism of carbohydrates, minerals, and sugar (glucose)
Manganese	2.3 mg	1.8 mg	Nuts, whole grains, vegetables, fruits	Enzyme activation; carbohydrate and fat production; sex hormone production; skeletal development
Molybdenum	**45 µg**	**45 µg**	Legumes, grain products, nuts	Functions as a cofactor for a limited number of enzymes in humans
Phosphorus	**700 mg**	**700 mg**	Fish, meat, poultry, eggs, grains	Bone development; important in protein, fat, and carbohydrate utilization
Potassium	4,700 mg	4,700 mg	Lean meat, vegetables, fruits	Fluid balance; controls activity of heart muscle, nervous system, and kidneys
Selenium	**55 µg**	**55 µg**	Seafood, organ meats, lean meats, grains	Protects body tissues against oxidative damage from radiation, pollution, and normal metabolic processing
Zinc	**11 mg**	**8 mg**	Lean meats, liver, eggs, seafood, whole grains	Involved in digestion and metabolism; important in development of reproductive system; aids in healing

* Recommended Dietary Allowances are presented in bold type; Adequate Intakes are presented in non-bolded type.

† RDAs and AIs given are for men aged 31–50 and nonpregnant, nonbreastfeeding women aged 31–50; mg = milligrams; µg = micrograms

minerals that do not have an established DRI, and will not be discussed in this chapter. Table 6-2 presents the DRIs for many minerals.

Macrominerals (Bulk Elements)

By definition, macrominerals are essential for adults in amounts of 100 mg/day or more.

Calcium

Calcium is the most abundant mineral in the human body and serves various functions, including mineralization of the bones and teeth, muscle contraction (including the heart), blood clotting, blood-pressure control, immunity, and possibly colon-cancer prevention (Mahan, Escott-Stump, & Raymond, 2011). Significant sources of calcium include dairy products, small fish with bones, green leafy vegetables, and legumes. Most people in the U.S. do not consume the recommended amounts of calcium from food sources. To help counter this problem, calcium supplements are often used to increase intake. Calcium deficiency in childhood and adolescence can contribute to decreased peak bone mass and suboptimal bone strength. Calcium deficiency in adulthood, particularly in postmenopausal women, can lead to osteomalacia, **osteopenia,** and/or osteoporosis. Calcium toxicity, particularly when combined with vitamin D toxicity, can lead to hypercalcemia and calcification of soft tissues, particularly of the kidneys. High calcium intake also interferes with the absorption of other minerals, including iron, zinc, and manganese. Relatively common effects of excessive calcium intake include constipation and kidney stones.

Phosphorus

Phosphorus is the second most abundant mineral in the body (Mahan, Escott-Stump, & Raymond, 2011). Like calcium, phosphorus plays a role in mineralization of bones and teeth. Phosphorous also helps filter out waste in the kidneys and contributes to energy production in the body by participating in the breakdown of carbohydrates, protein, and fats. It also may help reduce muscle pain after a strenuous workout. Phosphorus is needed for the growth, maintenance, and repair of all tissues and cells, and for the production of the genetic building blocks, DNA and **ribonucleic acid (RNA).** Phosphorus is also needed to balance and metabolize other vitamins and minerals, including vitamin D, calcium, iodine, magnesium, and zinc. Animal products such as meat, fish, poultry, eggs, and milk are excellent sources of phosphorus. As a general rule, any food high in protein is also high in phosphorus. The outer coating of many grains contains phosphorus, but in the form of phytic acid, a bound form of phosphorus that is not bioavailable. The leavening process during bread making unbinds the phosphorus, making leavened breads a good source of the mineral. Phosphorus is also present in sodas in the form of phosphoric acid. Deficiency of phosphorus is practically unheard of in the United States. In fact, most individuals consume much more than the DRI. People taking phosphate-binding medications (typically used in patients with chronic renal failure) may be at risk of deficiency, which can present with neuromuscular, skeletal, hematologic, and renal abnormalities and may be deadly. Excessive phosphorus intake interferes with calcium absorption and may lead to decreased bone mass and density.

Magnesium

Magnesium, which is present primarily in bone, muscle, soft tissue, and body fluids, is important for bone mineralization, protein production, muscle contraction, nerve conduction, enzyme function, and healthy teeth. Excellent food sources include nuts, legumes, whole grains, dark green leafy vegetables, and milk. In general, a diet high in vegetables and unrefined grains will include more than adequate amounts of magnesium. Unfortunately, most Americans eat a diet high in refined foods and meat and do not meet recommended magnesium intakes. High intakes of calcium, protein, vitamin D, and alcohol increase the body's magnesium requirements. Magnesium deficiency is very rare, but moderate depletion is fairly common, especially in the elderly. Magnesium depletion may contribute to many chronic illnesses and is associated with heart **arrhythmias** and **myocardial infarction.** Magnesium toxicity may prevent bone calcification, but toxicity is also very rare, even in cases of supplement overuse.

Sodium, Potassium, and Chloride

Known as **electrolytes**, these minerals exist as ions in the body and are extremely important for normal cellular function. All three electrolytes play at least four essential roles in the body: water balance and distribution, osmotic equilibrium [i.e., assuring that the negative ions (**anions**) balance with positive ions (**cations**) when electrolytes move in and out of cells], acid–base balance, and intracellular/extracellular differentials (i.e., assuring that the sodium and chloride stay mostly outside of the cell while potassium stays mostly inside the cell).

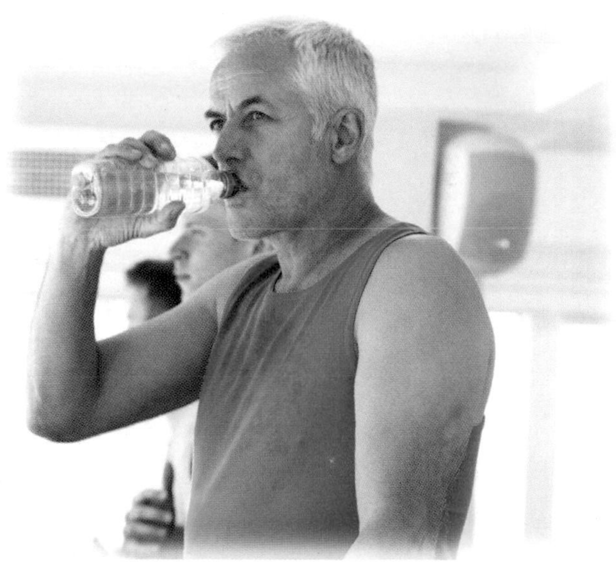

When electrolytes are out of balance, such as in a state of **dehydration** (leading to a high concentration of electrolytes) or **hyponatremia** (leading to a low concentration of electrolytes resulting from overhydration), serious consequences may occur. Symptoms of dehydration include nausea, vomiting, dizziness, disorientation, weakness, irritability, headache, cramps, chills, and decreased performance. Symptoms of hyponatremia include nausea, vomiting, dizziness, confusion, disorientation, coma, extreme fatigue, respiratory distress, and seizures. In severe cases, both conditions can result in death. Electrolytes are excreted in urine, feces, and sweat.

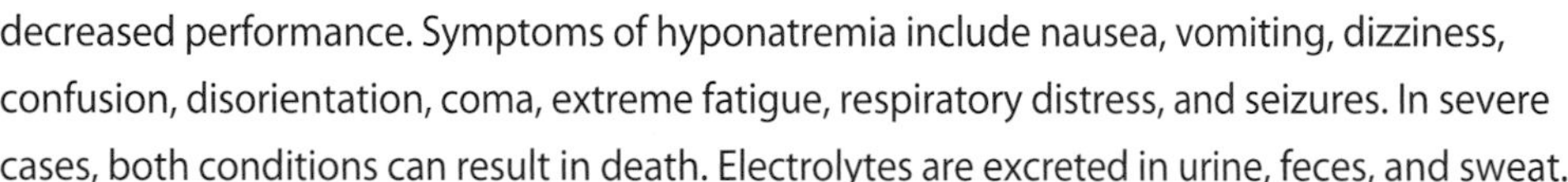

Generally, electrolyte deficiencies do not occur. In fact, sodium excess (and consequently, **hypertension**) is increasingly common given the typical American diet of highly processed and salty foods. *Note:* Hypertension related to sodium sensitivity has been more strongly linked to black and elderly populations (Champagne, 2006; Campese, 1994). Sodium excess may also contribute to osteoporosis, as high sodium increases calcium excretion. Potassium tends to be underconsumed, because most people do not consume enough fruits and vegetables. Insufficient potassium intake is linked to hypertension and osteoporosis.

Sulfur

Sulfur is an important component of several important bodily compounds, including two amino acids (cystine and methionine); three vitamins (thiamin, biotin, and pantothenic acid); and heparin, an anticoagulant found in the liver and other tissues. Meat, poultry, fish, eggs, dried beans, broccoli, and cauliflower are good food sources of the mineral. Sulfur deficiency is relatively uncommon and does not appear to cause any symptoms. Excess sulfur intake may lead to decreased bone mineralization, though sulfur toxicity is very rare.

Microminerals (Trace Elements)

Trace elements are found in minute amounts [less than 1 teaspoon (5 mL)] in the body. Despite the need for minimal doses of these minerals, they are critical for optimal growth, health, and development. RDAs have been established for only four trace elements: iron, iodine, selenium, and zinc.

Iron

Iron plays a very important role in normal human function. It is essential for the production of hemoglobin, the protein that carries inhaled oxygen from the lungs to the tissues, and myoglobin, the protein responsible for making oxygen available for muscle contraction. Iron also regulates cell growth and differentiation. It can be stored in the body for future use as the protein complex ferritin. Liver, oysters, seafood, kidney, heart, lean meat, poultry, and fish are excellent food sources, though many people use iron supplements to meet recommended intake amounts. Regardless of the source of iron intake, it is important to meet recommended intakes, as iron deficiency leads to fatigue, poor work performance, and decreased immunity. It is equally important to not exceed recommended intakes, as excess amounts can lead to accumulation of iron in the liver, causing toxicity, and sometimes even death.

Iodine

Iodine, a mineral stored in the thyroid gland and essential for normal growth and metabolism, is found naturally in seafood, though the most common source of iodine in the U.S. is iodized salt. Thanks to this fortification, iodine deficiency is rare in developed countries. However, in some developing countries, deficiency can cause goiter (enlargement of the thyroid gland) and mental retardation in children of mothers who were iodine-deficient during pregnancy. Excessive iodine intake also causes goiter and, potentially, thyroid disease.

Selenium

Selenium, an important antioxidant found mostly in plant foods grown in selenium-rich soil, is needed only in small amounts for optimal function. A lack of this mineral may lead to heart disease, hypothyroidism, and a weakened immune system. Too much selenium can lead to a condition called selonosis, which is manifested as gastrointestinal distress, hair loss, white blotchy nails, garlic breath odor, fatigue, irritability, and nerve damage.

Zinc

Zinc is found in almost every cell in the body and is the second most abundant trace element after iron. It stimulates the activity of enzymes, supports a healthy immune system, assists with wound healing, strengthens the senses (especially taste and smell), supports normal growth and development, and helps with DNA synthesis. Foods rich in zinc include meat, fish, poultry, milk products, and seafood such as oysters and other shellfish. Zinc deficiency causes delayed wound healing and immune-system dysfunction. Toxicity is rare in otherwise healthy individuals, although too much zinc as a result of overzealous supplementation can decrease healthy HDL cholesterol, interfere with copper absorption, and alter iron function [National Institutes of Health (NIH), 2011].

Antioxidants and Phytochemicals

Many of the vitamins and minerals already discussed, including vitamin A (in the form of beta-carotene), vitamin C, vitamin E, and selenium, function as antioxidants. Just as metal rusts over time when exposed to water and oxygen, cells are damaged from chronic oxygen exposure. This damage-causing process is called oxidation, and can set in motion various chemical reactions that at best cause aging and at worst cause cancer. Antioxidants function to prevent or repair oxidative damage. In the past, antioxidants were considered potent disease fighters. Subsequent research suggests that the agents not only fail to protect against disease, but also that, in excess, some of them may act to increase the risk of cancer, heart disease, and mortality in some individuals (Bjelakovic et al., 2007; Halliwell, 2007). Their true role in disease pathology is yet to be determined. What remains undisputed is that a diet high in fruits and vegetables is associated with a lower risk of developing chronic disease, such as heart disease, cancer, and possibly Alzheimer's disease. Their beneficial effects could be due to antioxidants, fiber, agents that stimulate the immune system, monounsaturated fatty acids, B vitamins, folic acid, or various other potential **phytochemicals**—substances in plants that are not necessarily required for normal functioning, but improve health and reduce the risk of disease.

Vitamins, Minerals, and Weight Management

Though vitamins and minerals are calorie-free (and thus are not a source of energy), they are essential for optimal health. Given the body's demands for vitamins and minerals and the relative caloric restriction many clients may follow in an effort to lose weight, it is especially important for clients to adopt a nutrient-dense, low-calorie eating plan. Not only should clients limit "empty calories" from nutrient-poor foods, but they should also pay special care to eat a balanced diet that includes all of the major food groups to ensure sufficient vitamin and mineral intake. Clients who restrict whole food groups or who have adopted a very restrictive eating plan should discuss the necessity of a daily multivitamin with their physicians.

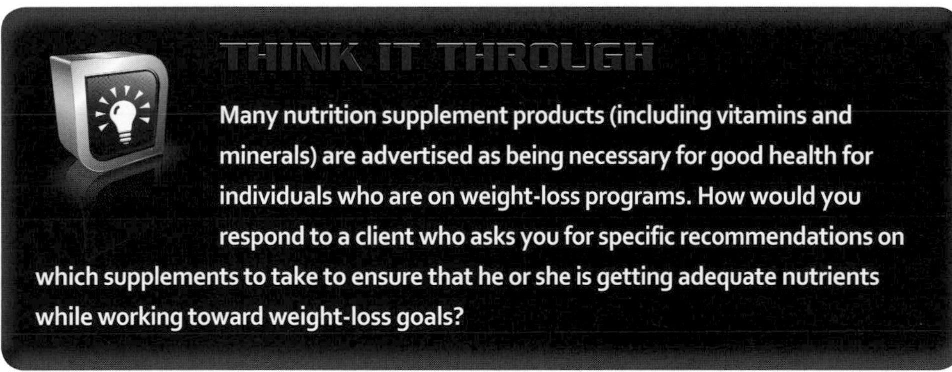

THINK IT THROUGH
Many nutrition supplement products (including vitamins and minerals) are advertised as being necessary for good health for individuals who are on weight-loss programs. How would you respond to a client who asks you for specific recommendations on which supplements to take to ensure that he or she is getting adequate nutrients while working toward weight-loss goals?

Water

When people think of nutrition, they often forget to think about water. Although it provides no calories and is inorganic in nature, it is as important as oxygen. Loss of only 20% of total body water could cause death. A 10% loss causes severe disorders (Figure 6-8). In general, adults can survive up to 10 days without water, while children can survive for up to five days (Mahan, Escott-Stump, & Raymond, 2011).

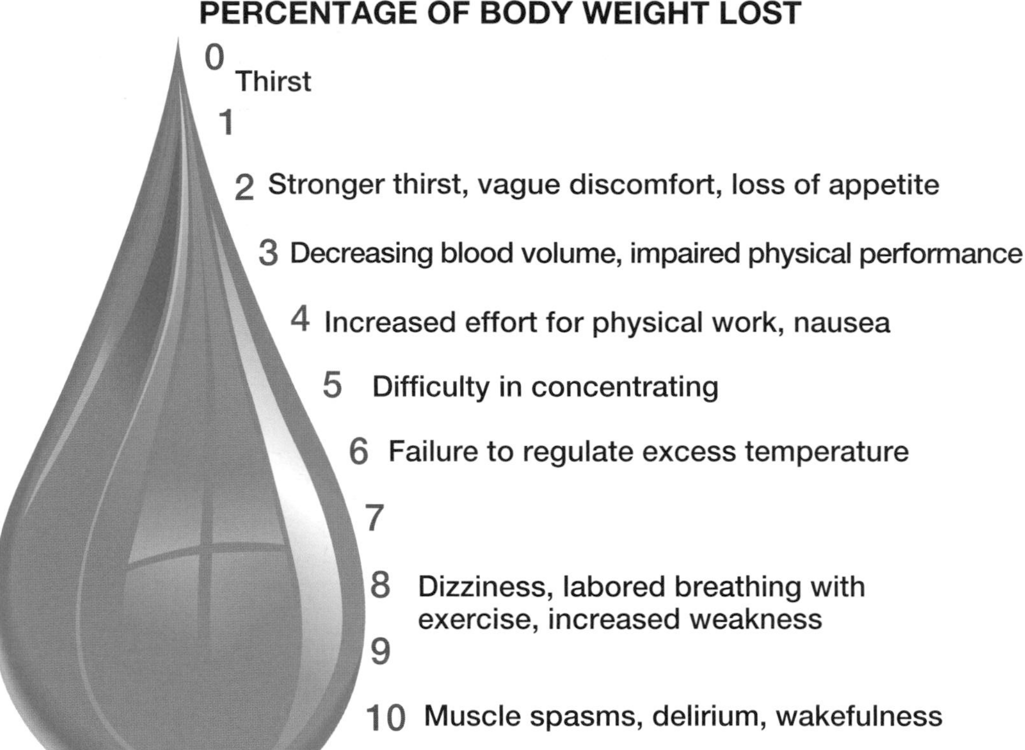

Figure 6-8
Adverse effects of dehydration

Reprinted with permission from Mahan, L.K., Escott-Stump, S., & Raymond, J.L. (2011). *Krause's Food and the Nutrition Care Process* (13th ed.). Philadelphia: W.B. Saunders Company.

Water is the single largest component of the human body, making up approximately 50 to 70% of body weight. In other words, about 85 to 119 pounds (39 to 54 kg) of a 170-pound (77-kg) man is water weight. Physiologically, water has many important functions, including regulating body temperature, protecting vital organs, providing a driving force for nutrient absorption, serving as a medium for all biochemical reactions, and maintaining an adequate blood volume for optimal athletic performance. In fact, total body water weight is higher in athletes compared to nonathletes and tends to decrease with age due to diminishing muscle mass.

Water volume can be influenced by a variety of factors, such as food and beverage intake; sweat, urine, and feces excretion; metabolic production of small amounts of water; and losses of water that occur with breathing. These factors play an especially important role during exercise when metabolism is increased. The generated body heat is released through sweat, which is a solution of water, sodium, and other electrolytes.

If fluid intake is not increased to replenish the lost fluid, the body attempts to compensate by retaining more water and excreting more concentrated urine. Under these conditions, the person is said to be dehydrated. Severe dehydration can lead to **heat exhaustion** and eventually **heat stroke.** On the other hand, if people ingest excessive amounts of fluid to compensate for minimal amounts of water lost in sweat, they may become overloaded with fluid, a condition called hyponatremia. When the blood's water-to-sodium ratio is severely elevated, excess water can leak into brain tissue, leading to encephalopathy, or brain swelling.

Fortunately, the human body is well-equipped to withstand dramatic variations in fluid intake during exercise and at rest with little or no detrimental health effects. Most recreational exercisers will never suffer from serious hyponatremia or dehydration. The latest recommendations are to follow individualized hydration regimens and let thirst be the guide—if thirsty, drink water (Rodriguez, DiMarco, & Langley, 2009; Sawka et al., 2007). Exceptions include infants, vigorously exercising athletes, hospitalized patients, and the sick and elderly, who may have a diminished thirst sensation. Because these individuals have higher water needs, they should be closely monitored.

APPLY WHAT YOU KNOW

Endurance Training and Hydration Status

Past headlines shared the unlikely but real tragedy of the 28-year-old novice Boston Marathon runner who suffered severe hyponatremia and later died en route to the hospital, as well as the story of the 24-year-old elite runner who collapsed from dehydration while exploring desolate trails in the Grand Canyon's summer heat without sufficient water. In all, a scattering of half-marathon and marathon deaths have drawn attention to the safety concerns of these endurance challenges.

Underlying heart conditions, dehydration, and overhydration (hyponatremia) most often are the causes of life-ending races in young athletes. Sadly, it turns out that not many runners are paying serious attention to hydration. In one study, a whopping 65% of the athletes studied were "not at all" concerned about keeping themselves hydrated (Brown et al., 2011). This indifference can come at a cost.

Drinking too little can lead to dehydration, which results from a sweat rate that is beyond fluid replenishment. Exercising at very high intensities, exercising in humid conditions, and low fluid intake all increase the likelihood of dehydration. Dehydration, along with high exercise intensity, hot and humid environmental conditions, poor fitness level, incomplete heat acclimatization, and a variety of other factors can all raise body temperature and together lead to heat stroke.

While dehydration is a serious concern, athletes should also be aware that drinking too much—out of fear of not drinking enough—could lead to hyponatremia, a less well known and less understood but equally frightening condition characterized by a low blood sodium level. Exertional hyponatremia results from excessive intake of low-sodium fluids during prolonged endurance activities—that is, drinking a greater volume of fluid than the volume lost in sweat—and possibly, to a lesser extent, from inappropriate fluid retention.

A study of 488 Boston Marathon runners published in the *New England Journal of Medicine* found that 13% (22% of women and 8% of men) had hyponatremia, and 0.6% had critical hyponatremia, at the end of the race. Runners with hyponatremia were more likely to be of low **body mass index (BMI),** consume fluids at every mile (and more than 3 liters total throughout the race), finish the race in more than four hours, and gain weight during the run. The greatest predictor of hyponatremia was weight gain, which researchers attributed to excessive fluid intake (Almond et al., 2005). But hyponatremia is not limited to runners. Anyone exercising at a low to moderate intensity for an extended period of time (generally four hours or more) while consuming too much water can be at risk.

Engineered Foods, Alcohol, Drugs, and Stimulants

While nature has produced an abundance of nutrient-rich foods for human consumption, man has developed an ability to alter the natural form to create engineered foods, various alcoholic beverages, drugs, **stimulants,** and other compounds. Scientists have learned to process foods to make them taste better (though in general, the greater the processing, the lesser the nutritional value). Humans genetically modify foods to make a more perfect and abundant plant, and they manufacture products to help people lose weight or gain muscle. The processed-food industry is huge, with people spending billions of dollars each year to reap the promised benefits.

> In January 2012, the American Dietetic Association (ADA) changed its name to the Academy of Nutrition and Dietetics (A.N.D.). Throughout this text, research conducted by the organization prior to this name change is cited to the ADA, while newer studies will be credited to the A.N.D. Refer to www.eatright.org for more information on the reasons behind the name change.

Some of these food products are considered **functional foods.** While various definitions exist, the American Dietetic Association (ADA) considers a functional food to be any whole food or fortified, enriched, or enhanced food that has a potentially beneficial effect on human health beyond basic nutrition (ADA, 2009). Whole foods such as phytochemical-containing fruits and vegetables are functional foods, as are modified foods that have been fortified with nutrients or phytochemicals. Because functional foods may play a role in decreasing signs of aging, altering disease prevalence and progression, and providing various other benefits, the public is willing to pay more for these products. As a result, many manufacturers and various other companies and individuals are interested in profiting from these products. At times, promises are made that are not backed by quality research or FDA approval. Health coaches play an important role in helping clients sift through the barrage of nutritional products to help them distinguish between quality products and hyped junk.

Clients also may be interested in learning how alcohol intake affects their weight-loss plans. Alcohol is a non-nutritive calorie-containing beverage (7 calories per gram). Moderate alcohol consumption (one drink per day for women and two drinks per day for men) provides many health benefits, such as increased HDL cholesterol and reduced risk for cardiovascular disease. However, too much alcohol may contribute to weight gain, regretful behavior, and serious accidents. In addition, alcohol use during pregnancy is linked to birth defects, and alcohol in excess can cause cirrhosis of the liver. Therefore, alcohol is best avoided altogether for those who are pregnant, cannot control intake, or are taking certain medications.

Herbal supplements, as well as legal and illicit drugs, have been used and abused in weight-loss efforts. While some herbs and other supplements may in fact have beneficial effects, consumers should purchase and use these products cautiously, as they are not regulated by the FDA. The **Dietary Supplement and Health Education Act (DSHEA)** dictates supplement production, marketing, and safety guidelines. The following are the highlights of the legislation.

Health coaches and their clients must be aware that savvy product manufacturers and marketing experts have found ingenious ways to get around some of the rules.

- A **dietary supplement** is defined as a product (other than tobacco) that functions to supplement the diet and contains one or more of the following ingredients: a vitamin, mineral, herb or other botanical, amino acid, a nutritional substance that increases total dietary intake, metabolite, constituent, or extract, or some combination of these ingredients.
- Safety standards provide that the Secretary of the Department of Health and Human Services may declare that a supplement poses imminent risk or hazard to public safety. A supplement is considered **adulterated** if it, or one of its ingredients, presents a "significant or unreasonable risk of illness or injury" when used as directed, or under normal

conditions. It may also be considered adulterated if too little information is known about the risk of an unstudied ingredient.

- Retailers are allowed to display "third-party" materials that provide information about the health-related benefits of dietary supplements. DSHEA stipulates the guidelines that this literature must follow, including the fact that it must not be false or misleading and cannot promote a specific supplement brand.
- Supplement labels cannot include claims that the product diagnoses, prevents, mitigates, treats, or cures a specific disease. Instead, they may describe the supplement's effects on the "structure or function" of the body or the "well-being" achieved by consuming the substance. Unlike other health claims, these nutritional support statements are not approved by the FDA prior to marketing the supplement.
- Supplements must contain an ingredient label, including the name and quantity of each dietary ingredient. The label must also identify the product as a "dietary supplement" (FDA, 1995).

Many clients experiment with various herbs and supplements during the course of their exercise and weight-loss programs. The websites of the FDA (www.fda.gov) and the National Institutes of Health Office of Dietary Supplements (www.ods.od.nih.gov) provide reputable, up-to-date information about numerous supplements and herbs that health coaches can reference.

Caffeine

One supplement that warrants specific mention is caffeine. Caffeine is a stimulant found in coffee, tea, soft drinks, chocolate, and various other foods and drinks. Over 90% of Americans admit to regular caffeine use (Frary, Johnson, & Wang, 2005); 20–30% take in a whopping 600 milligrams (equivalent to about 6 cups of coffee) or more each day (Armstrong et al., 2007).

Caffeine rapidly enters the bloodstream and reaches all organs of the body within 40 to 60 minutes, causing physiological changes that last for up to six hours (Table 6-3) (Keisler & Armsey,

Table 6-3

Physiological Effects of Caffeine by Organ System

Central Nervous System	Increased alertness and mood Decreased pain and fatigue
Metabolism	Increased oxygen uptake, fat breakdown, and glycogen sparing
Endocrine System	Increased catecholamines, endorphins, and cortisol
Skeletal Muscle	Increased endurance Possible increased power and speed
Cardiovascular System	Increased heart rate, stroke volume, and blood pressure
Respiratory System	Increased respiratory rate
Kidneys	Increased urine production Possible increased loss of urinary electrolytes No change in 24-hour electrolyte or water balance
Temperature Regulation	No change in sweat rate, skin blood flow, or rectal (core) temperature

Reprinted with permission from Armstrong, L.E. et al. (2007). Caffeine, fluid-electrolyte balance, temperature regulation, and exercise-heat tolerance. *Exercise and Sports Science Reviews,* 35, 3, 135–140.

2006). Due to its lipophilic, or "fat-loving," chemical structure, caffeine easily crosses the blood–brain barrier—the brain's security system aimed to prevent water-soluble toxins from damaging the all-important organ. To a nerve cell, caffeine resembles adenosine, a molecule that slows down the nervous system, dilates blood vessels, and allows sleep. The nerve's adenosine receptor cannot tell the difference between the two molecules, so caffeine and adenosine compete for receptor binding. When caffeine wins, the calming effects of adenosine are negated and an exaggerated stress response takes hold. The cell activity speeds up, the brain's blood vessels constrict, and neuron firing increases. The pituitary gland responds to the increased activity by sending a message to the adrenal glands to produce adrenaline, the "fight or flight" hormone. Pupils and bronchial tubes dilate. Heart rate increases. Blood flow redirects to the muscles. Blood pressure rises. Muscles contract. The liver releases extra glucose into the bloodstream to fuel the fight or flight reaction, thus sparing muscle glycogen stores (Keisler & Armsey, 2006).

Research findings are clear: caffeine enhances athletic performance. Caffeine sustains exercise duration, maximizes effort at 85% **$\dot{V}O_2$max** in cyclists, and quickens speed in an endurance event (Keisler & Armsey, 2006). Perceived exertion decreases and high-intensity efforts seem less taxing (Armstrong et al., 2007). The World Anti-Doping Agency (WADA) does not classify caffeine as a banned substance (www.wada-ama.org), while the National Collegiate Athletic Association (NCAA) allows intakes up to an approximately 800 mg dose, as measured by urine concentration of caffeine. There is a catch: performance-enhancing benefits of caffeine are stronger in nonusers (<50 mg/day) than regular users (>300 mg/day), as the brain adapts to chronic caffeine use by producing more adenosine receptors for adenosine binding. Caffeine's effects are lessened and the same dose produces fewer desirable physiological changes.

Some clients may also consider turning to caffeine to boost weight loss. The stimulant is a common ingredient in many weight-loss supplements. Caffeine may contribute to weight loss by suppressing appetite, increasing water loss (it is a **diuretic**), and potentially increasing resting metabolic rate. However, any effect on weight loss is likely to be minimal, and the risks of caffeine overconsumption and dependence that could develop are greater than a small weight-loss benefit.

Consider this scenario: A client attributes increased performance and some weight loss to caffeine. But despite maintaining the same caffeine intake, the perceived benefits diminish over time. Having developed a tolerance to caffeine, the client consumes more caffeine. While the extra caffeine binds up the newly created adenosine receptors, the brain gets back to work, increasing receptor production. As the dose continues to increase in pursuit of the invigorating caffeine jolt, risk of severe consequences multiply. *The U.S. News and World Report* reported that one teen spent the night in the pediatric intensive care unit after binging on caffeine pills and energy drinks to stay awake to play video games all night (Shute, 2007). A 19-year-old Connecticut man died of cardiac arrest from an overdose of 25 to 30 caffeine pills—the equivalent of about 30 cups of coffee (Shute, 2007). In addition to its toxicity at high doses, when combined with other substances like alcohol, ephedrine, or anti-inflammatory medications, even moderate caffeine use can be dangerous.

On top of tolerance, chronic caffeine use may contribute to high blood pressure, high blood sugar, decreased bone density in women, jittery nerves, sleeplessness (Doheny, 2007), and for many, the dreaded withdrawal symptoms after a brief respite from the stimulant, including headache, irritability, increased fatigue, drowsiness, decreased alertness, difficulty concentrating, and decreased energy and activity levels (Keisler & Armsey 2006).

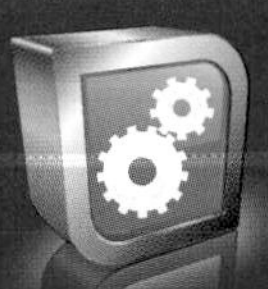

EXPAND YOUR KNOWLEDGE

Five-step Two-week Taper From Caffeine Use

The good news is that clients can moderate caffeine consumption to optimize its advantages and at the same time avoid caffeine dependence and the ensuing withdrawal after a stint of quitting caffeine cold turkey. The following five-step two-week taper offers one way to get started:

- Choose a two-week period of relative low stress. The taper may cause some tiredness—the key is to hit the sack, not the sodas. Aim for at least seven to eight hours of sleep each night.
- Tally daily caffeine intake from the first sip of coffee in the morning, to the lunch-time sodas, mid-afternoon energy drink, and evening tea. Remember to look beyond the nutrition label. The Center for Science in the Public Interest, a non-profit nutrition watchdog, and the American Medical Association have lobbied unsuccessfully for more than 10 years to convince the federal government to mandate caffeine information on nutrition labels. Sensing a possible shift in congress, many soda manufacturers now voluntarily include the caffeine content. But still, chances are that clients are going to have to search for the caffeine amounts in their favorite foods and drinks. Table 6-4 lists caffeine amounts in some common beverages.
- Substitute a caffeine-free beverage for one caffeinated beverage each day. Maintain this level of caffeine use for the week. The next week decrease by one more. Each week, decrease the total number of caffeinated beverages per day until total caffeine intake is less than 100 mg per day.
- Maintain a level of caffeine use less than or equal to 100 mg per day, the level below which dependency is unlikely to occur (Shapiro, 2007). Then try quitting cold turkey for three days. Research suggests withdrawal occurs around three days after quitting for new users and as quickly as 12 hours in regular users (Keisler & Armsey 2006). The onset of a caffeine headache indicates the baseline dose is not low enough. Continue the taper to a 25-mg maintenance dose (Lu et al., 2007) or endure the headache and within a few days the caffeine habit will be history.
- Get out of crisis mode. Not every day, deadline, or life event needs a caffeine boost to make it through. Choose wisely and carefully so that when the caffeine boost feels essential, the brain and body are prepared to give the maximal effect at the lowest possible dose.

Table 6-4

Caffeine Content of Popular Beverages

Substance	Caffeine per ounce (mg)
Coffee	13
Monster® Energy Drink	10
Red Bull® with caffeine	9
Full Throttle® energy drink	9
Starbucks® Mocha Frappucino	8
Iced Tea	6
Pepsi Max®	6
Mountain Dew®	5
Coca-Cola® (regular or diet)	4
Dr. Pepper®	3
Propel® Invigorating Water (coming soon)	3
Sprite®	0
Over-the-counter stimulants (e.g., NoDoz®)	100 (per capsule)
Clif Shot®: Strawberry, Mocha, Double Expresso	25, 50, 100 (per shot)

Sources: Caffeine content from product websites and www.energyfiend.com.

Summary

An individual's health is at least partially determined by the nutrients he or she chooses to consume. While each nutrient plays a specific role in the body's well-being, it is the balance among these different nutrients that allows the body to function optimally. As such, a balanced and varied diet is the foundation for good health. Health coaches should arm their clients with an understanding and appreciation of basic nutrition, digestion, and absorption to help them make proper choices and follow the path toward optimal health and well-being.

References

Almond, C.S.D. et al. (2005). Hyponatremia among runners in the Boston Marathon. *New England Journal of Medicine,* 352, 1550–1556.

American Dietetic Association (2009). Position of the American Dietetic Association: Functional foods. *Journal of the American Dietetic Association,* 109, 735–746.

Armstrong, L.E. et al. (2007). Caffeine, fluid-electrolyte balance, temperature regulation, and exercise-heat tolerance. *Exercise and Sports Science Reviews*, 35, 3, 135–140.

Bjelakovic, G. et al. (2007). Mortality in randomized trials of antioxidant supplements for primary and secondary prevention. *Journal of the American Medical Association,* 297, 842–857.

Brooks, G.A. (1987). Amino acid and protein metabolism during exercise and recovery. *Medicine & Science in Sports & Exercise,* 19, Suppl., S150–156.

Brown, S. et al. (2011). Lack of awareness of fluid needs among participants at a midwest marathon. *Sports Health: A Multidisciplinary Approach*, 3, 5, 451–454.

Campese, V. (1994). Salt sensitivity and hypertension: Renal and cardiovascular implications. *Hypertension,* 23, 531–550.

Champagne, C.M. (2006). Dietary interventions on blood pressure: The Dietary Approaches to Stop Hypertension (DASH) trials. *Nutrition Reviews*, 64, 2, (II), S53–S56.

Doheny, K. (2007). Pros and cons of the caffeine craze. *WebMD.* Retrieved November 9, 2011: www.webmd.com/diet/features/pros-and-cons-caffeine-craze?page=4

Duffey, K.J. & Popkin, B.M. (2008). High-fructose corn syrup: Is this what's for dinner? *American Journal of Clinical Nutrition,* 88, Suppl., 1722S–1732S.

Fischer, L.M. et al. (2010). Dietary choline requirements of women: Effects of estrogen and genetic variation. *American Journal of Clinical Nutrition*, 92, 1113–1119.

Food and Drug Administration (1995). *Dietary Supplement Health and Education Act of 1994.* http://www.cfsan.fda.gov/~dms/dietsupp.html

Frary, C.D., Johnson, R.K., & Wang, M.Q. (2005). Food sources and intakes of caffeine in the diets of persons in the United States. *Journal of the American Dietetic Association*, 105, 110–113.

Goyal, S.K., Samsher, I., & Goyal, R.K. (2010). Stevia (*Stevia rebaudiana)* a bio-sweetener: A review. *International Journal of Food Sciences and Nutrition,* 61, 1, 1–10.

Halliwell, B. (2007). Dietary polyphenols: Good, bad, or indifferent for your health? *Cardiovascular Research,* 73, 341–347.

Harris, W.S. (2010). Omega-6 and omega-3 fatty acids: Partners in prevention. *Current Opinions in Clinical Nutrition and Metabolic Care,* 13, 2, 125–129.

Harris, W.S. et al. (2009). Omega-6 fatty acids and risk for cardiovascular disease: A science advisory from the American Heart Association Nutrition Subcommittee of the Council on Nutrition, Physical Activity, and Metabolism; Council on Cardiovascular Nursing; and Council on Epidemiology and Prevention. *Circulation,* 119, 6, 902–990

Institute of Medicine, Food and Nutrition Board (2005). *Dietary Reference Intakes: Energy, Carbohydrates, Fiber, Fat, Fatty Acids,Cholesterol, Protein and Amino Acids*. Washington, D.C.: National Academies Press.

Keisler, B.D. & Armsey, T.D. (2006). Caffeine as ergogenic acid. *Current Sports Medicine Reports*, 5, 215–219.

Kobylewski, S. & Eckhert, C.D (2008). *Toxicology of Rebaudioside A: A Review.* Retrieved June 14, 2011: www.cspinet.org/new/pdf/stevia-report_final-8-14-08.pdf.

Lappé, F.M. (1992). *Diet for a Small Planet.* New York: Ballantine Books.

Lu, Y.P. et al. (2007). Voluntary exercise together with oral caffeine markedly stimulates UVB light-induced apoptosis and decreases tissue fat in SKH-1 mice. *Proceedings of the National Academy of Sciences*, 104, 31, 12936–12941.

Mahan, L.K., Escott-Stump, S., & Raymond, J.L. (2011). *Krause's Food and the Nutrition Care Process* (13th ed.). Philadelphia: W.B. Saunders Company.

Mattes, R.D. & Popkin, B.M. (2009). Nonnutritive sweetener consumption in humans: Effects on appetite and food intake and their putative mechanisms. *The American Journal of Clinical Nutrition,* 89, 1, 1–14.

McArdle, W.D., Katch, F.I., & Katch, V.L. (2008). *Sports and Exercise Nutrition* (3rd ed.). Philadelphia: Lippincott Williams & Wilkins.

McDaniel, M.A., Maier, S.F., & Einstein, G.O. (2003). "Brain-specific" nutrients: A memory cure? *Nutrition*, 19, 957–975.

Miller, M. et al. (2011). Triglycerides and cardiovascular disease: A scientific statement from the American Heart Association. *Circulation*, 123, 20, 2292–2333.

National Institutes of Health Office of Dietary Supplements (2011). *Dietary Supplement Fact Sheet: Zinc.* www.ods.od.nih.gov/factsheets/Zinc-QuickFacts/

Rabobank Group (2009). *New Sweetener May Hit Sweet Spot in U.S. Market.* www.rabobank.com/content/news/news_archive/076Newsweetenermayhitsweetspotin USmarket.jsp

Rizkalla, S.W. (2010). Health implications of fructose consumption: A review of recent data. *Nutrition and Metabolism (London)*, 7, 82.

Rodriguez, N.R., DiMarco, N.M., & Langley, S. (2009). Position of the American Dietetic Association, Dietitians of Canada, and the American College of Sports Medicine: Nutrition and athletic performance. *Journal of the American Dietetic Association*,109, 3, 509–527.

Sawka, M.N. et al. (2007). American College of Sports Medicine exercise and fluid replacement position stand. *Medicine & Science in Sports & Exercise*, 39, 2, 377–390.

Shapiro, R.E. (2007). Caffeine and headaches. *Neurological Science*, 28, S179–S183.

Shute, N. (2007). Over the limit? *U.S. News and World Report*, 142, 14, 60–68.

U.S. Department of Agriculture (2015). *2015-2020 Dietary Guidelines for Americans* (8th ed.). www.health.gov/dietaryguidelines

World Health Organization (2010). *Micronutrients.* www.who.int/nutrition/topics/micronutrients/en/index.html

Zeisel, S.H. & Niculescu, M.D. (2006). Perinatal choline influences brain structure and function. *Nutrition Reviews*, 64, 197–203.

Suggested Reading

Clark, N. (2008). *Nancy Clark's Sports Nutrition Guidebook.* Champaign, Ill.: Human Kinetics.

Institutes of Medicine (2005). *Dietary Reference Intakes.* www.iom.edu/CMS/3788/4574.aspx

National Institutes of Health, Office of Dietary Supplements: *Vitamin and Mineral Supplement Fact Sheets.* www.ods.od.nih.gov/Health_Information/Vitamin_and_Mineral_Supplement_Fact_Sheets.aspx

Rodriguez, N.R., DiMarco, N.M., & Langley, S. (2009). Position of the American Dietetic Association, Dietitians of Canada, and the American College of Sports Medicine: Nutrition and athletic performance. *Journal of the American Dietetic Association*,109, 3, 509–527.

U.S. Department of Agriculture (2015). *2015-2020 Dietary Guidelines for Americans* (8th ed.). www.health.gov/dietaryguidelines

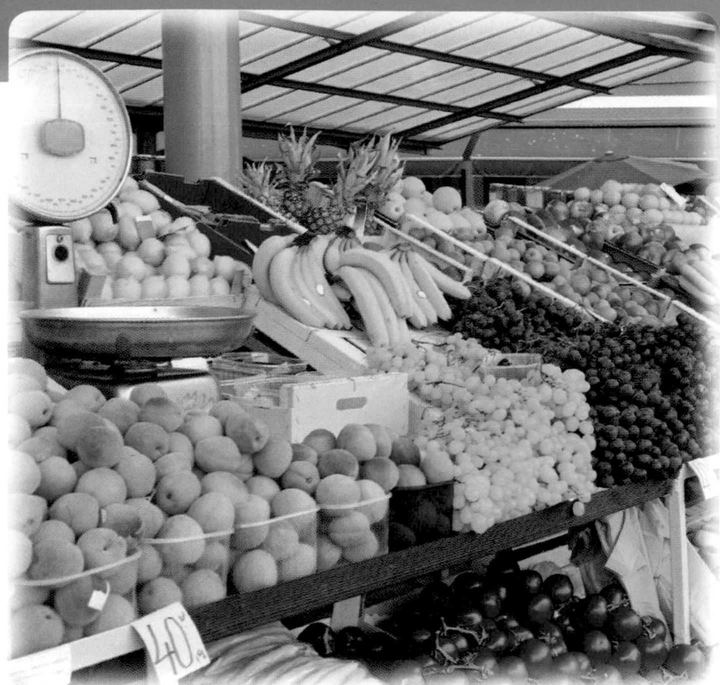

IN THIS CHAPTER:

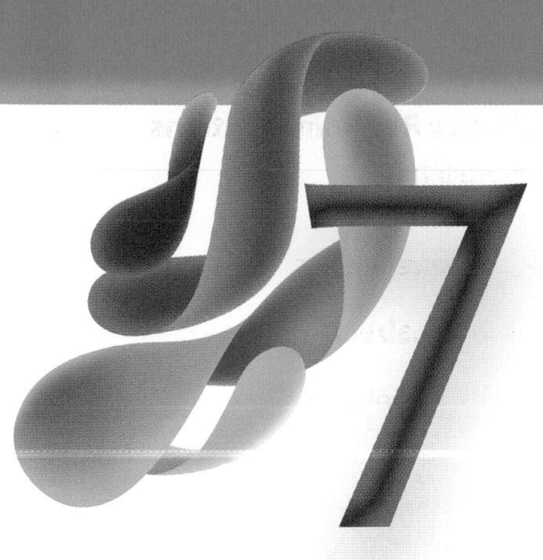

Application of Nutrition

NATALIE DIGATE MUTH

Natalie Digate Muth, M.D., M.P.H., R.D., is a pediatrician, registered dietitian, Board-Certified Specialist in Sports Dietetics (CSSD), and Senior Consultant - Nutrition for the American Council on Exercise (ACE). She is also an ACE-certified Personal Trainer and Group Fitness Instructor, an American College of Sports Medicine Health and Fitness Instructor, and a National Strength and Conditioning Association Certified Strength and Conditioning Specialist. She is author of more than 50 articles, books, and book chapters, including the books "Eat Your Vegetables!" and Other Mistakes Parents Make: Redefining How to Raise Healthy Eaters *(Healthy Learning, 2012) and the upcoming textbook* Sports Nutrition for Allied Health Professionals *(F.A. Davis, in press).*

ACE-certified Health Coaches provide nutrition guidance and recommendations to clients who have struggled with myriad challenges, health conditions, and weight-management successes and failures. To provide clients with the highest quality of care and help them achieve their goals, health coaches must have knowledge of the latest nutrition recommendations and guidelines for optimal health. But, more importantly, to empower clients to adopt healthful lifestyle changes, a health coach must be adept at translating nutrition knowledge into action. While diets come and go with the pounds lost and regained, healthful habits that are adopted, reinforced, and encouraged are the keys to a client's weight-management success.

Federal Dietary Recommendations

People require varying amounts of nutrients depending on gender, age, activity level, health status, and other factors. The federal government has taken this into consideration when developing recommended intakes. The *2015-2020 Dietary Guidelines for Americans,* MyPlate, and **Dietary Reference Intakes (DRIs)** provide individualized nutrition recommendations for a healthy diet.

Dietary Guidelines

Published every five years, the *Dietary Guidelines* are the government's best advice to Americans on how to eat to promote health (U.S. Department of Agriculture, 2015).

The *2015-2020 Dietary Guidelines,* which are available at www.health.gov/dietaryguidelines, offer five big-picture recommendations that are key to good nutrition. An overview of these five key recommendations is provided here.

Key Guideline 1: Follow a Healthy Eating Pattern Across the Lifespan

All food and beverage choices matter. Choose a healthy eating pattern at an appropriate calorie level to help achieve and maintain a healthy body weight, support nutrient adequacy, and reduce the risk of chronic disease.

The *Guidelines* make a point to emphasize overall eating patterns more so than individual nutrients, recognizing that the overall nutritional value of a person's diet is more than "the sum of its parts." The main components of a healthy eating pattern include:

- A variety of vegetables from five different groups—dark green, red and orange, legumes (beans and peas), starchy, and other
- Fruit
- Grains, primarily whole grains
- Fat-free or low-fat dairy, including milk yogurt, cheese, and/or fortified soy products
- A variety of foods rich in protein, including seafood, lean meats and poultry, eggs, legumes (beans and peas), nuts, seeds, and soy products
- Limited amounts of saturated fats and trans fats (less than 10% of calories), added sugars (less than 10% of calories), and sodium (less than 2,300 mg per day). If alcohol is consumed, it should be consumed in moderation, defined as up to one drink per day for women and two drinks per day for men.

Key Guideline 2: Focus on Variety, Nutrient Density, and Amount

To meet nutrient needs within calorie limits, choose a variety of nutrient-dense foods across and within all food groups in recommended amounts.

The *Guidelines* suggest that Americans are most likely to meet nutrient needs and manage weight by choosing nutrient-dense foods, which provide high levels of vitamins, minerals, and other nutrients that may have health benefits relative to caloric content. Categories of nutrient-dense foods include vegetables, fruits, grains, dairy, protein foods, and oils.

Key Guideline 3: Limit Calories from Added Sugars and Saturated Fats and Reduce Sodium Intake

Consume an eating pattern low in added sugars, saturated fats, and sodium. Cut back on foods and beverages higher in these components to amounts that fit within healthy eating patterns.

The *Guidelines* urge Americans to pay attention to—and limit—consumption of foods with low to no nutritional value, especially those that are, or may be, harmful to health such as added sugars, saturated fat, and sodium. New to the *2015-2020 Dietary Guidelines* compared to previous editions, dietary cholesterol is no longer noted as a nutrient to limit, as it is likely not harmful to health for most people.

Key Guideline 4: Shift to Healthier Food and Beverage Choices

Choose nutrient-dense foods and beverages across and within all food groups in place of less healthy choices. Consider cultural and personal preferences to make these shifts easier to accomplish and maintain.

While the *Guidelines* advocate an overall healthy and balanced nutrition pattern that is low in added sugars and sodium, the reality is that most Americans eat nothing like the eating patterns recommended by the *Guidelines*. By making shifts in dietary patterns, Americans can achieve and maintain a healthy body weight, meet nutrient needs, and decrease the risk of chronic disease.

Key Guideline 5: Support Healthy Eating Patterns for All

Everyone has a role in helping create and support healthy eating patterns in multiple settings nationwide, from home to school to work to communities.

The *Guidelines* charge all sectors of society to play an active role in the movement to make the United States healthier by developing coordinated partnerships, programs, and policies to support healthy eating.

MyPlate

The goal of MyPlate is to simplify the government's nutrition messages into an easily understood and implemented graphic—a dinner plate divided into four sections: fruits, vegetables, protein, and grains, with a glass of 1% or non-fat milk—and to encourage Americans to eat a more balanced diet that is made up of approximately 50% fruits and vegetables (Figure 7-1).

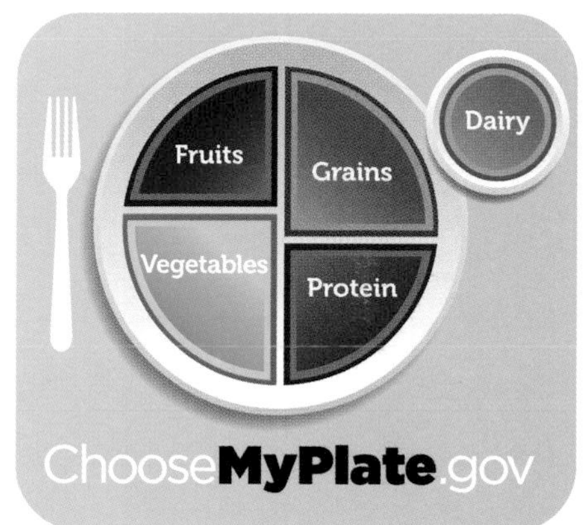

Figure 7-1
MyPlate

On the website www.ChooseMyPlate.gov, consumers can use the Super Tracker, which uses age, gender, height, weight, and physical-activity level to develop an individualized eating plan to meet their caloric needs. The program calculates **estimated energy requirement** based on this demographic information.

Within seconds, users are categorized into one of 12 different energy levels (anywhere from 1,000 to 3,200 calories) and are given the recommended number of **servings**—measured in cups and ounces—to eat from each of the five food groups (i.e., vegetables, fruit, protein, grains, and dairy). A set number of **empty calories** (i.e., calories from food components such as SoFAS that provide little nutritional value) is also allocated for that individual. By following these recommendations, users receive an optimal diet for disease prevention and weight maintenance based on their personalized needs.

In general, MyPlate encourages people to:

- Balance calories. People should only eat the amount of calories that the body needs. Physical activity helps to balance calories (this is the only place where physical activity is discussed in the new MyPlate talking points). Individual calorie recommendations are available at www.ChooseMyPlate.gov.
- Enjoy your food, but eat less. The key here is to slow down while eating to truly enjoy the food (and key in to the body's internal cues of hunger and **satiety**) and try to minimize distractions like television.
- Avoid oversized portions. MyPlate recommends smaller plates, smaller serving sizes, and more mindful eating.
- Eat more vegetables, fruits, whole grains, and fat-free or 1% milk dairy products for adequate potassium, calcium, vitamin D, and fiber.
- Make half your plate fruits and vegetables. Most Americans need nine servings of fruits and vegetables per day. Very few people get anywhere near that.
- Switch to fat-free or low-fat (1%) milk. Full-fat dairy products provide excess calories and saturated fat in exchange for no nutritional benefit over fat-free and low-fat versions.

- Make half your grains whole grains (ideally even more than that). This will help to ensure adequate fiber intake and decreased intake of highly processed foods.
- Eat fewer foods high in solid fat (typically saturated and **trans fat**), added sugars, and salt.
- Compare sodium in foods and then choose the lower sodium versions.
- Drink water instead of sugary drinks to help cut sugar and unnecessary, empty calories.

These messages will be emphasized during a multiyear campaign by the Let's Move initiative and the United States Department of Agriculture (USDA) to promote better eating. Online tools and how-to strategies will also become available (see www.ChooseMyPlate.gov to identify the tools currently available). Table 7-1 shows recommended daily amounts of each of the five food groups for a 2,000-calorie diet.

Table 7-1

MyPlate Recommended Daily Amounts for a 2,000-Calorie Diet

Food Group	Daily Average Over 1 Week
Grains	6.2 oz eq
Whole grains	3.8 oz eq
Refined grains	2.4 oz eq
Vegetables	2.6 cups
Vegetable subgroups (amount per week)	
Dark green	1.6 cups per week
Red/orange	5.6 cups
Starchy	5.1 cups
Beans and peas	1.6 cups
Other vegetables	4.1 cups
Fruits	2.1 cups
Dairy	3.1 cups
Protein foods	5.7 oz eq
Seafood	8.8 oz per week
Oils	29 grams
Calories from added fats and sugars	245 calories

Note: oz eq = Ounce equivalents

THINK IT THROUGH

Recently, your 62-year-old client, Charles, expressed an increased interest in making a commitment to eating healthier. Upon his request for your recommendation for a healthy eating plan, you direct him to the USDA website, www.ChooseMyPlate.gov. Charles agrees to check it out before your next session together. During his next visit, you discuss his thoughts about the website and discover that he feels intimidated by using the computer and that he gave up trying to use the interactive nutrition guidance tool because he found it difficult to navigate. How would you handle situations when clients are reluctant to use technology? What are some ways you can help them be successful with the use of helpful websites or applications so that they are encouraged to continue learning about healthy eating and physical activity?

Dietary Reference Intakes

In the past, only **Recommended Dietary Allowances (RDAs)** were published for the different nutrients based on age and gender. The RDAs are defined as "the levels of intake of essential nutrients that, on the basis of scientific knowledge, are judged by the Food and Nutrition Board to be adequate to meet the known needs of practically all healthy persons." Newer reference values, known as Dietary Reference Intakes (DRIs), are more descriptive. DRI is a generic term used to refer to three types of reference values:

- RDA
- **Estimated Average Requirement (EAR),** an adequate intake in 50% of an age- and gender-specific group
- **Tolerable Upper Intake Level (UL)**, the maximal intake that is unlikely to pose risk of adverse health effects to almost all individuals in an age- and gender-specific group

The term **Adequate Intake (AI)** is used when an RDA cannot be based on an EAR. Adequate intake is a recommended nutrient intake level that, based on research, appears to be sufficient for good health.

DRIs have been established for calcium, vitamin D, phosphorus, magnesium, and fluoride; folate and other B vitamins; **antioxidants** (vitamins C and E, and selenium); macronutrients (protein, carbohydrate, and fat); trace elements (vitamin A and K, iron, and zinc); **electrolytes** (sodium and potassium); and water. The complete set of DRIs is available at the website of the Institute of Medicine (IOM): www.iom.edu.

EXPAND YOUR KNOWLEDGE

How Much Should You Eat?

All of the abbreviations and their accompanying definitions that make up the DRIs can be confusing even for the most seasoned nutrition experts. In the past, the dietary recommendations were based simply on the RDA, or the amount of a particular nutrient that would be sufficient to prevent deficiency in 97 to 98% of the population. However, in 2000, the Food and Nutrition Board of the IOM released the complete set of DRIs to help nutrition professionals better assess and plan diets.

The RDA and the EAR should be considered together when designing and implementing a comprehensive nutrition plan. If a person's intake of a particular nutrient falls well below the EAR, it is likely that person does not consume enough of that nutrient. If the level is within the EAR and the RDA, then it is likely the client consumes enough of the nutrients. If the level is at or above the RDA, then the client almost certainly consumes a sufficient amount (since the RDA covers 97 to 98% of the population).

If the nutrient has not been adequately studied and too little information is available to determine an EAR (a level good enough for 50% of the population), then it is also not possible to determine an RDA (a level good enough for 97 to 98% of the population). In these cases, the AI is published. If a client's intake is at, or exceeds, the AI, then it is very likely that he or she consumes enough of the nutrient to prevent deficiency. If intake is below the AI, then it is possible (but not certain) that the client is deficient in that nutrient.

Comparing a person's usual intake of a nutrient to the UL helps determine whether a client is at risk of nutrient toxicity. The UL is set so that even the most sensitive people should not have an adverse effect of a nutrient below the UL. Thus, many people who have intakes above the UL may never experience a nutrient toxicity, though it is difficult to assess which clients may be at risk for a nutrient overdose.

Ultimately, "how much you should eat" is an approximation based on a series of probabilities that are known collectively as the DRIs.

Nutrition Facts Labels

For people to make healthy nutrition decisions, they first have to be able to understand what nutrients contribute to a healthy diet, and second, know which foods contain those nutrients. The nutrition facts label, a required component of nearly all packaged foods, can help people turn knowledge into action (Figure 7-2).

Health coaches can advise individuals to dissect a nutrition facts label by starting from the top with the serving size and the number of servings per container. In general, serving

Serving Size
The label presents serving sizes as the amount that most people actually consume in a sitting. This is not necessarily the same as how much one should eat per serving. All of the nutrition information on the label is based on one serving. If you eat one-half of the serving size shown here, cut the nutrient and calorie values in half.

Total Fat
Fat is calorie-dense and, if consumed in large portions, can increase the risk of weight problems. While once vilified, most fat, in and of itself, is not bad.

Cholesterol
Many foods that are high in cholesterol are also high in saturated fat, which can contribute to heart disease. Dietary cholesterol itself likely does not cause health problems.

Sodium
You call it "salt," the label calls it "sodium." Either way, it may add up to high blood pressure in some people. So, keep your sodium intake low—less than 2,300 mg each day. (The American Heart Association recommends no more than 3,000 mg of sodium per day for healthy adults.)

Sugars
Too much sugar contributes to weight gain and increased risk of diseases like diabetes and fatty liver disease. Foods like fruits and dairy products contain natural sugars (fructose and lactose), but also may contain added sugars. It is best to consume no more than 10% of total calories from added sugar, or a total of 50 g per day based on a 2,000-calorie eating plan.

Vitamins and Minerals
Your goal here is 100% of each for the day. Don't count on one food to do it all. Let a combination of foods add up to a winning score.

Nutrition Facts

4 Servings Per Container
Serving Size **1/2 cup (114g)**

Amount Per Serving	
Calories	**90**
	% Daily Value*
Total Fat 3g	**5%**
Saturated Fat 0g	**0%**
Trans Fat 0g	**0%**
Cholesterol 0mg	**0%**
Sodium 300mg	**13%**
Total Carbohydrate 13g	**4%**
Dietary Fiber 3g	**12%**
Total Sugars 12g	
Includes 10g Added Sugars	**20%**
Protein 3g	
Vitamin D 2mcg	10%
Calcium 260mg	20%
Iron 8mg	45%
Potassium 235mg	6%

* The % Daily Value (DV) tells you how much a nutrient in a serving of food contributes to a daily diet. 2,000 calories a day is used for general nutrition advice.

Daily Value
Daily Values are listed based on a 2,000-calorie daily eating plan. Your calorie and nutrient needs may be a little bit more or less based on your age, sex, and activity level (see https://fnic.nal.usda.gov/fnic/interactiveDRI/). For saturated fat, sugars and added sugars, and sodium, choose foods with a low % Daily Value. For dietary fiber, vitamins, and minerals, your Daily Value goal is to reach 100% of each.

Ingredients: *This portion of the label lists all of the foods and additives contained in a product, in order from the most prevalent ingredient to the least.*

Allergens: *This portion of the label identifies which of the most common allergens may be present in the product.*

(More nutrients may be listed on some labels)

mg = milligrams (1,000 mg = 1 g)
g = grams (about 28 g = 1 ounce)

Calories
Are you trying to lose weight? Cut back a little on calories. Look here to see how a serving of the food adds to your daily total. A 5'4", 138-lb active woman needs about 2,200 calories each day. A 5'10", 174-lb active man needs about 2,900.

Saturated Fat
Saturated fat is part of the total fat in food. It is listed separately because it is an important player in raising blood cholesterol and your risk of heart disease. Eat less!

Trans Fat
Trans fat works a lot like saturated fat, except it is worse. This fat starts out as a liquid unsaturated fat, but then food manufacturers add some hydrogen to it, turning it into a solid saturated fat (that is what "partially hydrogenated" means when you see it in the food ingredients). They do this to increase the shelf-life of the product, but in the body the trans fat damages the blood vessels and contributes to increasing blood cholesterol and the risk of heart disease.

Total Carbohydrate
Carbohydrates are in foods like bread, potatoes, fruits, and vegetables, as well as processed foods. Carbohydrate is further broken down into dietary fiber and sugars. Consume foods high in fiber often and those high in sugars, especially added sugars, less often.

Dietary Fiber
Grandmother called it "roughage," but her advice to eat more is still up-to-date! That goes for both soluble and insoluble kinds of dietary fiber. Fruits, vegetables, whole-grain foods, beans, and peas are all good sources and can help reduce the risk of heart disease and cancer.

Protein
Most Americans get more than they need. Eat small servings of lean meat, fish, and poultry. Use skim or low-fat milk, yogurt, and cheese. Try vegetable proteins like beans, grains, and cereals.

Figure 7-2
Nutrition facts label

sizes are standardized so that consumers can compare similar products, such as Triscuits® and Wheat Thins® or natural applesauce and sweetened applesauce. All of the nutrient amounts listed on the nutrition facts label are for one serving, so it is important to determine how many servings are actually being consumed to accurately assess nutrient intake. Next, consumers should look at the total calories. The calories indicate how much energy a person gets from a particular food. Americans tend to consume too many calories, and too many calories from fat, without meeting daily nutrient requirements. This part of the nutrition facts label is the most important factor for weight control. According to FDA food labeling requirements, 40 calories per serving is considered low, 100 calories is moderate, and 400 or more calories is considered high. The next two sections of the label note the nutrient content of the food product. Consumers should try to minimize their intake of fat (especially saturated and trans fat), sugars, and sodium and aim to consume adequate amounts of vitamins and minerals, especially fiber, vitamin A, vitamin C, calcium, and iron. The food label includes the total amount of sugars and specifies the amount of added sugars.

The **percent daily values (PDV)** are listed for key nutrients to make it easier to compare products (just make sure that the serving sizes are similar), evaluate nutrient content claims (does 1/3 reduced sugar cereal really contain less carbohydrate than a similar cereal of a different brand?), and make informed dietary trade-offs (e.g., balance consumption of a high-calorie product for lunch with lower-calorie products throughout the rest of the day). The *Dietary Guidelines for Americans* suggest that 5% daily value or less is considered low, while 20% daily value or more is considered high (USDA, 2010).

The footnote at the bottom of the label reminds consumers that all PDVs are based on a 2,000-calorie diet. Individuals who need more or fewer calories should adjust recommendations accordingly. For example, 3 grams of fat provides 5% of the recommended amount for someone on a 2,000-calorie diet, but 7% for someone on a 1,500-calorie diet. The footnote also includes daily values for nutrients to limit (total fat, saturated fat, trans fat, and sodium), recommended carbohydrate intake for a 2,000-calorie diet (60% of calories), and minimal fiber recommendations for 2,000- and 2,500-calorie diets.

Legislation also requires food manufacturers to list all potential food **allergens** on food packaging. The most common food allergens are fish, shellfish, soybean, wheat, eggs, milk, peanuts, and tree nuts. This information is included below the list of ingredients on the package. Note that the ingredient list is in decreasing order of substance weight in the product. That is, the ingredients that are listed first are the most abundant ingredients in the product. Health coaches can teach people to avoid foods with sugar, high-fructose corn syrup, bleached flour, or partially hydrogenated oils near the top of the ingredient list.

While the nutrition facts label is found on the side or the back of products, other health and nutrition claims are often visibly displayed on the front of the package. The Food and Drug Administration regulates these claims, which usually meet strict criteria. However, a loophole allowing **qualified health claims** has paved the way for manufacturers to claim unproven benefits to products, as long as the label states the claim is supported by very little scientific evidence (Table 7-2).

Table 7-2

Nutrient Content Claims

REQUIREMENTS FOR HEALTH CLAIMS

According to government requirements, foods must meet three criteria to carry a health claim:

- Not exceed specific levels for total fat, saturated fat, cholesterol, and sodium. These are the main nutrients that health professionals suggest consumers limit in their daily diets.
- Contain at least 10% of the daily value, before supplementation, for any one or all of the following: protein, dietary fiber, vitamin A, vitamin C, calcium, and iron. These are the nutrients that health professionals suggest consumers get adequate amounts of in their daily diets.
- Meet nutrient levels that are specific for each approved health claim.

ALLOWABLE HEALTH CLAIMS

Calcium and osteoporosis

The food or supplement must be "high" in calcium and must not contain more phosphorus than calcium. Claims must cite other risk factors; state the need for regular exercise and a healthful diet; explain that adequate calcium early in life helps reduce fracture risk later by increasing as much as genetically possible a person's peak bone mass; and indicate that those at greatest risk of developing osteoporosis later in life are white and Asian teenage and young adult women, who are in their bone-forming years. Claims for products with more than 400 mg of calcium per day must state that a daily intake over 2,000 mg offers no added known benefit to bone health.

Sodium and hypertension (high blood pressure)

Foods must meet criteria for "low sodium." Claims must use "sodium" and "high blood pressure" in discussing the nutrient-disease link.

Dietary fat and cancer

Foods must meet criteria for "low fat." Fish and game meats must meet criteria for "extra lean." Claims may not mention specific types of fats and must use "total fat" or "fat" and "some types of cancer" or "some cancers" in discussing the nutrient-disease link.

Dietary saturated fat and cholesterol and risk of coronary heart disease

Foods must meet criteria for "low saturated fat," "low cholesterol," and "low fat." Fish and game meats must meet criteria for "extra lean." Claims must use "saturated fat and cholesterol" and "coronary heart disease" or "heart disease" in discussing the nutrient-disease link.

Fiber-containing grain products, fruits, and vegetables and cancer

Foods must meet criteria for "low fat" and, without fortification, be a "good source" of dietary fiber. Claims must not specify types of fiber and must use "fiber," "dietary fiber," or "total dietary fiber" and "some types of cancer" or "some cancers" in discussing the nutrient-disease link.

Fruits, vegetables, and grain products that contain fiber, particularly soluble fiber, and risk of coronary heart disease

Foods must meet criteria for "low saturated fat," "low fat," and "low cholesterol." They must contain, without fortification, at least 0.6 g of soluble fiber per reference amount, and the soluble fiber content must be listed. Claims must use "fiber," "dietary fiber," "some types of dietary fiber," "some dietary fibers," or "some fibers" and "coronary heart disease" or "heart disease" in discussing the nutrient-disease link. The term "soluble fiber" may be added.

Fruits and vegetables and cancer

Foods must meet criteria for "low fat" and, without fortification, be a "good source" of fiber, vitamin A , or vitamin C. Claims must characterize fruits and vegetables as foods that are low in fat and may contain dietary fiber, vitamin A, or vitamin C; characterize the food itself as a "good source" of one or more of these nutrients, which must be listed; refrain from specifying types of fatty acids; and use "total fat" or "fat," "some types of cancer" or "some cancers," and "fiber," "dietary fiber," or "total dietary fiber" in discussing the nutrient-disease link.

Folate and neural tube birth defects

Foods must meet or exceed criteria for "good source" of folate—that is, at least 40µg of folic acid per serving (at least 10% of the Daily Value). A serving of food cannot contain more than 100% of the Daily Value for vitamin A and vitamin D because of their potential risk to fetuses. Claims must use "folate," "folic acid," or "folacin" and "neural tube defects," "birth defects spina bifida or anencephaly," "birth defects of the brain or spinal cord, anencephaly or spina bifida," "spina bifida and anencephaly, birth defects of the brain or spinal cord," "birth defects of the brain and spinal cord," or "brain or spinal cord birth defects" in discussing the nutrient-disease link. Folic acid content must be listed on the Nutrition Facts panel.

Dietary sugar alcohol and dental caries (cavities)

Foods must meet the criteria for "sugar free." The sugar alcohol must be xylitol, sorbitol, mannitol, maltitol, isomalt, lactitol, hydrogenated starch hydrolysates, hydrogenated glucose syrups, erythritol, or a combination of these. When the food contains a fermentable carbohydrate, such as sugar or flour, the food must not lower plaque pH in the mouth below 5.7 while it is being eaten or up to 30 minutes afterwards. Claims must use "sugar alcohol," "sugar alcohols," or the name(s) of the sugar alcohol present and "dental caries" or "tooth decay" in discussing the nutrient-disease link. Claims must state that the sugar alcohol present "does not promote," "may reduce the risk of," "is useful in not promoting," or "is expressly for not promoting" dental caries.

Dietary soluble fiber, such as that found in whole oats and psyllium seed husk, and coronary heart disease

Foods must meet criteria for "low saturated fat," "low cholesterol," and "low fat." Foods that contain whole oats must contain at least 0.75 g of soluble fiber per serving. Foods that contain psyllium seed husk must contain at least 1.7 g of soluble fiber per serving. The claim must specify the daily dietary intake of the soluble fiber source necessary to reduce the risk of heart disease and the contribution one serving of the product makes toward that intake level. Soluble fiber content must be stated on the nutrition label. Claims must use "soluble fiber" qualified by the name of the eligible source of soluble fiber and "heart disease" or "coronary heart disease" in discussing the nutrient-disease link. Because of the potential hazard of choking, foods containing dry or incompletely hydrated psyllium seed husk must carry a label statement telling consumers to drink adequate amounts of fluid, unless the manufacturer shows that a viscous adhesive mass is not formed when the food is exposed to fluid.

Source: Food and Drug Administration

DO THE MATH

Nutrition Facts Label Sample Problem

Using the nutrition facts label from Figure 7-2, determine (1) the number of calories per container; (2) the calories from carbohydrate, protein, and fat per serving; and (3) the percentage of calories from carbohydrate, protein, and fat.

1. 90 calories per serving x 4 servings per container = 360 calories per container
2. *Carbohydrate:* 13 grams carbohydrate per serving x 4 calories per gram = 52 calories per serving from carbohydrate
   Protein: 3 grams protein per serving x 4 calories per gram = 12 calories per serving from protein
   Fat: 3 grams fat per serving x 9 calories per gram = 27 calories per serving from fat
   [*Note:* The nutrition facts label does this calculation for you and lists the calories from fat on the label. On this label, it states that the product contains the rounded number 30 calories from fat vs. the calculated 27 calories from fat. Also note that the total calories for this food is 91 per the calculations (52 + 12 + 27), but the label rounds to 90.]
3. *Carbohydrate:* 52 calories from carbohydrate/91 calories = 57% carbohydrate
   Protein: 12 calories from protein/91 calories = 13% protein
   Fat: 27 calories from fat/91 calories = 30% fat

Food Safety and Selection

An important but often underestimated key to healthy eating is to avoid foods contaminated with harmful bacteria, viruses, parasites, and other microorganisms. About one in six Americans, or 48 million people, become sick each year from foodborne illness; 128,000 are hospitalized and approximately 3,000 die [Centers for Disease Control and Prevention (CDC), 2011a]. Special populations most at-risk include pregnant women, infants and young children, older adults, and people who are immunocompromised. The majority of foodborne illnesses are preventable with a few simple precautions (Table 7-3). Refer to www.fightbac.org, www.foodsafety.gov, or www.cdc.gov/foodsafety for more information.

Table 7-3
Steps to Safe Food Handling
To avoid microbial foodborne illness: • Clean hands, food contact surfaces, and fruits and vegetables. Meat and poultry should not be washed or rinsed. • Separate raw, cooked, and ready-to-eat foods while shopping, preparing, or storing foods. • Cook foods to a safe temperature to kill microorganisms [bacteria grow most rapidly between the temperatures of 40 and 140° F (4 and 60° C)]. Pregnant women should only eat certain deli meats and frankfurters that have been reheated to steaming hot. • Refrigerate perishable food promptly (within two hours) and defrost foods properly. Eat refrigerated leftovers within three or four days. • Avoid raw (unpasteurized) milk or any products made from unpasteurized milk, raw or partially cooked eggs, or foods containing raw eggs, raw or undercooked meat and poultry, unpasteurized juice, and raw sprouts. This is especially important for infants and young children, pregnant women, older adults, and those who are immunocompromised.

Reprinted from U.S. Department of Agriculture (2015). *2015-2020 Dietary Guidelines for Americans* (8th ed.). www.health.gov/dietaryguidelines

Advise clients to follow these tips while grocery shopping to reduce the risk of foodborne illnesses:

- Check produce for bruises, and feel and smell for ripeness.
- Look for a sell-by date for breads and baked goods, a use-by date on some packaged foods, an expiration date on yeast and baking powder, and a packaged date on canned and some packaged foods.
- Make sure packaged goods are not torn and cans are not dented, cracked, or bulging.
- Separate fish and poultry from other purchases by wrapping them separately in plastic bags.
- Pick up refrigerated and frozen foods last. Try to make sure all perishable items are refrigerated within one hour of purchase .

Nutrition and Hydration for Sports and Fitness

Optimal nutrition and hydration and athletic performance go hand in hand. Clients not only can optimize their health, but also improve their performance in a given sport or activity by following a few basic sports nutrition principles. Active adults require conscientious fueling and refueling to maintain optimal performance and overall health.

Determining Caloric Needs

Nutrition recommendations can be tailored to individual clients by determining their daily energy needs. For healthy adults, the most accurate estimation of **resting metabolic rate (RMR),** an approximation of the energy expended at rest each day, is the Mifflin-St. Jeor equation (Frankenfield, Routh-Yousey, & Compher, 2005):

For men: RMR = 9.99 x wt (kg) + 6.25 x ht (cm) – 4.92 x age (yrs) + 5

For women: RMR = 9.99 x wt (kg) + 6.25 x ht (cm) – 4.92 x age (yrs) – 161

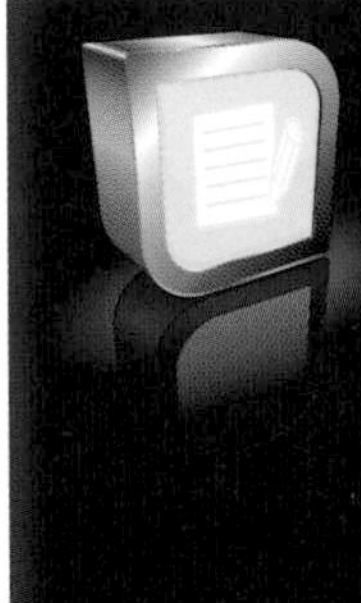

DO THE MATH

Moderately active people are generally advised to consume about 1.5 to 1.7 times the calculated RMR (Rodriguez, Di Marco, & Langley, 2009). For example, a 30-year-old female who is 5'6" (1.7 m), weighs 145 pounds (66 kg), and engages in 40 to 60 minutes of vigorous physical activity most days of the week would need approximately 2,200 calories per day for weight maintenance:

RMR = 9.99 x 66 kg + 6.25 x 170 cm – 4.92 x 30 – 161
= 659 + 1,063 – 148 – 161
= 1,413

Multiply by 1.5 to 1.7 = 2,120 to 2,402 calories per day

Once a client has determined the appropriate total number of calories to consume per day to maintain weight, together with a health coach, the client should determine performance and weight-management goals. Chapter 8 describes weight-management principles in detail, but in short, in order to burn 1 pound (0.45 kg) of fat, a client needs to create a 3,500-calorie deficit. This can come from increased energy expenditure through physical activity, decreased caloric intake through dietary changes, or both. Very active athletes may have opposite concerns, in which they need to make a focused effort to consume an adequate number of calories to fuel particularly prolonged or intense activity.

Daily caloric intake should be apportioned to carbohydrate, protein, and fat. The DRIs recommend that approximately 45 to 65% of calories come from carbohydrates, 10 to 35% from protein, and 20 to 35% from fats (IOM, 2005). Although active individuals require ample carbohydrates to maintain blood glucose during exercise and replace muscle **glycogen** expended during exercise, as well as increased protein for muscle repair, research suggests that active individuals do not need a greater *percentage* of calories from carbohydrate or protein than the average population. However, they are able meet increased nutrition demands via a greater overall caloric intake (Rodriguez, Di Marco, & Langley, 2009).

Carbohydrates and Sports Nutrition

The EAR for carbohydrates is 100 grams (about seven servings) for children and nonpregnant, non-lactating adults; 135 grams (about nine servings) for pregnant women; and 160 grams (about 11 servings) for lactating women. The American Dietetic Association (ADA) and the American College of Sports Medicine (ACSM) recommend that athletes consume 3 to 5 g/lb (6 to 10 g/kg) of body weight per day depending on their total daily energy expenditure, type of exercise performed, gender, and environmental conditions to maintain blood glucose levels during exercise and to replace depleted muscle glycogen (Rodriguez, Di Marco, & Langley, 2009).

In January 2012, the American Dietetic Association (ADA) changed its name to the Academy of Nutrition and Dietetics (A.N.D.). Throughout this text, research conducted by the organization prior to this name change is cited to the ADA, while newer studies will be credited to the A.N.D. Refer to www.eatright.org for more information on the reasons behind the name change.

Carbohydrate Loading

Individuals training for long-distance endurance events lasting more than 90 minutes, such as a marathon or triathlon, may benefit from **carbohydrate loading** in the days or weeks prior to competition. Eating more carbohydrates helps muscles store more carbohydrates in the form of glycogen. If more glycogen is stored, it will take longer to deplete the body's preferred energy source during a prolonged workout. This effort to maximize available glycogen on race day is the same reason that fitness professionals advise people to taper their workout duration as they approach an event. Health coaches may warn clients who are carbohydrate loading that they may gain a few pounds because carbohydrates require water for storage. Those individuals who are serious about optimizing sports performance may consider a consultation with a sports nutritionist to help them adopt the most appropriate dietary plan and carbohydrate-loading regimen.

While various carbohydrate-loading regimens exist, the following is a one-week sample plan:

- *Days 1–3:* Moderate-carbohydrate diet (50% of calories)
- *Days 4–6:* High-carbohydrate diet (80% of calories). This equates to about 4.5 grams of carbohydrate per pound (0.45 kg) of body weight. For a 170-lb (77.2-kg) man, that is 765 grams, or a whopping 3,000 calories from carbohydrates per day.
- *Day 7—Competitive event:* Pre-event meal (typically dinner the night before the event) with >80% of calories from carbohydrates

THINK IT THROUGH

One of your regular clients, Jamie, is a physically active college student. She performs the following workouts consistently each week:

- Running on a treadmill at 70% heart-rate reserve for 30 minutes on Monday, Wednesday, and Friday
- Lifting weights at a moderate intensity for all the major muscle groups on Tuesday, Thursday, and Saturday

One of Jamie's friends is a marathon runner and recently underwent a carbohydrate loading program to prepare for a race. While Jamie has no desire to run in endurance competitions, she is curious about the potential for carbohydrate loading to help her with her current training program. What would your advice to Jamie be regarding carbohydrate loading for the type of training program in which she currently engages?

Glycemic Index

As far as refueling goes, not all carbohydrates are created equal. Historically, much debate has centered on whether consumption of simple or complex carbohydrates is better for athletic performance. The role of a particular carbohydrate in athletic performance may be better determined by its **glycemic index (GI)** than its structure (i.e., whether it is simple or complex). GI ranks carbohydrates based on their blood glucose response. High-GI foods break down rapidly, causing a large glucose spike; low-GI foods are digested more slowly and cause a smaller increase in blood glucose (Table 7-4). **Glycemic load (GL)** accounts for GI as well as the amount of carbohydrate being consumed (GL = GI x grams of carbohydrate/100).

Table 7-4

Glycemic Index (GI) of Various Foods

High GI ≥70	Medium GI 56–69	Low GI ≤55
White bread	Rye bread	Pumpernickel bread
Corn Flakes®	Shredded Wheat®	All Bran®
Graham crackers	Ice cream	Plain yogurt
Dried fruit	Blueberries	Strawberries
Instant white rice	Refined pasta	Oatmeal

The role of glycemic index in exercise performance has been a source of ongoing research for the past two decades. Initial studies suggested that a low-GI diet prior to exercise improves performance. While this still seems to be true, further research found that this benefit is negated as soon as a carbohydrate-containing sports drink, gel, or bar is consumed during an exercise session (O'Reilly, Wong, & Chen, 2010). It seems logical that a high-GI diet would be more effective at replenishing glycogen stores after exercise. After all, carbohydrates with a high glycemic index, such as pancakes and bananas, are more rapidly absorbed and more quickly release sugar into the bloodstream. Thus, they should be more effective at replenishing energy stores than low-GI foods, which are broken down more slowly and take longer to release sugar into the bloodstream. While an early body of research supported this supposition, more recent studies have found that low-GI foods eaten before exercise may contribute to increased performance by increasing the availability of nonessential fatty acids during an exercise session (Stevenson et al., 2009; Trenell et al., 2008). Overall, despite years of research on the glycemic index and endurance performance, the jury is still out as to how glycemic index affects performance. In regards to overall health, several high-quality studies suggest that a low-GI eating plan may be better for weight loss and improvement in cholesterol levels (Thomas, Elliott, & Baur, 2007) and for people with diabetes (Brand-Miller et al., 2003).

Protein and Sports Nutrition

While low-carbohydrate/high-protein diets, such as the Atkins® or South Beach® plans, are no longer the hottest trend, "high-protein" diets (i.e., diets that contain a greater percentage of calories from protein than the standard 15 to 20%) seem to be just as good as, if not better than, high-carbohydrate diets for weight loss and health benefits (Gardner et al., 2007; Dansinger et al., 2005; Foster et al., 2003). A high-protein diet can even help optimize athletic performance (and muscle strengthening) due to the important role of protein in both endurance and resistance-training exercise. The two modes of exercise stimulate muscle protein synthesis, which is further enhanced if protein is consumed around the time of the physical activity. Eating protein immediately after exercising helps in the repair and synthesis of muscle proteins. Protein intake during exercise probably does not offer any additional performance benefit if sufficient amounts of carbohydrate—the body's preferred energy source—are consumed. However, for endurance athletes who need to consume adequate calories to fuel extended training sessions, or for any exerciser striving to lose weight, protein can help preserve lean muscle mass and ensure that most weight loss comes from fat rather than lean tissue.

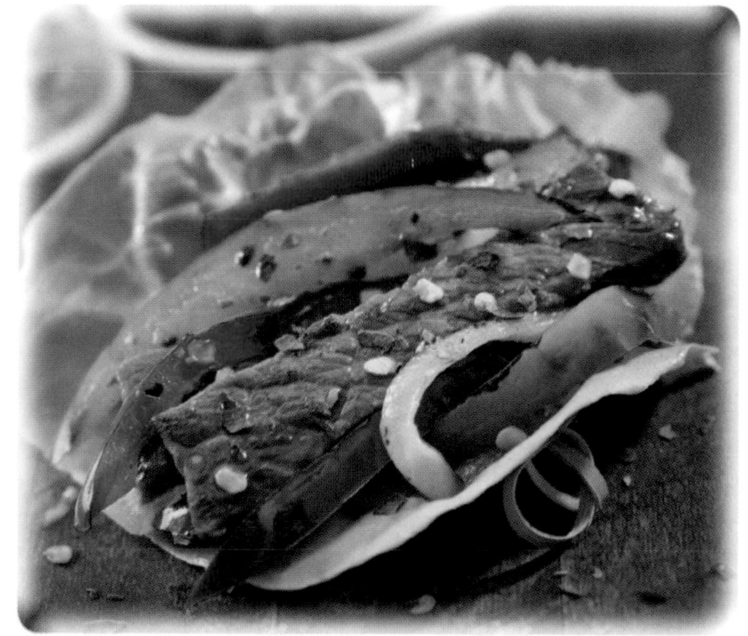

The average person requires 0.8 to 1.0 g/kg of body weight per day (0.4 to 0.5 g/lb). Athletes need anywhere from 1.2 to 1.7g/kg (0.5 to 0.8 g/lb) depending on gender, age, and type and intensity of the exercise (less for endurance athletes and more for strength-trained athletes) (Rodriguez, Di Marco, & Langley, 2009). Clients can ensure adequate protein consumption if recommendations are based on the **Acceptable Macronutrient Distribution Range (AMDR)** of 10 to 35% of daily energy intake (Wolfe & Miller, 2008; IOM, 2005). Table 7-5 shows the total protein intake at various levels of energy intake within the AMDR for protein.

Table 7-5				
Protein Intake (grams) at Various Levels of Energy Intake				
Energy intake (kcal/d)	Low-protein diet (<10% kcal)	Average diet (~15% kcal)	High-protein diet (≥20% kcal)	Very-high protein diet (≥30% kcal)
1,200	30	45	60	90
2,000	50	75	100	150
3,000	75	112	150	225

Note: Each gram of protein contains 4 calories.

Reprinted with permission from the American Heart Association, Inc.; St. Jeor, S.T. et al. (2001). Dietary protein and weight reduction: A statement for healthcare professionals from the nutrition committee of the Council on Nutrition, Physical Activity, and Metabolism of the American Heart Association. *Circulation,* 104, 1869-1874.

AND emphasizes that the recommended protein intakes are best met through diet, though many athletes do turn to **whey**- or **casein**-based protein powders and other supplements to boost protein intake and muscle regeneration (Rodriguez, Di Marco, & Langley, 2009).

ACE Position Statement on Nutritional Supplements

It is the position of the American Council on Exercise (ACE) that it is outside the defined scope of practice of a fitness professional to recommend, prescribe, sell, or supply nutritional supplements to clients. Recommending supplements without possessing the requisite qualifications [registered dietitian (R.D.)] can place the client's health at risk and possibly expose the fitness professional to disciplinary action and litigation. If a client wants to take supplements, a fitness professional should work in conjunction with a qualified R.D. or medical doctor to provide safe and effective nutritional education and recommendations.

ACE recognizes that some fitness and health clubs encourage or require their employees to sell nutritional supplements. If this is a condition of employment, fitness professionals should protect themselves by ensuring their employers possess adequate insurance coverage for them should a problem arise. Furthermore, ACE strongly encourages continuing education on diet and nutrition for all fitness professionals.

Several factors come into play when choosing the "best" type of protein, including protein quality, health benefits, dietary restrictions, cost, convenience, and taste. While no one type of protein is best for everyone, keep these considerations in mind:

- *Protein quality varies.* Similar to lean meats, poultry, and fish, whey, casein, egg, and soy contain all of the **essential amino acids** in amounts proportional to need and are easily digested and absorbed. Fruits, vegetables, grains, and nuts are incomplete proteins and must be combined throughout the day to ensure adequate intake of each of the essential amino acids.
- *Different types of proteins are better at different times.* Many athletes consume the milk proteins whey and casein in an effort to maximize muscle building. Whey protein—the

liquid remaining after milk has been curdled and strained—is rapidly digested, resulting in a short burst of amino acids into the bloodstream. Whey is known for its ability to stimulate muscle protein synthesis, even more so than casein and soy. Casein—the protein that gives milk its white color and accounts for the majority of milk protein—is slowly digested, resulting in a more prolonged release of amino acids lasting up to hours. If the goal is for amino acids to be readily available for muscle regeneration immediately following a workout, an athlete may consider timing protein intake accordingly to best maximize muscle building and repair (e.g., in theory, consuming casein-based proteins prior to exercise and whey-based proteins during and immediately following exercise should enhance performance, though the efficacy of this approach has not been confirmed.)

- *More is not always better.* Total daily protein intake should not be excessive. Protein consumption beyond recommended amounts is unlikely to result in further muscle gains because the body has a limited capacity to use amino acids to build muscle.

Ultimately, the jury is still out on the best amounts, mechanisms, and methods of protein intake. However, it seems that when combined with regular exercise and an overall healthy lifestyle, protein can help clients gain muscle, lose weight, and improve overall health.

Fats and Sports Nutrition

Fat is an important source of energy, fat-soluble vitamins, and essential fatty acids. Athletes should consume a comparable proportion of food from fat as the general population—that is, 20 to 25% of total calories. There is no evidence for performance benefit from a very low-fat diet (<15% of total calories) or from a high-fat diet (Rodriguez, Di Marco, & Langley, 2009). A complete discussion of the role of fat in maintaining optimal health and fat's impact on blood lipids is presented in Chapter 6.

Fueling Before, During, and After Exercise

Athletes need the right types and amounts of food before, during, and after exercise to maximize the amount of energy available to fuel optimal performance and minimize the amount of gastrointestinal distress. Sports nutrition strategies should address three exercise stages: pre-exercise, exercise, and post-exercise (Figure 7-3).

Figure 7-3
Sports nutrition strategies

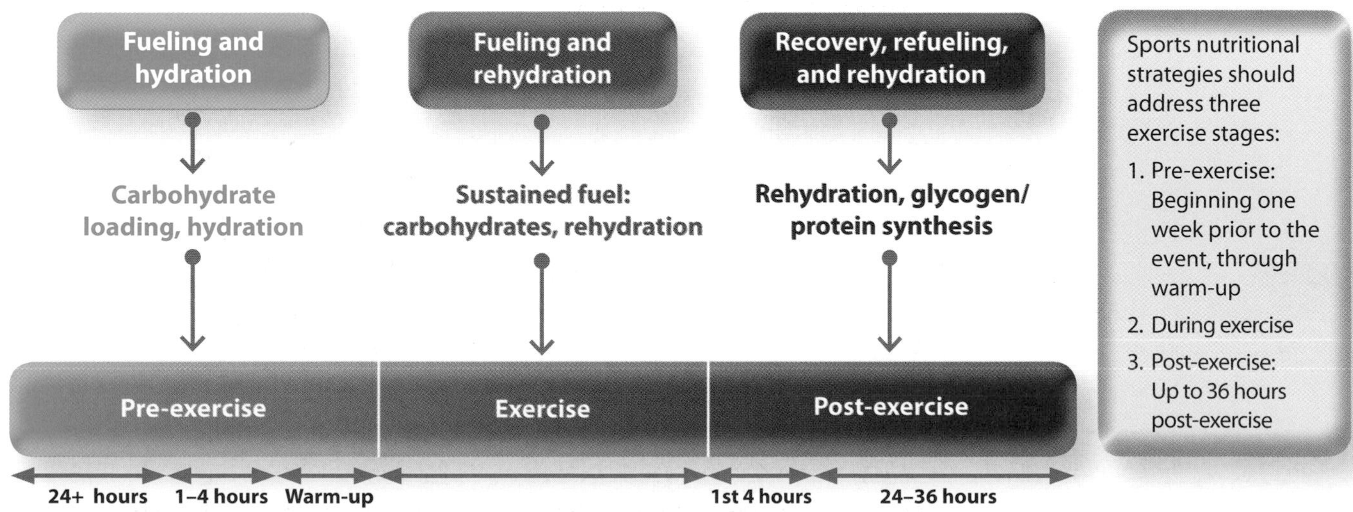

Pre-exercise

The two main goals of a pre-exercise snack are to optimize glucose availability and glycogen stores and provide the fuel needed for exercise performance. Keeping this in mind, in the days up to a week before a strenuous endurance effort, an athlete should consider what nutritional strategies might set the stage for optimal performance. For example, an athlete preparing for a long endurance event might consider the pros and cons of carbohydrate loading. On the day of the event or an important training session, the athlete should aim to eat a meal about four to six hours prior to the workout to minimize gastrointestinal distress and optimize performance. Four hours after eating, the food will already have been digested and absorbed; now liver and muscle glycogen levels are at their highest. To translate this into an everyday, practical recommendation, athletes who work out in the early afternoon should be certain to eat a wholesome carbohydrate-rich breakfast. Those who exercise in the early morning may benefit from a carbohydrate-rich snack before going to bed.

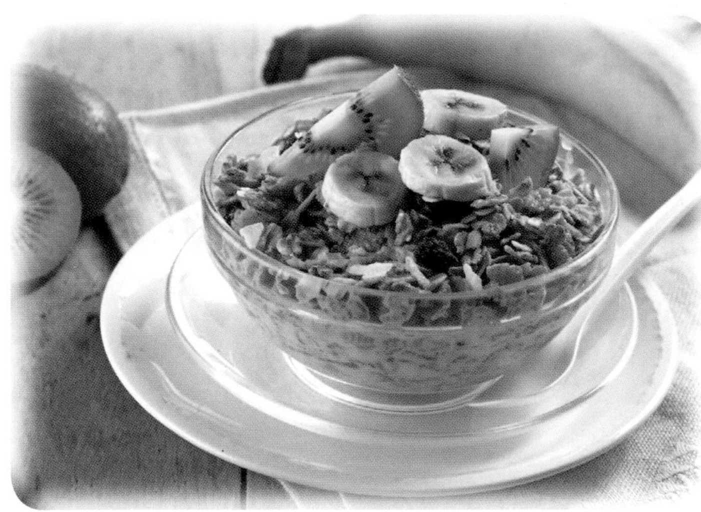

Some research also suggests that eating a relatively small carbohydrate- and protein-containing snack (e.g. 50 grams of carbohydrate and 5 to 10 grams of protein) 30 to 60 minutes before exercise helps increase glucose availability near the end of the workout and help to decrease exercise-induced protein catabolism (Kreider et al., 2010). The exact timing and size of the snack for peak performance will vary by athlete. As a general rule, athletes should try out any snacks or drinks with practice sessions prior to relying on them to help optimize athletic performance on the day of the event. In general, a pre-exercise meal or snack should be:

- Relatively high in carbohydrate to maximize blood glucose availability
- Relatively low in fat and fiber to minimize gastrointestinal distress and facilitate **gastric emptying**
- Moderate in protein
- Well-tolerated by the individual

Fueling During Exercise

The goal of fueling during exercise is to provide the body with the essential nutrients needed by muscle cells to maintain optimal blood glucose levels. During a prolonged endurance effort, such as a marathon, an athlete is at risk of "hitting the wall"—a phenomena often occurring around mile 20. This is when extreme fatigue sets in due to drained fuel stores. However, there are gradations on the physical demands of exercise based on the duration of the exercise session. Exercise lasting less than one hour can be adequately fueled with existing glucose and glycogen stores. No additional carbohydrate-containing drinks or foods are necessary. When exercise lasts longer than one hour, blood glucose levels begin to dwindle. After one to three hours of continuous moderate-intensity exercise (65 to 80% $\mathbf{\dot{V}O_2max}$), muscle glycogen stores may become depleted. If no glucose is consumed, blood glucose levels drop, resulting in further depletion of muscle glycogen. When this happens, regardless of the athlete's internal toughness or desire to maintain intensity, performance falters.

To maintain a ready energy supply during prolonged exercise sessions (>60 minutes), athletes should consume glucose-containing beverages and snacks. Athletes should consume 30 to 60 grams of carbohydrate per hour of training (Rodriguez, Di Marco, & Langley, 2009). This is especially important for prolonged exercise and exercise in extreme heat, cold, or high altitude; for athletes who did not consume adequate amounts of food or drink prior to the training session; and for athletes who did not carbohydrate load or who restricted energy intake for weight loss.

Carbohydrate consumption during prolonged exercise should begin shortly after the initiation of the workout. The carbohydrate will be more effective if the 30 to 60 grams per hour are consumed in small amounts in 15 to 20 minute intervals rather than as a large meal after two hours of exercise (Rodriguez, Di Marco, & Langley, 2009). Some believe that adding protein to carbohydrate during exercise will help to improve performance, but to date, the evidence is inconclusive.

Post-exercise Replenishment

The main goal of post-exercise fueling is to replenish glycogen stores and facilitate muscle repair. The average client training at moderate intensities every few days does not need any aggressive post-exercise replenishment. Normal dietary practices following exercise will facilitate recovery within 24 to 48 hours. Athletes following vigorous training regimens, especially those who will participate in multiple training sessions in a single day (like a triathlete), can benefit from strategic refueling. Studies show that the best post-workout meals include mostly carbohydrates accompanied by some protein (Kreider et al., 2010). Refueling should begin within 30 minutes after exercise and be followed by a high-carbohydrate meal within two hours (Kreider et al., 2010). The carbohydrates replenish the depleted energy that is normally stored as glycogen in muscle and liver. The protein helps to rebuild the muscles that were fatigued with exercise. A carbohydrate intake of 1.5g/kg of body weight is recommended in the first 30 minutes after exercise and then every two hours for four to six hours (Rodriguez, Di Marco, & Langley, 2009). After that, the athlete can resume his or her typical, balanced diet. Of course, the amount of refueling necessary depends on the intensity and duration of the training session. A long-duration, low-intensity workout may not require such vigorous replenishment.

Post-workout Snack and Meal Ideas

In the several hours following a prolonged and strenuous workout, consuming snacks and meals high in carbohydrates with some protein can set the stage for optimal glycogen replenishment and subsequent performance. Here are a few snack and meal ideas that fit the bill:

- *Snack 1:* In the first several minutes after exercise, consume 16 oz of Gatorade™ or other sports drink, a power gel such as a Clif Shot™ or GU™, and a medium banana. This quickly begins to replenish muscle glycogen stores. *Carbohydrates: 73 g; Protein: 1 g; Calories: 290*
- *Snack 2:* After cooling down and showering, grab another quick snack such as 12 oz of orange juice and ¼ cup of raisins. *Carbohydrates: 70 g; Protein 3 g; Calories: 295*

- *Small meal appetizer:* Enjoy a spinach salad with tomatoes, chickpeas, green beans, and tuna and a whole-grain baguette. *Carbohydrates: 70 g; Protein: 37 g; Calories: 489*
- *Small meal main course:* Replenish with whole-grain pasta with diced tomatoes. *Carbohydrates: 67 g; Protein: 2 g; Calories: 292*
- *Dessert:* After allowing ample time for the day's snacks and meals to digest, finish your refueling program with one cup of frozen yogurt and berries. *Carbohydrates: 61 g; Protein: 8 g; Calories: 280*

Hydration Before, During, and After Exercise

When it comes to fluid balance during exercise, it seems like the proverbial double-edged sword: Drinking too little can lead to **dehydration**—a scary condition exercisers have been cautioned against in every text, handout, and presentation on fluid replacement. But drinking too much—out of fear of not drinking enough—could lead to **hyponatremia,** a condition less well known and understood, but equally frightening. Here is the good news: The body is very good at handling and normalizing large variations in fluid intake. For this reason, severe hyponatremia and dehydration are rare and generally affect very specific high-risk populations, such as lighter-weight women in the case of hyponatremia and athletes with higher than average sweat rates in the case of dehydration, during specific types of activities (such as extended endurance activities like a marathon or intense activity in very humid conditions). Both conditions are highly preventable. To prevent dehydration and hyponatremia, the goal is to drink just the right amount of fluid before, during, and after exercise to maintain a state of **euhydration,** which is a state of "normal" body water content—the perfect balance between "too much" and "not enough" fluid intake. Athletes can estimate hydration status by monitoring the color of urine. Euhydration is when urine is light-yellow tinged. Very clear urine may indicate overhydration, while intensely yellow urine is a sign of dehydration.

Hydration Prior to Exercise

Most people begin exercise euhydrated with little need for a rigorous prehydration regimen. However, if fewer than eight to 12 hours have passed since the last intense training session or fluid intake has been inadequate, the athlete may benefit from a prehydration program.

An athlete should begin prehydrating about four hours prior to the exercise session. The athlete should aim to slowly consume about 5 to 7 mL (0.17 to 0.24 oz) of fluid per 1 kg (2.2 lb) of body weight. If after two hours of prehydration no urine is produced or if the urine is dark, the individual should aim to drink an additional 3 to 5 mL (0.10 to 0.17 oz) of fluid per 1 kg (2.2 lb) of body weight two hours before the event. Drinking fluid that contains 20 to 50 milliequivalents/liter (mEq/L) (460 to 1150 mg/L) of sodium or consuming salt-containing snacks at this time helps stimulate thirst and retain the consumed fluids (Sawka et al., 2007). Some athletes may try to hyperhydrate with glycerol-containing solutions that act to expand the extra- and intracellular spaces. While glycerol may be advantageous for certain athletes who meet specific criteria, glycerol is unlikely to be advantageous for athletes who will experience no to mild dehydration during exercise (loss of <2% body weight) and glycerol use may in fact contribute to increased risk of dilutional hyponatremia (van Rosendal et al., 2010).

Hydration During Exercise

The goal of fluid intake during exercise is to prevent performance-diminishing or health-altering effects from dehydration or hyponatremia. Health coaches can share the following guidelines with clients:

- *Aim for a 1:1 fluid replacement to fluid loss ratio.* Ideally, exercisers should consume the same amount of fluid as they lose in sweat. An easy way to assess post-exercise hydration is to compare pre- and post-exercise body weight. Perfect hydration has been accomplished when no weight is lost or gained during exercise. The goal is to avoid weight loss greater than 2%. There is no one-size-fits-all recommendation, though the ACSM position stand suggests that if determining individual needs is not feasible, athletes could consider aiming for a 0.4 to 0.8 L/h (8 to 16 oz/h) replenishment, with the higher rate for faster, heavier athletes in a hot and humid environment and the lower rate for slower, lighter athletes in a cool environment (Sawka et al., 2007). Because people sweat at varying rates and exercise at different intensities, this range may not be appropriate for everyone. However, when individual assessment is not possible, this recommendation works for most people.
- *Drink fluids with sodium during prolonged exercise sessions.* If an exercise session lasts longer than two hours or an athlete is participating in an event that stimulates heavy sodium loss (defined as more than 3 to 4 grams of sodium), then the athlete should consider consuming a sports drink that contains elevated levels of sodium. In one study, researchers did not find a benefit from sports drinks that contain only the 18 mmol/L (or 100 milligrams per 8 oz) of sodium typical of most sports drinks and thus concluded that higher levels would be needed to prevent hyponatremia during prolonged exercise (Almond et al., 2005). The IOM recommends that people exercising for prolonged periods in hot environments consume sports drinks that contain 20 to 30 mEq/L (450 to 700 mg/L) of sodium to stimulate thirst and replace sweat losses and 2 to 5 mEq/L (80 to 200 mg/L) of potassium to replace sweat losses (IOM, 2004). See Table 7-6 for the sodium content of some popular drinks. Alternatively, exercisers can consume extra sodium with meals and snacks prior to a lengthy exercise session or a day of extensive physical activity. Additional sodium or supplementation

Table 7-6

Evaluating Sports Drinks

Drink	Serving Size (oz)	Calories (kcal)	Sodium (mg)	Carbohydrate (g)	Carbohydrate Concentration (%)
Gatorade™	8	50	110	14	6
Gatorade Endurance™ Formula™	8	50	200	14	6
Powerade™	8	70	55	19	8
Ultima™	8	12.5	37	3	1
Power Bar Endurance™	8	70	160	17	7
Propel™	8	10	10	3	1
Zico™ coconut water	8	34	91	7.4	3

with salt tablets seems to be unnecessary based on the limited research to date on this topic (Hew-Butler et al., 2006; Speedy et al., 2002).

- *Drink carbohydrate-containing sports drinks to reduce fatigue*. Athletes exercising for longer than one hour should also consume carbohydrate with fluids. With prolonged exercise, muscle glycogen stores become depleted and blood glucose becomes a primary fuel source. To maintain performance levels and prevent fatigue, athletes should choose drinks and snacks that provide about 30 to 60 grams of rapidly absorbed carbohydrate for every hour of training. As long as the carbohydrate concentration is less than about 6 to 8%, it will have little effect on gastric emptying (Rodriguez, Di Marco, & Langley, 2009).

Sports drinks play an important role in replenishing fluids, glucose, and sodium lost during exercise lasting more than one hour. Although sports drinks may not completely protect against hyponatremia, they serve an important purpose in endurance exercise.

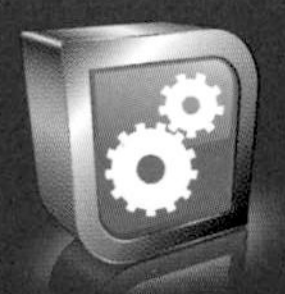

EXPAND YOUR KNOWLEDGE

Myth: Drinking Fluids Before and During Exercise Causes Gastrointestinal Distress

Logic: Since blood flow is diverted away from the gastrointestinal system during exercise, fluids consumed before or during exercise will just slosh around in the stomach during the workout.

The science: It is true that gastric emptying, or the speed with which the stomach empties its contents into the small intestine, slows down during exercise. This is largely because exercise-induced sympathetic stimulation diverts blood flow from the gastrointestinal (GI) system to the heart, lungs, and working muscles. As a result, athletes sometimes experience stomach cramps along with a variety of other uncomfortable GI issues such as reflux, heartburn, bloating, gas, nausea, vomiting, the urge to defecate, and diarrhea. It turns out that good hydration with the right fluids can help *increase* gastric emptying and lead to reduced GI problems with exercise. Gastric emptying is maximized when the amount of fluid in the stomach is high. On the other hand, high-intensity exercise (>70% $\dot{V}O_2$max), dehydration, hyperthermia, and consumption of high-energy, (>7% carbohydrate) hypertonic drinks (like juices and some soft drinks) slow gastric emptying.

Health coaches can recommend the following practical tips to prepare the gut for competition:

- Get acclimatized to heat.
- Stay hydrated.
- Practice drinking during training to improve event-day comfort.
- Avoid overnutrition before and during exercise.
- Avoid high-energy, hypertonic food (e.g., sugary candy) and drinks (e.g., fruit juice) before (within 30 to 60 minutes) exercise. Hypertonic food and drinks have greater than 8% of weight from carbohydrates. The high carbohydrate content pulls water into the intestine for digestion, which slows digestion and can cause cramping and gastrointestinal distress. Limit protein and fat intake before exercise.
- Ingest a high-energy, high-carbohydrate diet.
- Avoid high-fiber foods before exercise.
- Limit **nonsteroidal anti-inflammatory drugs (NSAIDs)** such as ibuprofen and naproxen, alcohol, caffeine, antibiotics, and nutritional supplements before and during exercise, as they can cause gastrointestinal discomfort. Clients should experiment during training to identify their triggers.
- Urinate and defecate prior to exercise.
- Consult a physician if GI problems persist, especially abdominal pain, diarrhea, or bloody stool.

Post-exercise Hydration

Following exercise, the athlete should aim to correct any fluid imbalances that occurred during the exercise session. This includes consuming water to restore hydration, carbohydrates to replenish glycogen stores, and electrolytes to speed rehydration. If the athlete will have at least 12 hours to recover before the next strenuous workout, rehydration with the usual meals, snacks, and water should be adequate. The sodium in the foods will help retain the fluid and stimulate thirst. If rehydration needs to occur quickly, then the athlete should drink about 1.5 L of fluid for each kilogram (or 0.75 L of fluid for each pound) of body weight lost (Sawka et al., 2007). This will be enough to restore lost fluid and also compensate for increased urine output that occurs with rapid consumption of large amounts of fluid. A severely dehydrated athlete (>7% body weight loss) with symptoms (nausea, vomiting, or diarrhea) may need intravenous fluid replacement. Those at greatest risk of hyponatremia should be careful not to consume too much water following exercise and instead should focus on replenishing sodium.

While fluid needs before, during, and after exercise vary by athlete depending on many factors (e.g., sweat rate, intensity of activity, outside humidity, age, and gender), the United States Track and Field Association suggests the general hydration recommendations shown in Table 7-7 to help maintain euhydration when calculating an individualized fluid regimen is not possible.

Table 7-7

Fluid-intake Recommendations During Exercise
2 hours prior to exercise, drink 500–600 mL (17–20 oz)
Every 10–20 minutes during exercise, drink 200–300 mL (7–10 oz) or, preferably, drink based on sweat losses
Following exercise, drink 450–675 mL for every 0.5 kg body weight lost (or 16–24 oz for every pound)

Source: Casa, D.J. et al. (2000). National Athletic Trainers' Association: Position statement: Fluid replacement for athletes. *Journal of Athletic Training,* 35, 212–224.

APPLY WHAT YOU KNOW

The Middle-aged Overweight Hiker

Risk Profile

Susan is a 55-year-old overweight teacher who is training to hike the Grand Canyon with her 17-year-old daughter and a guide. She is 5'2" and 180 pounds [**body mass index (BMI)** of 32.9 kg/m²]. She has hired a health coach to help her get in shape for this adventure. The trip is planned for late September, which is about three months from now. Susan anticipates that the 9.3-mile (15-km) trail down will take about six hours and the return up about nine hours. She plans to complete the trek over a three-day period.

1. Is this client more at risk for dehydration or hyponatremia? Explain.

She is more at risk for hyponatremia. Based on a study of marathon runners by Almond et al. (2005), hyponatremia was highest in athletes that had low BMI, consumed fluids at every mile (and more than 3 liters total throughout the race), finished the race in more than four hours, and gained weight during the run. The greatest predictor of hyponatremia was weight gain, which researchers attributed to excessive fluid intake. Though Susan is overweight, she has the other risk factors for hyponatremia. However, she still is at risk for dehydration, especially since it may be very hot in the Grand Canyon in September and there may be limited access to fluids other than what she carries with her.

Fluid Needs

On the morning of the training workout, Susan's pre-workout weight is 180.0 pounds.

The health coach chose to calculate sweat rate based on a one-hour hike. Susan does not drink anything during the hike and she does not urinate. At the completion of the workout she drank 16 ounces of water. Her post-workout weight is 179.4 pounds.

2. What is Susan's percent body-weight change?

179.4 lb/180lb = 0.9967. Thus her weight change is 1 – 0.9967 = 0.0033 = 0.3%

3. How much fluid does Susan need to drink per hour to maintain euhydration?

In one hour, Susan lost 0.6 lb (9.6 oz). In other words, she would have needed to drink an additional 9.6 oz to maintain perfect euyhdration and replace all lost fluids. Thus, sweat rate in 1 hour = 16 oz (amount of fluid she consumed) + 9.6 oz (extent of fluid deficit given the 0.6-lb weight loss) = 25.6 oz/hour.

Hydration recommendation before exercise

4. What hydration recommendations would you offer Susan in the days prior to the Grand Canyon hike?

Susan should aim for relatively clear urine in the days leading up to her hike by titrating her fluid intake. In the hours prior to exercise, she will need about 400 mL of fluid prior to exercise based on her weight of 180 pounds (5–7mL per 2.2 lb of body weight). Review "Hydration Prior to Exercise" on page 178. Answers may vary, but should include recommendations to ensure euhydration at the onset of an exercise session.

Hydration recommendation during exercise

5. What types of fluids would you recommend that Susan bring with her for her Grand Canyon hike, which is scheduled to occur over a three-day period?

Given the duration of Susan's exercise, she will need to balance fluid intake with a mixture of water and sodium- and carbohydrate-containing beverages and snacks. She should be sure to include a sports drink with moderate amounts of sodium (i.e., at least 50 mg per 8-oz serving), or at least be sure to bring sodium-containing snacks to minimize the risk of hyponatremia.

Hydration recommendation after exercise

6. What and how much would you advise Susan to drink in the 24 to 48 hours after she finishes her Grand Canyon hike?

Susan presumably will be resting and recovering for several days following her hike. Therefore, she does not need a strict refueling regimen, but she should be sure to drink fluids and eat a regular diet that will ensure adequate rehydration and glycogen replenishment over the course of her recovery period. One simple way to approximate hydration status is to assess urine color. If the urine is light yellow, then Susan can be certain that she is consuming adequate fluids. However, if the urine is more concentrated or yellow-colored, then Susan is not adequately hydrated (the darker the color, the greater the concern for significant dehydration).

Nutrition Applications in the Lifecycle

A well-balanced eating plan often extends beyond a one-size-fits-all dietary recommendation. At certain times, some individuals need slightly modified dietary recommendations to best meet their lifestyle, nutritional, and cultural needs.

While the USDA's *Dietary Guidelines* are intended for all Americans ages two and older, some stages of the human lifecycle require special nutritional needs. Health coaches can best serve their clients who are in the midst of these stages by tailoring recommendations to address their specific needs.

Nutrition in Childhood and Adolescence

The American Academy of Pediatrics (AAP) and the American Heart Association (AHA) recommend a diet rich in fruits, vegetables, whole grains, low-fat and nonfat dairy products, beans, fish, and lean meat for children and adolescents, as well as for adults (Gidding et al., 2005). Strategies to implement these recommendations are listed in Table 7-8.

Table 7-8

Dietary Strategies for Individuals >2 Years

- Balance dietary calories with physical activity to maintain normal growth.
- Perform 60 minutes of moderate to vigorous play or physical activity daily.
- Eat vegetables and fruits daily, and limit juice intake.
- Use vegetable oils and soft margarines low in saturated fat and trans fatty acids instead of butter or most other animal fats in the diet.
- Eat whole-grain breads and cereals rather than refined-grain products.
- Reduce the intake of sugar-sweetened beverages and foods.
- Use nonfat (skim) or low-fat milk and dairy products daily.
- Eat more fish, especially oily fish, broiled or baked.
- Reduce salt intake, including salt from processed foods.

Reprinted with permission from the American Heart Association et al. (2006). Dietary recommendations for children and adolescents: A guide for practitioners. *Pediatrics,* 117, 544–559.

Research confirms that a wide gap exists between nutrition recommendations for children and what children actually eat. Compared to the recent past, children and adolescents eat breakfast less often, away from home more often, a greater proportion of calories from snacks, more fried and nutrient-poor foods, greater portion sizes, fewer fruits and vegetables, excess sodium, more sweetened beverages, and fewer dairy products (Dwyer et al., 2010; French, Story, & Jeffrey, 2001). As a result, children and especially adolescents eat smaller amounts of many nutrients such as calcium and potassium than the recommended values.

AAP and AHA recommend that the family and cultural background of the child be considered when making nutrition recommendations (Gidding et al., 2005). Media messages, cultural beliefs that a chubby child is a healthy child, immediate access to inexpensive fast food, and motivation to change are all important determinants of a child's nutrition status. Health coaches are encouraged to adjust the recommendations presented in Table 7-9 as needed.

Table 7-9
Improving Nutrition in Young Children
• Parents choose meal times, not children.
• Provide a wide variety of nutrient-dense foods such as fruits and vegetables instead of high-energy-density/nutrient-poor foods such as salty snacks, ice cream, fried foods, cookies, and sweetened beverages.
• Pay attention to portion size; serve portions appropriate for the child's size and age.
• Use nonfat or low-fat dairy products as sources of calcium and protein.
• Limit snacking during sedentary behavior or in response to boredom and particularly restrict the use of sweet/sweetened beverages as snacks (e.g., juice, soda, and sports drinks).
• Limit sedentary behaviors, with no more than one to two hours per day of video screen/television and no television sets in children's bedrooms.
• Allow self-regulation of total caloric intake in the presence of normal BMI or weight for height.
• Have regular family meals to promote social interaction and role model food-related behavior.

Reprinted with permission from the American Heart Association, Inc.; American Heart Association et al. (2006). Dietary recommendations for children and adolescents: A guide for practitioners. *Pediatrics,* 117, 544–559.

Adolescents face unique nutritional challenges due to rapid bone growth and other maturational changes associated with the onset of puberty. While caloric and some micronutrient needs increase to support growth, adolescence is also a time of decreasing physical activity for many teens and increased independence when making food choices. Ready access to juice and sports drinks in schools, the prevalence of fast food restaurants, and peer and media pressure to eat fat- and sugar-laden foods make it easy for many teens to eat more calories than they expend, which puts them at greater risk for **obesity,** hypertension, and **type 2 diabetes.** While the *Dietary Guidelines* and the MyPlate Food Guidance System provide scientifically sound nutrition guidelines for teens, any nutrition advice offered must be individualized and consistent with the teen's readiness to change if it is to be successful.

Nutrition in Aging

Optimal nutrition choices are important for successful aging, which is defined as the ability to maintain a low risk of disease, high mental and physical function, and active engagement in life (Rowe & Kahn, 1998). Eating a nutritious diet, engaging in regular physical activity, and not smoking may be more important than genetics in helping people avoid the deteriorating effects of aging. After all, smoking, poor diet, and physical inactivity account for about 35% of U.S. deaths. These harmful health behaviors also are risk factors underlying the nation's leading killers, including heart disease, cancer, **stroke,** and diabetes (CDC, 2007).

While the U.S. suffers from an epidemic of obesity at least partly due to excessive caloric intake, many older adults are at risk of inadequate caloric intake to supply needed nutrients. Appetite often decreases with age and, as a result, many older adults do not consume enough of certain nutrients, such as calcium, zinc, iron, and B vitamins. The

decreased appetite is likely due to a combination of decreased taste and smell, as well as altered appetite and satiety regulation. Older adults are also at risk of age-related nutrient malabsorption and dehydration resulting from a blunted thirst sensation, decreased functioning of the kidneys, medication side effects, and other factors.

Though caloric intake may decrease with age, many older adults are overweight or obese because the age-related decrease in physical activity and metabolic rate is often more pronounced than the reduction in caloric intake. This scenario leads to a **positive energy balance** and weight gain.

The ADA recommends that older adults consume a variety of healthful foods to assure adequate nutrient intake and also adopt a healthful eating plan such as the DASH eating plan (see pages 189–190) to control chronic disease (ADA, 2005). Older adults are advised to pay particular attention to consuming foods high in fiber. Nutrient supplementation may be necessary for some older adults with poor dietary intake. In these situations, referral to a **registered dietitian (R.D.)** is prudent.

Nutrition and Special Considerations

Obesity

Obesity is described as a BMI of ≥30 kg/m^2, a measurement based on height and weight (see Chapter 11). While not a perfect measure of body fatness, it accurately categorizes most people. Obesity results from an imbalance of caloric intake and caloric expenditure. It makes sense that obesity treatments are aimed at either decreasing caloric intake (or in some cases, decreasing the absorption of calories consumed) or increasing caloric expenditure either via increased exercise or by revving up the body's metabolism. In all, there are four potential treatment options: dietary changes, lifestyle changes including exercise and behavioral modification, medications, and surgery. The dietary and lifestyle changes that help prevent or treat obesity are discussed earlier in this chapter.

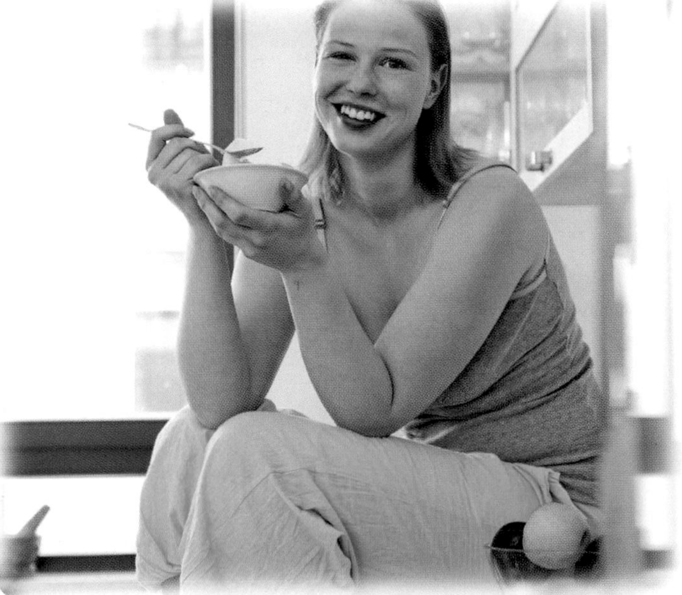

While medications used to treat obesity are never a "quick fix" for an unhealthy lifestyle, in some cases they may be beneficial for people who are not successful with improved eating and exercise habits. Research suggests that overweight or obese people who eat healthfully, exercise regularly, and take a weight-loss medication may lose more weight than those who use the drug alone or lifestyle treatment alone at one year (Wadden et al., 2005). The two most well-studied weight-loss medications are sibutramine and orlistat. Sibutramine (Meridia®) is available by prescription only and works by decreasing appetite. It costs about $100 per month, and on average leads to a 10-lb (4.4-kg) weight loss over the course of the program. Orlistat (Xenical® and Alli®) blocks fat absorption. While orlistat used to be available by prescription only, Alli can be purchased over the counter (see page 237 for more information on Alli). Weight loss is modest—about 6 pounds (2.7 kg)—and the cost reaches about $170 per month for the prescription version (Li et al., 2005). In general, an effective weight-loss medication will lead to a 4-lb (1.8-kg) loss within four weeks.

When dietary, lifestyle, and pharmacological approaches do not work, some people may benefit from weight-loss surgery. Ideal candidates are either severely obese (BMI >40) or have a BMI >35 with other high-risk conditions, such as diabetes, sleep apnea, or life-threatening cardiopulmonary problems; have an "acceptable" operative risk determined by age, degree of obesity, and other pre-existing medical conditions; have been previously unsuccessful at weight loss with a program integrating diet, exercise, behavioral modification, and psychological support; and are carefully selected by a multidisciplinary team that has medical, surgical, psychiatric, and nutritional expertise [National Heart, Lung, and Blood Institute (NHLBI), 1998; Consensus Development Conference Panel, 1991]. Weight-loss surgery is not recommended for the overweight or mildly obese person who is trying to lose 20 or 30 pounds (9.1 to 13.6 kg). Furthermore, only those individuals who are committed to permanent lifestyle changes—including regular physical activity and a healthy diet—are considered good candidates for surgery (NHLBI, 1998; Consensus Development Conference Panel, 1991).

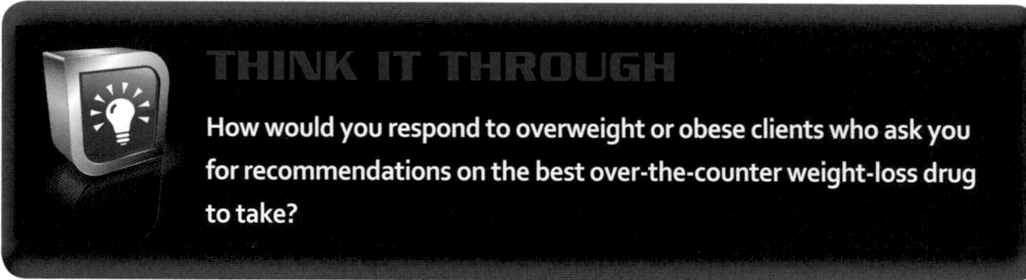

THINK IT THROUGH
How would you respond to overweight or obese clients who ask you for recommendations on the best over-the-counter weight-loss drug to take?

Childhood Obesity

It is no secret that the United States faces an epidemic of childhood obesity. Obesity prevalence among children increased from 5% in the 1960s to 17% in the 2000s (Ogden et al., 2012). African-American girls (24%), Mexican-American boys (24%), and children from lower-income communities with little access to healthful foods and physical-activity opportunities suffer the highest rates or obesity (Ogden et al., 2012). While genes and environment both contribute to obesity risk, the increasing prevalence of childhood obesity has occurred too rapidly to be explained by a genetic shift; rather, changes in physical activity and nutrition are responsible (Barlow et al., 2007).

As with adults, behavior-based weight loss and subsequent weight maintenance prove to be extremely challenging for children. In fact, obesity in childhood, especially among older children and those with the highest BMIs, is likely to persist into adulthood (Whitaker et al., 1997). Social marginalization, type 2 diabetes, **cardiovascular disease,** and myriad other morbidities are significant threats for overweight children both during childhood and as they move into adulthood (Lobstein, Baur, & Uauy, 2004). Alarmed by these sobering statistics, stakeholders—including fitness professionals—have responded with the development of numerous policies, programs, and interventions aimed at preventing childhood obesity. Nutrition recommendations for children are discussed in "Nutrition in Childhood and Adolescence" on page 183.

Cardiovascular Disease

Coronary heart disease (CHD), a leading killer of both men and women in the United States, develops from **atherosclerosis,** or an accumulation of fat and cholesterol in the lining of the arteries that supply oxygen and nutrients to the heart muscle. Over time, blood flow is reduced and oxygenation to the heart can become limited, leading to **angina** (chest pain) and **myocardial infarction** (heart attack). Though atherosclerosis usually is not deadly until middle age and beyond, it begins to develop in childhood (McMahan et al., 2006; Haust, 1990). High blood cholesterol levels—in particular, **low-density lipoprotein (LDL)**—and cholesterol's susceptibility to oxidation are main culprits in the development of atherosclerosis. Cholesterol, lipoproteins, and triglycerides—all factors important in the development of heart disease—are discussed in more detail in the "Fats" section that begins on page 130.

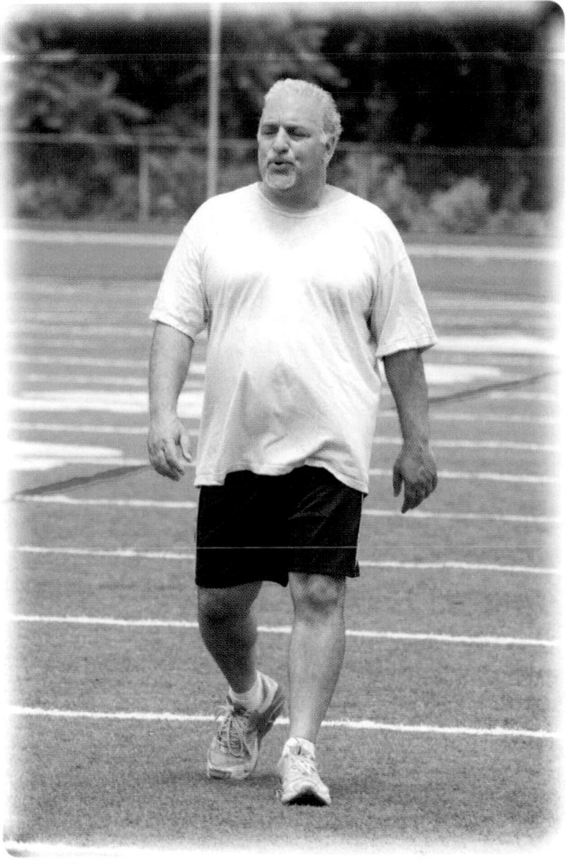

Health coaches can play an important role in helping people minimize their cardiovascular disease risk by educating them about risk factors and encouraging them to talk with their physicians about their own personal risk. It is important to emphasize the importance of keeping close tabs on risk factors not only for older adults who may have already developed one or more risk factors and now must vigorously work to reverse them, or at least prevent their progression, but also for younger individuals who appear to be perfectly healthy.

Regardless of a person's overall risk, everyone should be encouraged to follow these nutrition recommendations to optimize heart health:

- Eat a diet rich in fruits and vegetables, whole grains, and high-fiber foods.
- Consume fish (in particular oily fish like salmon, trout, and tuna) at least twice per week.
- Limit saturated fat to <10% of total caloric intake (preferably <7%), limit added sugars <10% of total caloric intake per day, alcohol to no more than one drink per day, and sodium intake to <2.3 g/day (1 tsp of salt).
- Keep trans fat intake as low as possible.

Studies have shown that following these basic dietary recommendations leads to beneficial changes in reported dietary intake as well as measurable decreases in blood pressure, total cholesterol, and LDL cholesterol (Brunner et al., 2007). Still, implementation is overwhelming and extremely difficult for many people. In fact, only 3% of Americans eat healthfully, engage in regular physical activity, maintain a healthy weight, and do not smoke (Sandmaier, 2007). MyPlate (www.ChooseMyPlate.gov) offers many resources to help people get started, but if this is not enough, health coaches should consider referring clients to an R.D.

EXPAND YOUR KNOWLEDGE

Does the Mediterranean Diet Increase Longevity?

The Greek island of Crete is famous for more than its stunning scenery and ancient roots. Fifty years ago, American scientist Ancel Keys, who himself lived to 100, attributed the exceptional longevity and miniscule rates of cardiovascular disease and cancer on the island to the "Cretan" Mediterranean diet—a diet rich in fruits, vegetables, legumes, whole grains, fish, and olive oil and moderate in red wine. Since then, a large body of research on the Mediterranean diet has accumulated, suggesting that adhering to a Mediterranean diet offers numerous benefits such as enhanced weight loss, heart health, and mental health, as well as a reduction in Alzheimer's disease, cancer, and Parkinson disease (Sofi et al., 2008). But is there enough evidence to support the assertion that adopting a Mediterranean diet may add years to your life?

Greek researchers from the University of Athens medical school set out to rigorously evaluate the assertion that adherence to a Mediterranean diet may improve longevity. They enrolled 22,043 adults in Greece who completed a comprehensive survey that included a food-frequency questionnaire aimed to evaluate how closely their current diet resembled the traditional Mediterranean diet. The researchers rated adherence to the Mediterranean diet on a nine-point scale that incorporated the diet's major features. They then checked up on the study participants 44 months later, during which 275 participants had died. A higher degree of adherence to the Mediterranean diet was associated with a lower likelihood of death from any cause as well as death from cardiovascular disease or cancer. Interestingly, associations between individual food groups within the Mediterranean diet and mortality were not significant. The authors concluded that adherence to the traditional Mediterranean diet is associated with a significant reduction in mortality and that greater adherence to a Mediterranean diet may be related to the increased longevity.

The authors evaluated adherence to a Mediterranean diet with a scale very similar to the one presented here. Health coaches can use this scale to assess how closely a client's typical diet resembles the Mediterranean diet. Clients get one point for each "yes." If they score 6 or higher, they are eating like they live in the Mediterranean.

	YES	NO
Vegetables (other than potatoes), 4 or more servings per day	☐	☐
Fruits, 4 or more servings per day	☐	☐
Whole grains, 2 or more servings per day	☐	☐
Beans (legumes), 2 or more servings per week	☐	☐
Nuts, 2 or more servings per week	☐	☐
Fish, 2 or more servings per week	☐	☐
Red and processed meat, 1 or fewer servings per day	☐	☐
Dairy foods, 1 or fewer servings per day	☐	☐
Alcohol, ½ to 1 drink per day for women, 1 to 2 for men	☐	☐

Source: Trichopoulou, A. et al. (2003). Adherence to a Mediterranean diet and survival in a Greek population. *New England Journal of Medicine*, 348, 2599–2608.

Hypertension

Hypertension is defined as having a **systolic blood pressure (SBP)** of ≥140 mmHg, a **diastolic blood pressure (DBP)** of ≥90 mmHg, and/or being on antihypertensive medication. According to these criteria, more than 30 percent of Americans older than 20 years old have hypertension (CDC, 2011b). Millions more are **prehypertensive,** with a blood pressure greater than 120/80 mmHg (CDC, 2011b). Hypertension is the leading cause of stroke in the United States; therefore, blood pressure should be carefully monitored and controlled. While prescription medications are highly effective in reducing blood pressure, nutrition and physical activity are also important in the treatment and prevention of hypertension. In fact, multiple studies have shown that the DASH eating plan combined with decreased salt intake can substantially reduce blood-pressure levels and potentially make blood-pressure medications unnecessary (Champagne, 2006).

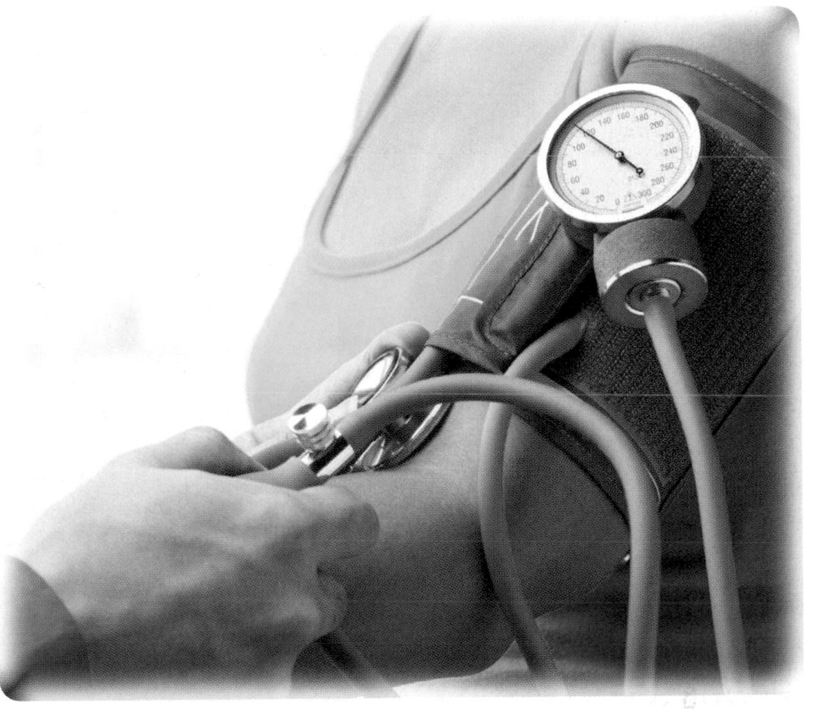

The DASH eating plan, while developed to reduce blood pressure, is an overall healthy eating plan that can be adopted by anyone regardless of whether he or she has elevated blood pressure. In fact, some studies suggest that the DASH eating plan may also reduce CHD risk by lowering total cholesterol and LDL cholesterol in addition to lowering blood pressure (Champagne, 2006). The DASH eating plan is low in saturated fat, cholesterol, and total fat. The staples of the eating plan are fruits, vegetables, and low-fat dairy products. Fish, poultry, nuts, and other unsaturated fats as well as whole grains are also encouraged. Red meat, sweets, and sugar-containing beverages are very limited (Table 7-10). The DASH eating plan recommends that men drink two or fewer and women drink one or fewer alcohol beverages per day. One drink is equivalent to 12 ounces of beer, 5 ounces of wine, or 1.5 ounces of hard liquor.

Diabetes

An estimated 21 million people in the United States have diabetes, with more than 6 million undiagnosed cases, while prevalence is approximately 7.0% of the population (CDC, 2011b). Diabetes mellitus is a condition that results from abnormal regulation of blood glucose. **Type 1 diabetes** results from the inability of the pancreas to secrete sufficient amounts of **insulin,** the **hormone** that allows the cells to take up glucose from the bloodstream. Type 2 diabetes results from the cells' decreased ability to respond to insulin. In most cases, the nutrition recommendations for individuals with diabetes closely resemble the *Dietary Guidelines.* However, it is especially important for people with diabetes to balance nutrition intake with exercise and insulin or other medications in order to maintain a regular blood sugar level throughout the day.

Table 7-10

The DASH Eating Plan

Food Group	Daily Servings (except as noted)	Serving Sizes	Examples and Note	Significance of Each Food Group to the DASH Eating Plan
Grains and grain products	7–8	1 slice bread 1 oz dry cereal* ½ cup cooked rice, pasta, or cereal	Whole-wheat bread, English muffin, pita bread, bagel, cereals, grits, oatmeal, crackers, unsalted pretzels, popcorn	Major sources of energy and fiber
Vegetables	4–5	1 cup raw leafy vegetable ½ cup cooked vegetable 6 oz vegetable juice	Tomatoes, potatoes, carrots, green peas, squash, broccoli, turnip greens, collards, kale, spinach, artichokes, green beans, lima beans, sweet potatoes	Rich sources of potassium, magnesium, and fiber
Fruits	4–5	6 oz fruit juice 1 medium fruit ¼ cup dried fruit ½ cup fresh, frozen, or canned fruit	Apricots, bananas, dates, grapes, orange juice, grapefruit, grapefruit juice, mangoes, melons, peaches, pineapples, prunes, raisins, strawberries, tangerines	Important sources of potassium, magnesium, and fiber
Low-fat or fat-free dairy foods	2–3	8 oz milk 1 cup yogurt 1½ oz cheese	Fat-free (skim) or low-fat (1%) milk, fat-free or low-fat buttermilk, fat-free or low-fat regular or frozen yogurt, low-fat and fat-free cheese	Major sources of calcium and protein
Meats, poultry, and fish	2 or less	3 oz cooked meats, poultry, or fish	Select only lean; trim away visible fats; broil, roast, or boil, instead of frying; remove skin from poultry	Rich sources of protein and magnesium
Nuts, seeds, and dry beans	4–5 per week	⅓ cup or 1½ oz nuts 2 Tbsp or ½ oz seeds ½ cup cooked dry beans	Almonds, filberts, mixed nuts, peanuts, walnuts, sunflower seeds, kidney beans, lentils, peas *Note:* All nuts should be unsalted.	Rich sources of energy, magnesium, potassium, protein, and fiber
Fats and oils†	2–3	1 tsp soft margarine 1 Tbsp low-fat mayonnaise 2 Tbsp light salad dressing 1 tsp vegetable oil	Soft margarine, low-fat mayonnaise, light salad dressing, vegetable oil (such as olive, corn, canola, or safflower)	DASH has 27% of calories as fat, including fat in or added to foods
Sweets	5 per week	1 Tbsp sugar 1 Tbsp jelly or jam ½ oz jelly beans 8 oz lemonade	Maple syrup, sugar, jelly, jam, fruit-flavored gelatin, jelly beans, hard candy, fruit punch, sorbet, ices	Sweets should be low in fat

* Equals ½–1¼ cups, depending on cereal type. Check the product's nutrition facts label.

† Fat content changes serving counts for fats and oils. For example, 1 Tbsp of regular salad dressing equals one serving; 1 Tbsp of a low-fat dressing equals ½ a serving; 1 Tbsp of a fat-free dressing equals 0 servings.

Source: National Heart, Lung, and Blood Institute (2006). *Your Guide to Lowering Your Blood Pressure With DASH.* Bethesda, Md.: National Heart, Lung, and Blood Institute.

In addition, people who have diabetes should consume five to six equally sized small meals to maintain healthy blood sugar levels throughout the day. All individuals with diabetes who have not already had a comprehensive nutrition consultation prior to beginning an exercise program should be referred to an R.D. for an evaluation and nutrition education.

Osteoporosis

Osteoporosis is characterized by weakness and susceptibility to bone fracture, specifically of the hip, spine, and wrist. It is estimated that more than 50% of all women and 20% of all men over the age of 50 will suffer an osteoporotic fracture at some time in their lives (U.S. Department of Health & Human Services, 2004). The disease most often affects elderly women, although it can occur in men and younger women. Nutrition therapy for the prevention and treatment of osteoporosis includes adequate calcium intake, which is modestly correlated with **bone mineral density,** and adequate vitamin D intake. Vitamin D deficiency is associated with higher bone turnover, reduced calcium absorption, and decreased bone mass. Adequate vitamin K (found primarily in green leafy vegetables and some vegetable oils) intake might also help decrease fracture risk (Cockayne et al., 2006). Smoking and a sedentary lifestyle also increase the risk of osteoporosis, while engaging in weight-bearing physical activity decreases the risk (National Institutes of Health, 2001).

Iron-deficiency Anemia

Up to 20% of women between the ages of 18 and 44 have **iron-deficiency anemia** (ADA, 2004). Iron is an important component of hemoglobin, the protein complex responsible for delivering oxygen to muscles and the body's other cells. With iron deficiency, less oxygen is available for cells to use to produce energy. As a result, iron deficiency decreases energy levels and endurance capacity. It also can induce preterm labor and result in low birth weight. Infants, adolescent girls, pregnant women, endurance athletes, and elderly women are at highest risk of iron-deficiency anemia (ADA, 2004). To prevent iron-deficiency anemia, advise clients to consume adequate amounts of iron-rich foods; consume a source of vitamin C at each meal to increase iron absorption; include a serving of meat, fish, poultry, beans, or legumes at each meal; and avoid drinking large amounts of coffee or tea, which contain tannins that interfere with iron absorption (Mahan, Escott-Stump, & Raymond, 2011).

Pregnancy and Lactation

Good nutrition habits during pregnancy optimize maternal health and reduce the risk for some birth defects, suboptimal fetal growth and development, and chronic health problems in the developing child. The key components of a health-promoting lifestyle during pregnancy include:

- *Appropriate weight gain:* The Institute of Medicine (2009) recommends that women with a BMI <18.5 gain 28 to 40 pounds (12.7 to 18.2 kg), a BMI of 18.5 to 24.9 gain 25 to 35 pounds (11.4 to 15.9 kg), a BMI of 25.9 to 29.9 gain 15 to 25 pounds (6.8 to 11.4 kg), and a BMI of >30 gain 11 to 20 pounds (5.0 to 9.1 kg).
- *Appropriate physical activity:* Pregnant women should aim to incorporate 30 minutes or more of moderate-intensity physical activity appropriate for pregnancy on most, if not all, days of the week (ADA, 2008).

- *Consumption of a variety of foods and calories in accordance with the* Dietary Guidelines for Americans: MyPlate offers specialized guidance for optimal nutrition for pregnant and lactating women (www.ChooseMyPlate.gov). Women do not have increased caloric needs until the second trimester, at which time needs increase by 340 calories per day. Women need an additional 450 calories above baseline during the third trimester.

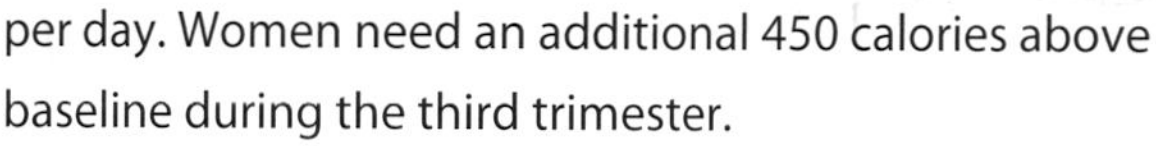

- *Appropriate and timely vitamin and mineral supplementation:* Pregnant women need 600 µg of folic acid daily from fortified foods or supplements in addition to food forms of folate (such as green leafy vegetables, broccoli, and lentils) from a varied diet (ADA, 2008). Folic acid reduces the risk of neural tube defects if taken prior to conception through the sixth week of pregnancy, and may reduce birth defects if taken later in pregnancy. Many pregnant women suffer from iron-deficiency anemia and may benefit from iron supplementation.
- *Avoidance of alcohol, tobacco, and other harmful substances:* Pregnant women and women who could become pregnant should avoid caffeine intakes above 300 mg/day due to increased risk of delayed conception, miscarriage, and low birth weight (ADA, 2008).

- *Safe food handling:* Pregnant women and their fetuses are at higher risk of developing foodborne illness and should take extra precautions to prevent consumption of contaminated foods by avoiding:
  - ✓ Soft cheeses not made with pasteurized milk
  - ✓ Deli meats, unless they have been reheated to steaming hot
  - ✓ Raw or unpasteurized milk or milk products, raw eggs, raw or undercooked meat, unpasteurized juice, raw sprouts, and raw or undercooked fish
  - ✓ Shark, swordfish, king mackerel, or tilefish. Pregnant women can safely consume 12 ounces or less of fish or shellfish per week, provided that it is low in mercury, such as shrimp, canned light tuna, salmon, pollock, and catfish. Consumption of albacore tuna should be limited to 6 ounces or less per week due to its slightly higher mercury content.

In addition to the previously mentioned foods, pregnant women should avoid cat litter boxes and handling pets while preparing foods.

Prior to the child's birth, most women will make the decision as to whether they plan to breastfeed. Breastfeeding provides optimal nutrition and health protection for the first six months of life. From six to 12 months, breastfeeding combined with the introduction of complementary foods is optimal. Women who breastfeed require approximately 500 additional calories per day for weight maintenance. Thus, breastfeeding generally quickens postpartum weight loss. Health coaches can help women return to pre-pregnancy weight

by reinforcing the positive nutrition changes made during pregnancy, such as increased fruit, vegetable, and whole-grain consumption. Also, health coaches should facilitate entry or re-entry into a regular physical-activity program.

Gluten-free Diet

Over the past several years, a growing number of people have experimented with gluten-free diets to help alleviate symptoms like abdominal pain, cramping, and generalized fatigue. While historically (and scientifically), a gluten-free diet only has been considered necessary for people with celiac disease (a condition defined by an allergy to gluten-containing products), many people who do not have celiac disease attest to the benefits of a gluten-free diet.

Gluten is a protein compound made of two proteins: gliadin and glutenin. Gluten is found joined with starch in the grains wheat, rye, and barley. People with celiac disease have a severe immune reaction when the gastrointestinal system is exposed to gliadin. Ultimately, the small intestine loses its capacity to effectively absorb nutrients, leading to vitamin deficiencies, anemia, weight loss, abdominal pain, diarrhea, and, in some cases, neurologic dysfunction. Anyone who suffers from the symptoms of celiac disease should be evaluated by a physician who can order laboratory testing and possibly arrange for a biopsy of the small intestine to confirm the diagnosis. The only definitive treatment for the disease is strict avoidance of gluten-containing foods.

Gluten sensitivity is much more common, and less understood, than celiac disease. This occurs when the body has a pronounced response to gluten-containing foods, leading to feelings of tiredness, abdominal pain, and other gastrointestinal symptoms like diarrhea or constipation. Many people report experiencing these symptoms after eating gluten-containing foods (or more commonly, they report these symptoms going away after avoiding gluten), but it is not exactly clear what causes these symptoms or the body's actual response to the gluten. It is very important for anyone who believes they might have a gluten sensitivity to see a physician and dietitian prior to adopting a gluten-free diet. The physician can test for celiac disease (the tests are not accurate if done after a person has eliminated gluten from the diet) and the dietitian can help develop a balanced eating plan. Typically, people with gluten sensitivity will test negative for celiac disease but still feel that gluten-containing foods make their symptoms worse.

Many foods contain gluten and, without appropriate dietary planning, complete elimination of gluten from the diet can lead to nutritional deficiency. The *Dietary Guidelines* recommend that most adults get anywhere from six to eight servings of grains per day. Grains are an excellent source of B vitamins and fiber. Most standard grains such as bread, cereal, and pasta contain wheat, rye, or barley and therefore include gluten. Complete elimination of gluten-containing grains can lead to nutritional deficiencies, including B vitamins, calcium, vitamin D, iron, zinc, magnesium, and fiber. In fact, a Swedish study of people with celiac disease who had been gluten-free for 10 years found that half of the patients had vitamin deficiencies, including low levels of vitamin B6, folate, or both (Hallert et al., 2002). Likewise, a survey of people on a gluten-free diet in the United States found that more than half had inadequate fiber, iron, and calcium intake (Thompson et al., 2005). Though it is true that a multivitamin may be able to provide "insurance" and protect from overt nutritional deficiencies, it is always ideal to get the body's needed nutrients from food sources whenever possible. While adhering

to a gluten-free diet is a challenge, thanks to the 2004 Food Allergen Labeling and Consumer Protection Act, nutrition facts labels must identify if they contain any of the top eight food allergens, which includes wheat (see Figure 7-2). While it is possible to buy gluten-free bread, pasta, cereal, and various other products, these tend to cost substantially more than their gluten-containing counterparts. However, many fresh and healthy fruits, vegetables, and unprocessed foods are affordable and naturally gluten-free. Other naturally gluten-free foods include rice, corn, soy, potato, tapioca, beans, quinoa, millet, buckwheat, flax, nut flours, uncontaminated oats, milk, butter, cheese, meat, fish, poultry, eggs, beans, and seeds.

Importantly, adopting a gluten-free diet is not recommended as a method to lose weight or to "become healthier." The diet is restrictive and, if poorly planned, could lead to serious vitamin deficiencies and contribute to disordered eating behaviors. In addition, unlike saturated and trans fat, for example, gluten itself is not inherently unhealthy.

Vegetarian Diets

A growing number of Americans are vegetarians, meaning that they do not eat meat, fish, poultry, or products containing these foods. Vegetarian diets come in several forms, all of which are healthful, nutritionally adequate, and effective in disease prevention if carefully planned. The main types of vegetarianism are:

- **Lacto-ovo-vegetarians,** who do not eat meat, fish, or poultry
- **Ovo-vegetarians,** who eat eggs but avoid dairy products
- **Lacto-vegetarians,** who eat dairy products, but do not eat eggs, meat, fish, or poultry
- **Vegans,** who do not consume any animal products, including dairy products such as milk and cheese

Vegetarian diets provide several health advantages. They are low in saturated fat, cholesterol, and animal protein and high in fiber, folate, vitamins C and E, carotenoids, and some **phytochemicals.** Compared to omnivores, vegetarians have lower rates of obesity, death from cardiovascular disease, hypertension, type 2 diabetes, and prostate and colon cancer. However, if poorly planned, vegetarian diets may include insufficient amounts of protein, iron, vitamin B12, vitamin D, calcium, and other nutrients (ADA, 2009).

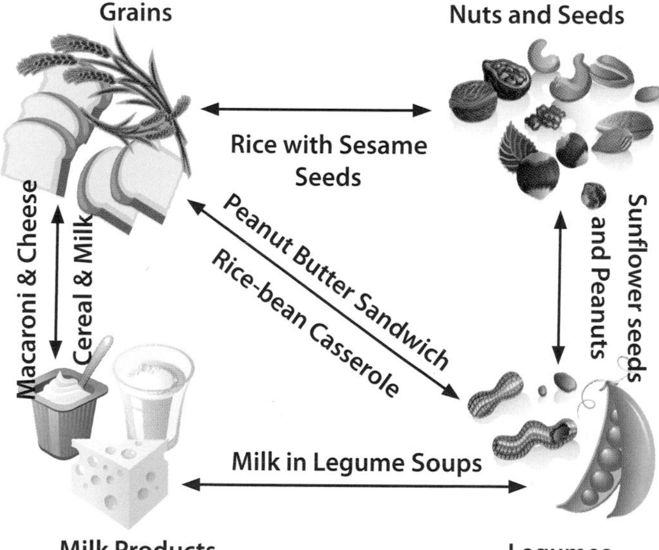

Figure 7-4
Protein complementarity chart

Adapted with permission from Lappé, F.M. (1992). *Diet for a Small Planet.* New York: Ballantine Books.

Quality protein intake is crucial for vegetarians. A main determinant of protein quality is whether a food contains all of the essential amino acids. Most meat-based products are higher-quality proteins because they have varying amounts of the essential amino acids, while plant proteins other than soy are incomplete proteins because they do not contain all eight to 10 essential amino acids (see page 128). However, complementary plant products such as rice and beans together provide all essential amino acids. Research suggests that most vegetarians consume adequate amounts of complementary plant proteins throughout the day to meet their protein needs (Figure 7-4). Thus, the complementary proteins do not need to be consumed in the same meal (ADA, 2009).

Too few well-conducted research studies exist to determine whether or not a vegetarian diet affects athletic performance (Venderley & Campbell, 2006). However, if vegetarian athletes do not consume enough calories to fuel exercise, performance may suffer. Some suggestions to increase caloric intake include the following:

- Eat more frequent meals and snacks
- Include meat alternatives, including soy, tofu, and legumes
- Add dried fruit, seeds, nuts, and other healthful calorie-dense foods

THINK IT THROUGH

Vegetarianism is becoming more of a common practice in today's society. Thus, health coaches will most likely encounter clients who choose to eat vegetarian diets. What will you do to educate and coach clients who choose to practice one of the many vegetarian eating plans about how to maintain adequate nutritional status while meeting their performance and weight-management goals?

Eating Disorders

Most health coaches will at some point face the challenge of helping someone overcome the powerful grips of an eating disorder such as **anorexia nervosa, bulimia nervosa, binge eating disorder,** or other disordered eating. Health coaches and coaches who work with young people and others at risk for eating disorders play a critically important role in helping prevent the onset of an obsession with weight, body image, and exercise. The National Eating Disorders Association (www.nationaleatingdisorders.org) offers the following tips that health coaches can use to help prevent eating disorders:

- Take warning signs seriously. If a health coach believes that someone may have an eating disorder, he or she should share those concerns in an open, direct, and sensitive manner, keeping in mind the following "don'ts" when confronting someone with a suspected eating or exercise disorder: Don't oversimplify, diagnose, become the person's therapist, provide exercise advice without first helping the individual get professional help, or get into a battle of wills if the person denies having a problem.
- De-emphasize weight. Health coaches should not weigh individuals they suspect may have an eating disorder. They should also eliminate comments about weight.
- Do not assume that reducing body fat or weight will improve performance.
- Help other fitness professionals recognize the signs of eating disorders and be prepared to address them.
- Provide accurate information about weight, weight loss, body composition, nutrition, and sports performance. Have a broad network of referrals (such as physicians and R.D.s) who may also be able to help educate individuals when appropriate.
- Emphasize the health risks of low weight, especially for female athletes with menstrual irregularities (in which case, referral to a physician, preferably one who specializes in eating disorders, is warranted).
- Avoid making any derogatory comments about weight or body composition to or about anyone.
- Do not restrict athletic performance and gym privileges to an athlete or exerciser who

is found to have eating problems unless medically necessary. Consider the individual's physical and emotional health and self-image when deciding how to modify exercise participation level.

- Strive to promote a positive self-image and self-esteem in exercisers and athletes.
- Carefully assess one's own assumptions and beliefs as they relate to self-image, body composition, exercise, and dieting.

In addition to being a source of help and **empathy**, health coaches can play an important role in developing structured exercise programs for people recovering from eating and exercise disorders who have already sought help from a qualified medical professional. An important first step is to develop a partnership with the individual's treating physician. Seek medical clearance and general recommendations from the physician regarding the maximal duration and intensity of exercise. Note that individuals with a BMI of less than 20 may not receive clearance to exercise until they gain a specified amount of weight. When working with the individual, emphasize the positive psychological and health benefits of appropriate exercise and minimize focus on appearances and weight. Health coaches should always strive to develop a balanced and well-rounded program that includes cardiovascular training, resistance training, and flexibility exercises. The goal is to help the individual learn how to exercise in moderation.

Cultural Considerations

Flavor, price, tradition, and the emotional and social meaning of food are critical factors to consider when providing dietary recommendations. It is important to recommend healthful food choices that are compatible with the client's typical eating patterns, cultural beliefs about food, and overall lifestyle. In most situations, retaining components of the individual's customary eating habits is recommended. After all, adopting a more Westernized diet often leads to increased intake of calories, refined carbohydrates, fat, processed foods, and sodium, in addition to reduced consumption of complex carbohydrates, fruits, and vegetables. Together, these changes lead to dramatic increases in obesity. However, some traditional eating patterns, such as the typical diet in the Southeastern United States, are typically less healthy than the standard American fare. In those cases, it may be advisable to help individuals adopt more mainstream eating habits, or better yet, make healthy substitutions for high-fat and low-nutrient-density foods in their traditional diets (Kumanyika, 2006).

Summary

Clients rely on health coaches to provide them with credible nutrition recommendations and advice to develop a healthy eating plan and lifestyle. While physically active individuals may have specific nutritional needs compared to the general population, a thorough understanding of federal dietary recommendations gives health coaches a basis from which to make general nutrition recommendations while staying within their professional scope of practice. Sources such as the *Dietary Guidelines* and MyPlate are helpful resources to consult when providing clients with nutrition information. Clients who request or require an individualized nutrition plan may benefit from a consultation with a registered dietitian. Ultimately, the health coach is uniquely positioned to help clients transform nutrition information and recommendations into action.

References

Almond, C.S.D. et al. (2005). Hyponatremia among runners in the Boston Marathon. *New England Journal of Medicine,* 352, 15, 1550–1556.

American Dietetic Association (2009). Position of the American Dietetic Association and Dietitians of Canada: Vegetarian diets. *Journal of the American Dietetic Association,* 109, 1266–1282.

American Dietetic Association (2008). Position of the American Dietetic Association: Nutrition and lifestyle for a healthy pregnancy outcome. *Journal of the American Dietetic Association,* 108, 3, 566–561.

American Dietetic Association (2005). Position of the American Dietetic Association: Nutrition across the spectrum of aging. *Journal of the American Dietetic Association,* 106, 616–633.

American Dietetic Association (2004). Position of the American Dietetic Association and Dietitians of Canada: Nutrition and women's health. *Journal of the American Dietetic Association,* 104, 6, 984–1001.

American Heart Association et al. (2006). Dietary recommendations for children and adolescents: A guide for practitioners. *Pediatrics,* 117, 544–559.

Barlow S.E. and the Expert Committee (2007). Expert committee recommendations regarding the prevention, assessment, and treatment of child and adolescent overweight and obesity: Summary report. *Pediatrics,* 120, S4, S164–S193.

Brand-Miller, J. et al. (2003). Low-glycemic index diets in the management of diabetes: A meta-analysis of randomized controlled trials. *Diabetes Care,* 26, 8, 2261–2267.

Brunner E.J. et al (2007). Dietary advice for reducing cardiovascular risk. *Cochrane Database of Systematic Reviews,* 4: CD002128.

Casa, D.J. et al. (2000). National Athletic Trainers' Association: Position statement: Fluid replacement for athletes. *Journal of Athletic Training,* 35, 212–224.

Centers for Disease Control and Prevention (2011a). *CDC Estimates of Foodborne Illness in the United States.* http://www.cdc.gov/foodborneburden/PDFs/FACTSHEET_A_FINDINGS_updated4-13.pdf . Retrieved on November 20, 2011.

Centers for Disease Control and Prevention (2011b). *Health, 2011 With Chartbook on Trends in the Health of Americans.* http://www.cdc.gov/nchs/data/hus/hus10.pdf#066. Retrieved on November 20, 2011.

Centers for Disease Control and Prevention (2007). *The State of Aging and Health in America 2007.* http://www.cdc.gov/aging/pdf/saha_2007.pdf

Champagne, C.M. (2006). Dietary interventions on blood pressure: The Dietary Approaches to Stop Hypertension (DASH) trials. *Nutrition Reviews,* 64, 2, (II), S53–S56.

Cockayne S. et al. (2006). Vitamin K and the prevention of fractures. *Archives of Internal Medicine,* 166, 1256–1261.

Consensus Development Conference Panel (1991). Gastrointestinal surgery for severe obesity. *Annals of Internal Medicine,* 115, 956–961.

Dansinger M.L. et al. (2005). Comparison of the Atkins, Ornish, Weight Watchers, and Zone diets for weight loss and heart disease risk reduction: A randomized trial. *Journal of the American Medical Association,* 293, 1, 43–53.

Dwyer, J.T. et al. (2010). Feeding infants and toddlers study 2008: Progress, continuing concerns, and implications. *Journal of the American Dietetic Association,* 110, S60–67.

Foster, G.D. et al. (2003). A randomized trial of a low-carbohydrate diet for obesity. *New England Journal of Medicine,* 348, 21, 2082–2090.

Frankenfield, D., Routh-Yousey, L., & Compher, C. (2005). Comparison of predictive equations of resting metabolic rates in healthy non-obese and obese adults: A systematic review. *Journal of the American Dietetic Association,* 105, 5, 775–789.

French, S.A., Story, M., & Jeffrey, R.W. (2001). Environmental influences on eating and physical activity. *Annual Reviews of Public Health,* 22, 309–335.

Gardner, C.D. et al. (2007). Comparison of the Atkins, Zone, Ornish, and LEARN diets for change in weight and related risk factors among overweight premenopausal women: The A TO Z Weight Loss Study: A randomized trial. *Journal of the American Medical Association,* 297, 9, 969–977.

Gidding, S.S. et al. (2005). American Heart Association & American Academy of Pediatrics:

Dietary recommendations for children and adolescents: A guide for practitioners: Consensus statement from the American Heart Association. *Circulation,* 112, 2061–2075 [published corrections appear in *Circulation,* 2005, 112, 2375 and *Circulation,* 2006, 113, e857].

Hallert C. et al. (2002). Evidence of poor vitamin status in celiac patients on a gluten-free diet for 10 years. *Alimentary Pharmacology & Therapeutics,* 16, 1333–1339.

Haust, M.D. (1990). The genesis of atherosclerosis in pediatric age-group. *Pediatric Pathology,* 10, 1–2, 253–271.

Hew-Butler, T.D. et al. (2006). Sodium supplementation is not required to maintain serum sodium concentrations during an Ironman triathlon. *British Journal of Sports Medicine,* 40, 3, 255–259.

Institute of Medicine (2009). *Weight Gain During Pregnancy.* Washington, D.C.: National Academy Press.

Institute of Medicine (2005). *Dietary Reference Intakes for Energy, Carbohydrate, Fiber, Fat, Fatty Acids, Cholesterol, Protein, and Amino Acids.* Washington, D.C.: National Academy Press.

Institute of Medicine (2004). *Dietary Reference Intakes for Calcium, Magnesium, Phosphorus, Vitamin D, and Fluoride.* Washington, D.C.: National Academy Press.

Kreider, R.B. et al (2010). ISSN exercise & sport nutrition review: Research & recommendations. *Journal of the International Society of Sports Nutrition,* 7, 7.

Kumanyika, S. (2006). Nutrition and chronic disease prevention: Priorities for U.S. minority groups. *Nutrition Reviews,* 64, 2, (II), S9–S14.

Lappé, F.M. (1992). *Diet for a Small Planet.* New York: Ballantine Books.

Li, Z. et al. (2005). Meta-analysis: Pharmacologic treatment of obesity. *Annals of Internal Medicine,* 5, 142, 532–546.

Lobstein, T., Baur, L., & Uauy, R. (2004). Obesity in children and young people: A crisis in public health. *Obesity Reviews,* 5, Suppl. 1, 4–85.

Mahan, L.K., Escott-Stump, S., & Raymond, J.L. (2011). *Krause's Food and the Nutrition Care Process* (13th ed.). Philadelphia, Pa.: W.B. Saunders Company.

McMahan, C.A. et al. (2006). Pathological determinants of atherosclerosis in youth risk scores are associated with early and advanced atherosclerosis. *Pediatrics,* 118, 4, 1447–1455.

National Heart, Lung, and Blood Institute (2006). *Your Guide to Lowering Your Blood Pressure With DASH.* Bethesda, Md.: National Heart, Lung, and Blood Institute.

National Heart, Lung, and Blood Institute (1998). *Clinical Guidelines on the Identification, Evaluation, and Treatment of Overweight and Obesity in Adults: The Evidence Report.* Bethesda, Md.: National Heart, Lung, and Blood Institute.

National Institutes of Health (2001). Osteoporosis prevention, diagnosis, and therapy. *Journal of the American Medical Association,* 285, 6, 785–795.

Ogden, C.L. et al. (2012). Prevalence of overweight and trends in body mass index among U.S. children and adolescents, 1999–2010. *Journal of the American Medical Association,* 307, 5, 483–490.

O'Reilly, J., Wong, S.H., & Chen, Y. (2010). Glycaemic index, glycaemic load and exercise performance. *Sports Medicine,* 40, 27–39.

Rodriguez, N.R., Di Marco, N.M., & Langley, S. (2009). American College of Sports Medicine position stand: Nutrition and athletic performance. *Medicine & Science in Sports & Exercise,* 41, 709–731.

Rowe, J.W. & Kahn R.L. (1998). *Successful Aging.* New York: Pantheon Books.

Sandmaier, M. (2007). *The Healthy Heart Handbook for Women.* Bethesda, Md.: U.S. Department of Health and Human Services: National Institutes of Health, National Heart, Lung, and Blood Institute. nhlbi.nih.gov/health/public/heart/other/hhw/hdbk_wmn.pdf. Retrieved on November 21, 2011.

Sawka, M.N. et al. (2007). American College of Sports Medicine position stand: Exercise and fluid replacement. *Medicine & Science in Sports & Exercise,* 39, 2, 377–390.

Sofi, F. et al. (2008). Adherence to Mediterranean diet and health status: Meta-analysis. *British Medical Journal,* 337, a1344.

Speedy, D.B. et al. (2002). Oral salt supplementation during ultradistance exercise. *Clinical Journal of Sport Medicine,* 12, 5, 279–284.

Stevenson, E.J. et al. (2009). Dietary glycemic index influences lipid oxidation but not muscle or liver glycogen oxidation during exercise. *American Journal of Physiology, Endocrinology, and Metabolism,* 296, E1140–1147.

St. Jeor, S.T. et al. (2001). Dietary protein and weight reduction: A statement for healthcare professionals from the nutrition committee of the Council on Nutrition, Physical Activity, and Metabolism of the American Heart Association. *Circulation,* 104, 1869–1874.

Thomas, D.E., Elliott, E., & Baur, L. (2007). Low glycemic index or low glycemic load diets for overweight and obesity. *Cochrane Database of Systematic Reviews,* 18, 3, CD005105.

Thompson, T. et al. (2005). Gluten-free diet survey: Are Americans with celiac disease consuming recommended amounts of fibre, iron, calcium and grain foods? *Journal of Human Nutrition and Dietetics,* 18, 163–169.

Trenell, M.I. et al. (2008). Effect of high and low glycaemic index recovery diets on intramuscular lipid oxidation during aerobic exercise. *British Journal of Nutrition,* 99, 326–332.

Trichopoulou, A. et al. (2003). Adherence to a Mediterranean diet and survival in a Greek population. *New England Journal of Medicine,* 348, 2599–2608.

U.S. Department of Agriculture (2015). *2015-2020 Dietary Guidelines for Americans* (8th ed.). www.health.gov/dietaryguidelines

U.S. Department of Health & Human Services (2004). *Bone Health and Osteoporosis: A Report of the Surgeon General.* Rockville, Md.: U.S. Department of Health & Human Services, Office of the Surgeon General.

van Rosendal S.P. et al. (2010). Guidelines for glycerol use in hyperhydration and rehydration associated with exercise. *Sports Medicine,*40, 2, 113–129.

Venderley, A.M. & Campbell, W.W. (2006). Vegetarian diets: Nutritional considerations for athletes. *Sports Medicine,* 36, 4, 293–305.

Wadden, T.A. et al. (2005). Randomized trial of lifestyle modification and pharmacotherapy for obesity. *New England Journal of Medicine,* 353, 2111–2120.

Whitaker, R.C. et al. (1997). Predicting obesity in young adulthood from childhood and parental obesity. *New England Journal of Medicine,* 337, 869–873.

Wolfe, R.R. & Miller, S.L. (2008). The recommended dietary allowance of protein: A misunderstood concept. *Journal of the American Medical Association,* 299, 24, 2891–2893.

Suggested Reading

Clark, N. (2008). *Nancy Clark's Sports Nutrition Guidebook* (4th ed.). Champaign, Ill.: Human Kinetics.

Dunford, M. & Doyle, J.A. (2011). *Nutrition for Sport and Exercise* (2nd ed.). Belmont, Calif.: Thomson Wadsworth.

McArdle, W.D., Katch, F.L., & Katch, V.L. (2008). *Sports and Exercise Nutrition* (3rd ed.). Baltimore, Md.: Lippincott Williams & Wilkins.

National Heart Lung and Blood Institute (2010). *The DASH Eating Plan.* www.nhlbi.nih.gov/health/health-topics/topics/dash/

Rodriguez, N.R., Di Marco, N.M., & Langley, S. (2009). American College of Sports Medicine position stand: Nutrition and athletic performance. *Medicine & Science in Sports & Exercise,* 41, 709–731.

Sawka, M.N. et al. (2007). American College of Sports Medicine position stand: Exercise and fluid replacement. *Medicine & Science in Sports & Exercise,* 39, 2, 377–390.

U.S. Department of Agriculture (2015). *2015-2020 Dietary Guidelines for Americans* (8th ed.). www.health.gov/dietaryguidelines

Williams, M. (2009). *Nutrition for Health, Fitness and Sport* (9th ed.). New York: McGraw-Hill.

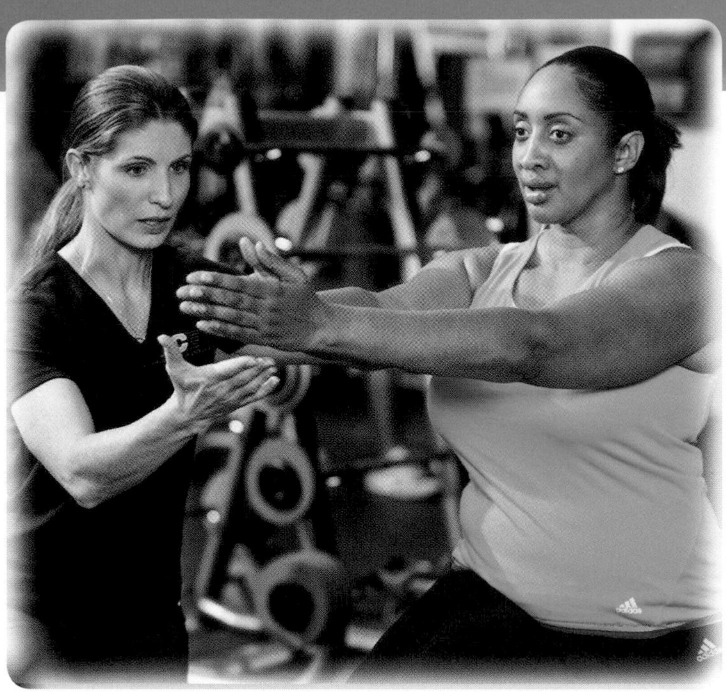

IN THIS CHAPTER:

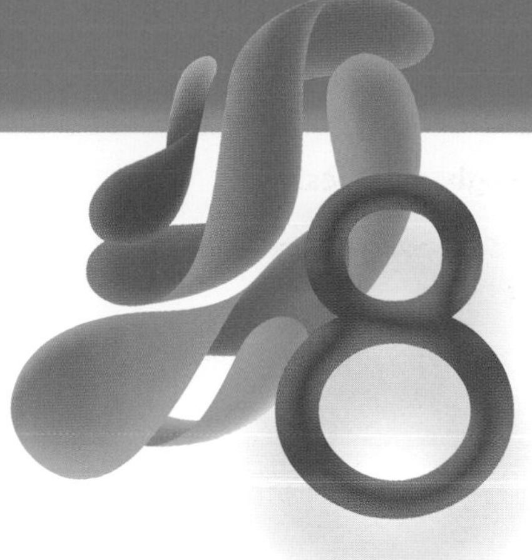

The Physiology of Obesity

KARA A. WITZKE

Kara A. Witzke, Ph.D., is an associate professor and department chair of Kinesiology at California State University, San Marcos. Her work in the fitness industry spans over 20 years and has included positions in personal training, cardiac rehabilitation, corporate fitness, fitness certification, weight management, education, and research. Her research focuses on the effects of exercise on the musculoskeletal and metabolic systems and she teaches classes related to exercise in the management of chronic disease.

O**besity** is the result of excess body-fat accumulation. This excess is associated with many adverse health outcomes, such as cardiovascular disease, metabolic disease, and cancer [National Heart, Lung, and Blood Institute (NHLBI), 1998]. Despite an increased awareness of these negative health risks, the prevalence of **overweight** and obesity is on the rise in the United States.

Unfortunately, the rise in childhood obesity has never been more rapid and a clear understanding of this complex disease is imperative. According to the Centers for Disease Control and Prevention (CDC) (2010), American society has become **obesogenic,** meaning that it is an environment that tends to generate or create a state of obesity. An increasingly convenient lifestyle, characterized by environments that promote unhealthy food intake and physical inactivity, has contributed to an increase in the percentage of obese adults from just 13.3% in 1960 to 35.7% in 2010 (Ogden et al., 2012). Adults categorized as overweight or obese has risen from 44.8% in 1960 to 68.3% in 2008 (Table 8-1). It is estimated that by 2015, more than 40% of U.S. adults will be obese (Flegal et al., 2012; Wang & Beydoun, 2007).

Unfortunately, the poor habits of American adults have been passed down to their children. Results from the 2007–2008 National Health and Nutrition Examination Survey (NHANES) using measures of **body mass index (BMI)** indicate that 16.9% of all children and adolescents ages 2 to 19 years are now obese (Figure 8-1) (Flegal et al., 2010). In the 1960s, this number was only 4.4%. The chance of having a BMI greater than 25 starts to rise around age 35 and declines around age 75 in both men and women. However, women are still more likely to be obese at all ages. Not surprisingly, these trends are similar for other countries throughout the world.

Table 8-1

Prevalence of Overweight and Obesity Among Children, Adolescents, and Adults in the U.S. From 1960 to 2010

Survey Year	Children 6–11 Obese* (%)	Adolescents 12–19 Obese* (%)	Adults 20–74 Overweight or Obese (%)	Adults 20–74 Overweight (%)	Adults 20–74 Obese (%)
1960-1962	—	—	44.8	31.5	13.3
1963-1965	4.2	—	—	—	—
1966-1970†	—	4.6	—	—	—
1971-1974	4.0	6.1	47.7	33.1	14.6
1976-1980	6.5	5.0	47.4	32.3	15.1
1988-1994	11.3	10.5	56.0	32.7	23.3
1999-2002	16.3	16.7	65.2	34.1	31.1
2003-2004	18.8	17.4	66.3	34.1	32.2
2005-2006	15.1	17.8	67.0	32.7	34.3
2007-2008	19.6	18.1	68.3	34.4	33.9
2009-2010	18.0	18.4	—	—	35.7

*Obesity among children and adolescents is defined as body mass index (BMI) greater than or equal to sex- and age-specific 95th percentile from the 2000 CDC Growth Charts.

†Data for 1966-1970 are for adolescents aged 12-17, not 12-19 years.

Sources: Ogden, C.L. et al (2012). *Prevalence of Obesity in the United States 2009-2010.* NHCS Data Brief, No. 82. Washington, D.C.: Centers for Disease Control and Prevention; Flegal, K.M. et al. (2010). Prevalence and trends in obesity among U.S. adults, 1999-2008. *Journal of the American Medical Association,* 303, 3, 235-241; Ogden, C.L. et al. (2010a). Prevalence of high body mass index in U.S. children and adolescents, 2007-2008. *Journal of the American Medical Association,* 303, 3, 242-249.

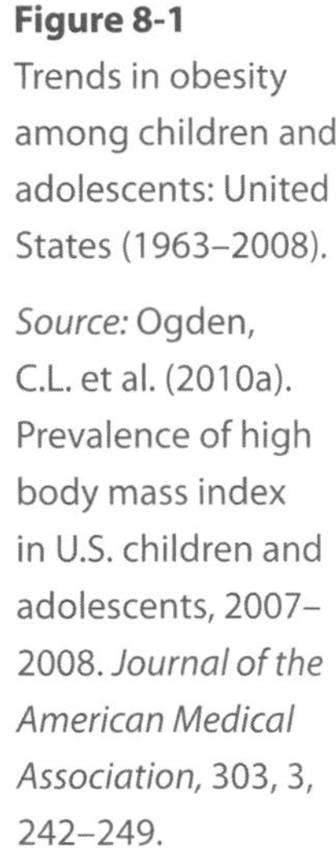

Figure 8-1
Trends in obesity among children and adolescents: United States (1963–2008).

Source: Ogden, C.L. et al. (2010a). Prevalence of high body mass index in U.S. children and adolescents, 2007–2008. *Journal of the American Medical Association,* 303, 3, 242–249.

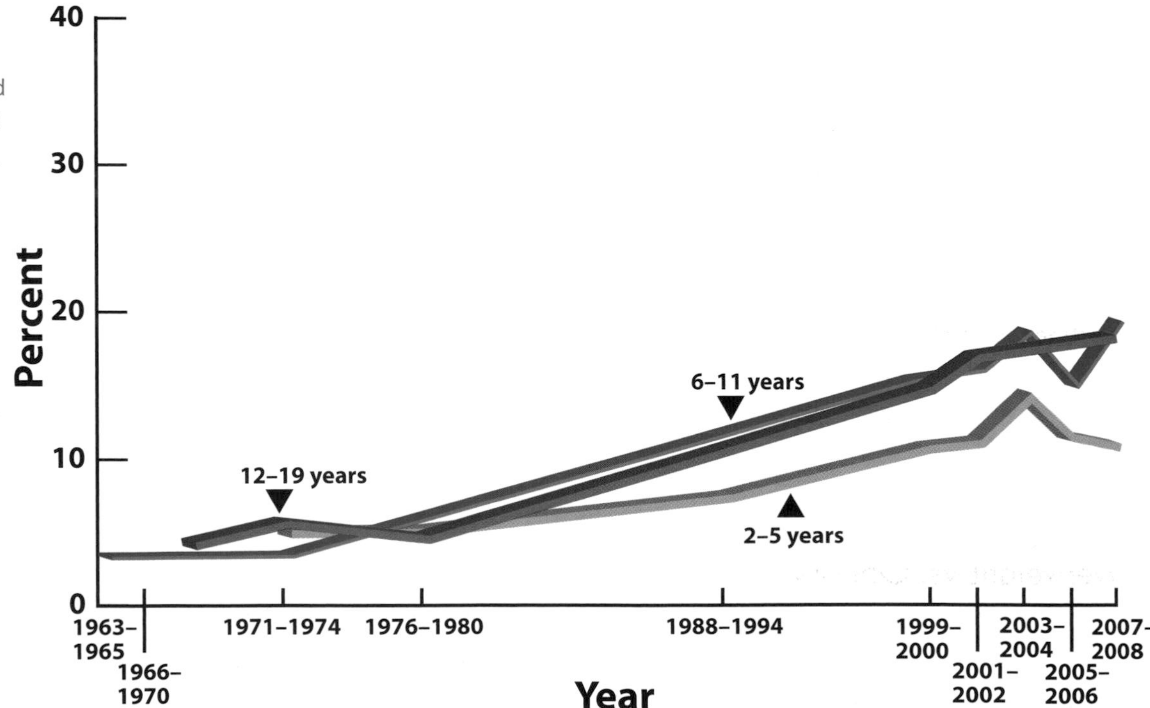

Note: Obesity is defined as body mass index (BMI) greater than or equal to sex- and age-specific 95th percentile from the 2000 CDC Growth Charts.

Sources: CDC/NCHS, National Health Examination Surveys II (ages 6–11), III (ages 12–17), and National Health and Nutrition Examination Surveys (NHANES) I–III, and NHANES 1999–2000, 2001–2002, 2003–2004, 2005–2006, and 2007–2008.

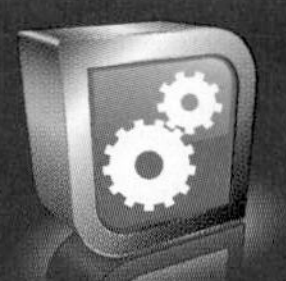

EXPAND YOUR KNOWLEDGE

Key Facts About Obesity

- Worldwide obesity has more than doubled since 1980.
- In 2008, 1.5 billion adults age 20 and older were overweight. Of these, more than 200 million men and nearly 300 million women were obese.
- Overall, more than one in 10 of the world's adult population is obese.
- 65% of the world's population lives in countries where overweight and obesity kill more people than underweight.
- Nearly 43 million children under the age of five were overweight in 2010.

Source: World Health Organization (2011). *Obesity and Overweight.* www.who.int/mediacentre/factsheets/fs311/en/

There are also differences in overweight and obesity prevalence by racial/ethnic group. It is estimated that 54% of non-Hispanic black women are considered obese, compared with 32% of Mexican-American and 30% of non-Hispanic white women of the same age. Among males, 34% of black males, compared to 31% of white and 32% of Mexican-American males, are obese (Ogden et al., 2006). Among children of color, these estimates are also alarming, with 24.5% of non-Hispanic black children and 22.1% of Mexican-American children now meeting the criteria for obesity (Ogden et al., 2010b).

These racial differences may be explained by a combination of genetics, food, and exercise habits, as well as cultural attitudes toward body weight. On average, non-Hispanic black women burn about 100 fewer calories each day during rest than white women, which translates into nearly 1 pound (0.45 kg) of body fat gained each month (Carpenter et al., 1998). Non-Hispanic black women also tend to experience a more dramatic lowering of **resting metabolic rate (RMR)** during dieting than white women, which may also help to explain why they tend to have greater difficulty in achieving and maintaining a goal body weight than overweight white women (Foster et al., 1999). Again, however, the trend toward increasing overweight and obesity continues to increase among all racial/ethnic and socio-economic groups.

Overweight vs. Obesity

There is some confusion around the precise meaning of the terms overweight, overfat, and obesity as they pertain to **body composition** and risk for health problems. In proper context, the term "overweight" simply refers to a body weight that exceeds some predetermined average for height. A person who is overweight has usually experienced an increase in body fat, but not always, as in the case of muscular athletes. The term "obesity" refers to the overfat condition that accompanies a host of comorbidities, including **glucose** intolerance, **insulin resistance, dyslipidemia, type 2 diabetes, hypertension,** elevated plasma **leptin** concentrations, increased **visceral fat** tissue, and increased risk of **coronary heart disease** and cancer. Available research indicates a much clearer relationship between these conditions and increased body fat, rather than merely an increase in body weight. It is certainly possible for an individual to be overweight or overfat, but not exhibit these comorbidities. In most medical literature, the term "overweight" is used to describe an "overfat" condition, even in the absence of accompanying body-fat measures. In this context, obesity then refers to individuals at the extreme end of the overweight continuum. This is the framework used to determine body fatness using BMI, which is the most common technique for estimating fatness.

Determination of Body Fatness Using BMI

BMI is calculated as the ratio of one's weight to height (see Chapter 11):

$$\text{BMI} = \text{Weight (kg)}/\text{Height}^2\ \text{(m)}$$

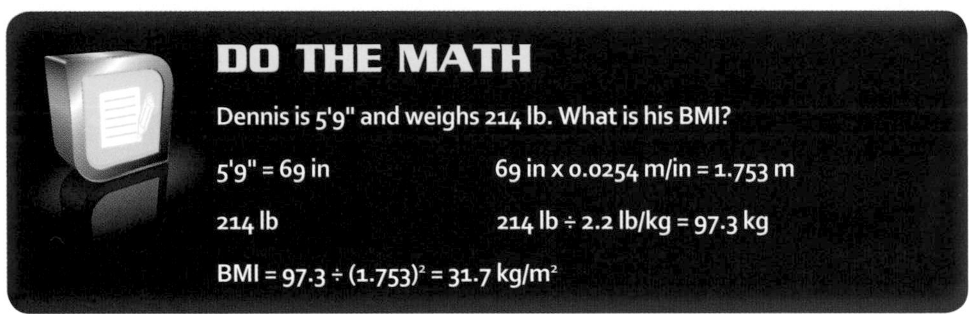

DO THE MATH

Dennis is 5'9" and weighs 214 lb. What is his BMI?

5'9" = 69 in — 69 in x 0.0254 m/in = 1.753 m

214 lb — 214 lb ÷ 2.2 lb/kg = 97.3 kg

BMI = 97.3 ÷ $(1.753)^2$ = 31.7 kg/m^2

Table 8-2 provides an easy way to determine BMI by intersecting an individual's height and weight in standard units. An easy-to-use BMI calculator is available on ACE's website at www.ACEfitness.org/calculators/default.aspx.

In 1997, the World Health Organization (WHO) developed guidelines that classified people with BMIs greater than 25 as overweight and those with BMIs greater than or equal to 30 as obese (WHO, 2000). Individuals who display BMIs greater than or equal to 40 are considered morbidly (extremely) obese (Table 8-3). These individuals clearly have a higher risk of death and disability due to their weight (Lavie, Milani, & Ventura, 2009). These standards place 97 million Americans in the overweight and obese categories, up from 72 million people using previously accepted standards.

Use of BMI in the Clinical Setting

While BMI does not measure body fat, it is considered one of the best ways to quickly approximate an individual's degree of body fatness, as opposed to looking at weight alone. It not only provides a simple baseline measure against which progress can be compared, but it also provides useful information about a client's potential health-risk factors. For example, if a client is classified as being overweight or obese using BMI, it would be a good idea for the ACE-certified Health Coach to inquire about the client's health history related to **blood pressure, cholesterol,** and heart health. At the very least, it does provide a platform from which to discuss the relationship between body fatness and chronic disease and provides both the client and the health coach with a starting point for more in-depth discussion.

Table 8-2
Body Mass Index

	19	20	21	22	23	24	25	26	27	28	29	30	35	40
Height (inches)	Weight (pounds)													
58	91	95	100	105	110	115	119	124	129	134	138	143	167	191
59	94	99	104	109	114	119	124	128	133	138	143	148	173	198
60	97	102	107	112	118	123	128	133	138	143	148	153	179	204
61	100	106	111	116	121	127	132	137	143	148	153	158	185	211
62	104	109	115	120	125	131	136	142	147	153	158	164	191	218
63	107	113	118	124	130	135	141	146	152	158	163	169	197	225
64	110	116	122	128	134	140	145	151	157	163	169	174	203	233
65	114	120	126	132	138	144	150	156	162	168	174	180	210	240
66	117	124	130	136	142	148	155	161	167	173	179	185	216	247
67	121	127	134	140	147	153	159	166	172	178	185	191	223	255
68	125	131	138	144	151	158	164	171	177	184	190	197	230	263
69	128	135	142	149	155	162	169	176	182	189	196	203	237	270
70	132	139	146	153	160	167	174	181	188	195	202	209	243	278
71	136	143	150	157	165	172	179	186	193	200	207	215	250	286
72	140	147	155	162	169	177	184	191	199	206	213	221	258	294
73	144	151	159	166	174	182	189	197	204	212	219	227	265	303
74	148	155	163	171	179	187	194	202	210	218	225	233	272	311
75	152	160	168	176	184	192	200	208	216	224	232	240	279	319
76	156	164	172	180	189	197	205	213	221	230	238	246	287	328

Note: Find your client's height in the far left column and move across the row to the weight that is closest to the client's weight. His or her body mass index will be at the top of that column.

Limitations of BMI

Despite its convenience and popularity, some researchers still consider BMI a relatively crude index of **adiposity,** since BMI fails to consider the body's proportional distribution of body fat and the composition of overall body weight. Healthy adults can be misdiagnosed by BMI as overweight or obese when fat mass is verified by a criterion method such as **dual-energy x-ray absorptiometry (DEXA)** or **hydrostatic weighing.** For instance, BMI may overestimate "fatness" in athletes and others who have a muscular build (false positive) and it may underestimate fatness in older persons and others who have lost muscle (false negative). The possibility of misclassifying someone as overweight using BMI standards applies particularly to large-size field athletes, bodybuilders, heavier wrestlers, and football players who tend to have large amounts of lean muscle mass, which weighs more than fat per unit volume but does not contribute to a higher percentage of body fat.

Table 8-3
Interpretation of Body Mass Index Scores

Body Mass Index Score	Interpretation
Less than 18	Underweight
18 to 24.9	Normal weight
25 to 29.9	Overweight
30 to 39.9	Obese
40 or higher	Morbidly obese

Source: National Heart, Lung, and Blood Institute (2012). *Calculate Your Body Mass Index.* www.nhlbisupport.com/bmi/

Although there are inherent problems with assessing fatness of an individual using the BMI method, it remains the method of choice for large-scale epidemiological studies due to the ease of obtaining the two measurements required for BMI calculation and its acceptable correlation with more technical measures (e.g., DEXA, hydrostatic weighing, and skinfold measurements). It should be emphasized, however, that the number obtained using BMI is *not* a measure of body composition (i.e., percent body fat) per se, but merely a calculated *ratio* using height and weight.

The measurement of body composition—whether using sophisticated methods such as hydrostatic weighing, DEXA, or **air displacement plethysmography** (e.g., BOD POD®) or less-sophisticated methods such as **bioelectrical impedance analysis,** skinfold measurements, or **near-infrared interactance**—produces *estimates* of the percentage of the body comprised of fat vs. fat-free mass. When working with *individuals*, body-composition measurement is considered a much better method of assessing overall fatness and risk for disease than BMI.

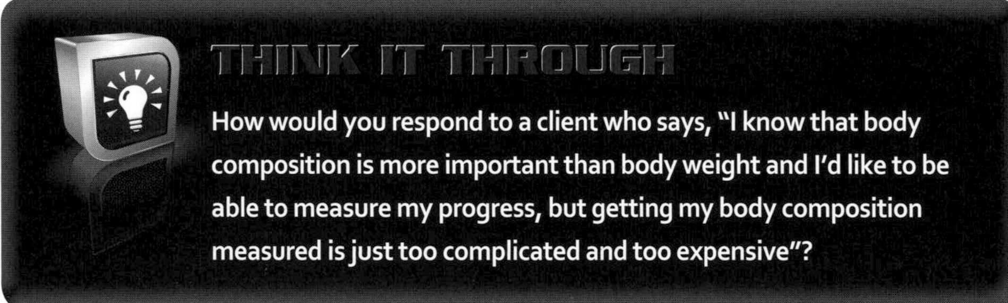

THINK IT THROUGH
How would you respond to a client who says, "I know that body composition is more important than body weight and I'd like to be able to measure my progress, but getting my body composition measured is just too complicated and too expensive"?

Fat Cell Size and Number: Hypertrophy vs. Hyperplasia

Obesity can also be classified by fat cell (**adipocyte**) size and number.

Fat cell **hypertrophy:** Existing fat cells enlarge or fill with fat

Fat cell **hyperplasia:** Total fat cell number increases

One technique for studying body fatness involves extracting small fragments of tissue through a syringe needle inserted directly into a fatty area on the body. Chemical treatment of the sample isolates the individual fat cells for counting. Dividing fat mass in the sample by fat cell number determines the average quantity of fat per cell.

Obesity that occurs early in life (before age one), during the adolescent growth spurt (ages nine through 13), or in adults with a BMI >40, can cause an increase in the number of adipocytes (fat cells), which is called hypercellular or hyperplastic obesity. This type of obesity can easily predispose an individual to obesity throughout adulthood, merely due to the increased numbers of adipose cells available to store and metabolize fat. In fact, children who are obese between the ages of six and nine have a 55% chance of becoming obese adults, which is 10 times the risk of children of normal weight. A child does not generally "outgrow" obesity fat cell (Whitaker et al., 1997). In fact, once established, the number of fat cells remains constant in spite of weight gain or loss. Reducing body fatness is especially difficult, though not impossible, for those with a high number of fat cells. Individuals with hyperplastic obesity are not easily treated with ordinary dietary and exercise regimens. When treated with a conventional low-energy diet, they seem to fail to lose weight after reaching a certain fat-cell size. Obese people who have lost weight by restricting energy intake are very prone to weight regain. Unfortunately for these individuals, no amount of dietary restriction or exercise can reduce fat-cell number (Vinten & Galbo, 1983). Therefore, lifestyle-modification plans that strive to reduce overall body fat will only reduce the amount of fat in each existing cell, which means that it will be more difficult to reduce body-fat percentage, and then to maintain any fat loss.

Obesity that occurs later in life, which is hypertrophic obesity, is associated with an enlargement of the existing fat cells, but a normal fat-cell number. This pattern is correlated with truncal fat distribution (an apple-shape) and health consequences later in life (McArdle, Katch, & Katch, 2010). Men, on average, gain between 0.4 and 1.8 pounds (0.2 and 0.8 kg) of fat each year until their 60s, despite a gradual decrease in food consumption. Approximately 14% of women gain more than 30 pounds (13.6 kg) between the ages of 25 and 34. Women in general have more fat cells than men (McArdle, Katch, & Katch, 2010). Figure 8-2 illustrates adipose cellularity in lean and obese individuals.

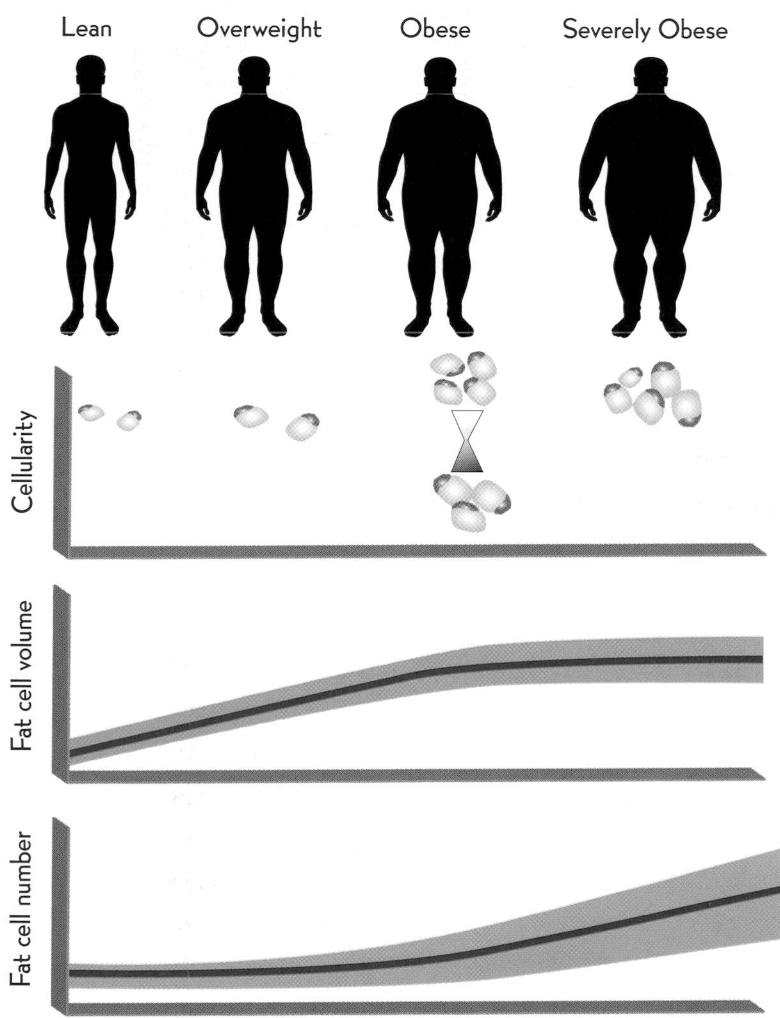

Figure 8-2
Adipose cellularity in lean and obese individuals

Reprinted with permission from Arner P. & Spalding K. (2010). Fat cell turnover in humans. *Biochemical and Biophysical Research Communications,* 396, 1, 101–104.

Health Consequences of Obesity

Adult obesity is linked to comorbidities that have been attributed to as many as 365,000 deaths annually in the United States (Mokdad et al., 2000). In two longitudinal analyses adjusted for smoking status, annual death risk among nonsmokers increased by 12 to 40% among overweight individuals and by 50 to 150% among obese individuals (Adams et al., 2006; Lawlor et al., 2006). Other studies have shown that obesity is an independent risk factor for coronary heart disease even when adjusted for the influences of other risk factors such as age, cholesterol, systolic blood pressure, smoking, left ventricular hypertrophy, and glucose intolerance (Hubert et al., 1983). Obesity is considered the second leading cause of preventable death in America, with smoking being the first (Allison et al., 1999). Obese individuals have an overall mortality rate almost twice that of normal-weight individuals, and being even moderately overweight is associated with a significant increase in the risk of premature death. Obesity reduces life expectancy by as much as 10 to 20 years, causing 280,000 to 325,000 premature deaths in the U.S. each year (Allison et al., 1999).

Obesity is associated with myriad health conditions (Table 8-4). Of special importance is the strong association between excess body fat and **diabetes mellitus.** Not surprisingly, overweight children are more prone to becoming overweight adults, especially if they have an obese parent (Guo & Chumlea, 1999; Whitaker et al., 1997). Obesity during adolescence is associated with many adverse health consequences in adulthood, even if the obesity does not persist (Must et al., 1992).

Table 8-4

Specific Health Risks of Excessive Body Fat

- Impaired cardiac function due to increased workload on the heart
- Hypertension
- Stroke
- Deep-vein thrombosis
- Increased insulin resistance in children and adults
- Renal disease
- Sleep apnea and pulmonary disease
- Problems receiving anesthesia during surgery
- Osteoarthritis, degenerative joint disease, and gout
- Endometrial, breast, prostate, and colon cancers
- Abnormal plasma lipid and cholesterol levels
- Menstrual irregularities
- Gallbladder disease
- Psychological distress, social stigma, and discrimination

Source: Adapted from McArdle, W.D., Katch, F.I., & Katch, V.L. (2010). Overweight, obesity, and weight control. In *Exercise Physiology: Energy, Nutrition, and Human Performance* (7th ed.). Philadelphia: Wolters Kluwer/Lippincott Williams & Wilkins.

According to the National Institutes of Health (NIH), obesity represents a chronic, degenerative disease, even at low levels of excessive body fat. A moderate 4 to 10% increase in body weight after the age of 20 correlates with a 50% greater risk of death from **coronary artery disease** and nonfatal heart attack (Rosengren et al., 1997). Even long-term body weight at the high-end of the normal range increases heart disease and cancer risk (Manson et al., 1995). In the Nurses Health Study, nurses of average weight experienced 30% more heart attacks compared to their thinnest counterparts, and the risk for a moderately overweight nurse was 80% higher (Manson et al., 1995). This means that a woman who gains only 20 pounds (9 kg) from her late teens to middle age doubles her risk of having a heart attack. Obesity is classified as an independent heart-disease risk factor, similar in nature to cigarette smoking, high cholesterol, and hypertension. It also appears to correspond to higher levels of arterial inflammation that slowly and progressively increases heart attack and **stroke** risk over many years.

The Importance of Body-fat Distribution Pattern

Where on the body a person tends to store body fat is also an important determinant of future health. Studies suggest that weight gain in the abdominal area, or **android obesity,** increases the risk for coronary heart disease, high blood pressure, diabetes, and stroke compared to individuals of the same overall body fat who tend to store fat in the **gynoid obesity** pattern, namely in the hips, buttocks, and thighs (Lee & Pratley, 2007; Wisse, 2004; Fasshauer & Paschke, 2003). The reason for this difference seems to be that fat in the abdomen is more easily released into the bloodstream, increasing the disease-related blood-fat levels. In general, men tend to gain weight in the android pattern, while women tend to store fat in the gynoid pattern, although any person (male or female) with android obesity carries increased health risks. To determine body-fat distribution pattern, a waist-to-hip ratio can be performed, whereby the girth of the waist at the smallest point at or near the navel is divided by the girth of the hip at the largest point around the buttocks (see Chapter 11). If the ratio exceeds 0.80 for women and 0.95 for men, this is indicative of a central body-fat distribution pattern (android) and therefore is associated with higher blood cholesterol, **triglycerides, insulin** levels, and blood pressure, and lower **high-density lipoprotein (HDL)** cholesterol, in addition to increased left ventricular wall thickness (Freedman et al., 1999).

Some clinicians use waist girth as a simple gauge of abdominal obesity and to complement measures of body fat for normal-weight individuals. Waist girth alone has been shown to correlate more strongly to direct measures of abdominal visceral fat accumulation and other heart-disease risks than the waist-to-hip ratio (Despres, 2001). Specifically, women with waist measurements higher than 30 inches (76.2 cm) develop heart disease twice as frequently as slimmer women. In general, men with waist circumferences above 40 inches (102 cm) and women with waist circumferences above 35 inches (86 cm) display elevated cardiovascular risk profiles (Expert Panel, 1998).

Etiology of Obesity

The exact cause of obesity remains a mystery. Unfortunately, obesity involves a complex interaction of many factors with psychological, environmental, evolutionary, biologic, and genetic causes. In its simplest context, the maintenance of body weight can be seen as involving three main factors: metabolic utilization of nutrients, dietary habits, and physical activity. In turn, these factors are affected by susceptibility genes, which may influence energy expenditure, fuel metabolism, muscle fiber function, and appetite or food choices. Certainly, the increasing rates of obesity cannot be explained solely by changes in the gene pool, but it is possible that genetic variants are more often triggered in modern society by an obesogenic environment that includes high availability of energy- and fat-dense foods and by people's increasingly **sedentary** lifestyles. The following sections review how excess energy intake, sedentary lifestyle, and genetics influence the presence of obesity.

Energy Intake

The most obvious theory of why individuals become obese is that they simply consume too many calories. Short-term overeating is a common habit that does little to adversely affect health, whereas overeating over long periods can create a health risk. Overeating can be either active or passive and can be induced by a number of conditions. Active overeating can be caused by a cognitive drive to consume too many calories (driven by internal or external cues), a physical defect in appetite and/or **satiety** regulation, or an inappropriate psychological response to stress. Passive overeating is a different phenomenon, in which the consumption of what would otherwise be a "normal" amount of food becomes excessive due to a sedentary, inactive lifestyle.

Whether overconsumption is accomplished through active or passive overeating, the result is the same; excessive intake of energy will be stored and can increase the size and/or number of adipocytes depending on the person's age and the size of existing adipocytes. While it is a common belief that "a calorie is a calorie" regardless of its nutrient composition, research indicates that not all of the **macronutrients** contribute to obesity equally. For instance, Flatt et al. (1985) and Schutz et al. (1989) demonstrated that a high-fat meal that provides more calories than are immediately necessary stimulates fat storage without a similar increase in fat utilization. This suggests that positive energy balance caused by excess fat intake will promote more fat storage. Furthermore, the storage of dietary fat into adipose tissue is associated with a very low metabolic cost (0 to 2%) (Jequier & Tappy, 1999) compared to the thermic effect for **carbohydrate** (6 to 8%) and **protein** (25 to 30%) (Jequier, 1995). Therefore, of the three macronutrients, it is more metabolically costly to convert and store dietary protein as fat than it is for either dietary carbohydrate or fat.

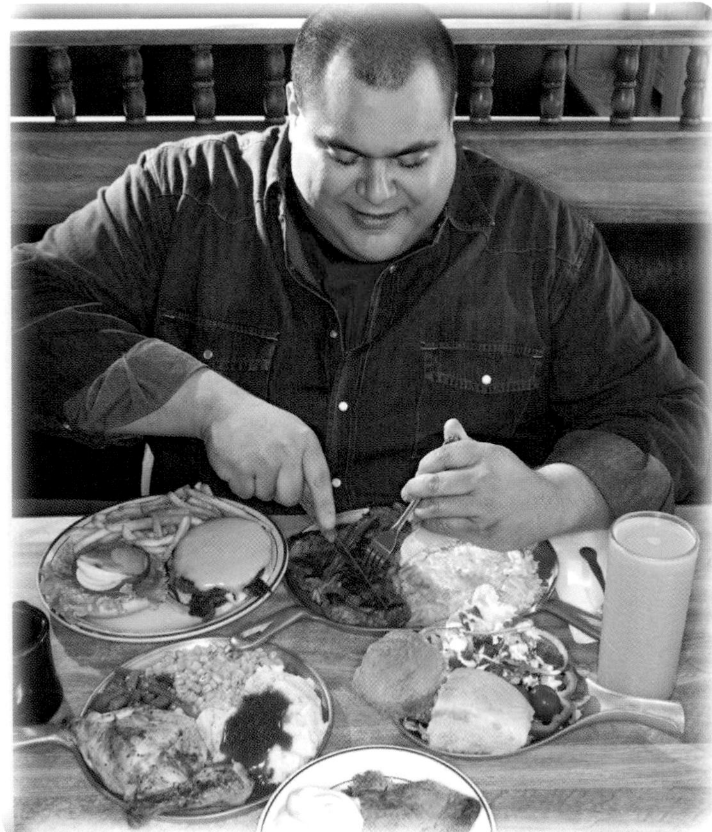

Many studies have also examined the effects on weight loss of varying macronutrient composition in diets with identical caloric content (see Chapter 9). In a study evaluating weight loss in participants consuming a low-calorie diet with high-protein vs. high-carbohydrate content, researchers concluded that the replacement of some dietary carbohydrate with protein improves weight and fat loss and spares protein loss by promoting lipid **oxidation** in the fasting state (Labayen et al., 2003). Randomized, controlled trials continue to show comparable or superior effects of high-protein diets on weight loss, preservation of lean body mass, and improvement in several cardiovascular risk factors for up to 12 months (Brehm & D'Alessio, 2008). Evidence that chronic high protein intake affects glucose metabolism, however, is inconclusive. Despite their appeal for weight loss, high-protein diets remain controversial due to questions about their safety, especially if consumed long-term. Diets with moderately increased protein and modestly restricted carbohydrate and fat contents (especially **saturated fat**), can have beneficial effects on body weight, body composition, and metabolic parameters. Key issues regarding long-term safety, however, warrant further study.

Active Overeating

Active overeating in humans can occur due to cultural norms that favor fatness and regard high body weight (in women in particular) as a symbol of affluence and attractiveness. In Western society, however, active overeating is mostly driven by marketing. Huge portion sizes and fast-food "combo" meals that are less expensive than the *a la carte* option provide an excessive amount of calories that bear no relationship to the single-meal energy requirement of most individuals. Dr. Barbara Rolls calls this phenomenon "volumetrics" (Rolls et al., 2007). In one study, 23 normal-weight men and women were presented standard-portion meals for 11 consecutive days and large-portion meals (additional 50%) for 11 days. When larger meals were an option, subjects consumed approximately 423 more calories per day. Therefore, it appears that the availability of larger portions contributed to energy overconsumption and excess body-weight gain (Rolls et al., 2007). However, evidence suggests that active overeating contributes to the obesity epidemic to a lesser degree in the general population than does passive overeating.

Passive Overeating

It is easy to demonstrate how increases in energy intake lead to positive energy balance and weight gain. In contrast, there is strong evidence to suggest that the modern sedentary lifestyle, and resultant low levels of energy expenditure, is the driving force behind the obesity epidemic. In fact, there is evidence to suggest that reduced energy expenditure increases a person's vulnerability to overeating, primarily due to the fat content of foods that provide excessive amounts of calories even though overall "portions" of these high-fat foods may be quite normal.

In an interesting study of this phenomenon, men were allowed to eat freely from seemingly identical diets that had been secretly manipulated to contain 20%, 40%, or 60% energy from fat. Regardless of the fat content of their diets, each group of men ate the same bulk of food. Therefore, the energy overload provided in the 60% fat diet was an "accidental" phenomenon (thus the term "passive overeating") (Prentice, 2001). The results showed a significantly higher fat balance in men consuming the highest fat diet (Lissner et al., 1987). Therefore, high-fat foods do not decrease consumption, but rather only serve as a source of unnecessary excessive calories.

Energy Expenditure

In the classic sense, there are three components of human daily energy expenditure: basal metabolic rate, **thermic effect of food,** and thermic effect of physical activity. Basal metabolic rate is the amount of energy required for vital, resting bodily functions without food. It accounts for about 60 to 75% of daily energy expenditure. Most of the variability across individuals is accounted for by differences in lean body mass, which is more metabolically active than fat mass. The thermic effect of food is the energy required to digest, absorb, and store ingested food energy, and accounts for about 10% of daily energy expenditure in most people. The remaining component, activity thermogenesis, represents between 15 and 30% of daily energy expenditure and can be further subdivided into exercise and **nonexercise activity thermogenesis (NEAT)** or spontaneous physical activity (Figure 8-3). In contrast to the other two components of energy expenditure, activity thermogenesis is highly variable across individuals and can easily vary by as much

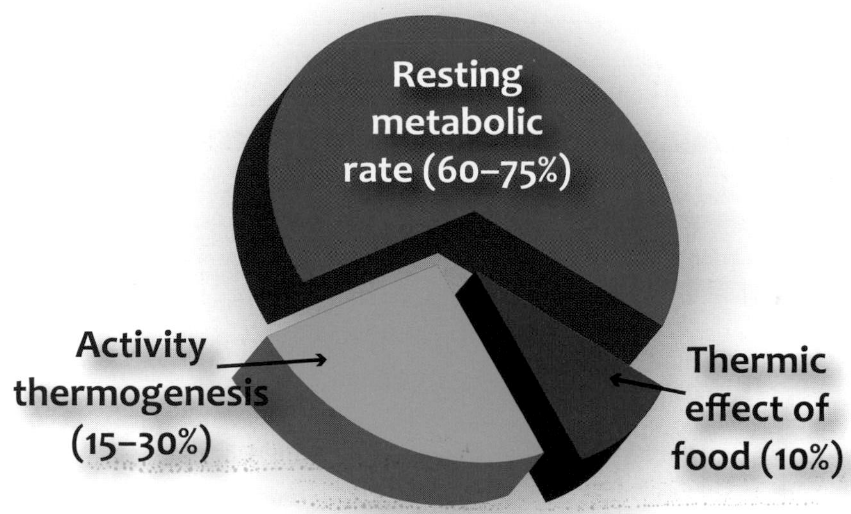

Figure 8-3
Three components of daily energy expenditure

as 2,000 kcal/day between individuals (Levine, 2007). The majority of individuals in the world do not participate in purposeful exercise for the sake of fitness, so for them, exercise thermogenesis is negligible. In those who do exercise, expenditure can be quite small, accounting for less than 100 kcal/day of energy expenditure. Therefore, it stands to reason that the variability between individuals for activity thermogenesis is largely accounted for by NEAT associated with occupation and leisure (e.g., going to work or school, performing household tasks, and ambulation). It also stands to reason that increasing energy expenditure by increasing NEAT may hold significant promise in combating the obesity epidemic.

The notion that obesity may be more related to energy expenditure related to NEAT than to energy expenditure related to exercise is supported by the literature. When positive energy balance is imposed through overfeeding, Levine and colleagues (1999) demonstrated that obese subjects sat 2.5 hours per day more than lean subjects. The lean sedentary volunteers stood and walked for more than 2 hours per day longer than obese sedentary subjects, even though all subjects lived and worked in similar environments. Therefore, those who voluntarily increase their NEAT the most (primarily through walking) gain the least fat, and those who consume excess calories but do not increase their NEAT gain the most fat (Levine et al., 1999). These researchers also calculated that if the obese subjects were to adopt the same activity patterns as the lean subjects, they could expend an additional 350 kcal/day due to their larger size. Thus, NEAT and specifically walking are of substantial energetic importance in obesity. It might seem obvious that because people with obesity are heavier, they sit more than lean people. However, these differences are not due to greater body weight alone, because when lean subjects gained weight through overfeeding their tendency to stand/ambulate persisted and when obese subjects became lighter, their tendency to sit did not change (Levine et al., 2005). Research in this area supports the notion that perhaps peoples' environments need to be reengineered to promote NEAT. This argument makes sense, especially given the fact that despite the best efforts nationally, participation in physical activity is at an all-time low and obesity rates are at an all-time high.

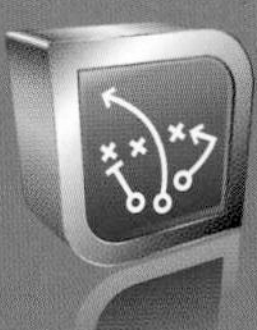

APPLY WHAT YOU KNOW

Incorporating Physical Activity Into the Daily Routine

In addition to purposeful physical activity and exercise routines, people need to make a conscious effort to "undo" their technologically geared and consequently sedentary lifestyles. While all of the modern conveniences people enjoy make working "easier," they have also successfully engineered physical activity right out of most people's lives. Putting it back in now requires behavioral change. The best advice that health coaches can offer to their clients is to sit less and move more. Many activities that involve sitting can be done while standing, pacing, or walking instead. The additional calories expended by doing these activities while not seated add up and contribute to an overall healthier lifestyle, not only because of the calories being burned, but also because of the thought process that people engage in when they make the choice to be active continuously throughout the day.

Clients can try the following methods to decrease their daily sitting time:

- Take a quick walk around the block before getting ready in the morning
- Walk 30 minutes at lunch
- Have a "walk and talk" meeting rather than sitting at a desk
- Pace when talking on the phone
- Work while standing rather than sitting (or better yet, convince your place of business to invest in an adjustable-height desk or even a "treadmill desk")
- Walk for 15 minutes right when arriving home, before getting preoccupied with home responsibilities
- Walk with their children and talk about their day
- When parking the car, choose the parking space farthest from the door
- Make it a general rule to avoid all labor-saving devices (e.g., escalators, elevators, and moving walkways).

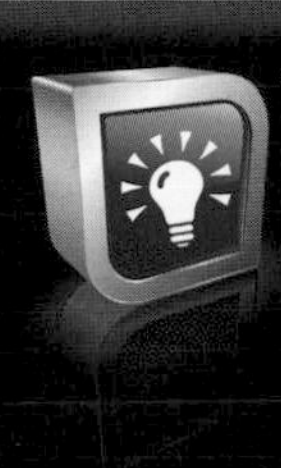

THINK IT THROUGH

A prospective client, who has always struggled with her weight, tells you, "There is just no way I can lose weight. I sit all day in an office and have to care for my family when I get home. When do I have time to exercise?" What quick tips could you give her to change her thinking about her opportunities for physical activity?

Possible Mechanisms of Obesity

In addition to the contributors to obesity mentioned previously, there are several **hormones** and genetic components that have been implicated in the **etiology** of obesity. Some of these have an effect on long-term control of energy intake (e.g., insulin and leptin). Signals that provide short-term information about hunger and satiety include gut hormones, such as **cholecystokinin, ghrelin,** and **peptide YY,** and signals from **vagal afferent neurons** within the gastrointestinal tract that respond to fullness, macronutrients, pH, tonicity, and hormones. Neural and humoral signals are then integrated in the arcuate nucleus, a group of cells in the hypothalamus, and are mediated by two types of neurons, the appetite-inhibiting **proopiomelanocortin (POMC)** and the appetite-stimulating **neuropeptide Y (NPY).** These neurons relay feedback signals to the hypothalamus via the **central nervous system,** the digestive tract, thyroid gland, adrenal glands, and the pancreas to signal the individual to either start or stop eating. The following section discusses the role that several key hormones, neuropeptides, and other factors may play in development of obesity.

Long-term Control of Energy Intake

Insulin

Insulin is a peptide hormone produced by the pancreatic β-cells and secreted in response to elevated blood glucose levels. Insulin is an anabolic hormone for both muscle and fat cells and plays an important role in the storage and utilization of energy in the adipocytes. Circulating levels of insulin rise rapidly after eating. Similar to leptin, insulin suppresses NPY and stimulates POMC to regulate feeding in response to the amount of stored calories. Through coordinated action on hypothalamic neurons that stimulate or inhibit feeding behavior, insulin and leptin function centrally as satiety signals to decrease food intake when energy levels are met and adipose tissue has been restored.

Leptin

Leptin is a **cytokine** hormone produced by the *ob* gene and is secreted by adipose tissue in direct proportion to the total amount of body fat. Leptin has been called a regulator of appetite, but more specifically, it is a hormone that acts on the hypothalamus in the brain via a negative feedback loop to regulate energy intake (Arch, 2005). In a normal situation, increases in triglyceride deposits into the adipocyte causes a release of leptin from the adipocyte, which in turn triggers the hypothalamus to reduce appetite and the drive to eat. Fasting induces a decrease in leptin produced in adipose tissue and a subsequent decrease in serum leptin levels, which stimulates hunger (Arch, 2005).

Although it was initially hypothesized in 1994 when leptin was discovered that obese individuals must have low leptin levels, research has now shown that most obese individuals actually have elevated blood plasma leptin levels (Arch, 2005). In obese children and adults, plasma leptin circulates in direct proportion to adipose tissue mass when weight is stable, in amounts four times higher than in lean individuals (Gutin et al., 1999). Analogous to insulin resistance in obese individuals with type 2 diabetes, it is now thought that perhaps obese individuals are "leptin resistant." This theory is supported by the observation that leptin transport across the blood-brain barrier is impaired in obese individuals.

Weight loss reduces leptin levels, and weight gain increases circulating levels. Even without significant weight loss, a prolonged state of negative caloric balance or fasting decreases circulating leptin concentrations and increases hunger sensations (Boden et al., 1996). Interestingly, neither short- nor long-term exercise significantly affects leptin independently. Injections of leptin in obese subjects who produce adequate amounts of leptin, but are resistant to it, do not stimulate an increase in fat loss. This may indicate that physiologically leptin may be more important as an indicator of energy deficiency and may be a possible mediator of an adaptation to starvation (Kelesidis et al., 2010).

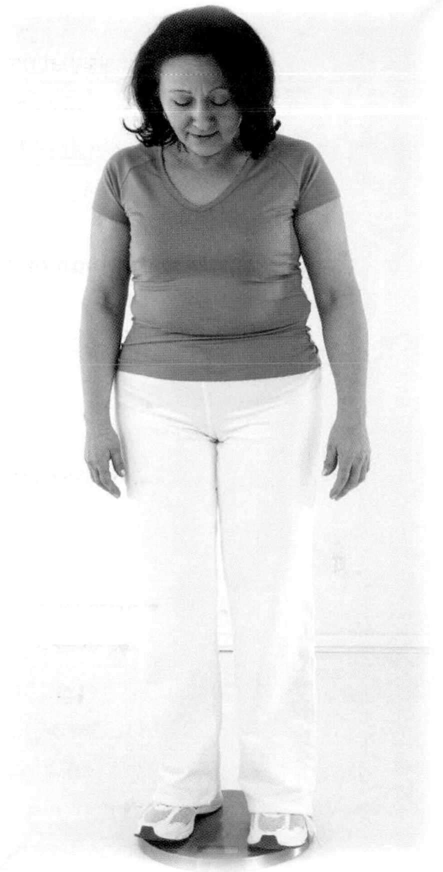

Leptin alone does not determine whether a person becomes obese, nor does it explain why some people can eat without restriction and maintain a stable body weight while others become overfat with the same caloric intake. It may, however, be a very important regulatory component of the obesity puzzle. For instance, leptin administration may have a clinical application in the treatment of weight-loss maintenance. Weight loss reduces leptin concentrations, which may activate neuroendocrine mechanisms that stimulate hunger and decrease energy expenditure by decreasing thyroid hormone levels, which slows metabolism (Rosenbaum et al., 2005). Thus, replacing leptin may reverse these neuroendocrine abnormalities and prevent the adverse effects of "yo-yo" dieting.

Short-term Control of Energy Intake

Cholecystokinin

Cholecystokinin (CCK) is a peptide hormone secreted in the **duodenum** and **jejunum** of the small intestine in response to digestive enzymes. It slows emptying of the stomach and sends satiety signals to the hypothalamus, which should inhibit food consumption. CCK administration reduces food intake, meal size, and meal duration when given to rodents and humans, but rodents compensate for the reduction in meal size by eating more frequently with no effect on overall body weight (Moran & Dailey, 2009). While its role in obesity is not known, there are currently drugs in development called CCK-A promoters that enhance the effects of CCK-A, an intestinal hormone that may inhibit appetite (Boguszewski et al., 2010).

Ghrelin

Ghrelin, a hormone discovered in 1999, is produced mainly in the stomach. It is responsible for stimulating appetite via stimulation of the NPY receptors and by stimulating growth hormone release from the pituitary gland. Ghrelin concentrations in the blood vary widely throughout the day, with higher levels during sleep and before meals and lower levels after meals. For this reason, ghrelin was thought to be a "hunger hormone" responsible for meal initiation, but it is more likely that ghrelin functions to prepare the body to deal with incoming food (Drazen et al., 2006). Ghrelin levels in the blood are inversely correlated with weight, meaning that high ghrelin levels are associated with low body weight.

Peptide YY

Peptide YY (PYY) is a hormone rapidly released from the descending colon and rectum in proportion to the number of calories consumed. PYY acts on the hypothalamus to suppress appetite, especially two to six hours after a meal, on the pancreas to increase its exocrine secretion of digestive juices, and on the gallbladder to stimulate the release of bile. The appetite suppression mediated by PYY works more slowly than that of cholecystokinin and more rapidly than that of leptin. Subjects given PYY were less hungry and ate less food over the next 12 hours than those who received a placebo (Batterham et al., 2003). In obese individuals, circulating levels of PYY are decreased, and release of PYY following a meal is lower than in normal-weight individuals, and therefore does not suppress appetite as much (Daniels, 2006). In addition, PYY also reduces ghrelin secretion, which may be an additional effect that promotes weight loss.

Influence of Genetics vs. Environment

Studies indicate that genetic factors that affect metabolism and appetite determine about 25% of the variation in body fatness, while a larger percentage is explained by environmental influences. The epidemic of obesity, begun decades ago, has occurred within a gene pool that has not changed in 100 years or more. Nonetheless, it is clear that genetic factors play an important role in one's susceptibility to becoming obese in an obesogenic environment rich with sedentary and stressful activities and ready access to inexpensive, large-portion, high-calorie, good-tasting food. Currently, researchers have established that genetics contributes to the development of obesity in two ways:

- *Single rare mutations in certain genes that wholly explain the development of obesity (monogenic obesity):* There are now at least 20 single-gene disorders that result in an autosomal form of obesity, but these forms are rare, very severe, and generally begin in childhood (e.g., lacking the gene that produces leptin) (O'Rahilly, 2009).
- *Several genetic variants that interact with an "at-risk" environment (polygenic obesity):* In this case, each gene, taken individually, would only contribute to body weight in a small way, and the cumulative effect of these genes would only become significant when there is an interaction with environmental factors that cause their expression (e.g., overeating and sedentary lifestyle).

The unique interaction between an individual's genetic composition and the environment in which his or her genes have an opportunity to express themselves makes it difficult to quantify the role of each in the development of obesity. While one's genes do not necessarily cause obesity, they may lower the threshold for its expression or manifestation in an individual. Researchers are just now starting to identify key genes and specific **deoxyribonucleic acid (DNA)** sequences that relate to the causes of appetite regulation and predispose a person to obesity. To date, more than 50 genes and **polymorphisms** have been tested and implicated in controlling food intake, energy expenditure, and fat and carbohydrate metabolism. While no conclusive role in obesity development has been established for these genes, certain variants are associated with different types of obesity (child- vs. adult-onset), metabolic and cardiovascular complications, appetite, and the interaction between excess body weight and physical activity (Clement, 2005). This area of research, however, is extremely complex, and progress in the knowledge of the human genome and the development of computing tools and new analysis strategies that can handle several hundreds of items of genetic and environmental information at once will be necessary to tackle these questions (Clement, 2005).

Genetic Factors

Many genes that are being targeted for their possible role in obesity development fall within two broad categories: genes affecting the central nervous system and those that operate peripherally via adipose tissue. Insightful information about the causes of obesity has come from the cloning of obesity genes in animals. Molecular and reverse genetic studies (using mouse "**knockouts**") have also helped to establish important pathways that regulate body fat and food intake. Leptin deficiency, produced by a single gene mutation as described earlier in this chapter, has shown us that true metabolic-gene pathways do exist (O'Rahilly, 2009). Similar deficiencies in genes that regulate food intake have been found, such as fat mass and obesity associated (FTO) and melanocortin-4 receptor (MC4R), where changes to the amino acid sequence of a key regulator of food intake causes uncontrolled appetite similar to that seen in leptin deficiency. These insights into biology have shown that body-fat regulation may be independent of willpower.

In a landmark study by Bouchard et al. (1990), the importance of genetics in body-weight regulation was clearly shown. Researchers intentionally overfed 12 pairs of male identical twins for 100 days (total overfeeding of 84,000 kcal) to observe differences within and between twin pairs. What they found was a striking similarity in the amount of weight gain, skinfold changes, and changes in BMI *within* the twin pairs, but three times more variance *between* twin pairs for these same variables. The within-pair similarity was particularly evident with respect to the changes in regional fat distribution and amount of abdominal visceral fat, with about six times as much variance between pairs as within pairs. They concluded that the most likely explanation for the similarity within pairs of twins in the adaptation to long-term overfeeding and for the large variations in weight changes and body-fat distribution between pairs of twins is that genetic factors were involved. These genetic factors may regulate a person's tendency to store extra calories as either fat or lean tissue and alter resting metabolism accordingly.

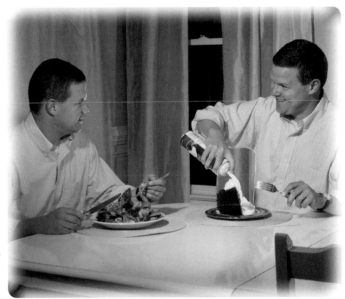

Environmental Factors

There has been an increasing interest in the role of the environment in the determination of dietary behavior among individuals (see Chapter 14). This "social ecological" view of health takes into account the fact that individuals interact with their environments, which ultimately influence their health behaviors (Giskes et al., 2007). Higher rates of obesity are found in those with the lowest incomes and the least education, especially among women and certain ethnic groups. This association may be partially explained by the relatively low cost of energy-dense, high-fat food, and the association of lower incomes and unavailability of fresh fruits and vegetables (Turrell et al., 2002). Observational studies in many different countries confirm that dietary patterns and obesity rates vary between neighborhoods, where living in a low-income neighborhood is independently associated with obesity and a poor diet (Cummins & Macintyre,

2006). These environmental influences on diet involve two pathways: access to foods for home consumption from supermarkets and grocery stores, and access to ready-made food from fast-food restaurants and convenience stores.

Studies on the built environment consistently show that the presence of supermarkets is associated with a lower prevalence of obesity. In the U.S. and Canada, "healthier" and more expensive foods are less available in poorer communities and access to supermarkets is more difficult in low-income neighborhoods, where independent stores dominate and tend to charge higher prices. Foods purchased from fast-food and other restaurants are becoming an increasingly important part of people's diets, especially in the U.S. These foods, which can be up to 65% more energy dense than the average diet, provide fewer nutrients and higher amounts of fat, and tend to be larger in portion size than foods consumed at home (Prentice & Jebb, 2003; Rolls, 2003). Several components of the food supply and food "environment" may be important determinants of obesity. Research on portion sizes or packages and servings clearly indicates that when more food is provided, more food is eaten (Diliberti et al., 2004). Portion sizes have increased dramatically in the past 40 years, and while containers do state that a particular package may contain more than one serving, it is common to consume food by the package and not by the serving size (see Chapter 15 for more information on serving sizes and typical portion sizes).

EXPAND YOUR KNOWLEDGE

Exposing the Myth of the Set Point Theory

The concept of a "set point" for body weight has been debated for many decades. Initially, this theory proposed that adult body weight is regulated at some predetermined or "preferred" level by a simple feedback control system regulated by the hypothalamus (Mrosovsky & Powley, 1977). This was based on studies of rats (Cohn & Joseph, 1962) and humans (Sims & Horton, 1968) that showed that weight gained or lost by over- or underfeeding was restored to the original control weight once feeding returned to normal. The homeostatic control mechanisms involved in this process were argued to include an adaptation in the energy economy of metabolic processes, whereby they became more or less wasteful in order to maintain fixed fat stores and body weight (Bennett, 1995). A low RMR is most often blamed for this phenomenon, but the simple notion that RMR is down-regulated during weight loss and therefore responsible for weight regain remains controversial (Weinsier, 2001). Roland Weinsier, a prominent obesity researcher, sought to answer the question, "Do adaptations in energy economy explain the weight-gain tendency of obesity-prone persons?" To fully answer this question, he and his colleagues designed a series of experiments that addressed five important research questions:

- *Is RMR reduced after weight loss to a post-obese state?* To address this question, 70 obese women were recruited, and through dietary restriction, lost approximately 16 to 17% of their body weight so that each woman had a BMI <25 kg/m^2. While RMR *did* decline after losing weight, RMR was *normal* when adjusting for changes in body composition. The researchers concluded that women were not more energy conservative in their post-obese state and did not have a lower body composition–adjusted RMR after losing weight (Weinsier et al., 2000).

- *Is RMR low in post-obese vs. never-obese women?* To address this question, the RMR of the post-obese group was compared with a group of matched never-obese women. The RMRs between the two groups were actually within 1 to 4% of each other and not statistically different, even after adjusting for small differences in body composition. The researchers concluded that RMRs were comparable between obesity-prone weight-reduced women and obesity-resistant women (Weinsier et al., 2000).
- *Does low RMR predict weight regain in post-obese women?* In the same study, women were followed for four years to observe their weight-gain patterns. The never-obese women had a mean BMI increase from 21.3 to 21.8, while the previously obese women went from an initial BMI of 28 to 23 during weight loss, and then regained to a BMI of 27 after four years. More importantly, body composition–adjusted RMR in the weight-reduced state did not correlate with the weight-regain patterns, nor was there a tendency for those with a lower RMR to regain more weight than those with a higher RMR. Therefore, the researchers concluded that factors other than variation in RMR were responsible for the weight regain of the obesity-prone women (Weinsier et al., 2000).
- *Are black women more energetically economical than white women?* To address this question, Byrne et al. (2003) studied 18 white and 22 matched black women in the overweight state, after weight reduction to normal weight (with diet only, no exercise), and after one year without intervention. What they found was that white and black women did not differ in their weight loss and subsequent regain, but RMR was higher in white women than black women. They attributed this, however, to differences in trunk lean body mass, possibly attributable to lower organ mass in the black women. Since organ tissue is more metabolically active than skeletal muscle tissue during rest, this could explain some of the variation in RMR.
- *Do differences in energy economy favor greater weight gain in black vs. white women?* In a study of 23 obese white and 23 matched obese black women and 38 never-obese controls, weight loss through diet alone was induced in the obese subjects. A host of metabolic measures were tracked, including activity energy expenditure, sleeping energy expenditure, free-living energy expenditure, body composition, and aerobic fitness. What they found was that weight-reduced white women increased their activity energy expenditure and consequently their aerobic fitness, while the black women appeared to produce a more obesity-prone sedentary state that favored weight relapse (Weinsier et al., 2002). Their earlier findings confirmed that after one year, black women tended to regain more weight than their weight-reduced white counterparts (Weinsier, 2001).

What this eloquent series of studies underscores is that the maintenance of a healthy body weight is achieved through a complex interaction among physical activity, food choice, and individual metabolism, and is influenced by hormonal, environmental, and genetic factors. One is not necessarily "programmed" to be a certain body weight, but people who have lost weight will naturally tend to return to their pre–weight loss state if the *behaviors* that led to the overweight state are not properly and permanently addressed.

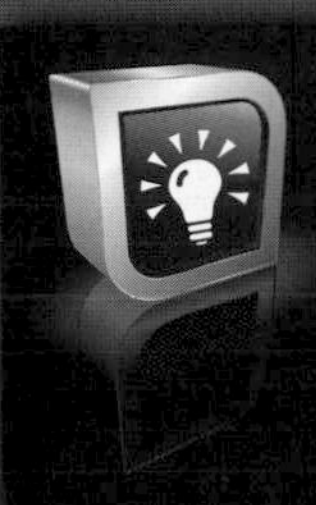

THINK IT THROUGH

You are training an African-American client who asks, "My whole family is overweight, including my parents, siblings, and my children. Isn't it true that African Americans are just genetically programmed to be heavy?" How would you respond to this client's question?

EXPAND YOUR KNOWLEDGE

Moving From Theory to Practice

Overweight and obesity are largely preventable. Individual choices are influenced by supportive communities and environments. Making healthy choices easier to act upon will go a long way in preventing obesity.

Individuals can reduce their obesity risk by:

- Engaging in daily physical activity according to the *2008 Physical Activity Guidelines* (U.S. Department of Health and Human Services, 2008)
- Limiting sedentary/inactive time
- Increasing consumption of fruits, vegetables, legumes, whole grains, and nuts
- Limiting sugar intake
- Achieving a healthy weight and maintaining energy balance

Society can help prevent obesity in individuals by:

- Supporting healthy decision-making through collaboration of public and private stakeholders
- Making regular physical activity and healthy diets affordable and accessible to all individuals, especially to members of groups with the largest health disparities

The food industry can promote healthy diets by:

- Reducing the fat, sugar, and salt content in processed foods
- Ensuring that nutritious food options are accessible to all
- Practicing responsible marketing

Source: Adapted from World Health Organization (2011). *Obesity and Overweight.* www.who.int/mediacentre/factsheet/fs311/en/

Summary

One of the lessons to be learned from the physiology of obesity is that overweight and obesity have numerous causes and effects in the human body. It is essential that health coaches avoid being—or even appearing—judgmental when working with their clients, many of whom will have struggled with weight-related issues for much of their lives. Instead, a health coach should serve as a resource for those clients seeking a deeper understanding of the "why" and "how" behind the development of obesity. In addition, health coaches should educate clients about the health consequences of obesity whenever it is appropriate and motivating to do so. By better understanding the causes of obesity and the countless influences on how, when, and what they eat, a health coach's clients will be better armed to make the behavioral changes needed to succeed with long-term weight management.

References

Adams, K.F. et al. (2006). Overweight, obesity, and mortality in a large prospective cohort of persons 50 to 71 years old. *The New England Journal of Medicine,* 355, 8, 763–778.

Allison, D.B. et al. (1999). Annual deaths attributable to obesity in the United States. *Journal of the American Medical Association,* 282, 16, 1530–1538.

Arch, J.R. (2005). Central regulation of energy balance: Inputs, outputs and leptin resistance. *The Proceedings of the Nutrition Society,* 64, 1, 39–46.

Arner P. & Spalding K. (2010). Fat cell turnover in humans. *Biochemical and Biophysical Research Communications,* 396, 1, 101–104.

Batterham, R.L. et al. (2003). Inhibition of food intake in obese subjects by peptide YY3-36. *The New England Journal of Medicine,* 349, 10, 941–948.

Bennett, W.I. (1995). Beyond overeating. *The New England Journal of Medicine,* 332, 10, 673–674.

Boden, G. et al. (1996). Effect of fasting on serum leptin in normal human subjects. *The Journal of Clinical Endocrinology and Metabolism,* 81, 9, 3419–3423.

Boguszewski, C.L. et al. (2010). Neuroendocrine body weight regulation: Integration between fat tissue, gastrointestinal tract, and the brain. *Endokrynologia Polska,* 61, 2, 194–206.

Bouchard, C. et al. (1990). The response to long-term overfeeding in identical twins. *New England Journal of Medicine,* 322, 21, 1477–1482.

Brehm, B.J. & D'Alessio, D.A. (2008). Benefits of high-protein weight loss diets: Enough evidence for practice? *Current Opinion in Endocrinology, Diabetes, and Obesity,* 15, 5, 416–421.

Byrne, N.M. et al. (2003). Influence of distribution of lean body mass on resting metabolic rate after weight loss and weight regain: Comparison of responses in white and black women. *The American Journal of Clinical Nutrition,* 77, 6, 1368–1373.

Carpenter, W.H. et al. (1998). Total daily energy expenditure in free-living older African-Americans and Caucasians. *American Journal of Physiology,* 274, 1, Pt 1, E96–101.

Centers for Disease Control and Prevention (2010). *What Are the Health Consequences of Living in an "Obesogenic" Society?* www.cdc.gov/speakers/subtopic/speechTopics.html

Clement, K. (2005). Genetics of human obesity. *Proceedings of the Nutrition Society,* 64, 2, 133–142.

Cohn, C. & Joseph, D. (1962). Influence of body weight and body fat on appetite of "normal" lean and obese rats. *The Yale Journal of Biology and Medicine,* 34, 598–607.

Cummins, S. & Macintyre, S. (2006). Food environments and obesity: Neighbourhood or nation? *International Journal of Epidemiology,* 35, 1, 100–104.

Daniels, J. (2006). Obesity: America's epidemic. *The American Journal of Nursing,* 106, 1, 40–50.

Despres, J.P. (2001). Health consequences of visceral obesity. *Annals of Medicine,* 33, 8, 534–541.

Diliberti, N. et al. (2004). Increased portion size leads to increased energy intake in a restaurant meal. *Obesity Research,* 12, 3, 562–568.

Drazen, D.L. et al. (2006). Effects of a fixed meal pattern on ghrelin secretion: Evidence for a learned response independent of nutrient status. *Endocrinology,* 147, 1, 23–30.

Expert Panel on the Identification, Evaluation, and Treatment of Overweight and Obesity in Adults (1998). Executive summary of the clinical guidelines on the identification, evaluation, and treatment of overweight and obesity in adults. *Archives of Internal Medicine,* 158, 17, 1855–1867.

Fasshauer, M. & Paschke, R. (2003). Regulation of adipocytokines and insulin resistance. *Diabetologia,* 46, 1594–1603.

Flatt, J.P. et al. (1985). Effects of dietary fat on postprandial substrate oxidation and on carbohydrate and fat balances. *The Journal of Clinical Investigation,* 76, 3, 1019–1024.

Flegal, K.M. et al. (2012). Prevalence of obesity and trends in the distribution of body mass index among US adults, 1999–2010. *Journal of the American Medical Association,* 307, 5, 491–497.

Flegal, K.M. et al. (2010). Prevalence and trends in obesity among US adults, 1999–2008. *Journal of the American Medical Association,* 303, 3, 235–241.

Foster, G.D. et al. (1999). Changes in resting energy expenditure after weight loss in obese African American and white women. *American Journal of Clinical Nutrition,* 69, 1, 13–17.

Freedman, D.S. et al. (1999). The relation of overweight to cardiovascular risk factors among children and adolescents: The Bogalusa Heart Study. *Pediatrics,* 103, 6, Pt 1, 1175–1182.

Giskes, K. et al. (2007). A systematic review of associations between environmental factors, energy and fat intakes among adults: Is there evidence for environments that encourage obesogenic dietary intakes? *Public Health Nutrition,* 10, 10, 1005–1017.

Guo, S.S. & Chumlea, W.C. (1999). Tracking of body mass index in children in relation to overweight in adulthood. *The American Journal of Clinical Nutrition,* 70, 1, 145S–148S.

Gutin, B. et al. (1999). Plasma leptin concentrations in obese children: Changes during 4-mo periods with and without physical training. *The American Journal of Clinical Nutrition,* 69, 3, 388–394.

Hubert, H.B. et al. (1983). Obesity as an independent risk factor for cardiovascular disease: A 26-year follow-up of participants in the Framingham Heart Study. *Circulation,* 67, 5, 968–977.

Jequier, E. (1995). Nutrient effects: Post-absorptive interactions. *The Proceedings of the Nutrition Society,* 54, 1, 253–265.

Jequier, E. & Tappy, L. (1999). Regulation of body weight in humans. *Physiological Reviews,* 79, 2, 451–480.

Kelesidis, T. et al. (2010). Narrative review: The role of leptin in human physiology: Emerging clinical applications. *Annals of Internal Medicine,* 152, 2, 93–100.

Labayen, I. et al. (2003). Effects of protein vs. carbohydrate-rich diets on fuel utilisation in obese women during weight loss. *Forum of Nutrition,* 56, 168–170.

Lavie, C.J., Milani, R.V., & Ventura, H.O. (2009). Obesity and cardiovascular disease: Risk factor, paradox, and impact of weight loss. *Journal of the American College of Cardiology,* 53, 1925–1932.

Lawlor, D.A. et al. (2006). Reverse causality and confounding and the associations of overweight and obesity with mortality. *Obesity,* 14, 12, 2294–2304.

Lee, Y.H. & Pratley, R.E. (2007). Abdominal obesity and cardiovascular disease risk: The emerging role of the adipocyte. *Journal of Cardiopulmonary Rehabilitation,* 27, 2–10.

Levine, J.A. (2007). Nonexercise activity thermogenesis: Liberating the life-force. *Journal of Internal Medicine,* 262, 3, 273–287.

Levine, J.A. et al. (2005). Interindividual variation in posture allocation: Possible role in human obesity. *Science,* 307, 5709, 584–586.

Levine, J.A. et al. (1999). Role of nonexercise activity thermogenesis in resistance to fat gain in humans. *Science,* 283, 5399, 212–214.

Lissner, L. et al. (1987). Dietary fat and the regulation of energy intake in human subjects. *The American Journal of Clinical Nutrition,* 46, 6, 886–892.

Manson, J.E. et al. (1995). Body weight and mortality among women. *New England Journal of Medicine,* 333, 11, 677–685.

McArdle, W.D., Katch, F.I., & Katch, V.L. (2010). Overweight, obesity, and weight control. In *Exercise Physiology: Energy, Nutrition, and Human Performance* (7th ed.). Philadelphia: Wolters Kluwer/Lippincott Williams & Wilkins.

Mokdad, A.H. et al. (2000). The continuing epidemic of obesity in the United States. *Journal of the American Medical Association,* 284, 13, 1650–1651.

Moran, T.H. & Dailey, M.J. (2009). Minireview: Gut peptides: Targets for antiobesity drug development? *Endocrinology,* 150, 6, 2526–2530.

Mrosovsky, N. & Powley, T.L. (1977). Set points for body weight and fat. *Behavioral Biology,* 20, 2, 205–223.

Must, A. et al. (1992). Long-term morbidity and mortality of overweight adolescents. A follow-up of the Harvard Growth Study of 1922 to 1935. *The New England Journal of Medicine,* 327, 19, 1350–1355.

National Heart, Lung and Blood Institute (2012). *Calculate Your Body Mass Index.* www.nhlbisupport.com/bmi/

National Heart, Lung and Blood Institute (1998). *Obesity Education Initiative Expert Panel: Clinical Guidelines on the Identification, Evaluation, and Treatment of Overweight and Obesity in Adults: The Evidence Report.* Bethesda, Md.: National Institutes of Health. NIH publication No. 98-4083.

O'Rahilly, S. (2009). Human genetics illuminates the paths to metabolic disease. *Nature,* 462, 7271, 307–314.

Ogden, C.L., et al (2012). *Prevalence of Obesity in the United States 2009–2010.* NHCS Data Brief, No. 82. Washington, D.C.: Centers for Disease Control and Prevention.

Ogden, C.L. et al. (2010a). Prevalence of high body mass index in U.S. children and adolescents, 2007–2008. *Journal of the American Medical Assocation*, 303, 3, 242–249.

Ogden, C.L. et al. (2010b). *Obesity and Socioeconomic Status in Adults: United States, 2005–2008. NCHS Data Brief, No. 50.* Washington, D.C.: Centers for Disease Control and Prevention.

Ogden, C.L. et al. (2006). Prevalence of overweight and obesity in the United States, 1999–2004. *Journal of the American Medical Association,* 295, 13, 1549–1555.

Prentice, A.M. (2001). Overeating: The health risks. *Obesity Research*, 9, Suppl 4, 234S–238S.

Prentice, A.M. & Jebb, S.A. (2003). Fast foods, energy density and obesity: A possible mechanistic link. *Obesity Review,* 4, 4, 187–194.

Rolls, B.J. (2003). The supersizing of America: Portion size and the obesity epidemic. *Nutrition Today*, 38, 2, 42–53.

Rolls, B.J. et al. (2007). The effect of large portion sizes on energy intake is sustained for 11 days. *Obesity,* 15, 6, 1535–1543.

Rosenbaum, M. et al. (2005). Low-dose leptin reverses skeletal muscle, autonomic, and neuroendocrine adaptations to maintenance of reduced weight. *The Journal of Clinical Investigation*, 115, 12, 3579–3586.

Rosengren, A. et al. (1997). Serum cholesterol and long-term prognosis in middle-aged men with myocardial infarction and angina pectoris: A 16-year follow-up of the Primary Prevention Study in Goteborg, Sweden. *European Heart Journal,* 18, 5, 754–761.

Schutz, Y. et al. (1989). Failure of dietary fat intake to promote fat oxidation: A factor favoring the development of obesity. *The American Journal of Clinical Nutrition*, 50, 2, 307–314.

Sims, E.A. & Horton, E.S. (1968). Endocrine and metabolic adaptation to obesity and starvation. *American Journal of Clinical Nutrition,* 21, 12, 1455–1470.

Turrell, G. et al. (2002). Socioeconomic differences in food purchasing behaviour and suggested implications for diet-related health promotion. *Journal of Human Nutrition and Dietetics*, 15, 5, 355–364.

U.S. Department of Health & Human Services (2008). *2008 Physical Activity Guidelines for Americans: Be Active, Healthy and Happy.* www.health.gov/paguidelines/pdf/paguide.pdf

Vinten, J. & Galbo, H. (1983). Effect of physical training on transport and metabolism of glucose in adipocytes. *American Journal of Physiology*, 244, 2, E129–134.

Wang, Y. & Beydoun, M.A. (2007). The obesity epidemic in the United States: Gender, age, socioeconomic, racial/ethnic, and geographic characteristics: A systematic review and meta-regression analysis. *Epidemiologic Reviews,* 29, 6–28.

Weinsier, R.L. (2001). Etiology of obesity: Methodological examination of the set-point theory. *Journal of Parenteral and Enteral Nutrition*, 25, 3, 103–110.

Weinsier, R.L. et al. (2002). Physical activity in free-living, overweight white and black women: Divergent responses by race to diet-induced weight loss. *American Journal of Clinical Nutrition*, 76, 4, 736–742.

Weinsier, R.L. et al. (2000). Do adaptive changes in metabolic rate favor weight regain in weight-reduced individuals? An examination of the set-point theory. *The American Journal of Clinical Nutrition*, 72, 5, 1088–1094.

Whitaker, R.C. et al. (1997). Predicting obesity in young adulthood from childhood and parental obesity. *New England Journal of Medicine,* 337, 13, 869–873.

Wisse, B.E. (2004). The inflammatory syndrome: The role of adipose tissue cytokines in metabolic disorders linked to obesity. *Journal of the American Society of Nephrology*, 15, 2792–2800.

World Health Organization (2011). *Obesity*

and Overweight. www.who.int/mediacentre/factsheets/fs311/en/

World Health Organization (2000). Obesity: Preventing and managing the global epidemic. In: *WHO Technical Report Series*. Geneva, Switzerland: World Health Organization.

Suggested Reading

Allison, D.B. et al. (2008). Obesity as a disease: A white paper on evidence and arguments commissioned by the council of the Obesity Society. *Obesity,* doi:10.1038/oby.2008.231

Donnelly, J.E. et al. (2009). Appropriate physical activity intervention strategies for weight loss and prevention of weight regain for adults. *Medicine & Science in Sports & Exercise,* 41, 2, 459–471.

Expert Panel on the Identification, Evaluation, and Treatment of Overweight and Obesity in Adults (1998). Executive summary of the clinical guidelines on the identification, evaluation, and treatment of overweight and obesity in adults. *Archives of Internal Medicine,* 158, 17, 1855–1867.

Gibbs, W. (1996). Gaining on fat. *Scientific American*, 275, 2, 88–94.

Heber, D. (2010). An integrative view of obesity. *American Journal of Clinical Nutrition,* 91, 280S–283S.

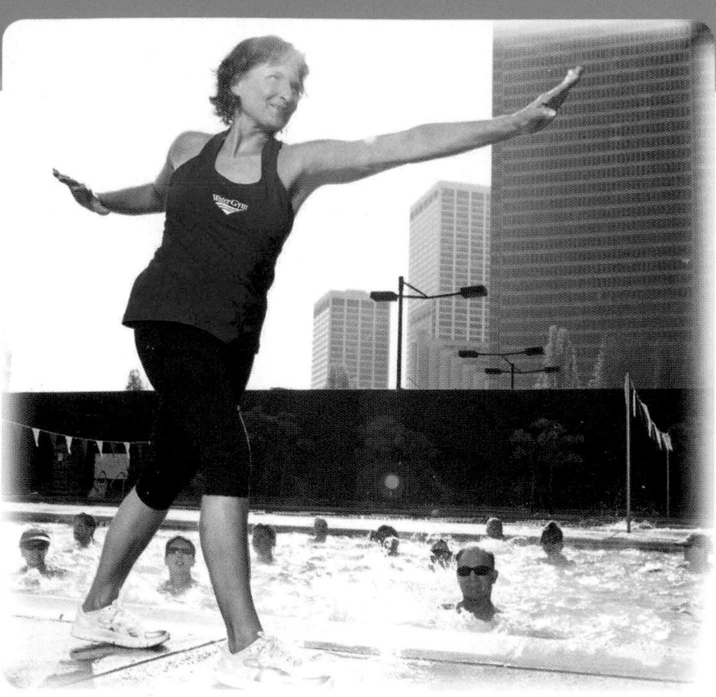

IN THIS CHAPTER:

Pamela M. Nisevich Bede, M.S., R.D., CSSD, is a board-certified specialist in sports dietetics and a nutrition consultant with Swim, Bike, Run, Eat! (www.swimbikeruneat.com). Nisevich Bede's areas of focus include sports nutrition, pediatrics, weight management, and healthy living. She earned her master's degree in medical dietetics at The Ohio State University and her bachelor's degree in dietetics from Miami University in Oxford, Ohio.

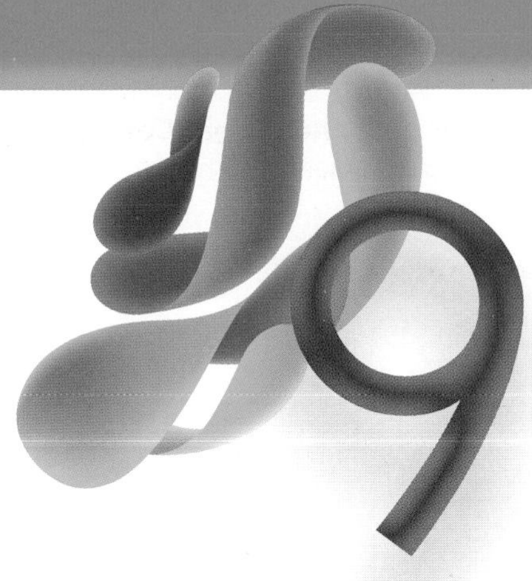

Current Concepts in Weight Management

PAMELA M. NISEVICH BEDE

& JENNA A. BELL

Jenna A. Bell, Ph.D., R.D., is a nutrition communications consultant in New York City, co-author of Energy to Burn: The Ultimate Food & Nutrition Guide to Fuel Your Active Lifestyle *(John Wiley & Sons, 2009) and* Launching Your Dietetics Career *(ADA, 2011), sports dietitian and blogger for www.runkeeper.com and www.swimbikeruneat.com, and member of the editorial advisory board for* Today's Dietitian. *She is the 2012–2013 chair-elect for the Sports, Cardiovascular and Wellness Nutrition Dietetic Practice Group of the Academy of Nutrition and Dietetics, and earned her doctorate in Health and Human Performance at the University of New Mexico (UNM), master's degree in nutrition and dietetic internship at UNM, and bachelor's degree in nutritional sciences from the University of New Hampshire.*

The number of **overweight** and obese individuals in the United States frequently makes headlines in both consumer magazines and scientific journals. Globally speaking, the United States does indeed claim the largest population of overweight and obese individuals (Popkin, 2010). However, this epidemic is not unique to the United States; a number of scholars and the World Health Organization (WHO) have documented that the globe's overweight population is greater than its underweight population (Popkin, 2008; WHO, 2003).

The growth in worldwide **obesity** numbers is rivaled only by the increase in weight-loss fads, from Internet programs to best-selling books. Health professionals are concerned and consumers are eager to find quick-fix solutions and remedies. This chapter reviews some popular diets and their associated health risks, details the slippery slope to eating disorders, and explains the health consequences of select eating disorders. To begin the discussion, a review of **energy balance**—the calories taken in compared to those expended—is provided. Chapter 8 offers a more detailed look at the development of obesity and the way in which the body regulates energy balance through hormones, genetics, and caloric intake.

Energy Balance and Weight Control

It is sometimes said that "life is a balancing act." Each day, financial statements are balanced, work is balanced against play, and individuals pursue a balance between their home lives and careers. Unbeknownst to many, the body is busy balancing energy as well. The balance between energy intake and energy output influences energy stores, such as **body fat** and **lean body mass.** This balance can be mathematically described with the following equations:

Energy balance = Energy intake – Energy output

Energy balance = Calories consumed – Calories expended

When an individual finds him- or herself in a state of **positive energy balance,** the intake of energy exceeds the amount expended. This state may be achieved by either consuming too many calories or by not using enough. Times of positive energy balance, during which an increase in calories is required, include phases of growth—infancy, childhood, and pregnancy. Otherwise, a positive energy balance results in weight gain. In general, an accrual of 3,500 calories in excess will result in the gain of 1 pound (0.45 kg) of body mass. Conversely, reducing energy intake and/or increasing energy expenditure by 3,500 calories will result in the loss of approximately 1 pound (0.45 kg) of body mass.

On the other hand, a **negative energy balance** reflects a state in which the number of calories expended is greater than what is taken in, thereby contributing to weight loss. For example, if an individual eats fewer calories than he or she works off through an exercise program and burns via basic metabolism and food digestion, he or she will experience a calorie deficit and weight loss will result. Indeed, according to the position paper from the American Dietetic Association (ADA) on the topic of weight management, fat stores can only be changed by a whole-body energy imbalance brought on by a change in energy intake, energy output, efficiency of energy use, or a combination of any of these components (ADA, 2009).

In January 2012, the American Dietetic Association (ADA) changed its name to the Academy of Nutrition and Dietetics (A.N.D.). Throughout this text, research conducted by the organization prior to this name change is cited to the ADA, while newer studies will be credited to the A.N.D. Refer to www.eatright.org for more information on the reasons behind the name change.

Finding a balance between intake and output throughout life is the cornerstone of maintaining a healthy weight and has been linked to numerous longevity-related benefits (Stubbs & Tolkamp, 2006). Achieving this balance, although seemingly straightforward, is very challenging over time, as evidenced by the growing number of overweight and obese individuals across the globe and the continual struggle to find the perfect diet.

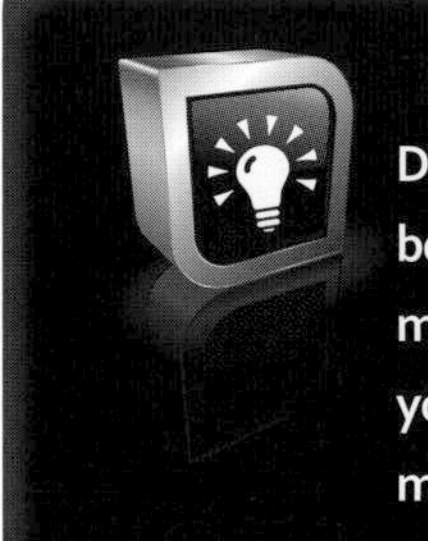

THINK IT THROUGH

Despite the volumes of evidence saying otherwise, many clients still believe that there must be some simple solution to their weight-management problems and seize onto every passing trend. How would you explain to resistant clients the simple fact that they need to expend more calories than they consume if they are going to lose weight?

Energy Requirements

The components of an individual's energy requirements must be considered to achieve weight loss, gain, and maintenance. An understanding of the factors that contribute to a person's overall energy (or calorie) requirements allows for an assessment of the efficacy of popular diets and answers questions regarding how an energy deficit can be created for weight loss. Factors that contribute to a person's energy requirements include controllable factors such as current weight and **body composition** (controllable to some degree) as well as physical-activity habits and environmental factors such as tobacco use and caffeine intake. Unalterable factors that affect energy requirements include age, gender, height, and the presence of disease or inflammation.

Energy Intake

The amount of food eaten in a day is dictated by a variety of factors. Availability, appetite, personal preferences, traditions, culture, social influences and value systems, psychological factors, and nutrition goals are on the long list of reasons why people eat what they do. In addition, agricultural advances, changes in technology and global economies, and other factors have led to a world where the energy of the food supply most frequently exceeds the opportunities for energy expenditure via physical activity (ADA, 2009). While the reasons behind intake vary widely, the primary reason for taking in food is to support the demands put on the body, from normal metabolism to physical work. This process has evolved over the centuries as the environment has changed. Food ingestion is imperative to survival and ecologists have studied the alterations that have occurred as eating has transitioned from being strictly survival-related to a behavioral response. Food establishments riddle major and minor roadways, eliminating the need for hunting and gathering meals. Therefore, the need to salvage and store intake has lessened. The environment may be overly dictating people's intake, thereby ameliorating the focus on food as a means of survival (see Chapter 8).

Energy Output

The determinants of calorie needs are influenced by energy output. This output includes calories "burned," or used, for normal metabolic functions, during physical activity and as a result of the **thermic effect of food (TEF).** Add these factors together and an estimate of **total energy expenditure (TEE)** can be determined.

Basal Metabolism

For all systems to work properly, a minimum amount of energy is required. This is referred to as basal metabolism, or **basal energy expenditure (BEE).** BEE allows the body to rest, maintain core temperature in ambient conditions, and survive. BEE, the calorie expenditure in a fasting state (12 to 14 hours after a meal), is influenced by several factors (Table 9-1), and makes up approximately 60 to 75% of the TEE.

Physical Activity

Energy is needed to sustain the work of physical activity. The calories expended above and beyond BMR via physical activity make up approximately 15 to 30% of TEE. The amount of physical activity varies from person to person, with many unfortunately choosing a **sedentary** lifestyle.

Physical activity is the most easily manipulated component of TEE, and therefore

Table 9-1		
Factors Affecting Basal Energy Expenditure (BEE)		
Factor	Affect on BEE	Comments
Age	↓	Metabolism declines with age; age-related loss of lean body mass likely contributes to this decline
Body temperature	↑	Seen with temperature extremes; fever and hypothermia (shivering)
Caffeine and nicotine	↑	Act as stimulants to increase BEE
Gender	↑ ↓	Males tend to have higher BEEs due to increases in lean body mass
Sympathetic nervous system activity	↑ ↓	Norepinephrine is associated with an increase in BEE
Nutritional status	↓	Reduced calorie intake can depress BEE
Pregnancy	↑	BEE increases gradually throughout pregnancy
Thyroid hormones	↑ ↓	People with too much thyroid hormone (hyperthyroidism) have increased RMR, and those (hypothryroidism) have decreased BEE

Note: ↑ = increase; ↓ = decrease; ↑ ↓ = variable

Sources: Shetty, P. (2005). Energy requirements of adults. Public Health Nutrition, 8, 7A, 994–1009; Byrd-Bredbenner, C. et al. (2008). *Wardlaw's Perspectives in Nutrition* (8th ed.). New York: McGraw-Hill.

plays a key role in creating an energy deficit when weight loss is desired. An individual can expend hundreds of calories on a daily basis by consistently engaging in physical activity.

Thermic Effect of Food

To digest and absorb **nutrients** from food, energy must be used. The total cost of this process makes up approximately 5 to 10% of TEE. Interestingly, the **macronutrient** composition of a meal can affect the thermic effect, or the number of calories required to digest and absorb it. The TEF associated with the consumption of a high-protein meal is significantly higher than it is following a high-carbohydrate or high-fat meal (Byrd-Bredbenner et al., 2008). The significance of this difference is still unclear in the long-term view of diet programs and weight-loss success.

Popular Diets and Associated Health Risks

If there is any question about whether diets are popular, simply typing the term "weight loss" into any online search engine will provide answers. It is likely that more than 100 million sites will pop up, many of which make grandiose claims and promises, and offer twists on similar themes. While a low-fat, reduced-calorie diet is the best studied weight-loss dietary strategy and is most frequently recommended by health professionals (ADA, 2009), the search for weight-loss solutions has not relented. Many popular weight-loss "solutions" fail to consider that the goals of weight management go well beyond the numbers on a scale, and that success in weight management encompasses the development of a healthful lifestyle along with behavioral modification for overall fitness and health (ADA, 2009). Regardless, investigations have continued, as individuals diligently pursue the easiest way to balance energy and lose weight. The following sections review popular diets and describe the health-related risks associated with each. Also, see Appendix C for additional information regarding the evaluation of popular diets.

Carbohydrate-restricted Diets

A number of popular diets with a variety of names and catchphrases fall under the umbrella of carbohydrate-restricted diets. Because of the plethora of diets touting themselves as carbohydrate-restricted plans, and with science testing a variety of carbohydrate levels, consumers are often confused by what carbohydrate restriction entails. There are carbohydrate-modified diets, such as Dr. Barry Sears' Zone® diet, the Carbohydrate Addict's Diet®, and the South Beach Diet®, but a low-carbohydrate diet is technically defined as an eating plan consisting of less than 20% of a day's calories from carbohydrate, or 20 to 60 grams per day (Last & Wilson, 2006). Arguably the most popular of its kind, the Atkins Diet® epitomizes this blend of low-carbohydrate eating with generous protein and fat.

Proponents of low-carbohydrate diets claim that by eliminating or restricting sugars and carbohydrates, weight loss will ensue. Physiologically, when carbohydrate content is decreased, **glycogen** stores are depleted and resultant **diuresis** produces an initial dramatic weight loss (ADA, 2009). Health professionals, including those in the American Dietetic Association and the American Heart Association, express concerns about the long-term safety of such diets and encourage individuals to tread lightly (St. Jeor et al., 2001; Stein, 2000). Reservations exist regarding the influence that carbohydrate restriction could have on chronic disease development, especially **cardiovascular disease** risk factors, **type 2 diabetes, osteoporosis,** and kidney disease, as well as nutrient deficiencies (ADA, 2009). Low-carbohydrate diets have been associated with deficiencies of vitamins A, B6, C, and E, as well as thiamin, folate, calcium, magnesium, iron, potassium, and fiber (Freedman, King, & Kennedy, 2001). Headaches and constipation are common complaints among people following a carbohydrate-restrictive diet (Astrup, Larsen, & Harper, 2004).

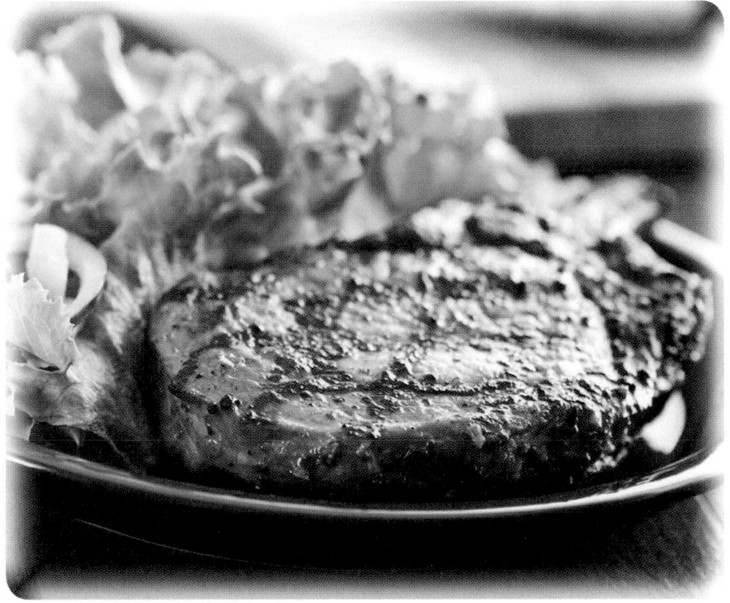

Several controlled trials have attempted to find answers to the following questions: Do carbohydrate-restricted diets promote weight loss? And more importantly, are they safe?

A randomized, controlled trial published in the *New England Journal of Medicine* sought to compare the traditional, higher-carbohydrate, energy-restricted diet to the Atkins low-carbohydrate plan. At six months, participants abiding by the Atkins principles showed a significantly greater weight loss (7.0%, SD 6.5) than those following the traditional plan (3.2%, SD 5.6). However, at 12 months, no difference between the groups could be detected (Foster et al., 2003).

Low-carbohydrate diets typically are below the **Acceptable Macronutrient Distribution Range** of 45 to 65% of total calories from carbohydrates (Krieger et al., 2006). A meta-regression was performed by Krieger and colleagues (2006) to see how low-carbohydrate diets performed during calorie restriction and to observe the effect that varying levels of protein have on body mass and composition. After sorting through the research, 87 studies were included in their analysis in an effort to delineate the predictors of weight and body composition. After researchers divided the data into quartiles of lower and higher intakes of protein and carbohydrate, protein was found to be a significant predictor of fat-free mass maintenance during a calorie-reduction plan [an average level of 1.05 g/kg/day as opposed to the 0.8 g/kg/day prescribed by the **Recommended Dietary Allowance (RDA)**]. The *lowest* levels of carbohydrate intake (less than 35 to 41.5% of total calories) were associated with a greater amount of body-weight loss and body-fat reduction. However, low-carbohydrate diets were also linked to a loss of fat-free mass that was greater than those seen with the low-fat diets. The authors concluded that a more generous amount of protein (>1.05 g/kg/day) may be beneficial during calorie restriction. It is important to note that this level of carbohydrate is above that suggested by the more restrictive carbohydrate diets, such as the Atkins Diet.

In an attempt to address the safety and efficacy concerns, Bravata and colleagues (2003) extensively reviewed the low-carbohydrate-related literature. Studies were evaluated for changes in weight, serum **lipids,** blood **glucose,** serum **insulin,** and **blood pressure** in outpatient settings. The researchers concluded that the data were insufficient to support the claim that low-carbohydrate diets promote weight loss better than traditional diets. As may be expected, diets that restricted calories and had a longer duration yielded improved weight-loss outcomes. Carbohydrate restriction alone was not associated with alterations in serum lipid, fasting glucose, or blood pressure.

Experts appear to agree that an insufficient amount of evidence is available to support the claim that carbohydrate restriction alone promotes weight loss. Despite the lack of certainty that such diets are the ideal approach to losing extra pounds, they appear to be safe in the short term. However, long-term studies are lacking.

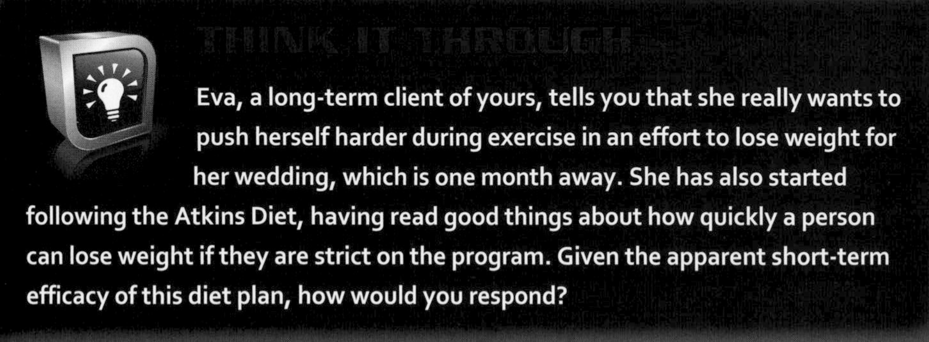

THINK IT THROUGH

Eva, a long-term client of yours, tells you that she really wants to push herself harder during exercise in an effort to lose weight for her wedding, which is one month away. She has also started following the Atkins Diet, having read good things about how quickly a person can lose weight if they are strict on the program. Given the apparent short-term efficacy of this diet plan, how would you respond?

High-fat Diets

Dietary fat has long been synonymous with "unhealthy" and "disease-promoting." It is often considered the root of obesity and assumed to be the greatest culprit in its development. As discussed in Chapter 6, dietary fat (or lipid) has specific and important purposes in the human body. Despite its necessity, consuming excess fat can be prohibitive in terms of an individual's efforts to lose weight. Remembering that energy balance is achieved through equalizing energy intake and output, keep in mind that fat, the most energy-dense macronutrient, provides 9 calories per gram, compared to the 4 calories per gram found in carbohydrates and protein. This additional energy can substantially influence the ability to create the negative caloric balance needed for weight reduction.

When considering the role that fat plays in the diet, experts review its affect on **satiety, thermogenesis,** and fat storage (Wenk, 2004; Westerterp-Plantenga, 2004). Simply put, satiety is the feeling of fullness after eating. If a person is satiated, it will be reflected in how much he or she chooses to eat after the meal. When assessed for its affect on satiety, as well as thermogenesis, a high-fat diet shows a lesser influence on satiety during the meal and throughout the day, and a lower thermogenic effect compared to a protein/carbohydrate diet (Westerterp-Plantenga, 2004). With less of an effect on how full a person feels, as well as a lower thermogenic effect, a high-fat diet could be an obstacle to weight loss.

In addition to its relatively limited effect on fullness and thermogenesis, dietary fat is easily stored as fat (Wenk, 2004). Forming body fat from dietary fat is a simpler process compared to doing so from carbohydrates and protein because of fat's high digestibility and metabolic efficiency. As a result of the aforementioned effects, a high-fat diet is generally incompatible with the quest to lose weight.

High-protein Diets

As discussed earlier in this chapter, deemphasizing carbohydrates, while promoting protein, has become a popular weight-loss technique. The promotion of protein dates back to the 1860s, when William Banting attributed his 46.2-pound (21-kg) weight loss to his ample protein intake, claiming that he did this without feeling hungry (Astrup, Larsen, & Harper, 2004). High-protein diets (above the 0.8 g/kg RDA) have received attention in the public, media, and among researchers.

Protein's role in weight maintenance stems from its potential for increasing satiety and thermogenesis, and its role in maintaining fat-free mass. During a period of caloric restriction, fat-free mass is lost and could potentially decrease calorie needs, thereby challenging even the most dedicated dieter.

Studies have supported the positive effects of protein on both satiety and thermogenesis (Westerterp-Plantenga & Lejeune, 2005). Individuals ingesting a greater amount of protein—approximately 30% of total calories—report less hunger and consume fewer calories. The thermogenic effect of protein is greater than that of carbohydrates and fat, which also shows its potential for weight-loss promotion.

Noakes and colleagues (2005) challenged this potential to see if improvements could be detected in weight loss, body composition, nutritional status, and markers for cardiovascular health in obese women. Subjects were assigned to one of two groups that were given the same number of calories. Their diets differed only by whether they were high in protein or carbohydrate. While both groups showed relatively similar reductions in body weight, individuals in the high-protein group with high **triacylglycerol** levels (a marker for cardiovascular disease) exhibited more fat loss and noticeable reductions in triacylglycerol levels. In their evaluation of nutritional status and renal function, the researchers found that the high-protein diet did not negatively affect measurements, leading them to state that a high-protein diet is a safe and viable option for weight loss.

Having already discussed carbohydrate-restrictive diets at levels below 20% of total calories, it is imperative to note that this particular study provided 34% of its energy from protein, 20% from fat, and 46% from carbohydrate in the high-protein group. The high-carbohydrate diet provided 17% protein, 20% fat, and 64% carbohydrate. While the aforementioned high-protein dietary protocol does not represent a **ketogenic**-inducing increase in protein intake, it is double that of the recommended level for protein intake and was found to be safe in this investigation (Noakes et al., 2005).

The ability to keep the weight off following a weight-loss program is an essential component of a successful program. Because of its role in satiety and thermogenesis, protein was assessed for its ability to moderate the reduction in energy expenditure associated with weight loss (Westerterp-Plantenga, 2004). After a four-week weight-loss program, subjects participated in a three-month follow-up for weight maintenance, with half the group receiving an additional 48.2 grams of protein per day (an approximate increase of 20% per day, or 18% vs. 15% of total calories from protein). Those who had a modest bump in their protein intake showed a 50% lower regain of body weight and reported feeling fuller. Interestingly, the weight gain was predominantly fat-free mass, not fat mass, in the protein group, leading to a lower percent of body fat. This data suggests that even moderate increases in protein intake can help keep the weight off after a short-term weight-loss program.

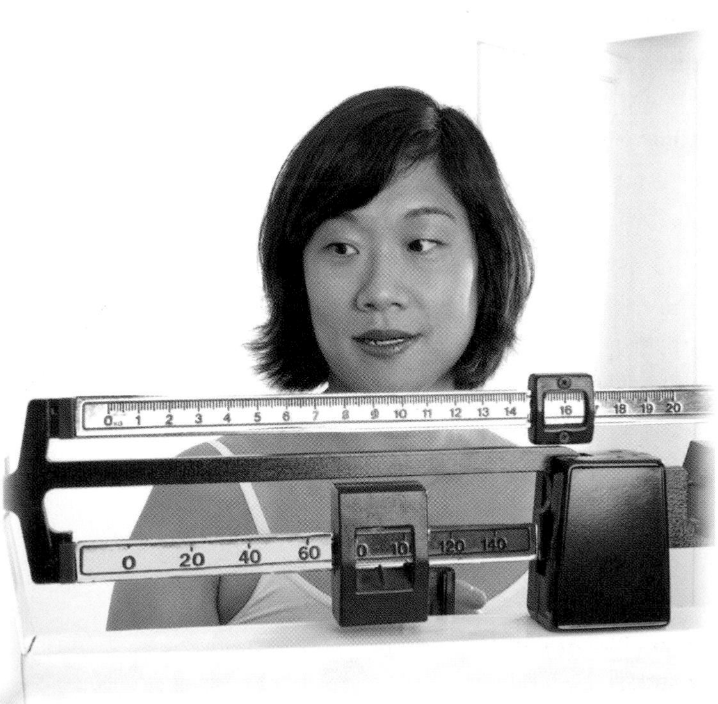

To date, ill health consequences have not been documented with the higher-protein diets described in this section. As discussed, a severe carbohydrate restriction cannot be safely recommended for weight loss, but a modest increase in protein may be beneficial in helping to maintain weight loss.

Detoxification Diets

The concept of detoxifying the body from the buildup of toxins is not new. Indeed, detoxification, cleansing, or purifying practices have been around for centuries and the popularity of these practices is cyclical, coming back into popularity every now and again. Historically, detoxification-type diets were based in religion or self-purifying and commonly involved fasting. Ancient Ayurvedic medicine, dating back prior to 400 BC, frequently recommended diets that cleansed the body of impurities by eliminating various food groups and instead focused on a plant-based diet.

Today, a diet is commonly classified as "detox" if it is a dietary regimen involving a change of eating patterns with the goal of ridding the body of the buildup of toxins. Detoxification diets are varied in nature but often involve fasts, avoidance of many food groups, or habitual drinking of cleansing beverages. Consequently, many individuals participate in such cleanses in an effort to lose weight. The premise behind detox diets is that by eliminating certain food groups, people also eliminate toxins commonly found within these foods, while also allowing the digestive system a break from foods such as meat, cheese, and processed items that are considered hard to digest and absorb. In theory, as a result of avoiding these food items, the body uses less energy for digestion and fighting off toxins, and therefore has more energy to direct toward healing. This healing and cleansing process often promises the dieter a renewed sense of self and overall better health. While not all detox diets are solely focused on weight loss, many purport a restrictive pattern of eating and accelerated weight loss often follows.

Generally speaking, this type of diet should be cautioned against. The many variations on detox diets, though they may facilitate weight loss in the short term, fail to bring about lifestyle changes such as improvements in nutrition and the inclusion of physical activity. It is likely that once the fast is completed, the client is bound to eventually go back to his or her old habits of eating poorly, and the lost weight is certain to return. According to a report in the *American Psychologist Journal,* researchers have found that while dieters can lose 5 to 10% of their weight in the first few months of a diet, more than 60% of people regain the weight they lost, and then some, within four or five years of ending the diet (Mann et al., 2007).

Experts would likely label any one of the available detoxification diets as a *food fad* or fad diet. A fad diet typically involves an unreasonable or exaggerated claim that by eating or avoiding specific foods, nutrients, or supplements, the consumer may experience special health benefits such as a cured chronic disease or weight loss (ADA, 2006). While the Federal Trade Commission (FTC), U.S. Food and Drug Administration (FDA), and other government bodies work to oversee many products and claims on the market, it is often difficult for federal regulations to keep pace with the proliferation of diet practices and related nutritional supplements.

Other concerns about fad diets or detoxification diets surround the fact that there are prohibitive costs to these diets—costs that are often unrelated to a consumer's bank account. Fads such as detox diets carry both long-term and short-term consequences. Short-term consequences can include physical harm from drug–nutrient interactions or potentially toxic components in cleansing products. Should the end user rely on a detox diet to treat a chronic disease, such as type 2 diabetes or another condition associated with obesity, the long-term costs are based on a potential delay of treatment, and may therefore involve the cost of intensive clinical therapy as well as the long-term cost of physical harm. Per the ADA (2006), other long-term costs surround psychological issues of dependency and diminished **self-efficacy** after one "fails" on a detox diet and then believes that no other diet or pattern of eating will promote better health, let alone weight loss.

Commercial Diets

While many individuals may turn to fad diets or detox diets in order to lose weight, still others turn to their healthcare practitioner (such as a **registered dietitian,** counselor, or physician) for assistance. Still others turn to commercial methods such as Weight Watchers®, Jenny Craig®, or online programs. Many commercial weight-loss programs, such as Weight Watchers, include weekly meetings that are led by trained instructors, are held in various locations (such as neighborhood meeting halls or workplace conference rooms), and require weekly weigh-ins and accountability. Commercial weight-loss programs and counseling provided by trained professionals can be effective in helping with weight management. A study published in the *British Journal of Medicine* found that individuals who seek out commercial programs can be just as successful at weight loss—if not more so—than if they had simply joined a health club or sought one-on-one counseling. This 12-week intervention compared the effects of six different weight-loss programs to a control group that was not counseled but was given access to a fitness center. The commercial programs included group-based weight-loss programs unique to the United Kingdom except for Weight Watchers. The other three weight-loss interventions included a dietetics professional–led group weight-loss program, a one-to-one nurse-led counseling program, and a one-to-one pharmacist-led program. At the end of 12 weeks, the study looked at weight loss and found that the commercial weight-loss programs resulted in the greatest amount of weight loss. Encouragingly, many participants sustained this weight loss for more than one year. The study authors suggest that perhaps the success of the group-based programs are due to the training of the counselors, the continuous nature of the programs, and the group atmosphere. The commercial programs were also less expensive compared to one-on-one sessions led by healthcare practitioners (Jolly, 2011).

Pharmacological Agents for Weight Loss

In an effort to decrease the health impact of obesity and provide individuals with pharmacological options for weight loss, medications have been developed to block fat absorption, increase energy expenditure, and suppress appetite. Pharmacological agents have not shown themselves to be "magic pills" and do not promote weight loss independently. Weight-loss drugs are constantly hitting the market—often as others disappear—and it is the responsibility of the ACE-certified Health Coach to be aware of what is happening on the pharmacological side of the weight-loss industry. The following sections provide a brief review of several weight-loss medications that have received a fair amount of attention in the marketplace.

Lipase Inhibition: Fat Malabsorption Agents

Orlistat (Xenical®)

Dietary fat provides more calories per gram than carbohydrates and protein, and can impede weight loss when consumed in excess. Because of fat's predominance in the diet and its effect on obesity development due to its relatively high caloric content, inhibiting fat digestion and absorption may help reduce intake and caloric contribution. Orlistat (Xenical) is a drug developed to inhibit gastric and pancreatic lipases in the gastrointestinal tract, thereby preventing **triglyceride** hydrolysis and resulting in the decreased absorption of dietary fats, which are consequently excreted through the feces (Steffen et al., 2010). Orlistat has been available by prescription as a weight-loss aid in the United States since 1999, and in 2007 orlistat was also approved by the FDA for nonprescription sales under the brand name Alli®.

A review of orlistat trials in humans reveals that weight loss was modestly greater in the groups receiving the recommended dosages of the drug as compared to a placebo (Halford, 2004).

Despite its success in promoting weight loss, orlistat's side effects cannot be overlooked. People taking orlistat report flatulence, oily stool, fecal urgency, incontinence, and abdominal pain prior to modifying their dietary fat intake. The absorption of **fat-soluble vitamins** is also decreased, thereby putting an individual at risk for deficiency if he or she does not take a vitamin supplement. However, few such cases have been reported (Halford, 2006).

The gastrointestinal distress experienced with orlistat use may also modify dietary intake. To avoid gastrointestinal distress, people taking the drug can reduce their fat intake. Unfortunately, human trials have revealed a compensatory increase in carbohydrate consumption—a response that could weaken this drug's weight-loss benefits (Halford, 2004).

EXPAND YOUR KNOWLEDGE

Alli

In June 2007, Alli became the first over-the-counter diet pill approved by the FDA. It remains the only FDA-approved weight-loss medication available over-the-counter (Steffen et al., 2010). It is a half-strength version of the prescription weight-loss drug Xenical (orlistat), approved for nonprescription use in the United States by overweight patients ages 18 and older who are also on a reduced-calorie, low-fat diet. For best results, Alli should be taken before every meal that contains fat. It works by decreasing the amount of fat absorbed by the gastrointestinal tract during the digestive process. When taken at the recommended dosage, Alli reduces dietary fat absorption by approximately 25% (Johnson et al., 2007; Zhi et al., 1994). Research has shown that when individuals use Alli in combination with diet and exercise, they lose up to 50% more weight on average compared to dieting and exercising alone. As with any drug, Alli has several documented side effects, including excessive flatulence, abdominal pain, and oily, difficult-to-control bowel movements. Those individuals hailing Alli as the next "magic bullet" for weight loss should bear in mind that most weight-loss experts contend that without the contributory effects of diet and exercise, Alli's beneficial weight-loss effects will be very limited.

EXPAND YOUR KNOWLEDGE

Alli Use and Eating Disorders

While weight loss–inducing pharmacological options exist for obese individuals in need of fat-absorption blockage, increased energy expenditure, and appetite suppression, the misuse of these pharmacological interventions does occur. Not uncommonly, patients with eating disorders misuse medications such as laxatives, diuretics, and diet pills to compensate for binge eating and/or to promote weight loss (Steffen et al., 2010). Steffen and colleagues surveyed 417 patients undergoing treatment for eating disorders to determine the frequency and characteristics of Alli use among these individuals. They found that 6.2% of responders reported a history of Alli use and, of those, nearly 58% met criteria for an eating disorder. The researchers also found that in the group with a history of Alli use, there was a higher percentage (not statistically significant) of patients who had used laxatives, diuretics, diet pills, syrup of Ipecac, and herbal weight-loss supplements, compared to the group who had not used Alli. Given these findings, it is worthwhile for health and fitness professionals to consider the possibility of, and monitor for, the misuse of this drug when working with someone who exhibits signs of, or is at risk for, an eating disorder.

Appetite Suppressants and Energy Expenditure–increasing Agents

Fen-Phen

In 1959, the FDA approved a drug called phentermine (Phen) for weight loss. It acted like an amphetamine and reduced appetite. A drug with a different mechanism, but similar results, called fenfluramine (Fen) was introduced and approved in 1973. Acting alone, these drugs suppressed appetite modestly and produced few safety issues. Researchers began investigating the combination of the two drugs to see if coupling enhanced results. They found that the combination caused further appetite suppression and weight loss. Although the combination was not approved by the FDA, their safety and effectiveness was assumed.

Following the prescription and use of "fen-phen," investigations and reports surfaced of a negative and dangerous synergistic effect. Reports of primary pulmonary hypertension and valvular heart disease began to emerge in people taking the fen-phen combination. Once a rare disorder, primary pulmonary hypertension increased in appearance following the fen-phen therapy. In addition, a thickening of the heart valves leading to valvular heart disease was discovered, with a greater incidence among users of the drug combination (Wellman & Maher, 1999). In July 1997, the FDA issued a warning regarding the safety of fen-phen, and two months later, removed it from the market.

Sibutramine

Efforts to find a way to decrease people's appetite for food are ongoing. Sibutramine (trade name is Meridia® in the United States and Reductal® in Europe) has been investigated as a tool to help reduce intake and hunger, as well as increase energy expenditure (Halford, 2004). Sibutramine acts to increase **norepinephrine** and **serotonin** activity in the brain by decreasing reuptake, thereby reducing feelings of hunger. The evidence supporting its role in enhancing energy expenditure is mixed. It has produced a stimulatory effect in rodent studies, but shows less of an impact when taken by humans (Halford, 2006).

As with most medications, side effects can be problematic. Patients report dry mouth, constipation, and insomnia, with some reporting mild increases in blood pressure and heart rate. In addition to its mild negative side effects, sibutramine appears to beneficially affect triglyceride, **high-density lipoprotein (HDL),** and blood glucose levels, therefore making it a viable option for obese individuals to use in combination with a diet and exercise program.

Glycemic Index

The use of the **glycemic index (GI)** as a weight-loss tool has been accepted in consumer publications and debated by the scientific community. GI is a value used to rate or categorize the impact that a carbohydrate-containing food has on blood glucose levels. Foods have been categorized as low, moderate, or high, compared to the reference food, which is glucose or white bread (Table 9-2).

Table 9-2

Glycemic Index (GI) of Various Foods

High GI ≥70	Medium GI 56–69	Low GI ≤55
White bread	Rye bread	Pumpernickel bread
Corn Flakes®	Shredded Wheat®	All Bran®
Graham crackers	Ice cream	Plain yogurt
Dried fruit	Blueberries	Strawberries
Instant white rice	Refined pasta	Oatmeal

The challenge lies in the fact that determining a food's GI is difficult without testing. GI is affected by cooking, ripeness, protein and fat content, and handling, and therefore cannot be easily determined by consumers. The GI of a food also does not reflect its overall nutritional value. A high-glycemic food is not necessarily "unhealthier" or less nutritious, nor is a low-glycemic food necessarily "healthier" or more nutritious.

It should also be noted that when these carbohydrates are combined with other nutrients, such as protein or fat, it changes the glycemic effect. For this reason, some experts consider the **glycemic load** to be a more realistic approach.

Glycemic load is a measure of the glycemic index, multiplied by the number of carbohydrates (CHO) consumed, divided by 100:

Glycemic load = Glycemic index x CHO (g)/100

The glycemic load is useful in that it represents how much a given amount of a food will affect blood sugar levels. The thinking behind glycemic index and glycemic load is that if blood sugar is rapidly increased, insulin levels will rise quickly and lead to increased fat deposition.

A link between the GI and weight loss may stem from epidemiological studies that show an inverse relationship between the intake of sugary, carbohydrate-containing foods and obesity (Saris, 2003). This relationship leads to speculation that even though carbohydrates, as a whole, promote a feeling of fullness, high-glycemic foods that cause a spike in blood glucose may instead lead to overeating and subsequent weight gain (Anderson & Woodend, 2003).

When the glycemic index is investigated for its effect on weight loss, the research is inconclusive at best. The ADA, in its position paper on weight management, suggests that low glycemic index foods can be incorporated, but are not essential for a diet to be efficacious in managing weight (ADA, 2009). Sloth et al. (2004) evaluated the influence of GI on appetite and body weight, as well as risk factors for type 2 diabetes over a 10-week intervention. After dividing groups into high-glycemic and low-glycemic diet programs, researchers assessed diet intake, body weight, and blood samples for lipids, glucose, and insulin. Upon completion, no differences in energy intake, body weight, or fat mass were detected. The low-glycemic group showed a significantly greater decrease in **low-density lipoproteins (LDL)** as the only change in blood levels. The results fail to support the assumption that a low-glycemic diet will be more satiating or that high-glycemic diets promote an increase in caloric intake (Sloth et al., 2004). The lack of difference in body weight and fat mass implies that the glycemic index alone is an ineffective tool for weight maintenance. In fact, experts agree that the evidence is insufficient to support the use of GI as an agent for weight loss (Saris, 2003).

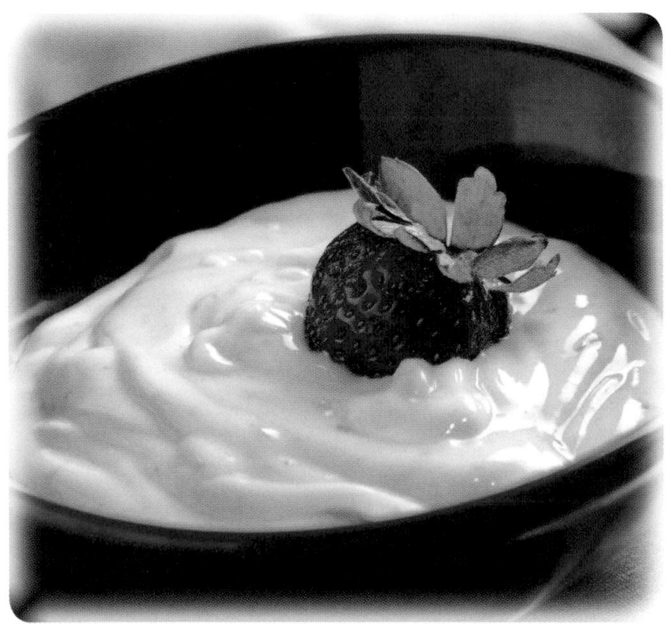

A controlled clinical trial was initiated to determine if diets with a low GI and high level of protein had a beneficial effect on weight loss in 129 overweight or obese young adults (McMillan-Price et al., 2006). The subjects were randomly assigned to one of three diet regimens:

- A reduced-fat, high-fiber diet
- A high-carbohydrate diet with either high- or low-GI carbohydrates
- A high-protein diet with either high- or low-GI carbohydrates

The results showed that although all participants lost similar amounts of weight (on average), there was a higher proportion of individuals that lost 5% or more of their body weight in the high-carbohydrate (55% of total calories), low-GI (40 GI, 75 glycemic load) and the high-protein (25% of total calories), high-GI (57 GI, 87 glycemic load) diets. These same two groups showed a greater loss of fat mass than those on the high-carbohydrate, high-GI diet. In review of the biomarkers for cardiovascular disease risk, the high-carbohydrate, low-GI diet group showed a decrease in LDL-cholesterol, although no differences were seen in lipid profiles between the other diet groups. The results of this study should be considered when encouraging people to consume more quality whole grains, thus moving toward a lower-GI diet composition (Liu, 2006). Researchers in both studies agree that further investigations are warranted.

Fasting

Many frustrated individuals turn to fasting as a means of kicking off a weight-loss plan. Fasting, or inadequate food intake to produce a negative energy balance, appears enticing, as weight can be lost rapidly. Unfortunately, the consequences of fasting may make sustained weight-loss efforts difficult and include unfavorable changes to the body.

Short-term calorie deficiencies lead to initial weight reductions, and can lead to changes in energy expenditure as they progress. As inadequate calorie intake continues, the body will make modifications to survive on the insufficient calories being supplied. This achievement of a new **steady state** can wreak havoc on a weight-loss plan. In the initial stages of a short-term calorie restriction, the body will rapidly lose weight. Glycogen reserves will decline, protein will be used to make glucose, and water will be lost (Kurpad, Muthayya, & Vaz, 2005). Fat loss occurs, but there will also be a decline in lean body tissue (i.e., muscle). During this time, the person can experience a drop in **basal metabolic rate (BMR),** thereby decreasing the number of calories needed to survive. Over time, if the energy deficiency persists, metabolic rate and total energy expenditure can plummet. Lean-body-mass loss continues and nutrient deficiencies can ensue.

Therefore, fasting is not recommended to create the negative energy balance required for weight loss. Increasing activity, with a modest restriction in calories, is still the most advisable way to tip the scale toward weight loss.

Surgical Interventions

Bariatric surgery, often considered the most effective tool for the treatment of severe obesity, poses both benefits and risks to the individuals. With its inherent structural change, surgery offers the benefit of long-term success in comparison with fad diets. Surgery is reserved, however, for patients who are at high risk for morbidity and mortality due to their weight and who have also failed at less invasive interventions. According to the criteria established by the National Institutes of Health (NIH), bariatric surgery is reserved for patients with a **body mass index (BMI)** >40 kg/m^2. In addition, a patient with a BMI of 35 to 40 kg/m^2 may also be a candidate if weight-related comorbidities including **diabetes, hypertension,** and sleep apnea are present (Weight Control Information Network, 2011).

For the morbidly obese, research indicates that bariatric surgery is the most effective therapy available and can result in improvement or even resolution of the weight-related comorbidities. While surgical procedures are ever-evolving, at this time there are four commonly used procedures, some of which restrict total caloric intake while others restrict caloric intake and promote malabsorption. Food intake may be reduced due to an adjustable band that allows only a small quantity of food to enter the stomach. This band can be adjusted following the procedure, allowing for greater, or lesser, intake. Other surgical procedures result in the removal of part of the stomach, resulting in a "gastric sleeve." Gastric bypass operations, such as the Roux-en-Y gastric bypass (RYGB), which is considered the gold standard of these surgical methods (Martins-Filho et al., 2008), and the more extensive gastric bypass, create a small pouch by stapling (or removing) a portion of the stomach, and also bypass the duodenum and other segments of the small intestine, thus resulting in malabsorption and restricted food intake.

For bariatric surgery to be considered a success, a weight loss of at least 50% of initial excess weight is the target. This weight loss typically occurs within 18 to 24 months post-surgery (Freire et al., 2011). In a meta-analysis of more than 22,000 patients who underwent RYGB, Buchwald and colleagues (2004) found that the loss of excess weight following surgery was between 56.7 and 66.5%. Diabetes, elevated blood lipid levels, and hypertension were resolved or improved in more than 70% of patients.

While procedures such as RYGB offer weight loss and improved quality of life, they are also linked to drastic changes in eating habits and higher risks of nutrient deficiencies. Because surgical interventions drastically change the capacity of the stomach or the organization of the digestive tract, changes to diet (i.e., quantity and quality) must follow the procedure. Many centers require nutrition intervention both prior to and following surgery.

While many patients achieve successful weight loss following surgery, weight regain is an important concern. The rate of regain ranges from 46 to 63% after the second year following surgery. Predictably, this weight regain is associated with the return of comorbidities, and deterioration of the individual's quality of life. It is not known exactly why the weight returns, but Freire and colleagues (2011) theorize that it may be related to factors such as psychological disorders, dilation of the gastric pouch as a result of increased food intake, or even the return of a sedentary lifestyle. With the goal of identifying predictive factors in weight loss and also weight regain, Freire et al. (2011) examined the lifestyle habits of 100 post-surgery patients. They found that weight regain increased over time and often as a result of poor diet quality (excess intake of calories and nutritionally poor choices), sedentary lifestyle, and lack of nutritional counseling follow-up. In support of this finding, Faria and colleagues (2010) found nutritional counseling reduced the weight of patients with previous weight regain and also led to a reduction in body fat, thus improving the perspective of weight maintenance in the future.

THINK IT THROUGH

As more and more individuals turn to bariatric surgery as the answer to their weight-loss needs, one must wonder, is this a step in the right direction? Does surgery truly address the issue at hand or is it simply a bandage on a gaping wound? While a smaller stomach or altered digestive tract might reduce one's weight, the question remains: Is the obesity a result of simply too much food or is it the result of a complexity of psychological issues, societal pressure, sedentary behavior, and other factors that cannot be resolved on the operating table?

Eating Disorders and Associated Health Risks

Eating disorders are defined as disturbances in eating behavior or methods to control weight that contribute to impairments in physical and mental health, and are not related to another medical or psychiatric disturbance (Klein & Walsh, 2004). Eating disorders are psychiatric disorders with diagnostic criteria based on psychological, behavioral, and physiological characteristics (ADA, 2011). The specific diagnostic criteria for eating disorders are currently under review and both the current criterion and the proposed revisions for the newest *Diagnostic and Statistical Manual of Mental Disorders (DSM)* edition are listed for each condition in the ADA (2011) report.

The frequency and distribution of individuals affected by eating disorders is unknown because the condition may exist for a considerable time period before clinical detection. That said, the National Comorbidity Survey Replication Study (Hudson et al., 2007) reported lifetime prevalence rates of 0.3% in men and 0.9% in women for **anorexia nervosa (AN),** 0.5% in men and 1.5% in women for **bulimia nervosa (BN),** and 2% in men and 3.5% in women for **binge eating disorder (BED).** Regardless of the specific disorder, medical complications can occur and, in extreme cases, result in death. The following sections review the clinical features and health complications associated with eating disorders.

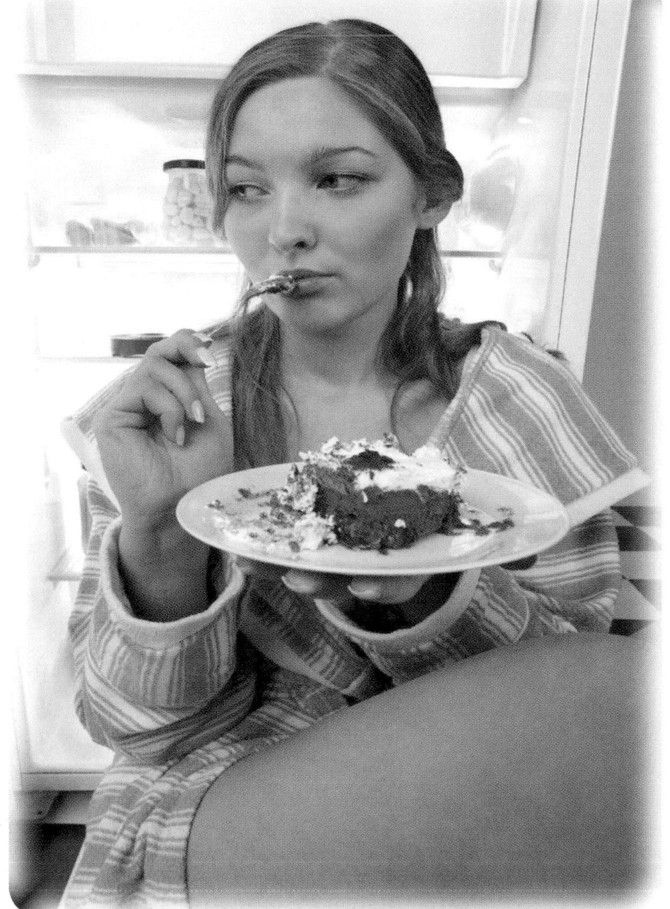

Binge Eating Disorder

Binge eating disorder is recognized as an increasingly common eating disorder. BED was initially considered an atypical eating disorder (Patrick, 2002). Characterized by recurrent episodes of binge eating, BED is not associated with compensatory episodes of purging, fasting, or excessive exercise, as is typical with BN. Individuals suffering from BED tend to eat more rapidly, until uncomfortably full, without physical hunger, alone, and with tremendous feelings of guilt and disgust after overeating (ADA, 2001). A diagnosis is given when someone partakes in this behavior more than two days a week over a six-month period. Proposed changes to these criteria include a diagnosis following repeated episodes of overconsumption of food with a sense of lack of control with a list of possible descriptors such as how much is eaten and the distress associated with the episode [American Psychiatric Association (APA), 2011]. Also, the proposed frequency for diagnosis is episodes occurring at least once a week for three months. BED is typically seen in the obese population and can impede weight loss due to its psychopathology.

Despite the consequent feelings of guilt and disgust following an episode, individuals with BED often seek comfort or attempt to dull feelings of **anxiety** and **depression** with bouts of overconsumption. Often a stressful situation or day will provoke an episode that is used as a means to cope. BED has therefore been described as a psychological dependence on food, as well as an addiction.

The **etiology** of BED continues to be investigated. Individuals suffering from BED are suspected to be unable to properly deal with their feelings or stressful situations. To cope with issues, they resort to overeating, and the cycle of binging and guilt/disgust persists. One area of interest is the impact that cortisol may have on the development of BED. Cortisol plays a role in the regulation of appetite, in addition to being released during stress. There is speculation that a chronic rise in cortisol may contribute to the consumption, or overconsumption, of "comfort foods" that are high in sugar and fat (Gluck, 2006).

The health consequences and psychological impact of BED mirror those of overweight and obesity. BED often prohibits success in weight-loss programs, because the reason for consumption is not being addressed. In addition, individuals with BED are unable to detect hunger. They are encouraged to seek assistance in dealing with their emotions and the underlying disturbance, while also learning to detect hunger and respond to feelings of fullness. Many self-help and support groups are available for BED, such as Overeaters Anonymous. Pharmaceutical interventions may also be warranted to relieve anxiety and/or depression.

Bulimia Nervosa

Like BED, BN is characterized by recurrent episodes of binge eating and feelings of a loss of control. Unlike BED, BN includes compensatory behavior such as vomiting, excessive exercise, fasting, or laxative use (despite its ineffectiveness in controlling calorie intake). The concern for weight gain and/or drive to lose weight is also a feature of BN, along with a preoccupation with food and an extreme desire to eat. Practitioners rely on the following resources to diagnose patients who suffer from BN: The *International Classification of Diseases,* 10th edition (*ICD-10*), *Diagnostic and Statistical Manual of Mental Disorders,* 4th edition (*DSM-IV*), and upcoming (proposed) changes to diagnostic criteria for BN (*DSM-V*). These classifications, as outlined by the APA and the World Health Organization, include the following (APA, 2011; Patrick, 2002):

- Recurrent episodes of overeating in a short period of time (for example, within any two-hour period), at least two times per week over three months
- Sense of a loss of control during episodes in combination with a strong desire to eat
- Recurrent, inappropriate compensatory behavior following overeating to prevent weight gain, including food restriction, self-induced vomiting, laxative or diuretic misuse, enemas, appetite suppressants, thyroid preparations, or medications to prevent weight gain. Diabetics with bulimia may modify their insulin treatment.
- Self-perception of being overweight and a morbid fear of becoming fat
- Behavior does not occur exclusively during episodes of BN
- Specific type: purging

The risk factors for BN range from a potential genetic link to a personality type. As with AN, family studies have identified an increase in lifetime risk for females with a family history of eating disorders (Klein & Walsh, 2003). Pinpointing the genetic marker for BN has yet to be done with consistency in the research, but is likely to be determined as investigations persist.

Personality, temperament, and environment each play a major role in the development of BN. It is quite common for people with BN to have a history of childhood obesity, as well as have experienced critical feedback from family regarding weight and body shape at an early age (Klein & Walsh, 2004). In a review of factors that make a person vulnerable to BN, Klein and Walsh (2004) point out the correlation between BN and anxiety and mood disorders, as well as personality traits common among patients. People with BN tend to be novelty-seeking and impulsive, and have a propensity for high negative emotionality and stress reactivity. Similarly, there is a three- to fourfold higher risk for substance abuse, and an increased rate of self-cutting and suicide attempts (Klein & Walsh, 2004; Patrick, 2002).

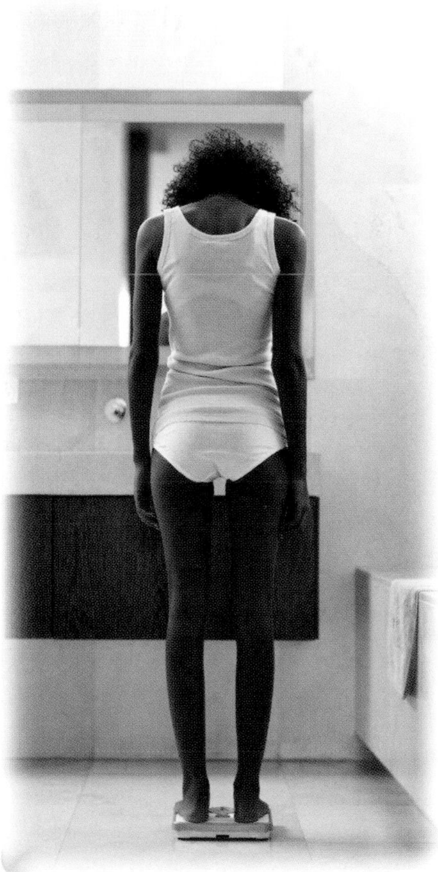

The health complications of BN far surpass the issue of weight loss. Individuals engaging in frequent vomiting or abuse of laxatives and diuretics are at risk for **electrolyte** disturbances, **dehydration,** muscle weakness, cardiac and kidney dysfunction, and gastrointestinal problems (Patrick, 2002; ADA, 2001). Of particular concern is the loss of potassium (**hypokalemia**), which can result in cardiac problems, as well as constipation, muscle myopathy, and kidney dysfunction. Cardiac abnormalities vary in severity, but can include **bradycardia** (heart rate below 60 beats per minute), low blood pressure (**hypotension**) leading to dizziness or fainting, electrocardiographic changes, and the potential for congestive heart failure, arrhythmias, and sudden death (Patrick, 2002; ADA, 2001). During recurring episodes of vomiting, the **esophagus** can become damaged and **gastroesophageal reflux disease (GERD)** may develop, as well as dental erosion (ADA, 2001).

The potential for serious medical complications with BN is high. Therefore, multidisciplinary intervention is imperative. Treatment varies, with many patients succeeding with outpatient care and others requiring hospitalization. The initial objectives are to control the compensatory behavior, especially the vomiting, and normalize eating behaviors. Medications may be prescribed for BN, and cognitive-behavioral therapy has been shown to be effective in treating individuals with BN.

Anorexia Nervosa

Cases of anorexia nervosa have been documented since the late 1800s (Klein & Walsh, 2003). Extreme weight loss and a drive for thinness are hallmark features of the disorder, and individuals with AN can suffer from myriad serious medical complications. More women are afflicted with AN than men—at a 10–20:1 ratio (females to males). An association with dance, fashion modeling, and some "weight-conscious" sports show greater numbers in both genders (Klein & Walsh, 2003). Of grave concern is the mortality rate for AN, as it is the highest among psychiatric disorders. In a review by Patrick (2002), AN is cited as a leading cause of death among females between the ages of 15 and 24 years, with suicide, infection, or chronic starvation being at fault.

The *DSM-IV* Diagnostic Criteria for AN outlined by the American Psychiatric Association and the World Health Organization's *ICD-10* classifications include the following (Patrick, 2002):

- Weight is at least 15% below normal for age/height or failure to gain weight during periods of growth, leading to less than 85% of expected weight
- Self-induced weight loss secondary to avoidance of high-calorie foods, impaired perception of body weight or shape, and intense fear of gaining weight accompanied by denial of the seriousness of low body weight
- In postmenarcheal females, presence of **amenorrhea** (absence of at least three consecutive menstrual cycles). In males, the hypothalamic-pituitary gonadal axis disturbance manifests as a loss of sexual interest and potency.
- Additional proposed criteria (for upcoming *DSM-V*) regarding the type of AN:
  - ✓ *Restricting type:* During the past three months, the person has not engaged in recurrent episodes of binge eating or purging behavior (i.e., self-induced vomiting or the misuse of laxatives, diuretics, or enemas).
  - ✓ *Binge-eating/purging type:* During the past three months, the person has engaged in recurrent episodes of binge eating or purging behavior (i.e., self-induced vomiting or the misuse of laxatives, diuretics, or enemas).

The development of AN is multifactorial. Genetics has emerged as a contributing factor to the risk for, and development of, AN. It is estimated that approximately 58 to 76% of variance in the occurrence of AN is due to genetic factors (Klein & Walsh, 2004). Environmental and personality factors explain the remainder of AN's development, with key contributors being socio-cultural influences and perfectionism. The impact of puberty is considered in the development of AN, as it rarely occurs prepuberty and may be the psychological response to the "growing pains" associated with the maturing body (Klein & Walsh, 2004).

A culture that accepts and promotes "dieting" has long been considered a contributing factor. Young women and men are influenced by the barrage of advertisements, discussions, and media attention on the topics of dieting and body image. During vulnerable years, in combination with any emotional instability and/or genetic factors, the socio-cultural influence can be great.

Typically, the first sign of AN to family and friends is weight loss. However, there are behavioral changes that present before weight loss occurs. Common alterations in behaviors surrounding food include the elimination of particular foods or food groups, focus on low- or no-calorie items, delineation of "safe" foods, and increased consumption of noncaloric beverages (Klein & Walsh, 2004). Early stages of AN combine the intense fear of fatness, a strong desire for thinness, hunger denial, and a focus on food as a mechanism of control. As the disorder progresses and the weight declines, individuals with AN will often mask their changes with loose-fitting clothing and withdrawal from social gatherings.

The consequences of starvation will eventually lead to decreased mental acuity, difficulty concentrating, and mood swings.

The medical symptoms and consequences can be quite serious as the disorder progresses. The following list presents the potentially devastating results from untreated AN (Patrick 2002; ADA, 2001):

- *Physical changes:* Lanugo hair (fine, downy hair) on the face and trunk, brittle hair, **cyanosis** of the hands and feet, and dry skin
- *Electrolyte disturbances:* As with BN, potassium levels can drop, accompanied by low magnesium. Resulting conditions include muscle weakness, loss of concentration, muscular cramping, arrythmias, and memory loss.
- *Cardiovascular abnormalities:* Bradycardia, hypotension, reduced heart mass, and postural hypotension. These effects can stem from electrolyte disturbances and can often lead to death.
- *Gastrointestinal issues:* When the gut is left unfed, it can **atrophy** and have reduced motility, incomplete gastric emptying, and constipation; increased transit time; diminished **peristalsis;** and irritable bowel syndrome
- Amenorrhea
- **Osteopenia** or osteoporosis
- Vitamin and mineral deficiencies

A multidisciplinary approach to AN care is integral. Whether it is inpatient or outpatient care will depend on the severity of the disorder. Body weight is the primary outcome measure for AN treatment, but comprehensive care requires a behavioral, nutritional, and psychiatric approach. Careful attention needs to be paid to the refeeding component of the plan, as rapid refeeding can lead to deadly changes in phosphate levels, drops in potassium and magnesium, alterations in glucose tolerance, and diminished gastrointestinal and heart function.

Eating Disorder Resources for the Health Coach

If a health coach suspects that a client has an eating disorder and requires a referral for both psychological and nutritional care, the Internet can provide some help if he or she is unaware of experts in the area:

www.edreferral.com: A continuously updated site of treatment centers and eating-disorder resources

www.eating-disorder-referral.com: Lists treatment centers by location

www.nationaleatingdisorders.org: Provides information and referral services

Anxiety and Eating Disorders

The link between eating disorders and other psychiatric disorders has long been recognized. Obsessive-compulsive disorders have been linked to risk for, and progression of, both AN and BN. As mentioned previously, particular personality traits are associated with eating disorders, and family history of these traits is influential as well. Anxiety disorder has been associated with AN and BN, and its influence has been investigated. Kaye et al. (2004) sought to assess the frequency of anxiety disorders among individuals with AN and BN, and to characterize its influence. After interviewing 282 individuals with BN and 293 with AN with a standardized tool for measuring anxiety, perfectionism, and obsessionality, researchers detected a significantly higher prevalence of anxiety disorder among the AN and BN subjects than is found in the overall population. The researchers concluded that anxiety disorder is not only linked to AN and BN, but may also be a warning sign for its development and should be considered during treatment.

Depression, Disordered Eating, and Obesity

Behavioral and social factors contribute to the development of obesity and eating disorders (Dubois & Girard, 2006). In addition, depression or self-esteem issues may play a role in the development and perpetuation of a disorder. The factors that affect weight status were evaluated in 2,101 tenth-grade Turkish adolescents (Ozmen et al., 2007). A self-esteem measurement and the Children's Depression Inventory revealed that body dissatisfaction was related to low self-esteem and depression, although not correlated with obesity or overweight. There was a relationship, however, between perceptions of being overweight and low self-esteem. A similar investigation of children between seven and 13 years of age showed that those who were overweight or obese were more concerned about their body weights and shapes than those with healthy weights, and had lower self-esteem ratings, greater body dissatisfaction, and higher depression ratings (Allen et al., 2006). Goodman and Whitaker (2002) discovered a similar result in a prospective study of the role of depression in the development and persistence of adolescent obesity, indicating that depressed mood at baseline was a predictor of obesity, whereas the participants who were obese at baseline did not predict depression. The researchers indicated that depressed adolescents are at an increased risk for developing obesity.

Psychological issues have been identified as comorbidities for eating disorders such as BN and AN (Blinder, Cumella, & Sanathara, 2006). In a sample of 2,436 inpatient females with a primary diagnosis of BN, AN, or eating disorders not otherwise specified, it was found that those with BN were more likely to suffer from alcohol abuse and polysubstance abuse. Those with AN and binge-purge anorexia were more likely to suffer from obsessive-compulsive disorder, post-traumatic stress disorder, schizophrenia, and/or other psychoses. All of those individuals with eating disorders suffered from depression. The evidence has implications for the prevention and treatment of all types of eating disorders, and supports the use of a multidisciplinary team approach.

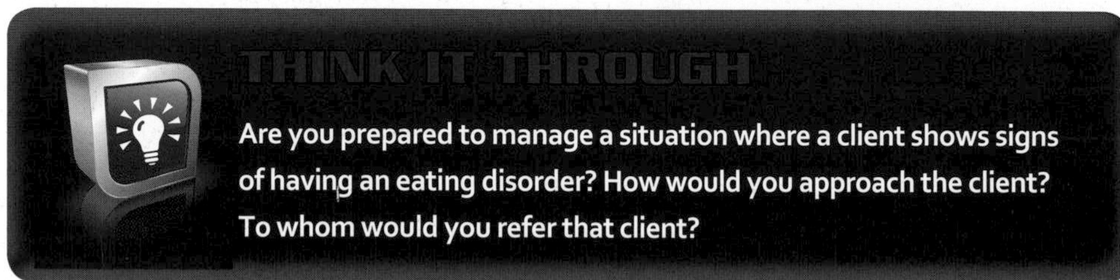

THINK IT THROUGH
Are you prepared to manage a situation where a client shows signs of having an eating disorder? How would you approach the client? To whom would you refer that client?

Eating Disorders in Athletes

It is not uncommon for athletes to focus on weight management as a tool to achieve a new personal best race time or improved performance in their sport. Dieting typically precedes a clinical eating disorder as an athlete restricts energy intake in order to achieve a lower body weight, perhaps for improved performance or appearance, or to gain access to a specific weight class. Energy restriction in athletes tends to occur most often in sports that encourage a lean physique such as running, dance, ballet, and wrestling. Studies involving young female dancers, elite figure skaters, and gymnasts found that average energy intakes were 50 to 80% of recommended energy intake and average intakes of the micronutrients calcium, zinc, and magnesium were also below the recommended levels (Croll et al., 2006; Sundgot-Borgen 1993).

In female athletes, the interrelationships between energy availability, menstrual function, and **bone mineral density (BMD)** may lead to the symptoms of amenorrhea, disordered eating, and osteoporosis known as the **female athlete triad.** The prevalence of the female athlete triad varies widely. The athletes at greatest risk are those who restrict overall energy intake, athletes who exercise for prolonged periods, vegetarian athletes, and athletes who limit the type of food they will eat [American College of Sports Medicine (ACSM), 2007]. In order to increase awareness and prevent the female athlete triad, the entire healthcare team and athletic administration must be in line. Education in the area of nutritional needs and requirements should be provided. Athletes with menstrual disorders and/or low energy availability should be educated about bone health, including stress fractures. Support and referrals should be made for those athletes at risk for, or suffering from, the female athlete triad.

THINK IT THROUGH

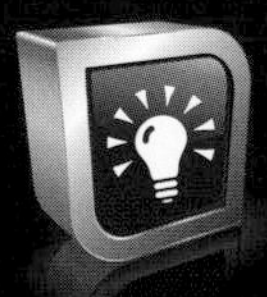

Female High School Athlete

One of your young clients, Sarah, is the team captain for her high school volleyball team. Sarah has worked with you for the past couple of months to help her make better nutrition choices and lose excess body fat so that she can become a better volleyball player. Sarah reports that at last week's physical, she was excited to learn that she had dropped 3 pounds (1.4 kg) over the past seven days. At her current height of 5'8" and body weight of 123 lb (56 kg), Sarah's BMI is 18.7 kg/m^2—still within the healthy range. Today, during your appointment, she mentions that she has been experiencing pain in her shins. You know that volleyball players, like gymnasts and other athletes who participate in sports in which leanness and body image are of importance, are at higher risk for eating disorders. Upon questioning Sarah about her current eating habits, she reveals that she rarely dines with the team. In addition, you ask if her menstrual cycle is regular. She reports that she has not had a period in a few months.

- You suspect that Sarah may be using some unsafe weight-loss practices. How would you approach this?
- Sarah is a vegetarian and is unsure about what to eat for protein. What are some good sources of protein for an athlete Sarah's age?
- Sarah would like to know if she should be taking a vitamin supplement to help her shins heal. What do you tell her?
- Do you think Sarah may be at risk for the female athlete triad? If so, what is your next step?

Summary

Weight management is largely a matter of energy intake versus energy output, and finding an appropriate long-term balance between the two will be the central challenge for most clients. It is important for health coaches to understand the many diets and pharmacological agents that continue to flood the marketplace, including both the potential effectiveness and the health risks and side effects associated with each. Having a solid foundation of up-to-date knowledge in this area is essential for health coaches who wish to present themselves as experts to their clients. Finally, health coaches must be able to identify the signs of various eating disorders and explain the associated health risks to their clients. While diagnosing and treating eating disorders falls outside of a health coach's scope of practice, health coaches are often among the first to discuss the topic with individuals who are at risk or are already coping with eating disorders, so it is vital for health coaches to approach this topic with compassion and basic knowledge of common eating disorders.

References

Allen, K.L. et al. (2006). Why do some overweight children experience psychological problems? The role of weight and shape concern. *International Journal of Pediatric Obesity,* 1, 4, 239–247.

American College of Sports Medicine (2007). ACSM Position Statement: The female athlete triad. *Medicine & Science in Sports & Exercise,* 39, 10, 1867–1882.

American Dietetic Association (2011). Position of the American Dietetic Association: Nutrition intervention in the treatment of Eating Disorders. *Journal of the American Dietetic Association*, 111, 8, 1236–1241.

American Dietetic Association (2009). Position of the American Dietetic Association: Weight management. *Journal of the American Dietetic Association*, 109, 2, 330–346.

American Dietetic Association (2006). Position of the American Dietetic Association: Food and nutrition misinformation. *Journal of the American Dietetic Association,* 106, 4, 601–607.

American Dietetic Association (2001). Position of the American Dietetic Association: Nutrition intervention in the treatment of anorexia nervosa, bulimia nervosa, and eating disorders not otherwise specified (EDNOS). *Journal of the American Dietetic Association*, 101, 7, 810–819.

American Psychiatric Association (2011). *DSM-V Development: Eating Disorders.* Accessed November 1, 2011: www.dsm5.org/ProposedRevision/Pages/proposedrevision.aspx?rid=372

Anderson, G.H. & Woodend, D. (2003). Effect of glycemic carbohydrates on short-term satiety and food intake. *Nutrition Reviews,* 61, 5, S17–S26.

Astrup, A., Larsen, T.M., & Harper, A. (2004). Atkins and other low-carbohydrate diets: Hoax or an effective tool for weight loss? *Lancet,* 364, 897–899.

Blinder B.J., Cumella E.J., & Sanathara V.A. (2006). Psychiatric comorbidities of female inpatients with eating disorders. *Psychosomatic Medicine,* 68, 3, 454–462.

Bravata, D.M. et al. (2003). Efficacy and safety of low-carbohydrate diets: A systematic review. *Journal of the American Medical Association,* 289, 14, 1837–1850.

Buchwald H. et al. (2004). Bariatric surgery: A systematic review and meta-analysis. *Journal of the American Medical Association,* 292, 1724–1737.

Byrd-Bredbenner, C. et al. (2008). *Wardlaw's Perspectives in Nutrition* (8th ed.). New York: McGraw-Hill.

Croll, J.K. et al. (2006). Adolescents involved in weight-related and power team sports have better eating patterns and nutrients intakes than non-sport-involved adolescents. *Journal of the American Dietetic Association,* 106, 709–717.

Dubois, L. & Girard, M. (2006). Early determinants of overweight at 4.5 years in a population-based longitudinal study. *International Journal of Obesity,* 30, 4, 610–617.

Faria, S.L. et al. (2010). Nutritional management of weight regain after bariatric surgery. *Obesity Surgery,* 20, 2, 135–139.

Foster, G.D. et al. (2003). A randomized trial of a low-carbohydrate diet for obesity. *New England Journal of Medicine,* 348, 2082–2090.

Freedman, M.R., King, J., & Kennedy, E. (2001). Popular diets: A scientific review. *Obesity Research,* 9 (Suppl): 1S–40S.

Freire R.H. et al. (2011). Food quality, physical activity, and nutritional follow-up as a determinant of weight regain after Roux-en-Y gastric bypass. *Nutrition,* doi:10.1016/j.nut.2011.01.011

Gluck, M.E. (2006). Stress response and binge eating disorder. *Appetite,* 46, 1, 26–30.

Goodman E. & Whitaker R.C. (2002). A prospective study of the role of depression in the development and persistence of adolescent obesity. *Pediatrics,* 110, 3, 497–504.

Halford, J. (2006). Pharmacotherapy for obesity. *Appetite,* 46, 1, 6–10.

Halford, J. (2004). Clinical pharmacotherapy for obesity: Current drugs and those in advanced development. *Current Drug Targets,* 5, 637–646.

Hudson, J.I. et al. (2007). The prevalence and correlates of eating disorders in the National Comorbidity Survey Replication. *Biological Psychiatry,* 61, 348–358.

Johnson S. et al. (2007). A predictive model for gastrointestinal side effects due to dietary fat with orlistat [abstract 010-27]. In: *2007 IFT Annual Meeting Technical Program Book of Abstracts*. Chicago, Ill.: Institute of Food Technologists.

Jolly, K. et al. (2011). Comparison of range of commercial or primary care led weight reduction programmes with minimal intervention control for weight loss in obesity: Lighten Up randomised controlled trial. *British Medical Journal,* 343:d6500 doi: 10.1136/bmj.d6500

Kaye, W.H. et al. (2004). Comorbidity of anxiety disorders with anorexia and bulimia nervosa. *American Journal of Psychiatry,* 161, 2215–2221.

Klein, D.A. & Walsh, B.T. (2004). Eating disorders: Clinical features and pathophysiology. *Physiology and Behavior,* 81, 2, 359–374.

Klein, D.A. & Walsh, B.T. (2003). Eating disorders. *International Review of Psychiatry,* 15, 205–216.

Krieger, J.W. et al. (2006). Effects of variation in protein and carbohydrate intake on body mass and composition during energy restriction: A metaregression. *American Journal of Clinical Nutrition,* 83, 2, 260–274.

Kurpad, A.V., Muthayya, S., & Vaz, M. (2005). Consequences of inadequate food energy and negative energy balance in humans. *Public Health Nutrition,* 8, 7A, 1053–1076.

Last, A.R. & Wilson, S.A. (2006). Low-carbohydrate diets. *American Family Physician,* 73, 11, 1942–1948.

Liu, S. (2006). Lowering dietary glycemic load for weight control and cardiovascular health: A matter of quality. *Archives of Internal Medicine,* 166, 1438–1439.

Mann, T. et al. (2007). Medicare's search for effective obesity treatments: Diets are not the answer. *American Psychologist,* 62, 3, 220–233.

Martins-Filho, E.D. et al. (2008). Evaluations of risk factors in superobese patients submitted to conventional Fobi-Capella surgery. *Archives of Gastroenterology,* 45, 3–10.

McMillan-Price, J. et al. (2006). Comparison of four diets of varying glycemic load on weight loss and cardiovascular risk reduction in overweight and obese young adults: A randomized controlled trial. *Archives of Internal Medicine,* 166, 1466–1475.

Noakes, M. et al. (2005). Effect of an energy-restricted, high-protein, low-fat diet relative to a conventional high-carbohydrate, low-fat diet on weight loss, body composition, nutritional status, and markers of cardiovascular health in obese women. *American Journal of Clinical Nutrition,* 81, 6, 1298–1306.

Ozmen, D. et al. (2007). The association of self-esteem, depression and body satisfaction with obesity among Turkish adolescents. *BMC Public Health,* 16, 7, 80.

Patrick, L. (2002). Eating disorders: A review of the literature with emphasis on medical complications and clinical nutrition. *Alternative Medicine Review,* 7, 3, 184–202.

Popkin, B.M. (2010). Recent dynamics suggest selected countries catching up to U.S. obesity. *American Journal of Clinical Nutrition,* 91, 1, 284S–288S.

Popkin, B.M. (2008). *The World Is Fat: The Fads, Trends, Policies, and Products that Are Fattening the Human Race.* New York: Avery-Penguin Group.

Saris, W.H.M. (2003). Glycemic carbohydrate and body weight regulation. *Nutrition Reviews,* 61, 5, S10–S16.

Shetty, P. (2005). Energy requirements of adults. *Public Health Nutrition,* 8, 7A, 994–1009.

Sloth, B. et al. (2004). No difference in body weight decrease between a low-glycemic-index and a high-glycemic-index diet but reduced LDL cholesterol after 10-wk ad libitum intake of the low-glycemic-index diet. *American Journal of Clinical Nutrition,* 80, 2, 337–347.

Steffen, K.J. et al. (2010). A prevalence study and description of Alli use by patients with eating disorders. *International Journal of Eating Disorders,* 43, 472–479.

Stein, K. (2000). High-protein, low-carbohydrate diets: Do they work? *Journal of the American Dietetic Association,* 100, 760–761.

St. Jeor, S.T. et al. (2001). Dietary protein and weight reduction: A statement for healthcare professionals from the Nutrition Committee of the Council on Nutrition, Physical Activity, and Metabolism of the American Heart Association. *Circulation,* 104, 1869–1874.

Stubbs, R.J. & Tolkamp, B.J. (2006). Control of energy balance in relation to energy intake and energy expenditure in animals and man: An ecological perspective. *British Journal of Nutrition,* 95, 4, 657–676.

Sundgot-Borgen, J. (1993). Prevalence of eating disorders in elite female gymnasts. *International Journal of Sports Nutrition,* 3, 29-40.

Weight Control Information Network: United States Department of Health and Human Services, National Institutes of Health, National Institute of Diabetes and Digestive and Kidney Diseases (2011). *Bariatric Surgery for Severe Obesity.* NIH Publication No. 08–4006, March 2009 (Updated June 2011). www.win.niddk.nih.gov/publications/PDFs/Bariatric_Surgery_508.pdf

Wellman, P.J. & Maher, T.J. (1999). Synergistic interactions between fenfluramine and phentermine. *International Journal of Obesity,* 23, 723–732.

Wenk, C. (2004). Implications of dietary fat for nutrition and energy balance. *Physiology and Behavior,* 83, 4, 564–571.

Westerterp-Plantenga, M.S. (2004). Fat intake and energy-balance effects. *Physiology and Behavior,* 83, 4, 579–585.

Westerterp-Plantenga, M.S. & Lejeune, M.P. (2005). Protein intake and body-weight regulation. *Appetite,* 45, 187–190.

World Health Organization (2003). *Diet, Nutrition, and the Prevention of Chronic Diseases: WHO Technical Report Series.* Geneva, Switzerland: World Health Organization.

Zhi, J. et al. (1994). Retrospective population-based analysis of the dose-response (fecal fat excretion) relationship of orlistat in normal and obese volunteers. *Clinical Pharmacology and Therapeutics,* 56, 82–85.

Suggested Reading

American Heart Association (2005). *American Heart Association No-Fad Diet: A Personal Plan for Healthy Weight Loss.* New York: Clarkson Potter/ Publishers.

Bauer, J. (2005). *The Complete Idiot's Guide to Total Nutrition* (4th ed.). Indianapolis, Ind.: Alpha Books.

Consumer Reports (June 2005). Rating the diets from Atkins to the Zone. 18–22.

Dansigner, M.L. et al. (2005). Comparison of the Atkins, Ornish, Weight Watchers, and Zone diets for weight loss and heart disease risk reduction: A randomized trial. *Journal of the American Medical Association,* 293, 1, 43–53.

Duyff, R.L. (2007). *American Dietetic Association Complete Food and Nutrition Guide* (3rd ed.). Indianapolis, Ind.: Wiley Higher Education.

Howard, B.V. et al. (2006). Low-fat dietary pattern and weight change over seven years: The Women's Health Initiative Dietary Modification Trial. *Journal of the American Medical Association,* 295, 39–49.

Nordmann, A.J. et al. (2006). Effects of low-carbohydrate vs. low-fat diets on weight loss and cardiovascular risk factors: A meta-analysis of randomized controlled trials. *Archives of Internal Medicine,* 166, 285–293.

Parikh, P. et al. (2005). Diets and cardiovascular disease: An evidence-based assessment. *Journal of the American College of Cardiology,* 45, 9, 1979–1987.

Sports, Cardiovascular and Wellness Nutritionists DPG & Dunford, M. (2006). *Sports Nutrition: A Practice Manual for Professionals* (4th ed.). Chicago, Ill.: American Dietetic Association.

Whitney, E.N. & Rolfes, S.R. (2010). *Understanding Nutrition.* (12th ed.). Belmont, Calif.: Wadsworth Publishing Company.

Yager, J. & Anderson, A. (2005). Anorexia nervosa. *New England Journal of Medicine,* 353, 14, 1481–1488.

SECTION IV

SCREENING AND ASSESSMENT

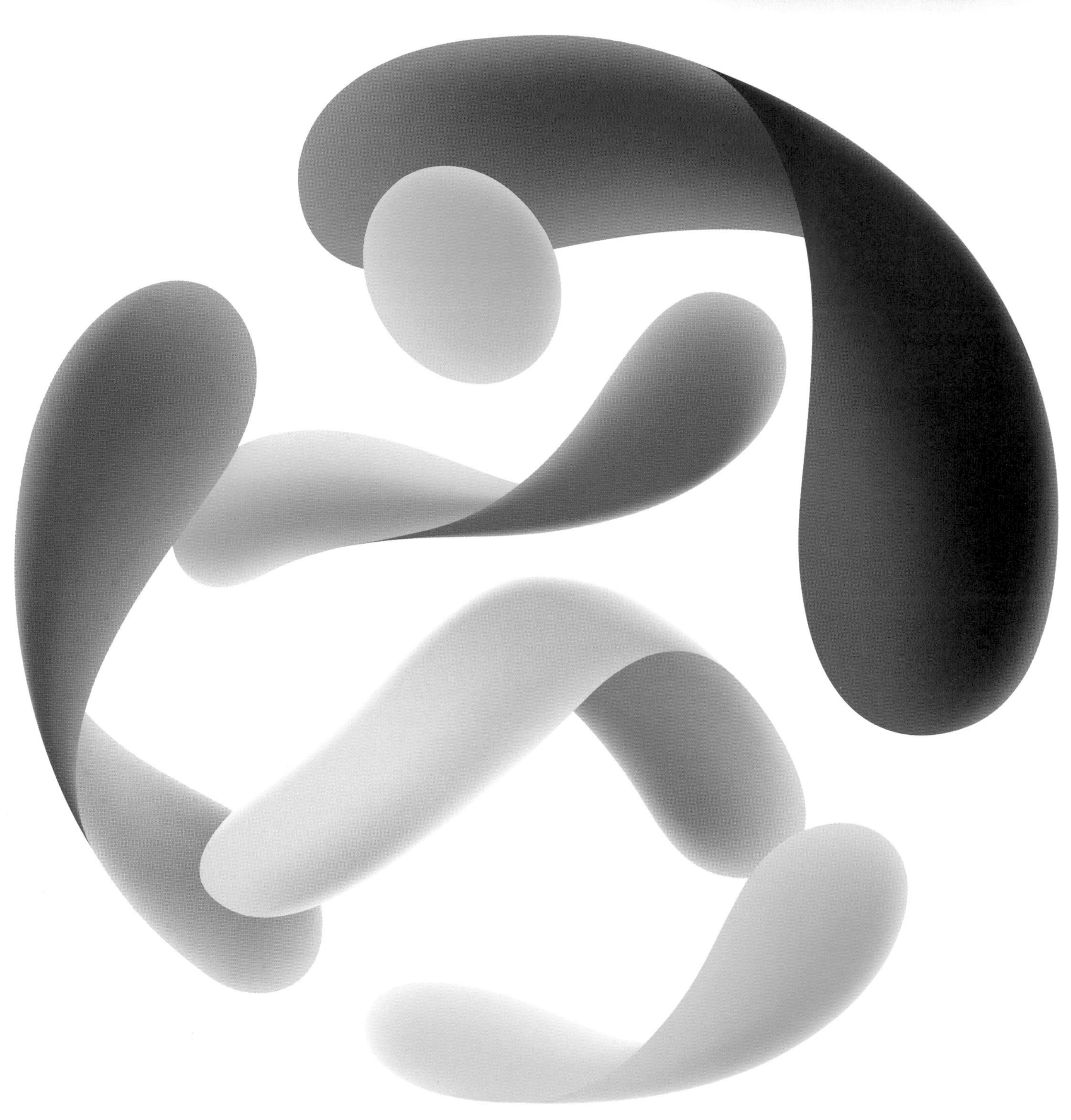

Chapter 10
Initial Interview and Client Screening

Chapter 11
Body-composition Assessment and Evaluation

Chapter 12
Physical-fitness Assessments

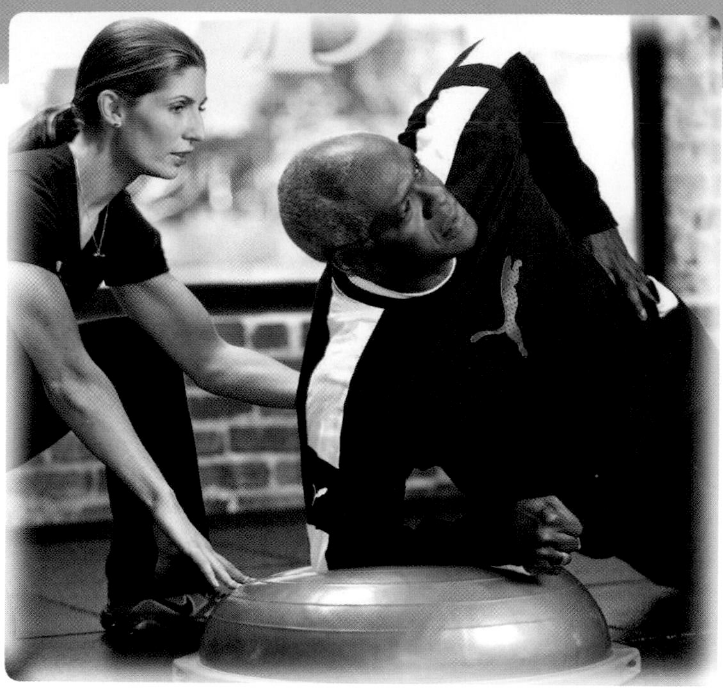

IN THIS CHAPTER:

Richard T. Cotton, M.A., is the national director of certification for the American College of Sports Medicine (ACSM). Cotton is the former chief exercise physiologist for the Scripps Clinic & Research Foundation as well as for the American Council on Exercise, where he also served as a media spokesperson and technical editor. He is certified by ACSM as both a Clinical Exercise Specialist and Preventive and Rehabilitative Program Director.

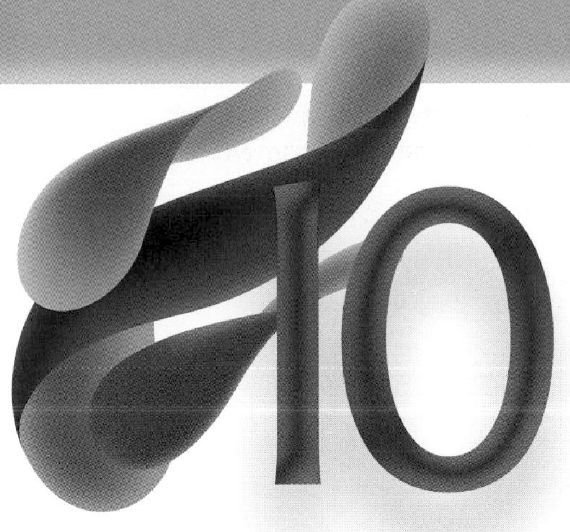

Initial Interview and Client Screening

RICHARD T. COTTON

& TRACIE ROGERS

Tracie Rogers, Ph.D., is a sport and exercise psychology specialist and the director of the MS Human Movement Program at A.T. Still University. She is also the owner of BAR Fitness, located in Phoenix, Arizona. Dr. Rogers teaches, speaks, and writes on psychological constructs related to physical-activity participation and adherence.

ACE-certified Health Coaches offer a valuable service, combining information from nutritional, behavioral, and exercise sciences to help clients manage their weight. The hallmark of health coaches is their ability to promote safe and effective lifestyle changes for a wide variety of individuals. However, not all clients who seek the services of a health coach can and should be treated by one. The purpose of this chapter is to assist health coaches in screening for potential contraindications to weight-loss treatment and provide a framework for the assessment of potential clients.

Health coaches should identify their goals for collecting assessments before any assessment is conducted. The goal should not be to add an additional session to the program or to gather information just for the purpose of keeping it in a client file. The goal of any assessment should always be to aid in the development of a safe and effective exercise program, and beyond the traditional meanings of this phrase, it could be argued that an effective program is best defined as one to which the client adheres. It is important for health coaches to be mindful of this goal in all of their assessment and program planning. Assessments can actually have a negative effect on a client if they are not conducted with care. For example, if a client undergoes an entire session of assessments (and is aware that this is the purpose of the session), the client knows that he or she is being judged, measured, or compared in some way. Many new clients are overweight with low fitness levels and, thus, score very poorly on nearly any assessment conducted. From a behavioral change and motivation standpoint, what is the value of starting a new program with an entire session of perceived failures? Assessments need to have purpose, be delivered in a manner that is not viewed as a test to the client, and, often times, the results, in terms of how the client is classified (e.g., fitness or strength level), should not immediately be shared with the client (especially at the start of a program). Most people who are starting a new program know that they are overweight and out of shape. Conducting a full session of body measurements and strength and cardiovascular tests is only going to prove this point and likely be a negative experience. In other words, newcomers to a lifestyle-modification program are essentially going to "fail" every assessment, and starting a new program with an entire session of "failure" is not beneficial to **self-efficacy, rapport,** or program enthusiasm.

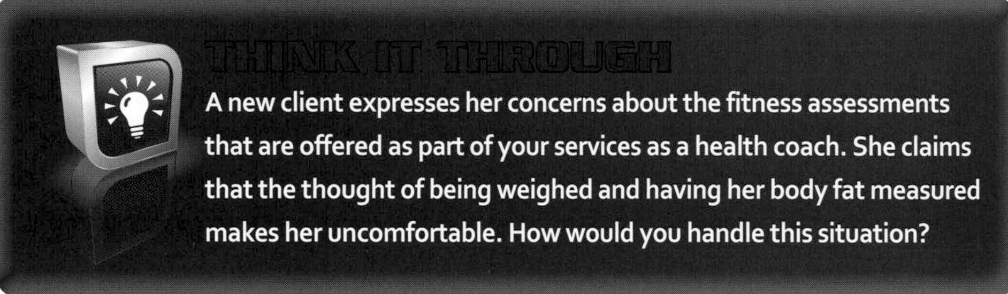

THINK IT THROUGH
A new client expresses her concerns about the fitness assessments that are offered as part of your services as a health coach. She claims that the thought of being weighed and having her body fat measured makes her uncomfortable. How would you handle this situation?

Instead, at the start of each new program, health coaches should determine what information is absolutely necessary to design a safe and effective program or what is specifically requested by the client. This critical information should then be gathered, and everything else should be left for another time. Health coaches should be mindful of the fact that when selected in this framework, many traditional assessments will not be completed, and as much as the health coach may want a baseline body-fat number (for example), it is unnecessary for the design of the program and may be harmful to the psychological readiness and efficacy of the client. The same is true with behavioral assessments. Presenting a "paper and pencil" inventory to assess each psychological construct is typically not the most beneficial approach to gathering information, as it creates a false sense of truth and takes the responsibility off of the health coach. Health coaches are not trained mental health professionals and should not attempt to label, diagnosis, or classify an individual into any particular mental health category. Additionally, paper-and-pencil inventories are impersonal and will never provide the same insight as quality communication. The behavioral assessment process should revolve around gathering information to create a program that meets the unique needs of the client.

The Importance of a Thorough Screening and Assessment

Many factors influence whether an individual will become overweight. Identifying underlying contributors to a client's weight problem is important, because they will influence the type of recommended treatment. Consider the following example: Joe is the chief counsel in a large law firm. His work takes him on the road often and for several weeks at a time. Before a trial, Joe works long days for weeks and does not get to relax until a couple of weeks after a trial. Though once a highly fit, athletic individual, Joe has gained about 50 pounds (23 kg) over the past

10 years. It is likely that Joe's long work hours, high stress level, frequent meals in restaurants, and lack of regular exercise are major contributors to his weight-management problems.

On the other hand, consider Sam, who is the chief operating officer of a major manufacturing plant. Recently separated from his wife, he is finding it increasingly difficult to return to an empty apartment each evening and has begun to work longer hours each day without taking a break for lunch or dinner. Once home, he finds himself consumed with thoughts of eating and binges nearly every night on food and alcohol. As a result, he has gained nearly 50 pounds (23 kg) in nine months. He confides that his eating is out of control and he feels powerless to stop his destructive behavior.

Both Joe and Sam need to lose similar amounts of weight. The excess 50 pounds (23 kg) each man carries pose a significant health risk, and their weight gain is likely to continue unless specific changes are made.

Joe's lifestyle is clearly affecting his weight. More appropriate food choices and behavioral strategies to reduce his calorie and fat consumption, combined with a regular program of physical activity, will be the cornerstone of his weight-management program. By contrast, Sam's weight difficulties appear more complex. His weight problem results from more than careless eating patterns or a **sedentary** lifestyle (though these may be important factors for later weight maintenance). The health coach may suspect that Sam has high levels of depressive symptoms in response to his current stressor (the separation), which expresses itself in a nightly pattern of excessive eating and drinking. **Depression,** current major stressors, and uncontrolled binging are potential contraindications for weight loss and may require the assistance of a mental-health professional before attempting weight-loss strategies. To best meet the needs of an overweight client, it is important to match his or her needs with the appropriate level of care.

Types of Obesity-treatment Programs

Many clients will require minimal direct involvement from healthcare professionals. However, to work with some clients, a health coach may need to seek support from healthcare providers, such as physicians, mental health specialists (e.g., psychologists, psychiatrists, and social workers), **registered dietitians (R.D.s),** and physical therapists.

To understand when outside help is needed and who to involve in a client's care, it is helpful to be familiar with the spectrum of services available for treating overweight persons. The various approaches to obesity treatment can be broadly broken down into three categories: self-help programs, nonclinical programs, and clinical approaches [Institute of Medicine (IOM), 1995]. While clients without special medical or psychological issues can be treated within the parameters of any of these three categories, some clients may be better served by working with licensed professionals in more intensive clinical programs.

Self-help programs are widely used and vary in format. Examples may include the use of meal-replacement shakes or frozen entrees, participation in support or self-help groups (e.g., Overeaters Anonymous and church-based groups), popular diet books, manuals, magazine articles, or increased exercise. The safety, effectiveness, and quality of such approaches vary greatly. In general, in self-help programs, one basic approach is recommended for everyone, with little or no individualization.

Nonclinical programs are typically more structured and tailored than self-help programs. Most nonclinical programs are commercial-based franchises. The parent company provides the structure, materials and, in some cases, the food for clients to utilize. Coaches are then employed to present the program to participants. The training levels of these coaches vary widely. In some cases, they are simply program graduates who have received additional training from the company. Coaches may or may not be supervised by experienced weight-loss professionals. While some attempts may be made to individualize treatment programs, most allow only minimal deviation from a well-defined plan.

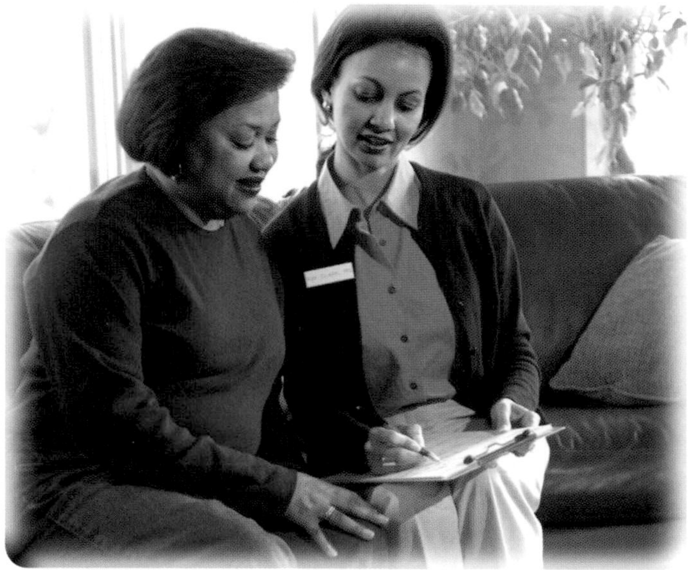

In clinical programs, treatment is provided largely by licensed professionals, such as psychologists, registered dietitians, and physicians. The clinician may work alone and refer patients to allied health professionals as needed, or, more often, be a part of a multidisciplinary team. Clinical programs are typically affiliated with a hospital or university. They generally begin with a thorough medical and psychological assessment and are best suited to treat complicated or severe cases of obesity. Treatment may be highly individualized to meet the unique medical and psychological needs of the participants.

Standards of Care for Weight-management Programs

New "diets" that promise fast, easy, and significant weight loss have been a part of American culture for decades. A quick, informal survey of the covers of top health and fitness and women's magazines shows that they all feature at least one article about diet and weight loss. New weight-loss books are often found among the top 10 best-sellers. Clearly, the weight-loss industry has grown tremendously, and with this growth has come the need to oversee the safety and efficacy of various approaches. Several regulatory bodies have developed guidelines to regulate the practices and advertising claims of weight-loss providers.

The Department of Consumer Affairs (DCA) of New York City was the first agency to document the deceptive practices of many rapid-weight-loss centers. These practices range from working with inappropriate candidates (i.e., underweight individuals) and offering false and misleading claims to outright quackery (Winner, 1991). The result was the first "Truth-in-Dieting" regulation, which mandated specific requirements for all centers promoting rapid weight loss [e.g., more than 1.5 to 2 pounds (0.7 to 0.9 kg) per week, or the loss of more than 1% of body weight per week after the second week of participation]. Specifically, such centers were required to post a "Weight-loss Consumers' Bill of Rights" and provide all consumers with a wallet-size card outlining them (Table 10-1). In addition, programs were required to disclose all costs and the recommended length of treatment.

Table 10-1
The Weight-loss Consumers' Bill of Rights
• WARNING: Rapid weight loss may cause serious health problems. (Rapid weight loss is weight loss of more than 1 ½ to 2 pounds per week, or weight loss of more than 1% of body weight per week after the second week of participation in a weight-loss program.)
• Only permanent lifestyle changes—such as making healthful food choices and increasing physical activity—promote long-term weight loss.
• Consult your personal physician before starting any weight-loss program.
• Qualifications of this provider's staff are available upon request.
• You have a right to ◦ Ask questions about the potential health risks of this program, its nutritional content, and its psychological support and educational components ◦ Know the price of treatment, including the price of extra products, services, supplements, and laboratory tests ◦ Know the program duration that is being recommended for you

Source: New York Department of Consumer Affairs

At about the same time, the Michigan Department of Public Health developed its own set of guidelines for weight-loss programs (Drewnowski, 1990). The Michigan Guidelines applied to all nonclinical and clinical programs and were even more detailed than those developed in New York City. The Michigan Guidelines made these key recommendations:

- All clients must be screened to verify that they have no medical or psychological conditions that could make weight loss inappropriate. Depending on the client, such screening would range from a simple health checklist to a complete physical exam.
- All clients must be classified not only by excess body weight, but also by overall health risks, to ensure that the individual receives the appropriate level of care. Level I is intended for low-risk clients, Level II is for moderate-risk clients who require medical monitoring, and Level III is reserved for very obese or high-risk individuals.
- Care should be given by trained individuals. The qualifications of weight-loss staff should be commensurate with the health-risk level of the client. Thus, programs that accept clients with high health risks require highly trained healthcare professionals.

Specific recommendations were made concerning daily caloric intake, dietary composition, use of appetite-suppressant drugs, and the inclusion of exercise. An emphasis was also placed on individualizing the programs and including a maintenance phase to promote long-term weight management.

At a national level, the Food and Nutrition Board of the IOM commissioned a committee to develop criteria for evaluating the effectiveness of weight-loss approaches to prevent and treat obesity. World-renowned researchers in nutrition, psychology, medicine, and exercise science sat on the committee. The book summarizing their results, *Weighing the Options: Criteria for Evaluating Weight-Management Programs* (IOM, 1995), set forth three primary criteria (Table 10-2).

Table 10-2		
Criteria for Evaluating Weight-management Programs		
Criterion	Program	Person
The match between program and consumer	Who is appropriate for this program?	Should I be in this program given my goals and characteristics?
The soundness and safety of the program	Is my program based on sound biological and behavioral principles, and is it safe for its intended participants?	Is the program safe for me?
Outcomes of the program	What is the evidence of success of my program?	Are the benefits I am likely to achieve from the program worth the effort and cost?

Source: Institute of Medicine (1995). *Weighing the Options: Criteria for Evaluating Weight-Management Programs.* Washington, D.C.: National Academy Press.

Criterion 1 of the IOM recommendations—the match between program and consumer—addresses the importance of matching individuals to appropriate treatment strategies. Treatment for weight disorders range from the least invasive and most economical strategies to those requiring intensive and/or expensive professional care. To better match their specific needs and treatment options, a **stepped-care model** was developed (IOM, 1995). Stepped-care models are widely used in medicine and are based on the premise that treatment can be cumulative or incremental.

As shown in Figure 10-1, step 1 utilizes a low-fat diet, physical activity, and lifestyle change to promote a healthy and reasonable weight loss of up to 10 pounds (4.5 kg). Step

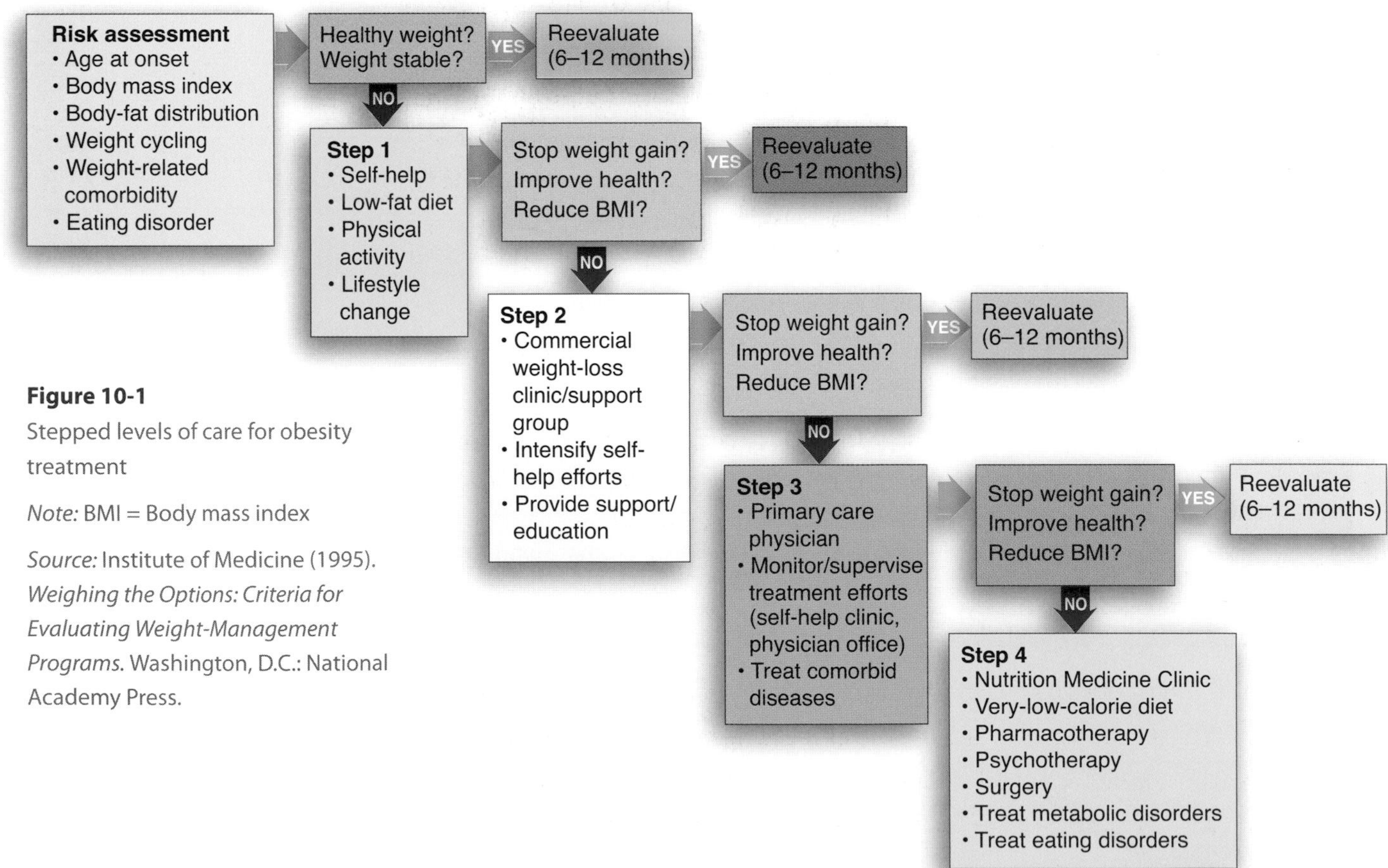

Figure 10-1
Stepped levels of care for obesity treatment

Note: BMI = Body mass index

Source: Institute of Medicine (1995). *Weighing the Options: Criteria for Evaluating Weight-Management Programs.* Washington, D.C.: National Academy Press.

2 involves a more detailed assessment of health risks and utilizes more intensive efforts to help clients change their lifestyles while promoting a larger weight loss. When individuals are diagnosed with comorbid disease or are at a high risk for weight-related diseases, more intensive monitoring of the individual is required, as shown in step 3. The client's primary care physician may also participate more actively in the weight-management program through supervision and monitoring. Step 4 provides the most intensive and aggressive interventions for weight loss, including the use of **very-low-calorie diets**, medication, psychotherapy, and even surgery as indicated. Step 4 incorporates all of the goals of steps 1 through 3, while maximizing the loss of excess body fat and enhancing metabolic fitness.

Where does the work of a health coach fit within the stepped model? It is possible that a health coach may work with clients through all four steps, depending on the setting, the level of professional support available, and the health coach's level of education and experience. However, a health coach is ideally suited to promote lifestyle change in steps 1, 2, and 3 through education, support, and structure. Also, as healthcare becomes increasingly oriented toward the prevention of illness, a health coach can potentially assume a primary role in working with individuals at step 1—that is, clients who are at risk for becoming overweight and developing obesity-related illnesses, but are currently free of such problems.

THINK IT THROUGH

As a health coach, within which areas of the stepped care model do you feel comfortable working? Will you focus on one area—such as prevention—and specialize your services, or will you try to reach individuals in all four steps? How will you attract clients in these different areas (e.g., networking with other healthcare professionals or advancing your education)?

Criterion 2 of the IOM recommendations—the soundness and safety of the program—proposes **standards of care,** or minimum expectations of a credible weight-loss approach. Specifically, the following four areas are identified:

- Assessment of physical health and psychological status (including assessment of a client's knowledge and attitudes related to weight and a periodic reassessment to see if the client is still committed to losing weight and learning the needed information and skills to succeed)
- Attention to diet
- Attention to physical activity
- Ensuring program safety

The IOM offers two additional recommendations supporting the importance of small weight losses to reduce health risks while emphasizing long-term maintenance of weight loss. "We recommend that...the goal of obesity treatment should be refocused from weight loss alone, which is often aimed at appearance, to weight management, [or] achieving the best weight possible in the context of overall health. [Weight-loss programs] should be judged more by their effects on the overall health of participants than by their effects on weight alone" (IOM, 1995, p. 5). Similar recommendations were incorporated into the National Institutes of Health (NIH) guidelines for healthcare providers on the identification, evaluation, and treatment of obesity (NIH, 1998).

How can a health coach ensure the soundness and safety of his or her program for potential clients? A structured guideline-based assessment of physical and psychological health (which may or may not involve the client's personal physician) is an important beginning. Attention needs to be given to dietary intake and physical activity to safely promote either an appropriate energy deficit (for weight loss) or **energy balance** (for weight maintenance). The IOM and NIH recommend that reassessment of diet and activity patterns be conducted at the beginning and end of the weight-loss phase of treatment, and every six months during the maintenance phase.

A health coach must also be aware of the known and potential risks associated with any weight-loss attempt. In general, the more restrictive the diet, the greater the associated risks. For example, the risk of gallbladder disease is greatest with low-calorie diets and rapid weight loss. Diets with a caloric intake of fewer than 1,200 kcal/day may not meet nutritional guidelines, have not been shown to have long-term efficacy, and should not be promoted. Very-low-calorie diets of fewer than 800 kcal/day must only be used under a physician's supervision (IOM, 1995). For significantly obese individuals [i.e., **body mass index (BMI)** >40 or BMI >35 in the presence of additional risk factors], bariatric surgery appears to offer the best long-term results (NIH, 1998). However, it should be noted that randomized, controlled studies comparing morbidly obese subjects who undergo either bariatric surgery or conventional treatment have not been conducted because of the difficulty of randomizing subjects, and there is a tendency for significant weight regain to occur over time after the surgery (Shah, Simha, & Garg, 2006). More research is needed in this area.

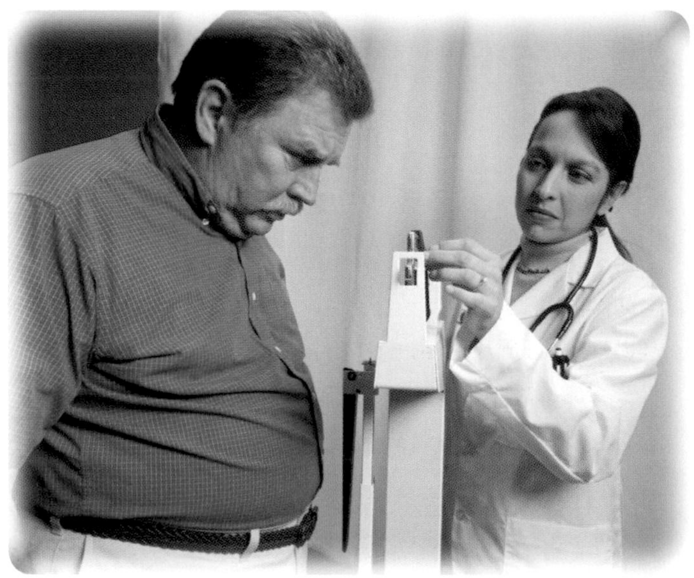

Criterion 3 of the IOM recommendations—outcomes of the program—focuses on four components of a successful program (IOM, 1995):

- Long-term weight loss
- Improvement in obesity-related risk factors
- Improved health practices (e.g., increased physical activity and improved eating habits)
- Monitoring of adverse effects that might result from the program

To successfully monitor outcome, it is critical that the initial and subsequent client assessments are thorough and well-documented. In the interest of consumer protection, the IOM suggests that all details of a weight-loss program be disclosed. This includes rate of weight loss, an outline of the treatment plan, cost estimates, the professional credentials of program staff, and the risks associated with treatment. Claims that weight losses will be maintained over time should be backed up with scientifically valid documentation, not "satisfied client" claims.

Screening Issues

Many factors must be considered when assessing the suitability of a potential client, including medical and psychological status, motivation, readiness to change, and timing. For example, think back to the examples of Joe and Sam. Even though Joe (the lawyer) appears to be a good candidate for the services of a health coach, if the timing is inappropriate (e.g., he is just beginning a lengthy trial out of town), the lack of control over his environment and an inability to meet frequently are significant barriers to success. Certain factors may clearly signal that a potential client is not well-suited for the services of a health coach. It is important that a health coach carefully screens, assesses, and documents the relevant components of physical and psychological health in all clients with whom he or she plans to work.

The initial screening process allows a health coach to separate individuals who may benefit from his or her services from those who clearly will not. The health coach uses the process of assessment to determine the significance or importance of various factors that contribute to, or complicate, a client's weight-management needs. A thorough screening and assessment process protects both the health coach and the consumer. It ensures that the needs of a potential client can be safely met by the services that a health coach can legitimately and ethically provide.

Is This Client Appropriate for This Setting?

The degree of overweight, the type of treatment or program, and client characteristics are all factors to be considered when matching individuals with treatment protocols (NIH, 1998; IOM, 1995). A chief responsibility of a health coach is to be able to determine the appropriateness of a program for a client. Though health coaches may be found in all types of settings, the greatest responsibility lies with the health coach who is essentially practicing without the formal support of an allied healthcare professional. Examples of this situation include health coaches who work independently or provide services in a health club or commercial franchise setting.

Assessment Issues

An assessment of medical and psychological status, diet, and activity level is strongly advised for all clients. The scope and depth of the assessment will vary with the program setting and the level of care provided. This section presents information on the basic or minimum evaluation of physical and psychological health, readiness to exercise, fitness parameters, and motivation or readiness to change.

Assessing Physical Health

Since weight-management practices can potentially help or harm the health of clients (IOM, 1995), some type of physical and psychological health assessment is required for all individuals with whom a health coach will work. Physical health can only be assessed by a physician. Physicians, physician assistants, and nurse practitioners are best trained to review a health history and conduct a physical exam to detect obesity-related illnesses and suitability for a diet and exercise program.

Criteria for Medical Clearance

Though it is recommended that all clients receive a physician's clearance before beginning a weight-management program, it is especially important for individuals with the following health conditions:

- Hypertension
- Elevated **cholesterol** or **triglyceride** levels
- **Diabetes**
- Significant emotional problems
- BMI greater than 30
- Chronic kidney failure
- Liver disease
- Cardiovascular disease, including **angina, arrhythmias,** and **congestive heart failure**
- Pregnancy—present or planned
- **Hyperthyroidism** or **hypothyroidism**
- Substance abuse
- Extreme obesity

Visit www.ACEfitness.org/HealthCoachResources to download a free PDF of a medical release form, lifestyle and health-history questionnaire, and musculoskeletal health questionnaire, as well as other forms and assessment tools that you can use throughout your career as a health coach.

The Basic Health Screen

For apparently healthy clients who report no significant current or past medical problems, it may be sufficient to obtain the following health data (National Task Force on the Prevention and Treatment of Obesity, 2000; NIH, 1998):

- BMI or body composition (percent body fat)
- **Waist circumference**
- Blood pressure and resting heart rate
- Current medications
- History of chronic illnesses
- Current medical history
- Family health history
- Health habits (e.g., cigarette, alcohol, and recreational drug use)
- Assessment of obesity-related risk factors

Height–weight tables are sometimes used to get a rough estimate of "ideal" body weight. A more useful estimate of appropriate body weight can be obtained by adjusting weight for height or stature and calculating a height-normalized index called the body mass index. Body mass index is highly predictive of the relative health risk associated with a person's body weight. (See Chapter 11 for information on the calculation and interpretation of body mass index and other body-composition testing methods.)

Dr. Nicholas DiNubile, in his book *FrameWork: Your 7-Step Program for Healthy Muscles, Bones, and Joints*, provides a self-test to determine an individual's musculoskeletal fitness and uncover what he terms "potential time bombs" (DiNubile & Patrick, 2005). Health coaches can use this book as a resource when working with clients to assess their musculoskeletal health. In addition, Figure 10-2 presents a musculoskeletal health questionnaire that should be used as part of every client's initial assessment. Having clients complete such forms and obtain physician clearance (if necessary) prior to the first meeting saves time during the initial consultation. Health coaches must review all of this information with the client present to ensure that nothing has been omitted. This meeting also provides an excellent opportunity to identify and record risk factors of which the client may or may not be aware.

Musculoskeletal Health Questionnaire

1. Have you had to see a doctor in the past three years for any bone, joint, or spine problems?
   - ❑ No
   - ❑ One or two visits, but no problems now
   - ❑ Do doctors give frequent-flyer miles?

2. Have you ever had an orthopedic injury severe enough to result in one of the following?
   - Kept you out of sports or exercise for a month?
   - Required crutches for two or more weeks?
   - Required surgery?

   ❑ No ❑ Yes (to any of the questions)

3. Have you ever dislocated or separated your shoulder?

   ❑ No ❑ Yes

   If yes, please explain.______________________

4. Do you have joint swelling? ❑ No ❑ Yes

5. Have you lost mobility (range of motion) in any joint? For example, can you fully straighten (extend) and fully bend (flex)? Compare right to left.
   - ❑ No
   - ❑ A little stiff at times, but motion is full
   - ❑ Motion is limited in one or two major joints or the spine

6. Do your knees creak or make noise when you are going up or down stairs?
   - ❑ No
   - ❑ Yes, but no discomfort or pain
   - ❑ Yes, and does cause discomfort and/or pain

7. Do you have trouble actually ascending or descending stairs?
   - ❑ No
   - ❑ Only after going up and down multiple times, especially while carrying heavier items
   - ❑ Yes

8. Do you have stiffness in any joints associated with any of the following conditions?
   - Upon awakening (i.e., until showering or moving for about 15–20 minutes)
   - After sitting still for more than 30 minutes
   - For no apparent reason

   ❑ No
   ❑ Only the day after a hard workout
   ❑ Yes

9. Does high barometric pressure (i.e., damp, rainy weather) make your joints ache?
   - ❑ No
   - ❑ Rarely
   - ❑ Friends consult me instead of the weatherman

10. Have you ever had an episode of lower-back or neck pain or spasm?
    - ❑ No
    - ❑ Yes, it kept me off my feet for less than 24 hours
    - ❑ Yes, I miss work due to recurrent episodes

11. Do you have pain while lying on either shoulder at night in bed?
    - ❑ No
    - ❑ Rarely
    - ❑ Almost nightly; tossing and turning to get comfy

12. Do you have difficulty falling asleep at night or awaken during the night because of any joint or muscle discomfort?
    - ❑ No
    - ❑ Rarely or minor difficulty
    - ❑ Yes

13. Do you awaken at night with your hands or fingers "asleep"?
    - ❑ No
    - ❑ Rarely and I easily shake it off
    - ❑ My hands get more sleep than I do

Note: If a client answers "Yes" to any of the items, this may suggest a musculoskeletal issue that warrants further evaluation. Be sure to refer to an appropriate healthcare professional as needed.

Figure 10-2

Sample musculoskeletal health questionnaire

Reprinted with permission from *FrameWork* by Nicholas A. DiNubile, M.D., with William Patrick

Measuring Blood Pressure and Resting Heart Rate

The health coach can also effectively screen for two more components: resting blood pressure and resting heart rate. Blood pressure reflects the force of the heartbeat and the resistance of the arteries to the pumping action of the heart. Health coaches must use an appropriate-sized cuff, as overweight clients may have falsely elevated blood-pressure readings when standard-sized cuffs are used. Refer to Chapter 12 for guidelines on how to measure resting blood pressure. Normative values for blood pressure readings are presented in Table 10-3.

Table 10-3

Classification of Blood Pressure for Adults Age 18 and Older[*]

Category	Systolic (mmHg)		Diastolic (mmHg)
Normal[†]	<120	and	<80
Prehypertension	120–139	or	80–89
Hypertension[‡]			
Stage 1	140–159	or	90–99
Stage 2	≥160	or	≥100

[*] Not taking antihypertensive drugs and not acutely ill. When systolic and diastolic blood pressures fall into different categories, the higher category should be selected to classify the individual's blood pressure status. For example, 140/82 mmHg should be classified as stage 1 hypertension, and 154/102 mmHg should be classified as stage 2 hypertension. In addition to classifying stages of hypertension on the basis of average blood pressure levels, clinicians should specify presence or absence of target organ disease and additional risk factors. This specificity is important for risk classification and treatment.

[†] Normal blood pressure with respect to cardiovascular risk is below 120/80 mmHg. However, unusually low readings should be evaluated for clinical significance.

[‡] Based on the average of two or more readings taken at each of two or more visits after an initial screening.

Source: National Institutes of Health (2003). *The Seventh Report of the Joint Committee on Prevention, Detection, Evaluation, and Treatment of High Blood Pressure.* NIH Publication No. 03-5233.

Resting heart rate also is considered to be a marker of physical health and cardiovascular fitness (see Chapter 12). The average resting heart rate is 72 beats per minute (bpm) with a normal range of 60 to 100 bpm. Generally, the more fit an individual is, the lower the resting heart rate. However, it is important to recognize that certain medications, such as **beta blockers,** may slow both resting and non-resting heart rates.

Determining a Reasonable Weight

For many significantly overweight individuals, lost weight is often regained. Research has shown that individuals who lose large amounts of weight regain approximately two-thirds of it within one year and almost all of it within five years (Wing & Phelan, 2005; Wadden et al., 1989). In response to such disappointing outcomes, recommendations no longer focus on the attainment of an **ideal weight.**

Obesity experts have suggested a weight loss of 10% of body weight over six months as an initial goal (NIH, 1998; IOM, 1995). Once this goal has been achieved, clients can be encouraged to focus on maintaining the initial weight loss. Alternatively, individuals who remain motivated may set an interval goal of losing additional weight, with reevaluation after each successive interval. While in many cases modest losses will not bring clients to their ideal weight, even small losses (e.g., 10%) produce important health benefits and may be more likely to be sustained over time. The results of body-composition testing can also be used to determine a reasonable weight or to set an initial goal based on lowering percent fat to a healthier level (see Chapter 11).

It is important to understand that muscle weight can increase even when exercise participation is limited to aerobic activity. Body composition should be assessed periodically throughout an exercise program. This can provide motivating information, especially when fat weight loss appears to have reached a plateau.

Assessing Psychological Health

The psychological health of all potential clients should be evaluated prior to beginning a weight-loss program. This is especially important since several psychiatric disorders, such as eating disorders, anxiety disorders, and clinical depression, can initially appear to be weight-related difficulties. In reality, though food is involved in the expression of symptoms (e.g., under- or overeating), eating disorders are classified as mental disorders that can be potentially life-threatening and require specialized interventions by skilled mental-health professionals.

Obtaining a psychological history is an important first step. A health coach should ask all clients whether they have any concerns about how frequently they experience high levels of stress, worry excessively, or feel down for more than a few days at a time. For clients who admit having any of these feelings, it may be wise to ask if they would consider counseling, are currently in therapy, or have previously received counseling. Keep a record of all counseling experiences, including the therapist's name, dates of treatment, and reasons for seeking therapy. If the client is currently receiving counseling, it may be helpful to contact the therapist (after obtaining the client's written permission) and mutually determine whether weight loss is appropriate at this time. Review the list of medications that each client is presently taking. Certain **psychotropic medications,** such as antidepressants, anti-anxiety medications, or mood stabilizers all signal the presence of psychological conditions, and many psychotropic medications may facilitate or significantly hamper weight loss.

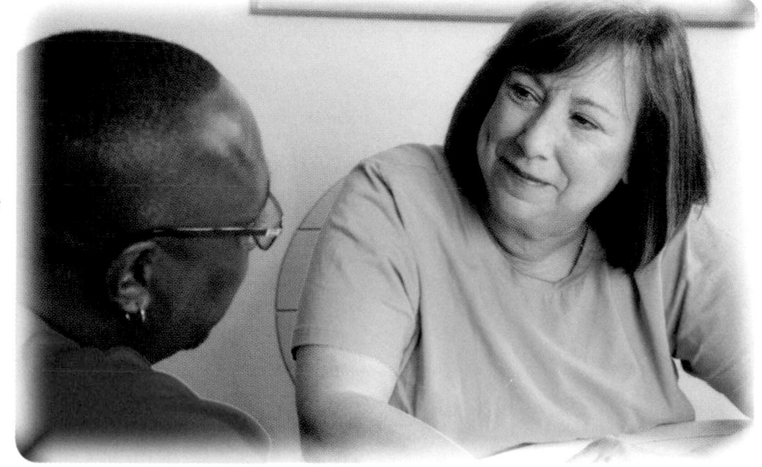

Specific training in psychology, psychiatry, medicine, or social work is required to adequately evaluate psychological symptoms. However, by exploring their current sense of well-being with potential clients, a health coach can obtain some indication of the person's likelihood of succeeding at weight loss and determine whether a more comprehensive psychological evaluation is indicated. Several psychological conditions, such as clinical depression and eating disorders (i.e., **anorexia nervosa, bulimia nervosa,** and **binge eating disorder**), are clear contraindications for weight loss (see Chapter 7).

Depression

Depression is a psychological disorder in which the person experiences pervasive feelings of sadness, hopelessness, helplessness, and worthlessness. Signs of depression include sleep disturbance (e.g., **hypersomnia** or **insomnia**), eating difficulties (overeating or lack of interest in eating), excessive guilt, and tearfulness or crying spells. Individuals who are depressed also may have difficulty concentrating, remembering, or thinking clearly [American Psychiatric Association (APA), 2000].

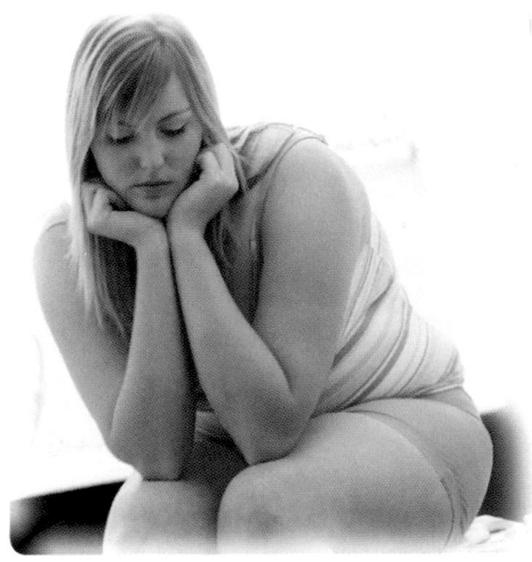

Depression is increasingly viewed, in part, as being related to a chemical imbalance in the brain. Effective treatments for depression include psychotherapy alone or in combination with medication and exercise. Weight loss is never an appropriate treatment for depression and, in fact, most obesity specialists believe that depression is a contraindication for weight-loss treatment (NIH, 1998; IOM, 1995). Some persons who are both overweight and depressed believe that the former causes the latter, but that would be oversimplifying potentially serious underlying problems. It is important to be able to identify signs of clinical depression and refer the individual to a mental-health specialist for further evaluation.

Eating Disorders

Anorexia nervosa is characterized by the refusal to maintain a minimally healthy body weight (i.e., at least 85% of ideal body weight), a morbid fear of gaining weight, **amenorrhea,** and disturbances in the way in which weight and shape are experienced or evaluated by the individual (APA, 2000). Bulimia nervosa is characterized by recurrent episodes of binge eating in which the individual experiences a loss of control over eating, followed by compensatory behaviors aimed at avoiding weight gain (e.g., vomiting, laxative or **diuretic** abuse, fasting, or excessive exercise) (APA, 2000). As with anorexia nervosa, self-evaluation is unduly influenced by weight and shape. Individuals with bulimia nervosa are often of normal weight or slightly overweight. In binge eating disorder, which is classified as "eating disorder not otherwise specified" (EDNOS), the individual also experiences episodes of bingeing coupled with a sense of loss of control over eating. However, there is no active attempt at compensating for the binges (APA, 2000). Individuals with binge eating disorder tend to be overweight or obese.

It is important to identify eating disorders in potential clients, because these individuals are more likely to suffer from other psychological disorders as well (Bruce & Wilfley, 1996). Weight loss or maintenance of an abnormally low body weight is never appropriate for an individual with anorexia nervosa. This is important to remember when working with athletes by whom a low body weight is coveted, such as bodybuilders, gymnasts, dancers, and runners. Weight loss is only appropriate in individuals with bulimia when it is accompanied by ongoing psychotherapy (or follows a successful course of therapy). Recovery from binge eating disorder also appears to require psychotherapy specifically aimed at reducing binge eating (Bruce & Wilfley, 1996). It is unclear whether dieting complicates or facilitates recovery from binge eating disorder. If a health coach suspects that a potential client may suffer from binge eating disorder, it is important to consider referral to an eating disorders specialist before starting to train the individual. Cognitive behavioral psychotherapy may increase the client's ability to lose weight and maximize the likelihood of successful maintenance of a lower body weight.

Assessing Exercise Readiness

For most people, physical activity will not pose any health problems. However, the primary purpose of any pre-exercise health screening is to identify individuals who may have health or medical conditions that could put them at risk during physical testing and exercise. The American Council on Exercise (ACE), the American College of Sports Medicine (ACSM), and other professional organizations for exercise professionals have determined that pre-exercise screening is an important part of the duties of a fitness professional. According to Heyward (2010), the pretest health screening of clients that a fitness professional should minimally complete before exercise testing and participation commence must include the following:

- The **Physical Activity Readiness Questionnaire (PAR-Q)**
- Identification of signs and symptoms of disease, if present
- Evaluation of the coronary risk profile
- Classification of heart disease risk factors

The Physical Activity Readiness Questionnaire

Individuals participating in self-guided activity should at least complete a general health-risk appraisal. The PAR-Q has been used successfully when a short, simple medical/health questionnaire is needed (Figure 10-3). Experts recognize the PAR-Q as a *minimal,* yet safe, pre-exercise screening measure for low-to-moderate, but not vigorous, exercise training:

- It serves as a minimal health-risk appraisal prerequisite.
- It is quick, easy, and non-invasive to administer.
- It is, however, limited by its lack of detail and may overlook important health conditions, medications, and past injuries.

If someone is identified by the PAR-Q as having multiple health risks, it is recommended that a more detailed health-risk appraisal that gathers more in-depth information relative to cardiovascular disease and dysfunctions be used.

> Visit www.ACEfitness.org/HealthCoachResources to download a free PDF of the PAR-Q, as well as other forms and assessment tools that you can use throughout your career as a health coach.

Risk Stratification

The American College of Sports Medicine (ACSM) has established recommendations concerning the need for a medical examination and exercise testing prior to participation in an exercise program (ACSM, 2014). The basis for performing a risk stratification prior to engaging in a physical-activity program is to determine the following (ACSM, 2014):

- The presence or absence of known cardiovascular, pulmonary, and/or metabolic disease
- The presence or absence of cardiovascular risk factors
- The presence or absence of signs or symptoms suggestive of cardiovascular, pulmonary, and/or metabolic disease

Risk stratification is important because someone with only one positive risk factor will be treated differently than someone with several positive risk factors. Recommendations for physical activity/exercise, medical examinations or exercise testing, and medically supervised exercise are based on the number of associated risks; risk stratification is categorized as low, moderate, or high.

Physical Activity Readiness Questionnaire - PAR-Q (revised 2002)

PAR-Q & YOU

(A Questionnaire for People Aged 15 to 69)

Regular physical activity is fun and healthy, and increasingly more people are starting to become more active every day. Being more active is very safe for most people. However, some people should check with their doctor before they start becoming much more physically active.

If you are planning to become much more physically active than you are now, start by answering the seven questions in the box below. If you are between the ages of 15 and 69, the PAR-Q will tell you if you should check with your doctor before you start. If you are over 69 years of age, and you are not used to being very active, check with your doctor.

Common sense is your best guide when you answer these questions. Please read the questions carefully and answer each one honestly: check YES or NO.

YES	NO	
☐	☐	**1. Has your doctor ever said that you have a heart condition and that you should only do physical activity recommended by a doctor?**
☐	☐	**2. Do you feel pain in your chest when you do physical activity?**
☐	☐	**3. In the past month, have you had chest pain when you were not doing physical activity?**
☐	☐	**4. Do you lose your balance because of dizziness or do you ever lose consciousness?**
☐	☐	**5. Do you have a bone or joint problem (for example, back, knee or hip) that could be made worse by a change in your physical activity?**
☐	☐	**6. Is your doctor currently prescribing drugs (for example, water pills) for your blood pressure or heart condition?**
☐	☐	**7. Do you know of any other reason why you should not do physical activity?**

If you answered

YES to one or more questions

Talk with your doctor by phone or in person BEFORE you start becoming much more physically active or BEFORE you have a fitness appraisal. Tell your doctor about the PAR-Q and which questions you answered YES.

- You may be able to do any activity you want — as long as you start slowly and build up gradually. Or, you may need to restrict your activities to those which are safe for you. Talk with your doctor about the kinds of activities you wish to participate in and follow his/her advice.
- Find out which community programs are safe and helpful for you.

NO to all questions

If you answered NO honestly to all PAR-Q questions, you can be reasonably sure that you can:

- start becoming much more physically active – begin slowly and build up gradually. This is the safest and easiest way to go.
- take part in a fitness appraisal – this is an excellent way to determine your basic fitness so that you can plan the best way for you to live actively. It is also highly recommended that you have your blood pressure evaluated. If your reading is over 144/94, talk with your doctor before you start becoming much more physically active.

DELAY BECOMING MUCH MORE ACTIVE:

- if you are not feeling well because of a temporary illness such as a cold or a fever – wait until you feel better; or
- if you are or may be pregnant – talk to your doctor before you start becoming more active.

PLEASE NOTE: If your health changes so that you then answer YES to any of the above questions, tell your fitness or health professional. Ask whether you should change your physical activity plan.

Informed Use of the PAR-Q: The Canadian Society for Exercise Physiology, Health Canada, and their agents assume no liability for persons who undertake physical activity, and if in doubt after completing this questionnaire, consult your doctor prior to physical activity.

No changes permitted. You are encouraged to photocopy the PAR-Q but only if you use the entire form.

NOTE: If the PAR-Q is being given to a person before he or she participates in a physical activity program or a fitness appraisal, this section may be used for legal or administrative purposes.

"I have read, understood and completed this questionnaire. Any questions I had were answered to my full satisfaction."

NAME ________________________________

SIGNATURE ________________________________ DATE ________________________________

SIGNATURE OF PARENT ________________________________ WITNESS ________________________________
or GUARDIAN (for participants under the age of majority)

Note: This physical activity clearance is valid for a maximum of 12 months from the date it is completed and becomes invalid if your condition changes so that you would answer YES to any of the seven questions.

CSEP SCPE © Canadian Society for Exercise Physiology   Supported by: Health Canada Santé Canada

Figure 10-3
The Physical Activity Readiness Questionnaire

This process involves three basic steps that should be followed chronologically:

- Identifying **coronary artery disease (CAD)** risk factors
- Performing a risk stratification based on CAD risk factors
- Determining the need for a medical exam/clearance and medical supervision

The worksheet presented in Table 10-4 presents clinically relevant CAD health risks that should be used to identify the total number of positive risk factors an individual possesses. Each positive risk factor category equals one point. There is also a negative risk factor for a high level of **high-density lipoprotein (HDL),** as a point is subtracted if the individual has an HDL cholesterol score that is equal to, or exceeds, 60 mg/dL. It is the total number of risk factors and the presence or absence of signs or symptoms that ultimately categorizes an individual's CAD risk during exercise and/or physical activity (ACSM, 2014). The health coach should add up the total number of risk factors for a client, subtracting one point for higher HDL cholesterol if appropriate, and use this score to stratify the client's risk (Figure 10-4).

Signs or symptoms are also included in risk stratification, but given the need for specialized training to make a diagnosis, and respecting the **scope of practice** of health coaches, these signs and symptoms must only be interpreted by a qualified licensed professional within the context in which they appear.

These signs and symptoms include pain (tightness) or discomfort in the chest, neck, jaw, arms, or other areas that may result from ischemia, shortness of breath, or difficulty breathing at rest or with mild exertion (dyspnea), orthopnea (dyspnea in a reclined position), ankle edema, palpitations or tachycardia, intermittent claudication (pain sensations or cramping in the lower extremities associated with inadequate blood supply), known heart murmur, unusual fatigue or difficulty breathing with usual activities, and dizziness or syncope, most commonly caused by reduced perfusion to the brain (ACSM, 2014).

Assessing Physical Fitness

Experts have had a difficult time agreeing on a definition of physical fitness over the years. However, most exercise scientists agree that four components are involved in physical fitness:

- Aerobic fitness
- Muscle and joint **flexibility**
- Muscular strength and endurance
- Body composition

A fitness assessment provides the opportunity to analyze each of these components and is used for any or all of the following (see Chapter 12):

- To assess current fitness levels in relation to age and sex
- To aid in the development of exercise programs
- To identify areas of health and injury risk and the need for possible referral to the appropriate healthcare professional
- To establish realistic, attainable goals and provide motivation
- To educate the client about physical fitness
- To evaluate the success of the fitness program through follow-up assessments

Many clients may request that a fitness evaluation be part of their early work with a

Table 10-4

Atherosclerotic Cardiovascular Disease Risk Factor Thresholds for Use With ACSM Risk Stratification

Positive Risk Factors	Defining Criteria	Points
Age	Men ≥45 years Women ≥55 years	+1
Family history	Myocardial infarction, coronary revascularization, or sudden death before 55 years of age in father or other first-degree male relative, or before 65 years of age in mother or other first-degree female relative	+1
Cigarette smoking	Current cigarette smoker or those who quit within the previous six months, or exposure to environmental tobacco smoke (i.e., secondhand smoke)	+1
Sedentary lifestyle	Not participating in at least 30 minutes of moderate-intensity physical activity (40 to <60% $\dot{V}O_2R$) on at least three days/week for at least three months	+1
Obesity	Body mass index ≥30 kg/m^2 or waist girth >102 cm (40 inches) for men and >88 cm (35 inches) for women	+1
Hypertension	Systolic blood pressure ≥140 mmHg and/or diastolic blood pressure ≥90 mmHg, confirmed by measurements on at least two separate occasions, or currently on antihypertensive medications	+1
Dyslipidemia	Low-density lipoprotein (LDL) cholesterol ≥130 mg/dL (3.37 mmol/L) or high-density lipoprotein (HDL) cholesterol <40 mg/dL (1.04 mmol/L) or on lipid-lowering medication; If total serum cholesterol is all that is available, use serum cholesterol ≥200 mg/dL (5.18 mmol/L)	+1
Prediabetes*	Fasting plasma glucose ≥100 mg/dL (5.55 mmol/L), but ≤125 mg/dL (6.94 mmol/L) or impaired glucose tolerance (IGT) where a two-hour oral glucose tolerance test (OGTT) value is ≥140 mg/dL (7.77 mmol/L), but ≤199 mg/dL (11.04 mmol/L), confirmed by measurements on at least two separate occasions	+1
Negative Risk Factor	**Defining Criteria**	**Points**
HDL cholesterol†	≥60 mg/dL (1.55 mmol/L)	–1
	Total Score:	

*If the presence or absence of a CVD risk factor is not disclosed or is not available, that CVD risk factor should be counted as a risk factor except for prediabetes. If the prediabetes criteria are missing or unknown, prediabetes should be counted as a risk factor for those ≥45 years old, especially for those with a body mass index (BMI) ≥25 kg/m^2, and those <45 years old with a BMI ≥25 kg/m^2 and additional CVD risk factors for prediabetes. The number of positive risk factors is then summed.

†High HDL is considered a negative risk factor. For individuals having high HDL ≥60 mg/dL (1.55 mmol/L), one positive risk factor is subtracted from the sum of positive risk factors.

Note: $\dot{V}O_2R$ = $\dot{V}O_2$reserve

Reprinted with permission from American College of Sports Medicine (2014). *ACSM's Guidelines for Exercise Testing and Prescription* (9th ed.). Philadelphia: Wolters Kluwer/Lippincott Williams & Wilkins.

health coach. Others may feel frightened or embarrassed to undergo such an assessment. Still others may be overwhelmed and discouraged by the potentially negative feedback of baseline testing results. It is important to respect a client's sensitivity to, and interest in, a thorough fitness assessment. However, the minimum evaluation that the health coach should undertake in assessing readiness for aerobic exercise involves assessing cardiovascular risk factors (see Chapter 12). Health coaches should also explore each client's activity history, attitudes toward exercise, and stated fitness goals. A sample Exercise History and Attitude Questionnaire is shown in Figure 10-5.

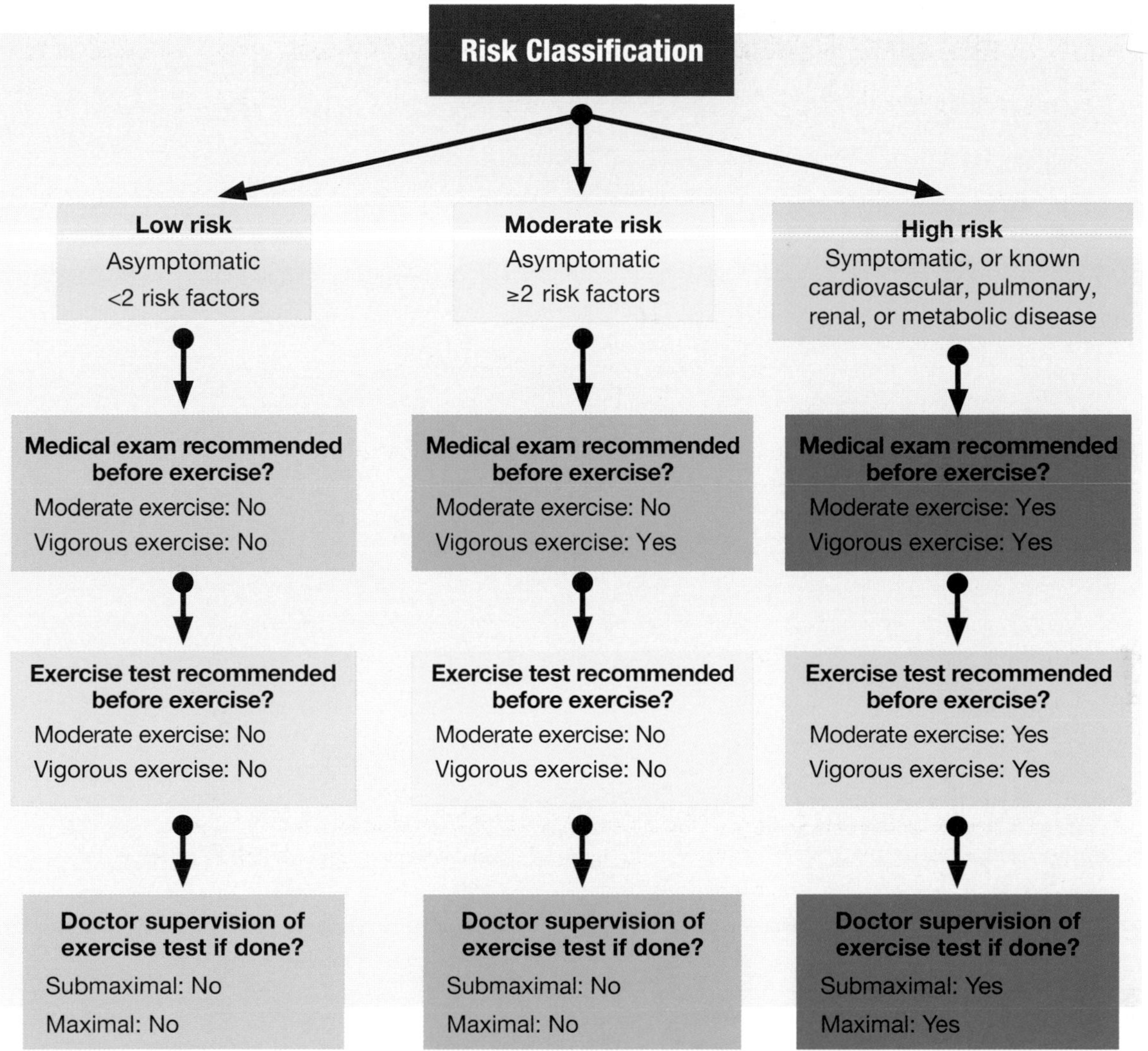

Medical examination, exercise testing, and supervision of exercise testing preparticipation recommendations based on classification of risk

Moderate exercise: 40% to <60% $\dot{V}O_2R$; 3 to <6 METs; "An intensity that causes noticeable increases in heart rate and breathing"

Vigorous exercise: ≥60% $\dot{V}O_2R$; ≥6 METs; "An intensity that causes substantial increase in heart rate and breathing"

Not recommended: Reflects the notion that a medical examination, exercise test, and physician supervision of exercise testing are not recommended in the preparticipation screening; however, they may be considered when there are concerns about risk, more information is needed for the exercise test, and/or are requested by the patient or client.

Recommended: Reflects the notion that a medical examination, exercise test, and physician supervision are recommended in the preparticipation health screening process.

Note: $\dot{V}O_2R = \dot{V}O_2$reserve; METs = Metabolic equivalents; Cardiovascular disease = Cardiac, peripheral artery, or cerebrovascular disease; Pulmonary disease = Chronic obstructive pulmonary disease (COPD), cystic fibrosis, interstitial lung disease, or asthma; Metabolic disease = Diabetes mellitus (type 1 or 2) and thyroid disorders; Renal disease = Kidney disease

Reprinted with permission from the American College of Sports Medicine (2014). *ACSM's Guidelines for Exercise Testing and Prescription* (9th ed.). Philadelphia: Wolters Kluwer/Lippincott Williams & Wilkins.

Visit www.ACEfitness.org/HealthCoachResources to download a free PDF of the exercise history and attitude questionnaire, as well as other forms and assessment tools that you can use throughout your career as a health coach.

Exercise History and Attitude Questionnaire

Name ______________________________ Date ____________

General Instructions: Please fill out this form as completely as possible. If you have any questions, DO NOT GUESS; ask your health coach for assistance.

1. Please rate your exercise level on a scale of 1 to 5 (5 indicating very strenuous) for each age range through your present age:

   15–20 _____ 21–30 _____ 31–40 _____ 41–50 _____ 51+_____

2. Were you a high school and/or college athlete?

   ❑ Yes ❑ No If yes, please specify ______________________________

3. Do you have any negative feelings toward, or have you had any bad experience with, physical-activity programs?

   ❑ Yes ❑ No If yes, please explain______________________________

4. Do you have any negative feelings toward, or have you had any bad experience with, fitness testing and evaluation?

   ❑ Yes ❑ No If yes, please explain______________________________

5. Rate yourself on a scale of 1 to 5 (1 indicating the lowest value and 5 the highest).

	Circle the number that best applies.				
Characterize your present athletic ability.	1	2	3	4	5
When you exercise, how important is competition?	1	2	3	4	5
Characterize your present cardiovascular capacity.	1	2	3	4	5
Characterize your present muscular capacity.	1	2	3	4	5
Characterize your present flexibility capacity.	1	2	3	4	5

6. Do you start exercise programs but then find yourself unable to stick with them? ❑ Yes ❑ No

7. How much time are you willing to devote to an exercise program? ________ minutes/day ________ days/week

8. Are you currently involved in regular endurance (cardiovascular) exercise?

   ❑ Yes ❑ No If yes, specify the type of exercise(s) ______________________________

   ________ minutes/day ________ days/week

   Rate your perception of the exertion of your exercise program (check the box):

   ❑ Light ❑ Fairly light ❑ Somewhat hard ❑ Hard

9. How long have you been exercising regularly?________ months ________ years

10. What other exercise, sport, or recreational activities have you participated in?

    In the past 6 months?______________________________

    In the past 5 years? ______________________________

11. Can you exercise during your work day? ❑ Yes ❑ No

12. Would an exercise program interfere with your job? ❑ Yes ❑ No

13. Would an exercise program benefit your job? ❑ Yes ❑ No

Figure 10-5
Sample exercise history and attitude questionnaire

14. What types of exercise interest you?

❑ Walking	❑ Jogging	❑ Swimming	❑ Cycling
❑ Aerobics	❑ Strength training	❑ Stationary biking	❑ Rowing
❑ Racquetball	❑ Tennis	❑ Other aerobic activity	❑ Stretching

15. Rank your goals in undertaking exercise: What do you want exercise to do for you? Use the following scale to rate each goal separately.

	Not at all important			Somewhat important				Extremely important		
a. Improve cardiovascular fitness	1	2	3	4	5	6	7	8	9	10
b. Facilitate body-fat weight loss	1	2	3	4	5	6	7	8	9	10
c. Reshape or tone my body	1	2	3	4	5	6	7	8	9	10
d. Improve performance for a specific sport	1	2	3	4	5	6	7	8	9	10
e. Improve moods and ability to cope with stress	1	2	3	4	5	6	7	8	9	10
f. Improve flexibility	1	2	3	4	5	6	7	8	9	10
g. Increase strength	1	2	3	4	5	6	7	8	9	10
h. Increase energy level	1	2	3	4	5	6	7	8	9	10
i. Feel better	1	2	3	4	5	6	7	8	9	10
j. Increase enjoyment	1	2	3	4	5	6	7	8	9	10
k. Other	1	2	3	4	5	6	7	8	9	10

16. By how much would you like to change your current weight?

(+) ________ lb (–) ________ lb

Readiness to Change

A key factor to assess is whether a client is at the right time in life to make a serious attempt at losing weight. Readiness to change is a complex phenomenon that encompasses an individual's motivation to lose weight, commitment to restructuring his or life, and surrounding circumstances. Chances for success increase when a client's readiness to change is high (Brownell, 2000). Ideally, clients have carefully thought through these issues before meeting the health coach. Realistically, however, many factors will lead people to seek help, including the need to please others (e.g., spouse or physician) or to find a quick fix for major problems.

Readiness to change can be assessed in several ways. The simplest way is to have clients evaluate what benefits may be obtained through weight loss against the sacrifices they need to make. Two psychologists, Dr. James Prochaska and Dr. Carlo DiClemente (1984), developed a sophisticated model in which they identify discrete stages of change (see Chapter 3). The **transtheoretical model of behavioral change (TTM)** suggests that a complicated period of psychological preparation precedes true readiness to commit to lifestyle change. Thus, even though clients may not be fully committed to losing weight, for many their motivation increases early on from seeing success and witnessing the benefits of making a lifestyle change. The American Dietetic Association has developed a Weight-Loss Readiness Quiz that addresses attitudes toward weight loss (Figure 10-6).

In January 2012, the American Dietetic Association (ADA) changed its name to the Academy of Nutrition and Dietetics (A.N.D.). Throughout this text, research conducted by the organization prior to this name change is cited to the ADA, while newer studies will be credited to the A.N.D. Refer to www.eatright.org for more information on the reasons behind the name change.

Figure 10-6
Sample weight-loss readiness quiz

Weight-loss Readiness Quiz

Are you ready to lose weight? Your attitude about weight loss affects your ability to succeed. Take this Weight-loss Readiness Quiz to learn if you need to make any attitude adjustments before you begin. Mark each item true or false. Please be honest! It's important that these answers reflect the way you really are, not how you would like to be. A method for interpreting your readiness for weight loss follows:

1. ____ I have thought a lot about my eating habits and physical activities to pinpoint what I need to change.
2. ____ I have accepted the idea that I need to make permanent, not temporary, changes in my eating and activities to be successful.
3. ____ I will only feel successful if I lose a lot of weight.
4. ____ I accept the idea that it's best if I lose weight slowly.
5. ____ I'm thinking of losing weight now because I really want to, not because someone else thinks I should.
6. ____ I think losing weight will solve other problems in my life.
7. ____ I am willing and able to increase my regular physical activity.
8. ____ I can lose weight successfully if I have no "slip-ups."
9. ____ I am ready to commit some time and effort each week to organizing and planning my food and activity programs.
10. ____ Once I lose some initial weight, I usually lose the motivation to keep going until I reach my goal.
11. ____ I want to start a weight-loss program, even though my life is unusually stressful right now.

Visit www.ACEfitness.org/HealthCoachResources to download a free PDF of the weight-loss readiness quiz, as well as other forms and assessment tools that you can use throughout your career as a health coach.

Scoring the Weight-loss Readiness Quiz

To score the quiz, look at your answers next to items 1, 2, 4, 5, 7, and 9. Score "1" if you answered "true" and "0" if you answered "false."

For items 3, 6, 8, 10, and 11, score "0" for each true answer and "1" for each false answer.

To get your total score, add the scores of all questions.

No one score indicates for sure whether you are ready to start losing weight. However, the higher your total score, the more characteristics you have that contribute to success. As a rough guide, consider the following recommendations:

1. If you scored 8 or higher, you probably have good reasons for wanting to lose weight now and a good understanding of the steps needed to succeed. Still, you might want to learn more about the areas where you scored a "0" (see "Interpretation of Quiz Items").
2. If you scored 5 to 7, you may need to reevaluate your reasons for losing weight and the methods you would use to do so. To get a start, read the advice given on page 279 for those quiz items where you received a score of "0."
3. If you scored 4 or less, now may not be the right time for you to lose weight. While you might be successful in losing weight initially, your answers suggest that you are unlikely to sustain sufficient effort to lose all the weight you want, or keep off the weight that you do lose. You need to reconsider your weight-loss motivations and methods and perhaps learn more about the pros and cons of different approaches to reducing. To do so, read the advice on page 279 for those quiz items where you scored "0."

Figure 10-6
continued

Interpretation of Quiz Items

Your answers to the quiz can clue you in to potential stumbling blocks to your weight-loss success. Any item score of "0" indicates a misconception about weight loss, or a potential problem area. While no individual item score of "0" is important enough to scuttle your weight-loss plans, you should consider the meaning of those items so that you can best prepare yourself for the challenges ahead. The numbers below correspond to the question numbers.

1. It has been said that you can't change what you don't understand. You might benefit from keeping records for a week to help pinpoint when, what, why, and how much you eat. This tool also is useful in identifying obstacles to regular physical activity.
2. Making drastic or highly restrictive changes in your eating habits may allow you to lose weight in the short-run, but be too hard to live with permanently. Similarly, your program of regular physical activity should be one you can sustain. Both your food plan and activity program should be healthful and enjoyable.
3. Most people have fantasies of reaching a weight considerably lower than they can realistically maintain. Rethink your meaning of "success." A successful, realistic weight loss is one that can be comfortably maintained through sensible eating and regular activity. Take your body type into consideration. Then set smaller, achievable goals. Your first goal may be to lose a small amount of weight while you learn eating habits and activity patterns to help you maintain it.
4. If you equate success with fast weight loss, you will have problems maintaining your weight. This "quick fix" attitude can backfire when you face the challenges of weight maintenance. It's best—and healthiest—to lose weight slowly, while learning the strategies that allow you to keep the weight off permanently.
5. The desire for, and commitment to, weight loss must come from you. People who lose and maintain weight successfully take responsibility for their own desires and decide the best way to achieve them. Once this step is taken, friends and family are an important source of support, not motivation.
6. While being overweight may contribute to a number of social problems, it is rarely the single cause. Anticipating that all of your problems will be solved through weight loss is unrealistic and may set you up for disappointment. Instead, realize that successful weight loss will make you feel more self-confident and empowered, and that the skills you develop to deal with your weight can be applied to other areas of your life.
7. Studies have shown that people who develop the habit of regular, moderate physical activity are most successful at maintaining their weight. Exercise does not have to be strenuous to be effective for weight control. Any moderate physical activity that you enjoy and will do regularly counts. Just get moving!
8. While most people don't expect perfection of themselves in everyday life, many feel that they must stick to a weight-loss program perfectly. This is unrealistic. Rather than expecting lapses and viewing them as catastrophes, recognize them as valuable opportunities to identify problem triggers and develop strategies for the future.
9. Successful weight loss is not possible without taking the time to think about yourself, assess your problem areas, and develop strategies to deal with them. Success takes time. You must commit to planning and organizing your weight loss.
10. Do not ignore your concerns about "going the distance," because they may indicate a potential problem. Think about past efforts and why they failed. Pinpoint any reasons, and work on developing motivational strategies to get you over those hurdles. Take your effort one day at a time; a plateau of weight maintenance within an ongoing weight-loss program is perfectly okay.
11. Weight loss itself is a source of stress, so if you are already under stress, it may be difficult to successfully implement a weight-loss program at this time. Try to resolve other stressors in your life before you begin a weight-loss effort.

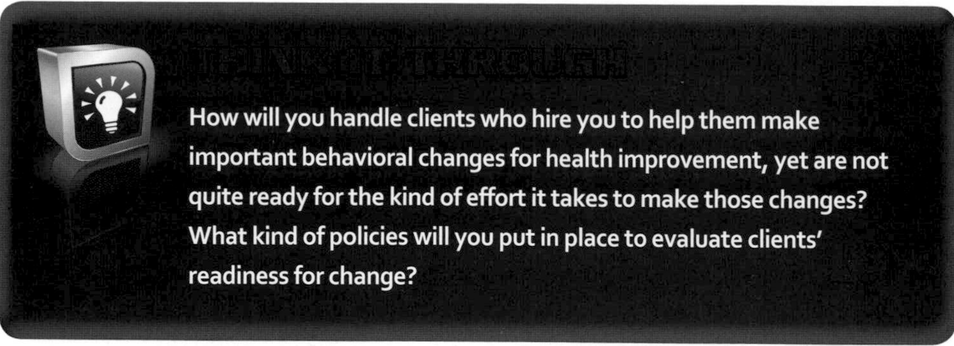

How will you handle clients who hire you to help them make important behavioral changes for health improvement, yet are not quite ready for the kind of effort it takes to make those changes? What kind of policies will you put in place to evaluate clients' readiness for change?

Behavioral Assessments

Assessments play an important part of exercise and lifestyle-modification program design. This topic is discussed in countless texts and articles, and there are numerous protocols from which to choose. Most fitness professionals have their preferences for which tools to use when it comes to assessing cardiovascular fitness, strength, flexibility, and dietary habits, which are commonly viewed as key components of any lifestyle-modification program. Many of the available assessments are objective measurements and are frequently used to gather information on a variety of fitness- and health-related constructs that are used to establish baseline values, identify areas of need for program design and modification, and demonstrate progress. While few fitness and health professionals would disagree with the fact that most often it is the behavioral and psychological factors that are most strongly linked to program success, much less is known about how to assess these constructs in a straightforward and objective manner. Assessing behavioral and psychological variables warrants caution, as most health coaches are not mental health professionals and, as with any assessment, the purpose must be to gather information for the program, and not to diagnose, analyze, or label a client's physical or mental state.

The goal of any lifestyle-modification program is, of course, to change behavior. Therefore, the focus of health coaches during program development is often on adopting and maintaining the target or goal behavior (healthy behaviors), and much less attention is typically given to the old behaviors (unhealthy behaviors) that must be replaced. In other words, it is common for health coaches to be excited about creating a new program, setting goals, and getting started, and, beyond a general conversation during an initial meeting, little focus is typically given to understanding the challenges associated with the process of replacing old, less desirable behaviors with the goal behaviors.

Effective behavioral assessment plays a key role in program design, adoption, and long-term program adherence, and the process must start by understanding what functions are being served by the existing behaviors (Groden, 1989). For example, in order to adopt healthy eating habits, the first step is to understand the current eating habits and the role those habits play in the client's life. It is easy to tell the client what he or she should and should not be eating, but just presenting this information is not enough to elicit long-term behavioral change. Instead, the health coach must develop a more comprehensive understanding of client behavior, including where the client typically exhibits the unwanted behavior and the times of day at which the negative behaviors are at their worst. All behaviors and habits serve some purpose in a client's life, so it is important for health coaches to try to understand how the client benefits from the negative behaviors (e.g., instant gratification or avoidance) and to identify the triggers in the environment, social network, or emotional state that lead to the negative behaviors. As a result, a functional assessment of behavior that is in line with the physical assessments that are conducted will increase the likelihood of designing a successful lifestyle-modification program (Sarafino, 2012).

Functional Assessments

Functional assessments in the exercise context are typically thought of in terms of evaluating movement patterns and capabilities. However, a functional assessment of behavior can also be conducted as part of a lifestyle-modification program. Functional behavioral assessments are a common part of the education literature (O'Neill et al., 1997). However, they serve an important purpose in the health behavioral change realm as well. The goal of a behavioral functional assessment is to identify connections between behaviors and the **antecedents** and **consequences** associated with the behaviors (Cone, 1997). This is called the principle of **operant conditioning** (see Chapter 3), and the process of identifying these elements can be informal. In the lifestyle-modification context, health coaches will be dealing with identifying **behavioral excess**, which is an undesirable behavior that is performed too often (e.g., unhealthy eating habits) and with **behavioral deficit**, which is a desirable behavior that is not performed often enough (e.g., physical activity). When dealing with behavioral excess issues, the goal is to identify the triggers and reinforcements that exist in the clients' environment related to the behavior. When dealing with behavioral deficit, the focus should be on identifying times and situations when the positive behavior can occur in the client's life and environment (Sarafino, 2012). For example, a client who is struggling with his choices and portions when he eats out for lunch, which he does three or four days each week, is dealing with behavioral excess. Simply telling this client to pack a lunch or to make better choices is not the best option. Instead, the health coach must take the time to learn about the client and then educate him about healthy restaurant and food selections so that he is better prepared to deal with the cues and triggers in the environment and make healthy selections.

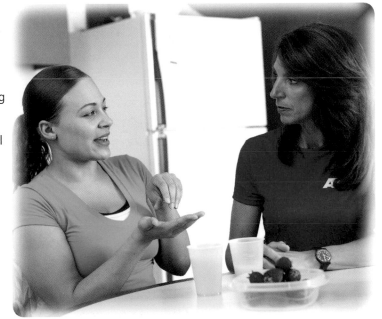

An example of behavioral deficit is a client who is struggling to meet her physical-activity goals and the health coach learns that her only weekly physical activity is the one scheduled and supervised session that is part of her program. She is failing to engage in outside activity on the other days of the week. She expresses that she is having a hard time finding the motivation to work out on her own, but that she cannot afford to purchase additional weekly sessions. The health coach must be prepared to provide program options that include others, build support, and are enjoyable to this client.

With both behavioral excess and deficit, it is important for health coaches to remember that simply instructing the client to eat better or exercise more is not an effective solution. Those behaviors are the goal outcomes and it is up to health coaches to provide the education, structure, and support to help ensure those outcomes become a reality.

Health coaches will most effectively conduct functional behavioral assessments indirectly, as information is going to be collected through conversations or "interviews" with the client. While some of the information regarding target behaviors (both excess and deficit) will be collected during initial consultations, other information and understanding will be gathered over time as rapport and relationships develop throughout the program. This is important for health coaches to remember, because attempting to gather too much information from the start can be counterproductive to program adoption and **adherence.**

Nevertheless, there are certain things that health coaches should work to understand from the start of a program (Sarafino, 2012). The first step in a functional assessment is to identify the target behavior(s), which in the lifestyle-modification context are typically dietary and physical-activity behaviors. In doing so, the starting point of the target behaviors (i.e., current dietary habits and physical-activity levels) can be established, as well as the goal behaviors for the program. Next, the health coach should work to understand the situations and circumstances that trigger or prevent the goal behaviors from occurring, as well as what the client is getting out of performing the target behaviors at their current levels. For example, it is common for unhealthy dietary habits and lack of physical activity to be related to clients avoiding or escaping from dealing with the truth about their health status or the work required to live a healthy lifestyle. It is also common that the instant gratification of the unhealthy habits has previously outweighed the willingness to make a change, or for the client's self-efficacy related to healthy behavior to be so low that it is a safer and less threatening alternative to continue to engage in the unhealthy/inactive behaviors. Regardless of the "rewards" that a client is receiving from the old habits, it is helpful for the health coach to gather this information.

Next, health coaches should gather the preferences of clients. Understanding clients' likes and dislikes is important when creating effective positive reinforcements for the behavior-change program. According to the principle of operant conditioning, every behavior has a consequence, which will determine the likelihood of the behavior happening again. Therefore, health coaches should work from the start of a program to understand client preferences in order to effectively create positive reinforcements that will increase the chance of continued activity or healthy eating. The best positive reinforcements for a health coach to create at the start of a program are enjoyment and mastery. In other words, the primary goal should be to create a comfortable and fun environment for clients, and for clients to leave with the feeling of accomplishment and success. This means that the exercise should be basic and straightforward and should allow clients to successfully learn something new. Also, the experience and environment should be engaging and fun. If new clients can associate exercise behavior with enjoyment and mastery and have positive interactions with the health coach, then they will be more likely to engage in the behavior again, as these are positive reinforcements that they will have the desire to duplicate.

The final component of the initial functional assessment process is determining what attempts the client has made in the past to live a healthy lifestyle and the outcomes of those previous attempts. Understanding previous successes and failures will provide important insight into program-design decisions, client motivation, client support systems, and readiness to change. For example, if a client succeeded in the past on a very structured program that left few opportunities for choice, but instead provided specific direction for behavior, the health coach should realize that a more structured program with detailed information may be needed, especially at the start. Another client may have had difficulties in the past with structured programs because she did not like the limited program options. For this client, the health coach is going to have to incorporate more opportunities for choice and options that capture the client's attention and interest. Additionally, if clients express lack of support in the past as an issue for adherence, the health coach needs to be creative in program design and include opportunities for social interaction with others during program participation. Each client will bring unique past experiences and health coaches must be flexible within the program design to meet client needs in order to maximize the likelihood of successful program adoption.

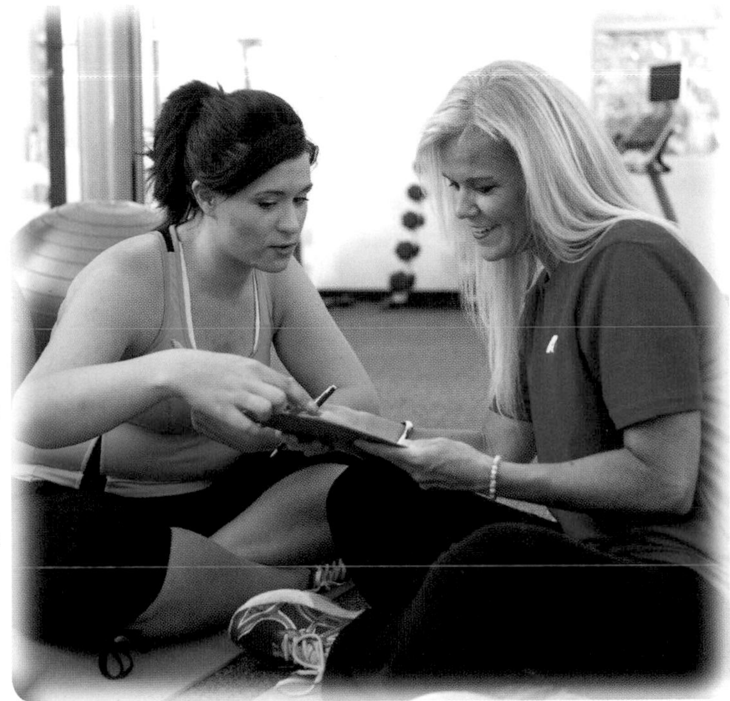

The most effective technique for gathering this behavioral assessment information is through conversation and effective communication (see Chapter 5). The health coach should not record every response as the client is talking, but should instead take brief and quick notes as necessary during the conversation, followed by a more detailed description after the consultation has ended. An effective way to organize this information is in a one-page behavioral outline that summarizes the key details and behaviors of the client. This outline should be customized by the health coach to meet his or her needs. Figure 10-7 presents a sample behavioral outline.

Motivation

Through the functional assessment process, it is important to make an effort to understand why the client wants to start the program. Most commonly, clients have at least some external forces serving as motivation to adopt a healthy lifestyle. Whether it is to look better for an upcoming event or due to the advice of a doctor, it is common for external factors to trigger the client's acknowledgement of the need or desire to make lifestyle modifications. At the start of the program, it is less important for health coaches to make judgments about a client's motivation, and more important to embrace the fact that, regardless of the reasons, he or she

<table>
<tr><th colspan="2">Behavioral Outline</th></tr>
<tr><td colspan="2">Target behaviors</td></tr>
<tr><td rowspan="2">Current daily behaviors (starting points)</td><td>Behavioral excess</td></tr>
<tr><td>Behavioral deficits</td></tr>
<tr><td colspan="2">Things triggering current behavior or preventing goal behavior?</td></tr>
<tr><td>Self-efficacy</td><td>Stage of behavioral change</td></tr>
<tr><td rowspan="2">Client Preferences</td><td>Dietary</td></tr>
<tr><td>Activity</td></tr>
<tr><td rowspan="2">Past Experiences</td><td>Dietary</td></tr>
<tr><td>Activity</td></tr>
</table>

Figure 10-7

Sample behavioral outline

Visit www.ACEfitness.org/HealthCoachResources to download a free PDF of this sample behavioral outline, as well as other forms and assessment tools that you can use throughout your career as a health coach.

is showing at least some willingness to make a change. Additionally, an understanding of what motivates a client to start a program will likely lead to the understanding of why that client has previously lacked the motivation to adhere long-term.

As previously discussed, all habits and behaviors serve a purpose in one's life, even if the purpose or motivation is to avoid another behavior or emotion. It is possible that the client has been avoiding an exercise and healthy eating program because of the effort required or even because of fear of failure. Such fear will be a very real part of the client's psychological participation in the program and will present itself as doubt, hesitancy, and low self-efficacy, which should be recognized by the health coach so that strategies to combat these issues can be implemented at the very beginning of the program. Ignoring such information and starting a program without considering client apprehensions is a mistake that will greatly jeopardize the chance of successful program adoption and adherence.

During the initial assessment, health coaches should not work to change or judge motivation levels, but instead should just focus on understanding what factors are driving the client to start the program. These factors should then be considered in the program design to create immediate moments of success, trust, and accomplishment, along with a sense of ownership and self- responsibility in the lifestyle-modification program. Positive and enjoyable experiences, quality support networks, and accomplishments (no matter how small) all work to increase **intrinsic motivation** for program adoption and maintenance.

Tools for Behavioral Assessment

The word "assessment" typically triggers thoughts of structured protocols, written questionnaires, and objective syntheses of outcomes related to some norm that can be looked up in a textbook. However, behavioral assessments, as used by health coaches, should not have these characteristics, but should instead revolve around quality communication, sharing, and understanding of clients' needs, goals, and experiences. Health coaches must be cautious when assessing behavioral and psychological constructs not to diagnosis or label a client's psychological state, as this would be out of the scope of practice. The most critical component of any lifestyle-modification program is the client, and any attempt to standardize and label one's thoughts, feelings, beliefs, and experiences into a scale can alter the personalization of the program and ultimately damage the rapport of the relationship. Creating an environment that is more focused on the program and less focused on the client is a barrier to successful program adoption and adherence. Health coaches must take the time to build rapport with clients, so that behavioral assessment can occur with a foundation of trust.

Numerous questionnaire-type inventories exist to measure readiness to change, motivation, personality type, social support, and history of exercise participation. Some questionnaires have been used in research and others have been created by practitioners seeking an easy way to gather information. Regardless of origin, health coaches should be cautious of using and interpreting information from such tools, as the reliability and validity of them is sometimes questionable. In other words, it is likely that if the client took the same inventory one week later, he or she may respond completely differently. Thus, depending on these tools for such critical information can be problematic. Additionally, in a one-on-one or small-group setting, health coaches should have the opportunity to build relationships and have conversations in which the important behavioral and psychological variables can be assessed. Because the goal of behavioral assessment in the health coach context is to better understand the client with the purpose of creating a safe and effective lifestyle-modification program that will trigger long-term adherence and success, and not to diagnose or even analyze these constructs, quality and structured communication can provide health coaches with the information needed to develop customized programs that meet the needs of individual clients.

Communication

The core of a functioning lifestyle-modification program is effective, consistent communication and understanding between the health coach and the client. Communication serves many purposes in the creation, implementation, and maintenance of a program, as it is the centerpiece of the client–health coach relationship. The most effective tool for behavioral assessment is structured and purposeful communication. Health coaches should be prepared and know what information they need to obtain from the client through conversation. They should then be able to use the principles of communication and rapport to gather that information in an informal setting. This type of purposeful communication requires practice, confidence, and patience, but gathering behavioral and psychological information in this manner is much more beneficial in terms of rapport and long-term success. Health coaches should approach each client with the knowledge that he or she is an individual and will bring unique experiences, expectations, and demands to the program. Any attempt to standardize the needs and motivations of clients will not benefit the health coach or the client.

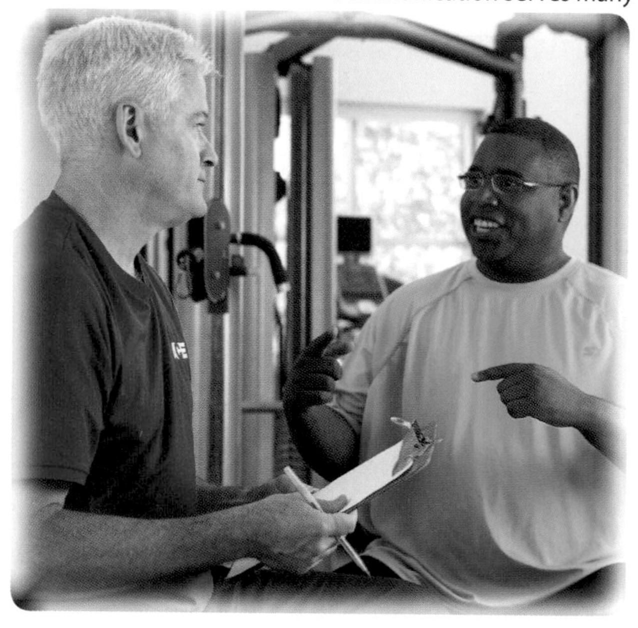

An effective practice for health coaches is to use Figure 10-7 to guide initial communication. This outline should not be a script and does not need to be followed exactly or in any particular order, but it should lay out the key pieces of information that the health coach wants to gather and provide purpose and direction for communication. It is probably most effective to take notes based on the outline and then complete the final outline after the conversation is over. Some clients may be so eager to share that they go off on tangents and the conversation, although lengthy, does not end up being productive or focused on the program. Others may be reserved and hesitant to share anything. In either situation, a prepared and effective health coach should use leadership and communication skills to keep the conversation focused and build rapport while gathering the needed information. This type of communication will always be the most effective technique for gaining an understanding of clients.

APPLY WHAT YOU KNOW

A 35-Year-Old Mother of Three

Ana, a 35-year-old mother of three, is ready to do something for herself and make a lifestyle change. She has been unable to effectively engage in an activity program since she had children and she is 25 pounds (11.4 kg) heavier than her pre-pregnancy (and current target) weight. She has finally made her health a priority and is starting a program with a health coach. She states that she is very nervous about starting a workout program and does not feel "fit" enough to exercise. She has not formally worked out in eight years, and when she did, she primarily engaged in group fitness activities. She says that she wants to lose at least 20 pounds (9.1 kg) and is eager to change the eating habits of her family, but admits that she needs help in identifying exactly what that means. She currently walks a couple of mornings each week with a friend and, while she tries to make healthy meals for her family, she struggles with breakfast and admits that they all snack too much most evenings. She has simply lost the energy to argue with her kids about making healthier choices. She states several times that she is ready to feel strong and healthy.

Based on this simple profile, what do you know about Ana and her needs in an exercise program? Try to fill in the information on a sample outline form (see Figure 10-7). What other information would you like to have? What additional questions would you ask?

Summary

Health coaches offer an important service that encompasses principles of nutrition, exercise science, and behavioral modification to promote lifestyle change for a wide variety of clients. Health coaches have an ethical and professional responsibility to adequately screen clients to assess relevant medical and psychological factors and fitness parameters, and refer clients to allied health professionals when indicated. In addition, the information that is gathered during the assessment phase provides an important foundation for establishing an individualized, safe, and effective weight-management program.

References

American College of Sports Medicine (2014). *ACSM's Guidelines for Exercise Testing and Prescription* (9th ed.). Philadelphia: Wolters Kluwer/ Lippincott Williams & Wilkins.

American Psychiatric Association (2000). *Diagnostic and Statistical Manual of Mental Disorders* (4th ed.). Washington, D.C.: American Psychiatric Association.

Brownell, K.D. (2000). *The LEARN Program for Weight Management* (10th ed.). Dallas: American Health.

Bruce, B. & Wilfley, D. (1996). Binge eating among the overweight population: A serious and prevalent problem. *Journal of the American Dietetic Association,* 96, 58–61.

Cone, J.D. (1997). Issues in functional analysis in behavioral assessment. *Behavior Research and Therapy,* 35, 259–275.

DiNubile, N.A. & Patrick, W. (2005). *FrameWork: Your 7-Step Program for Healthy Muscles, Bones, and Joints.* Emmaus, Pa.: Rodale Press.

Drewnowksi, A. (1990). *Toward Safe Weight Loss: Recommendations for Adult Weight Loss Programs in Michigan. Final Report of the Task Force to Establish Weight Loss Guidelines.* East Lansing, Mich.: Michigan Health Council.

Groden, G. (1989). A guide for conducting a comprehensive behavioral analysis of a target behavior. *Journal of Behavior Therapy and Experimental Psychiatry,* 20, 163–169.

Heyward, V.H. (2010). *Advanced Fitness Assessment & Exercise Prescription* (4th ed.). Champaign, Ill.: Human Kinetics.

Institute of Medicine (1995). *Weighing the Options: Criteria for Evaluating Weight-Management Programs.* Washington, D.C.: National Academy Press.

National Institutes of Health (2003). *The Seventh Report of the Joint Committee on Prevention, Detection, Evaluation, and Treatment of High Blood Pressure.* NIH Publication No. 03-5233.

National Institutes of Health (1998). Clinical guidelines on the identification, evaluation, and treatment of overweight and obesity in adults: The evidence report. *Obesity Research,* 6 (Suppl.), 51S–209S.

National Task Force on the Prevention and Treatment of Obesity (2000). Overweight, obesity, and health risk. *Archives of Internal Medicine,* 160, 898–904.

O'Neill, R.E. et al. (1997). *Functional Assessment and Program Development for Problem Behavior: A Practical Handbook* (2nd ed.). Pacific Grove, Calif.: Brooks/Cole.

Prochaska, J.O. & DiClemente, C.C. (1984). *The Transtheoretical Approach: Crossing Traditional Boundaries of Therapy.* Homewood, Ill.: Dow Jones/Irwin.

Sarafino, E.P. (2012). *Applied Behavioral Analysis: Principles and Procedures for Modifying Behavior.* Hoboken, N.J.: John Wiley & Sons.

Shah, M. , Simha, V. , & Garg, A. (2006). Long-term impact of bariatric surgery on body weight, comorbidities, and nutritional status. *Journal of Clinical Endocrinology & Metabolism,* 91, 4223–4231.

Wadden, T.A. et al. (1989). Treatment of obesity by very-low-calorie diets, behavior therapy, and their combination: A five-year perspective. *International Journal of Obesity,* 13, 2, 39–46.

Wing, R.R & Phelan, S. (2005). Long-term weight loss maintenance. *American Journal of Clinical Nutrition,* 82, 1, 222S–225S.

Winner, K. (1991). *A Weighty Issue: Dangers and Deceptions of the Weight Loss Industry.* New York: Department of Consumer Affairs.

Suggested Reading

Bellack, A.S. & Hersen, M. (Eds.). (1998). *Behavioral Assessment: A Practical Handbook* (4th ed.). New York: Allyn & Bacon.

Bryant, C.X., Franklin, B.A., & Merrill, S. (2011). *ACE's Guide to Exercise Testing and Program Design: A Fitness Professional's Handbook* (2nd ed.). Monterey, Calif.: Healthy Learning.

Heyward, V.H. (2010). *Advanced Fitness Assessment & Exercise Prescription* (4th ed.). Champaign, Ill.: Human Kinetics.

Hoffman, J. (2006). *Norms for Fitness, Performance, and Health.* Champaign, Ill.: Human Kinetics.

Martin, G. & Pear, J. (2010). *Behavior Modification: What Is It and How To Do It* (9th ed.). Upper Saddle River, N.J.: Pearson Prentice Hall.

Morrow, J.R. et al. (2011). *Measurement and Evaluation in Human Performance* (4th ed.). Champaign, Ill.: Human Kinetics.

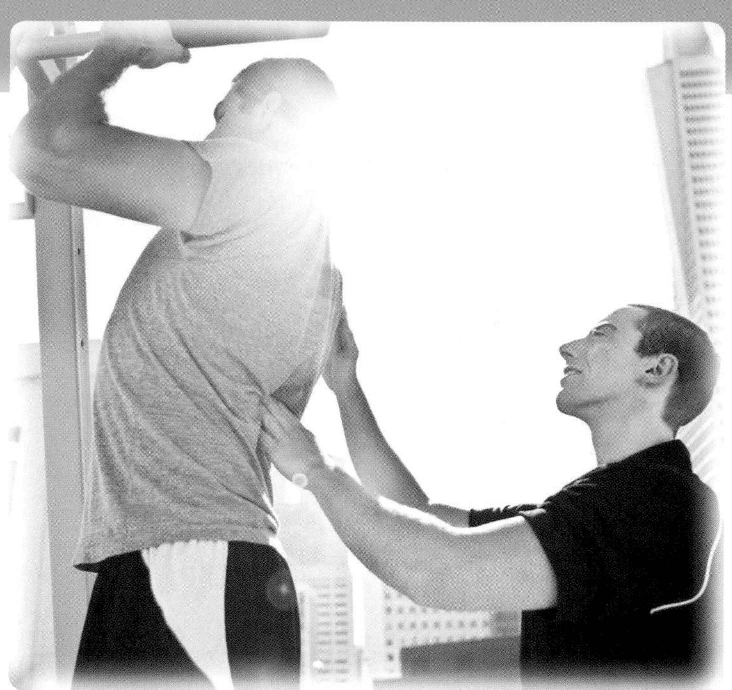

IN THIS CHAPTER:

Scott Roberts, Ph.D., is professor and chair of the Department of Kinesiology, California State University Chico. He is a fellow of the American College of Sports Medicine and the American Association of Cardiovascular and Pulmonary Rehabilitation. He is a widely published author and coauthor and an editor for several publications, including ACSM's Exercise Management for Persons with Chronic Diseases and Disabilities, *3rd edition.*

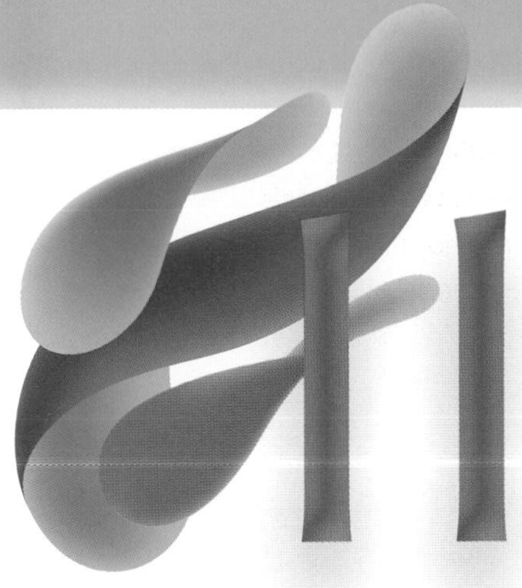

Body-composition Assessment and Evaluation

SCOTT ROBERTS &

KELLY SPIVEY

Kelly Spivey, Ph.D., has a doctorate in Natural Health and a master's degree in Fitness Management. She has an extensive career in the health and fitness arena, ranging from cardiopulmonary rehabilitation manager to owner/operator of three medically based fitness centers. Dr. Spivey is a Territory Manager for Freemotion Fitness, works with the University of Tampa in the Health Science & Human Performance Department, and serves as a subject matter expert for ACE. She has authored chapters in both the ACE Personal Trainer Manual *and the* ACE Advanced Health & Fitness Specialist Manual.

Achieving and maintaining a healthy body weight and **body composition** are central goals of good health. This issue also has become a national public-health priority, as nearly 36% of American adults and 18% of American children and adolescents are obese (Ogden et al., 2012). **Obesity** reduces quality of health and life, and increases the risk for developing numerous **chronic diseases,** including heart disease, **stroke, hypertension, type 2 diabetes,** certain types of cancer, gout, sleep apnea, and **osteoarthritis.**

Many Americans are becoming more skeptical of bathroom scales and **body mass index (BMI)** charts. Most people understand that there is a difference between fat weight and body weight, and that the only way to find out the difference is to have their body composition analyzed.

The term body composition refers to the ratio of the various components of the body that, when combined, make up a person's total **body mass (BM).** Body-composition analysis is a process used to determine the percentage of an individual's total body weight that is composed of **fat mass (FM)** versus **fat-free mass (FFM).** Body composition is typically expressed as **percent body fat (%BF),** or the ratio of fat mass to total BM. Scales and charts can only determine whether someone is above or below a recommended weight for his or her age, sex, and/or height, but cannot determine the percentage of body weight that is accounted for by FM versus FFM. Without a body-composition assessment, it is impossible to know whether weight lost or gained after starting a diet or exercise program is the result of a change in FM or FFM.

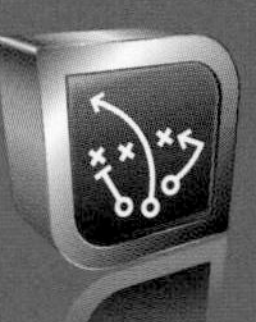

APPLY WHAT YOU KNOW

Discussing Body Composition Using Non-scientific Language

Terms such as mass, densitometry, and lean body tissue may sound like a foreign language to many people. At the same time, ACE-certified Health Coaches have to project a strong sense of professionalism, expertise, and knowledge in what they say and do to attract and keep good clients. The key is in learning how to communicate with clients based on their education levels, fitness knowledge, and previous exercise experiences. A good rule is to assume that new clients have little, if any, fitness and exercise background, and proceed from there.

Before defining body composition, make certain that clients understand that weight scales, height–weight charts, and BMI charts only consider total body weight, or total body weight in proportion to height, to indicate if individuals are of ideal weight, **overweight,** or obese. Anyone trying to lose weight needs to understand that they are really trying to lose fat, not necessarily weight. Charts are not a good indication of **ideal body weight (IBW)** for general health or for athletic performance. During a weight-loss program combining diet and exercise, there are going to be times when the rate or amount of weight loss slows, stops, or even reverses, and yet individuals can still be losing fat and gaining **lean body mass (LBM).** The only way to know for sure is through periodic body-composition assessments.

There are several ways to define body composition using non-scientific language. Clients should continually be reeducated about exercise-science principles and terminology as they become more comfortable and experienced with their training. Using the classic two-component model, body composition is typically defined as the ratio of fat mass or fat-free body mass to total body mass. LBM is sometimes used in place of FFM. Both versions are correct, with the only difference being that LBM includes a small amount of essential lipids, whereas FFM does not.

The following examples are ways to explain body composition in lay terms:

- "Body-composition testing measures how much body fat you have in proportion to the weight of your muscles, bones, and other tissues."
- "Body-composition testing is an estimate of the percentage of your weight that is fat, compared to "fat-free" weight, which is made up of muscles, bones, and organs."

Understanding Body Composition

For the average person, the most common way to monitor body weight, not body composition, is to step on the bathroom scale. Scales, however, only measure the mass (weight in pounds or kilograms) of a person, and are unable to differentiate between FM and FFM. Using scale weight alone, some people appear overweight, even if they are not necessarily overfat. Conversely, a person could appear to be normal weight, but have a high %BF level. The only way to know for sure if a person's body weight reflects an ideal %BF level is to assess body composition.

Having an understanding of, and being able to accurately determine, a person's body composition is especially useful if that individual is dieting to lose weight. Simply knowing how many pounds an individual has lost does not reveal a full or meaningful picture, because dieting frequently results in a loss of significant amounts of fat-free weight and water. Considerable research suggests, however, that individuals who are trying to lose weight should focus their efforts on losing body fat—as opposed to fat-free weight and/or water. As such, a sound weight-control program must involve modifying an individual's physical-activity and dietary habits to reach an appropriate level of body fat. In that regard, one of the critical steps is to be able to accurately assess an individual's body-fat level to determine changes in body composition.

Body composition, as an important part of a comprehensive fitness assessment, helps establish the degree of risk associated with being under or over the ideal body weight or of having a body composition that is not considered optimal for health, fitness, and athletic performance. Routine assessment of body composition is perhaps the best way of showing clients how effective changes in lifestyle can be (Table 11-1).

Table 11-1

Purpose of Body-composition Assessment

- To get baseline information
- To document for program assessment
- To use as a motivational tool
- To monitor development- and age-related changes in body composition
- To help formulate dietary recommendations
- To monitor changes in body composition that are associated with certain diseases
- To identify a client's health risk for excessively high or low levels of body fat
- To promote a client's understanding of body fat
- To monitor changes in body composition
- To assess the effectiveness of nutrition and exercise choices
- To help estimate healthy body weight for clients and athletes
- To assist in exercise programming

Body-composition Models

Body-composition analysis divides the human body into different components. The two-component model of body composition divides total body weight into FM and FFM. FM includes fat stored in the body, including both essential and non-essential body fat. **Essential fat** is fat that is necessary for normal functioning of the body and is incorporated into the nerves, brain, heart, lungs, liver, and mammary glands. Normal values for essential fat are 2 to 5% for men and 10 to 13% for women. Nonessential fat is composed mainly of **triglycerides,** which can be stored around vital organs and within muscle tissue, as well as directly beneath the skin. FFM includes organic compounds, tissues, water, muscle, bone, connective tissues, and internal organs.

Determinants of Body Composition

Genetics, lifestyle, heredity, bone structure, and body type explain most of the variation in body weight and body composition among people. **Energy balance** (caloric intake versus caloric expenditure) plays a significant role in regulating body composition. A healthy diet and daily exercise are the two most important habits affecting the ability to reach and sustain an ideal body weight and %BF level. Genetics, however, plays a crucial role in determining the extent to which body composition can be changed. Unfortunately, most people simply do not possess "media-body" genes, nor do they have the fortitude and time to develop a lean, muscular body with "six-pack abs," no matter how hard they try. Therefore, the primary focus of body-composition assessment should be to establish realistic and achievable goals that lead to a healthy and sustainable body weight.

Body Composition and Health Risks

Overweight refers to a total body weight above the recommended range for good health, whereas obesity refers to severe overweight and a high body-fat percentage. Both overweight and obesity increase the risk of **diabetes,** heart disease, and hypertension, as well as other chronic health conditions (Table 11-2). When reviewing an individual's health-assessment data, it is important to consider what proportion of a person's total body weight is fat (%BF).

Table 11-2

Increased Risk of Obesity-related Diseases with Higher BMI

	BMI			
Disease	<25	25–30	30–35	>35
Arthritis	1.00	1.56	1.87	2.39
Heart disease	1.00	1.39	1.86	1.67
Diabetes (type 2)	1.00	2.42	3.35	6.16
Gallstones	1.00	1.97	3.30	5.48
Hypertension	1.00	1.92	2.82	3.77
Stroke	1.00	1.53	1.59	1.75

Note: A value of 1.00 equals a standard level of risk, while values exceeding 1.00 represent increased risk. For example, a value of 1.87 means that the individual is at an 87% greater level of risk.

Source: Centers for Disease Control and Prevention. Third National Health and Nutrition Examination Survey. Analysis by The Lewin Group, 1999.

The location of excess storage fat is also significant. People who gain weight in the abdominal area (i.e., **android obesity** or "apple-shaped") are at an increased risk of developing coronary heart disease, high blood pressure, diabetes, and stroke compared to people who gain weight in the hip area (i.e., **gynoid obesity** or "pear-shaped").

Assessing **waist circumference** and **waist-to-hip ratio (WHR)** are simple ways to determine fat distribution. Body-composition analysis provides additional information that waist circumference and WHR cannot measure, such as FM, LBM, and %BF level.

EXPAND YOUR KNOWLEDGE

Normal-weight Obesity

Research conducted by the Mayo Clinic found that half of those considered to be of normal weight, according to BMI tables, were found to have excessive amounts of body fat (Romero-Corral et al., 2010). Those with "normal-weight obesity" are at risk for many of the same conditions found in those ranking higher on the BMI tables. Specifically, those with a normal BMI but a higher body fat percentage were found to be at risk for:

- Altered blood lipids, especially high **cholesterol**
- High levels of the hormone **leptin,** which is responsible for appetite regulation
- Increased risk of the **metabolic syndrome,** which predisposes many people to diabetes and heart disease

These findings conflict with the widely held belief that maintaining a normal body weight automatically guards against metabolic disorders. Thus, instead of tracking weight and BMI only, public health measures to prevent heart disease might benefit more from conducting waist circumference measurements or by assessing percentage of body fat as more reliable risk factors of cardiometabolic disease. This information further validates the importance of a thorough assessment of body composition and fat distribution.

Desirable Body Weight and Percent Body Fat

Many clients will ask health coaches to define what percentage of BF is acceptable, too low, or too high. A person's %BF will vary depending on his or her sex, age, race, physical-activity level, and health status. In addition, hormonal changes in women due to pregnancy, menopause, and menstruation can cause water retention that can account for variations in outcomes between tests. The minimum %BF that is essential for normal physiological functioning is roughly 2 to 5% for males and 10 to 13% for females. Some athletes get close to or below minimal ranges for %BF for brief periods due to their training and higher-than-average FFM. Low %BF levels may be appropriate for some athletes, as long as they are otherwise in good health and are getting all of their daily nutritional requirements. However, a low %BF alone is not a guarantee of athletic success. Female athletes with very low %BF levels are at risk for developing **osteoporosis,** eating disorders, and **amenorrhea,** which are together known as the **female athlete triad.** To try to achieve a low %BF level just to "look good" has potentially serious long-term physiological and psychological health risks.

Table 11-3 provides established %BF norms for men and women based on various categories of health and fitness. Whether someone's %BF is too high for good health depends on a number of variables. For example, some people may fall into in the high range of acceptability for %BF, but otherwise be healthy and physically active. Others may have acceptable %BF levels, but have an elevated risk for chronic illness and disease due to poor lifestyle choices. A person's overall health and lifestyle choices should be taken into account before making a decision about whether their %BF is acceptable or unacceptable. There is a large and convincing body of literature that confirms an increased risk of chronic illness and disease with high %BF levels of >32% in women and >25% in men (Wolf, 2002).

Table 11-3

Percent Body Fat Norms for Men and Women

Description	Women	Men
Essential fat	10–13%	2–5%
Athletes	14–20%	6–13%
Fitness	21–24%	14–17%
Acceptable	25–31%	18–24%
Obesity	≥32%	≥25%

APPLY WHAT YOU KNOW

How Often Should Body-composition Assessment Be Performed?

Assessing body composition on a frequent basis does not necessarily improve accuracy, and may cause more apprehension than motivation once people figure out that changes in body composition occur slowly. There are no definitive guidelines on how often body composition should be performed in a given population, because there are simply too many variables to consider. Practically speaking, there is little value in having it performed more frequently than monthly. For most people, two or three times a year should be adequate. Body composition may need to be assessed on a more frequent basis with a client who has a chronic disease or an eating disorder. In such cases, monitoring weight and lean body mass is essential to the medical therapy and treatment goals.

Calculating Ideal Body Weight

As previously discussed, determination of body composition is an essential skill for a health coach who is designing a personalized exercise program, especially if the client's primary goal is either weight loss or weight gain. Body-composition values can also be used to determine a goal weight. This calculation is based on the assumption that throughout the fitness program, LBM will not change. It should be noted that with any weight loss or gain, there is typically a change in the amount of both LBM and FM. Once %BF has been determined, ideal body weight can be predicted.

Body-composition Assessment of Morbidly Obese Clients

Body-composition assessment equipment and the associated prediction equations are limited in terms of how effectively they can be used with severely obese clients. In addition, issues such as self-esteem and body image play a role in deciding when, if, and how to assess body composition in this population (see Chapter 10). In some situations, it is not practical or possible to assess body composition in severely obese clients. Alternatives to body-composition assessment include weight and circumference measurements.

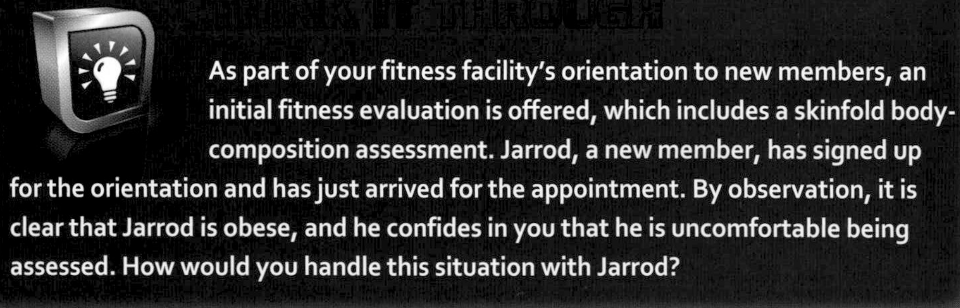

THINK IT THROUGH

As part of your fitness facility's orientation to new members, an initial fitness evaluation is offered, which includes a skinfold body-composition assessment. Jarrod, a new member, has signed up for the orientation and has just arrived for the appointment. By observation, it is clear that Jarrod is obese, and he confides in you that he is uncomfortable being assessed. How would you handle this situation with Jarrod?

Before deciding on an assessment method, health coaches must ensure that there are published prediction equations available, and that the equipment selected has been validated for use with a particular client. **Bioelectrical impedance analysis (BIA)** would seem like a good choice to use with obese clients, but most of the research published using BIA with this population tends to underestimate %BF (Coppini et al., 2005). It is important to keep in mind that an accurate measurement of body composition is not needed, nor a priority in many cases, when working with severely obese clients.

Body-composition Assessment Techniques

Most adults initiate an exercise program in an attempt to lose weight. Accordingly, it is important to be able to accurately assess a person's body composition to determine a reasonable body-weight goal and to develop a safe and effective exercise program to reach it. An accurate body-composition assessment measures the relative percentages of fat-free mass and fat mass within a particular individual.

The misunderstood term "ideal body weight" has historically been determined without concern for body composition and has involved the use of the standardized height–weight tables. In these circumstances, ideal body weight is estimated only from height and frame size, without consideration of the composition of the weight. As a result, a muscular athlete would most likely be considered overweight, while another person could fall within the accepted "ideal" body weight range and actually be overfat according to reasonable body-composition criteria.

Furthermore, it is not uncommon for an exerciser to lose fat weight and gain muscle weight without any change in total body weight. In reality, such a transformation would be very favorable from an overall health perspective. On the other hand, without an accurate assessment of a person's level of body composition, this positive change could go undetected and possibly lead to frustration on the part of the exerciser. A number of body-composition assessment techniques for identifying such a change are available. Among the more commonly used methods of estimating or assessing body composition are height–weight measurements, BMI, anthropometric measurements, BIA, and hydrostatic weighing.

Visit www.ACEfitness.org/HealthCoachResources to download a free PDF of a body-composition assessment form that you can use to record the results of all assessments introduced in this chapter, as well as other forms and assessment tools that you can use throughout your career as a health coach.

APPLY WHAT YOU KNOW

Calculating Ideal or Desired Body Weight

Consider a 47-year-old man who weighs 212 pounds (96 kg) and has an estimated body-fat percentage of 21.3%. His goal is to reach a body-fat percentage of 14 to 17%, which is the range for men desiring optimal fitness. To calculate this man's weight for the desired range, his lean mass must first be calculated. Since 21.3% of his body weight is fat mass, 78.7% of his weight is lean mass (100% – 21.3% = 78.7%). The decimal form of the percentage figures are used to derive a lean mass of 167 pounds (76 kg):

- Step 1: 100% – Body-fat percentage = Lean mass percentage
  - ✓ 100% – 21.3 = 78.7%
- Step 2: Body weight x Lean mass percentage = Lean mass
  - ✓ 212 pounds x 0.787 = 167 pounds (76 kg)
- Step 3: 100 – Desired body-fat percentage = Desired lean mass percent
  - ✓ Upper limit: 100% – 17% = 83%
  - ✓ Lower limit: 100% – 14% = 86%
- Step 4: Lean body mass/Desired lean body mass percentage = Desired body weight
  - ✓ 167/0.83 = 201 pounds (91 kg)
  - ✓ 167/0.86 = 194 pounds (88 kg)

The weight range corresponding to a desired body-fat percentage of 14 to 17% is 194 to 201 pounds (88 to 91 kg). With regular aerobic activity, resistance training, and dietary management, this man would need to lose a minimum of 11 pounds (5 kg) of fat weight (212 – 201 = 11 pounds; 96 – 91 = 5 kg).

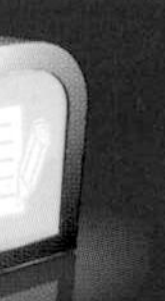

DO THE MATH

Your client weighs 220 lb (100 kg) and has 25% body fat. His goal is to achieve a weight loss that will put him at 12% body fat. How much will he weigh when he reaches his goal?

- Lean mass percentage: 100% – 25% = 75%
- Lean mass: 220 lb x 0.75 = 165 lb (75 kg)
- Desired body weight at goal body-fat percentage: 165 lb ÷ (100% – 12%) = 187.5 lb (85.2 kg)

THINK IT THROUGH

Holden, a 19-year-old client who has listed weight loss as his primary goal, is frustrated when he reaches a plateau after about six months of training. A body-composition analysis reveals that, while his body weight has remained nearly steady for the previous two months, he has lost body fat. How would you explain this to Holden in a way that refocuses his efforts? How might you reframe his goal now that he has seen some initial success and showed the ability to adhere to the program?

Height–Weight Tables

Again, the usual way that weight-conscious people track their body weight (not body composition) is to step on the bathroom scale. If the scale reads less than the last time, most people feel relieved. If the scale reading is higher than before, which is often the case, many people may decide to focus on weight loss. Periodically weighing oneself on a scale can help track weight gain or loss over time, but doing so provides no information about FM or LBM changes over time.

In 1943, the Metropolitan Life Insurance Company gave scale weight more meaning when it published desirable weight tables for men and women (Metropolitan Life Insurance Company, 1959). The tables, which are based on people who applied for life insurance policies, identify desirable weights based on height and frame size. For the Metropolitan Life Insurance Company, the tables determined the policy applicants with the lowest mortality rates. The tables became known as height–weight tables and eventually became a universal standard for deciding desirable weight for anyone, not just life insurance applicants. When the tables were revised in 1983, all of the weight ranges increased (Metropolitan Life Insurance Company, 1983). The term ideal weight gradually became associated with these tables, although the word "ideal" was never specifically used in this context.

Body Mass Index

More useful estimates of body composition can be obtained by adjusting weight for height or stature and calculating a height-normalized index. The most commonly used index is BMI, which is calculated as follows:

$$\text{BMI} = \text{Weight (kg)}/\text{Height}^2\ \text{(m)}$$

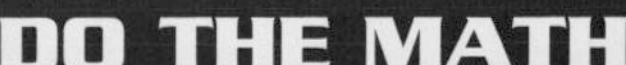

Calculate the BMI for a 209-pound man who is 5'8".

- Convert weight from pounds to kilograms by dividing by 2.2:
  - ✓209 lb/2.2 = 95 kg
- Convert height from inches to centimeters, and then to meters, by multiplying by 2.54 and then dividing by 100:
  - ✓68 inches x 2.54 = 173 cm
  - ✓173 cm/100 = 1.73 m
- BMI = $95/(1.73)^2 = 31.7$

Use Table 11-4 to determine BMI. People in a normal weight range usually have a BMI between 18.5 and 24.9 (Table 11-5). In 2008, approximately 68.3% of U.S. adults aged 20 years and older were either overweight or obese; 34.4% were overweight, defined as having a BMI of 25.0 to 29.9 kg/m^2; and 33.9% were obese, with a BMI of 30 kg/m^2 or higher (Flegal et al., 2010) (see Table 8-1, page 202).

Table 11-4

Body Mass Index

	19	20	21	22	23	24	25	26	27	28	29	30	35	40
Height (inches)							Weight (pounds)							
58	91	95	100	105	110	115	119	124	129	134	138	143	167	191
59	94	99	104	109	114	119	124	128	133	138	143	148	173	198
60	97	102	107	112	118	123	128	133	138	143	148	153	179	204
61	100	106	111	116	121	127	132	137	143	148	153	158	185	211
62	104	109	115	120	125	131	136	142	147	153	158	164	191	218
63	107	113	118	124	130	135	141	146	152	158	163	169	197	225
64	110	116	122	128	134	140	145	151	157	163	169	174	203	233
65	114	120	126	132	138	144	150	156	162	168	174	180	210	240
66	117	124	130	136	142	148	155	161	167	173	179	185	216	247
67	121	127	134	140	147	153	159	166	172	178	185	191	223	255
68	125	131	138	144	151	158	164	171	177	184	190	197	230	263
69	128	135	142	149	155	162	169	176	182	189	196	203	237	270
70	132	139	146	153	160	167	174	181	188	195	202	209	243	278
71	136	143	150	157	165	172	179	186	193	200	207	215	250	286
72	140	147	155	162	169	177	184	191	199	206	213	221	258	294
73	144	151	159	166	174	182	189	197	204	212	219	227	265	303
74	148	155	163	171	179	187	194	202	210	218	225	233	272	311
75	152	160	168	176	184	192	200	208	216	224	232	240	279	319
76	156	164	172	180	189	197	205	213	221	230	238	246	287	328

Note: Find your client's height in the far left column and move across the row to the weight that is closest to the client's weight. His or her body mass index will be at the top of that column.

Table 11-5

BMI Reference Chart

Weight Range	BMI Category
Underweight	<18.5
Normal weight	18.5–24.9
Overweight	25.0–29.9
Grade I Obesity	30.0–34.9
Grade II Obesity	35.0–39.9
Grade III Obesity	>40

Since BMI uses total body weight (i.e., not estimates of fat and lean body mass separately) in the calculation, it does not discriminate between the overfat and the athletic or more muscular body type. Therefore, BMI should ideally be used in conjunction with other body-composition assessments.

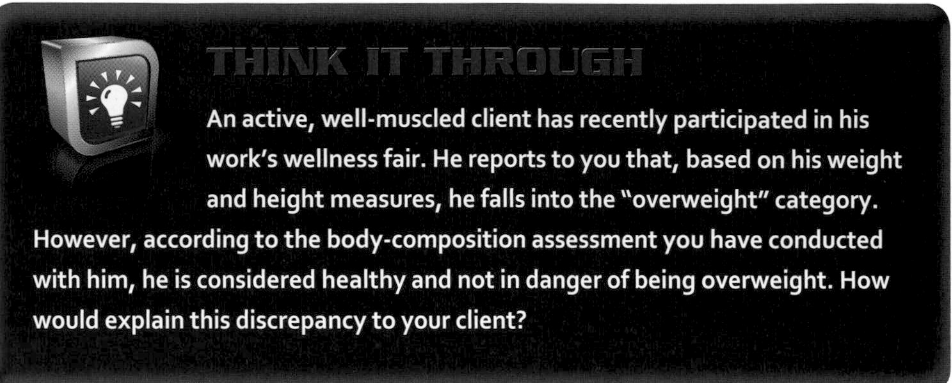

THINK IT THROUGH
An active, well-muscled client has recently participated in his work's wellness fair. He reports to you that, based on his weight and height measures, he falls into the "overweight" category. However, according to the body-composition assessment you have conducted with him, he is considered healthy and not in danger of being overweight. How would explain this discrepancy to your client?

Anthropometric Measurements

Anthropometric assessments of body composition are perhaps the easiest and least expensive methods for assessing body composition. These include circumference and skinfold measures, which are readily used in the field. Anthropometric measures also can be used to estimate body fat and its distribution (i.e., central vs. peripheral, upper body vs. lower body).

Circumference Measures

Circumference measures can easily be used to assess body composition, even with significantly overweight clients. However, to ensure accuracy, the health coach must use exact anatomical landmarks for taking each circumference measurement (Table 11-6 and Figures 11-1 through 11-4). A thorough review of anthropometric measurement sites and techniques for optimizing accuracy is presented in Lohman, Roche, & Martorell (1988).

Table 11-6

Anatomic Locations of Circumference Measurement Sites

Circumference	Anatomic Site
Abdomen	At the level of the umbilicus
Hips	The largest circumference at the posterior extension of the gluteals
Iliac	Level with the uppermost portion of the iliac crests
Waist	The narrowest part of the torso, or at the midpoint between the base of the sternum and the umbilicus

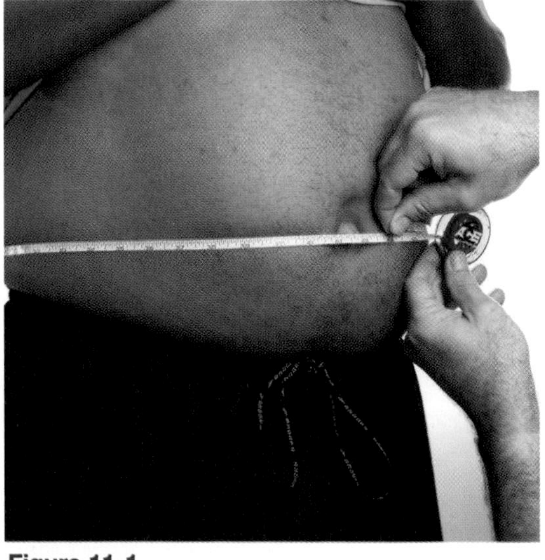

Figure 11-1
Abdominal circumference

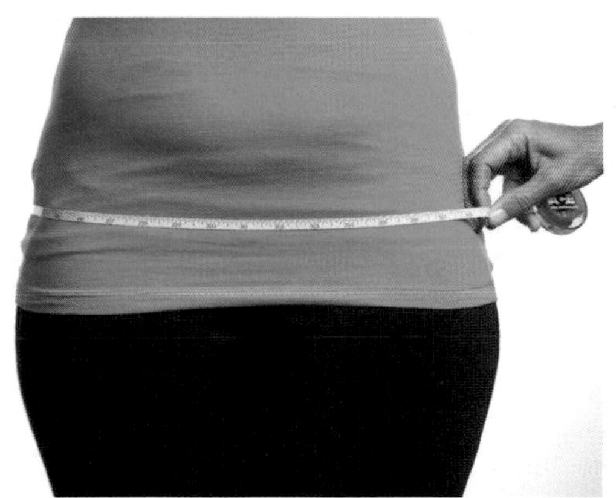

Figure 11-2
Hip circumference

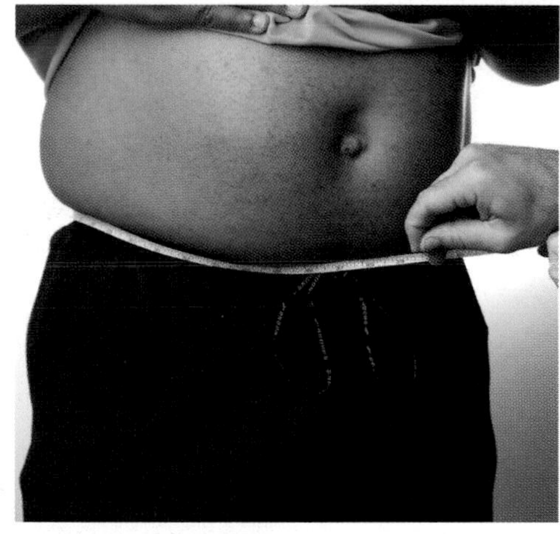

Figure 11-3
Iliac circumference

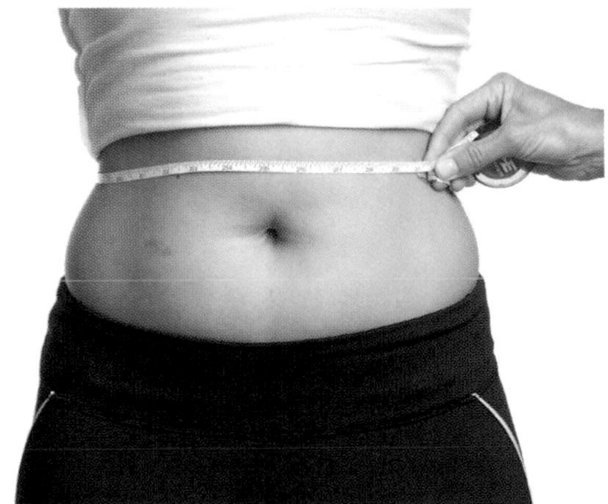

Figure 11-4
Waist circumference

> Many overweight and obese clients find the process of having their circumference measurements taken to be an unpleasant and demotivating experience. To help alleviate their uneasiness, health coaches should consider using an alternative technique that eliminates the numerical values that many clients find so upsetting. For example, health coaches can use a ribbon to measure the circumferences, cutting the ribbon at the appropriate lengths. Then, when these measurements are repeated later in the program (and the ribbons are noticeably shorter), the health coach has a very clear visual representation of the progress made.

A cloth or fiberglass (i.e., non-elastic) measurement tape must be used. The tape should be periodically calibrated against a meter stick to ensure that it has not been stretched. When assessing significantly overweight clients, be sure to use a long enough tape so as to avoid embarrassing the client. Pull the tape tight enough to keep it in position without causing an indentation of the skin. There are tapes available that have a gauge that indicates the correct tension.

Estimating Body Fat From Circumference Measures

Body density (BD) for women and men can be predicted from generalized equations that use girth measurements (Tran & Weltman, 1989; Tran, Weltman, & Seip, 1988):

$$\text{BD for women} = 1.168297 - (0.002824 \times \text{abdomen}) + (0.0000122098 \times \text{abdomen}^2) - (0.000733128 \times \text{hips}) + (0.000510477 \times \text{height}) - (0.000216161 \times \text{age})$$

$$\text{BD for men} = 1.21142 + (0.00085 \times \text{weight}) - (0.00050 \times \text{iliac}) - (0.00061 \times \text{hip}) - (0.00138 \times \text{abdomen})$$

Body density can then be converted to percent fat by using the following formula (Siri, 1961): Percent fat = (495/BD) – 450

Note: All measurements are done in centimeters; weight is measured in kilograms.

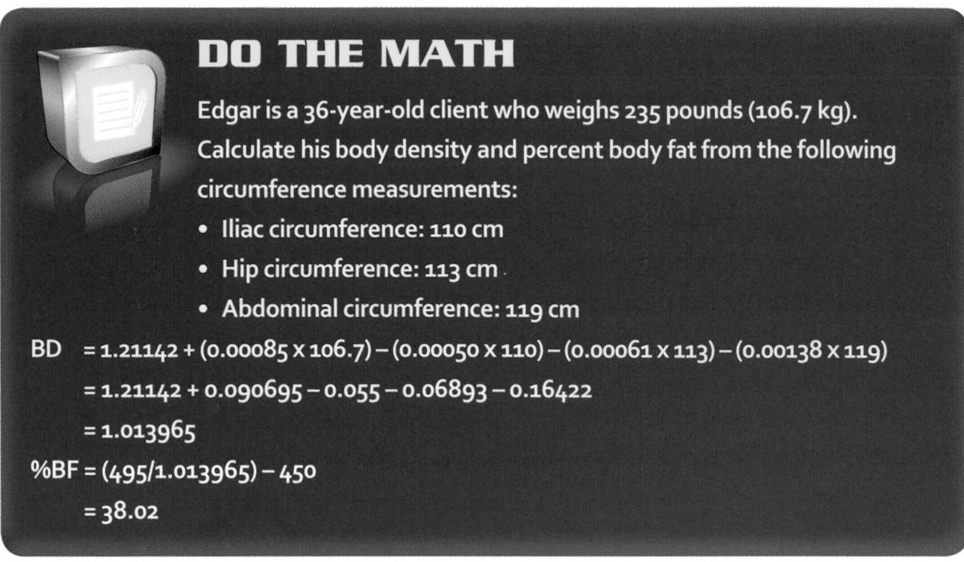

DO THE MATH

Edgar is a 36-year-old client who weighs 235 pounds (106.7 kg). Calculate his body density and percent body fat from the following circumference measurements:

- Iliac circumference: 110 cm
- Hip circumference: 113 cm
- Abdominal circumference: 119 cm

$$BD = 1.21142 + (0.00085 \times 106.7) - (0.00050 \times 110) - (0.00061 \times 113) - (0.00138 \times 119)$$
$$= 1.21142 + 0.090695 - 0.055 - 0.06893 - 0.16422$$
$$= 1.013965$$
$$\%BF = (495/1.013965) - 450$$
$$= 38.02$$

Estimating Body-fat Distribution

Upper-body or abdominal obesity is known to increase health risk (e.g., type 2 diabetes, hypertension, and **hypercholesterolemia**). A quick and reliable technique for determining body-fat distribution is the WHR ratio. To calculate WHR, divide the waist measurement by the hip measurement. Table 11-7 presents the relative risk ratings for WHR. It should also be noted that waist circumference is a reliable and easily measured indicator of abdominal obesity [Klein et al., 2007; National Heart, Lung, and Blood Institute (NHLBI), 1998]. Waist circumferences of greater than 40 inches (102 cm) in men and 35 inches (89 cm) in women are considered strong indicators of abdominal obesity.

Table 11-7

Waist-to-Hip Ratio (WHR) Norms

Gender	Excellent	Good	Average	At Risk
Males	<0.85	0.85–0.89	0.90–0.95	≥0.95
Females	<0.75	0.75–0.79	0.80–0.86	≥0.86

Source: Bray, G.A. & Gray, D.S. (1988). Obesity: Part I: Pathogenesis. *Western Journal of Medicine,* 149, 429–441.

Skinfold Measurements

Skinfold measurements are a relatively inexpensive way to assess body composition, and, if the measurements are taken properly, the results are both valid and reliable. The standard error associated with this method is ±3.5%, depending on the equation applied. This is compared to a ±2.7% error associated with hydrostatic weighing. Skinfold measurement involves measuring the thickness of the skinfolds at standardized sites; this is a reliable technique based on the belief that approximately 50% of total body fat lies under the skin. These measurements are summed and applied to one of many equations available. Skinfold calculations are derived from extensive research using hydrostatic weighing techniques. The calculation is often simplified through the use of a table or nomogram. Calipers specifically designed for skinfold measurement are the only equipment needed for this method of body-fat assessment, and range in cost from $20 to $600 (Table 11-8).

Table 11-8

Popular Skinfold Calipers

Make/Model	Details	Cost
Slim Guide	Reliable, low-end caliper; durable with large caliper opening (80 mm)	$20-25
Lafayette Skinfold Caliper II	Lightweight and durable; large caliper opening (100 mm)	$99
Trimmeter	LED digital screen; easiest to use on obese populations due to large jaw opening (90 mm)	$150
Skyndex II	Same caliper as Skyndex I (see below), but without the computer; digital readout with "hold" feature	$198-210
Lange	Best correlated with Jackson-Pollock skinfold formulas (see pages 307-308)	$220
Sanny	Newer version of Harpenden; dial gauge accuracy is ±0.1 mm	$260
Harpenden	Standard within research community due to consistent jaw pressure; accuracy is ±0.2 mm	$360
Skyndex I	Built-in computer calculates % fat; contains several formulas	$503-580

The procedure for measuring skinfolds is as follows:

- Take all measurements on the right side of the body. Identify the anatomical location of the skinfold. (*Optional:* Mark the site with an eyebrow pencil to expedite site relocation in repeated measures.)
- Grasp the skinfold firmly with the thumb and index finger of the left hand.
- Holding the calipers perpendicular to the site, place the pads of the calipers approximately 1⁄4 inch (0.6 cm) from the thumb and forefinger.
- Approximately one or two seconds after the trigger has been released, read the dial to the nearest 0.5 mm.
- A minimum of two measurements should be taken at each site, with at least 15 seconds between measurements to allow the fat to return to its normal thickness.
- Continue to take measurements until two measurements vary by less than 1 mm.

Improper site determination and measurement technique are the two primary sources of error when using this method. The technique is best learned by locating and measuring the standard sites numerous times and comparing results with those of a well-trained associate. Skinfold measurements should not be taken after exercise because the transfer of fluid to the skin could result in overestimations.

Of the many equations for estimating body composition, two developed by Jackson and Pollock (1985) have the smallest margin of error for the general population. These equations are based on the sum of measurements taken at three sites. For men, the skinfold sites are as follows:

- Chest (Figure 11-5): A diagonal skinfold taken midway between the anterior axillary line (crease of the underarm) and the nipple
- Thigh (Figure 11-6): A vertical skinfold taken midway between the hip and the top of the patella on the front of the thigh. Weight should be shifted to the left leg.
- Abdomen (Figure 11-7): A vertical skinfold taken 1 inch lateral to the umbilicus

For women, the skinfold sites are as follows:

- Triceps (Figure 11-8): A vertical fold on the back of the upper arm taken halfway between the acromion (shoulder) and olecranon (elbow) processes
- Thigh (Figure 11-9): A vertical skinfold taken midway between the hip and the top of the patella on the front of the thigh. Weight should be shifted to the left leg.
- Suprailium (Figure 11-10): A diagonal fold taken at, or just anterior to, the crest of the ilium

Figure 11-5
Chest skinfold measurement for men

Locate the site midway between the anterior axillary line and the nipple.

Grasp a diagonal fold and pull it away from the muscle.

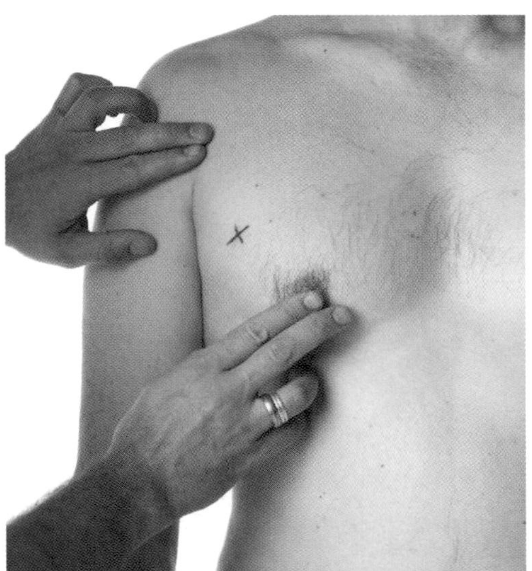

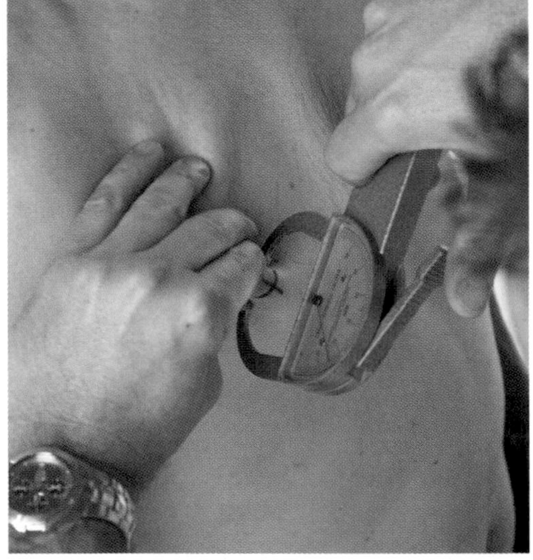

Figure 11-6
Thigh skinfold measurement for men

Locate the hip and the top of the patella and find the midpoint on the top of the thigh.

Grasp a vertical skinfold and pull it away from the muscle.

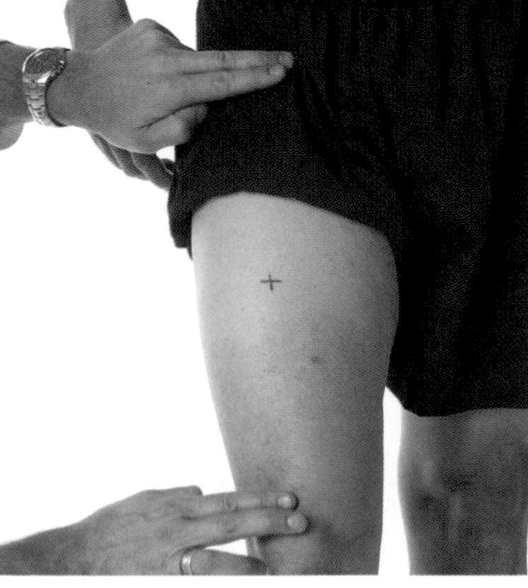

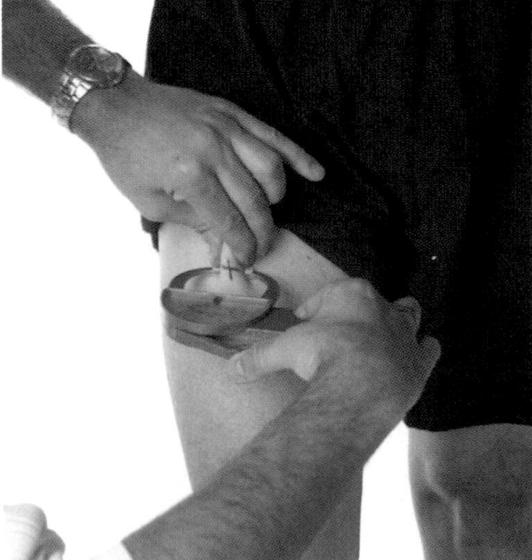

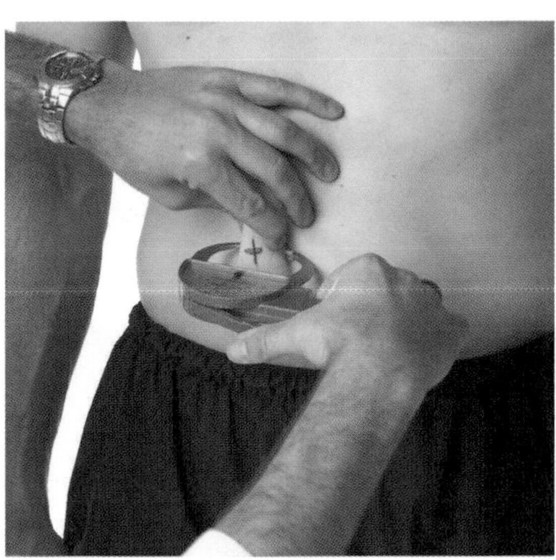

Figure 11-7
Abdominal skinfold measurement for men

Grasp a vertical skinfold one inch to the right of the umbilicus.

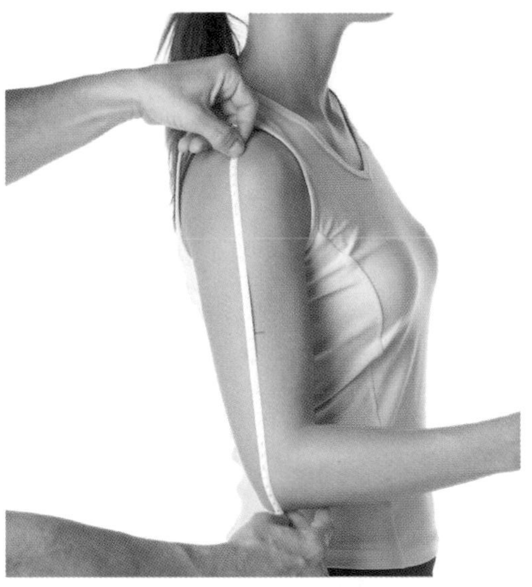

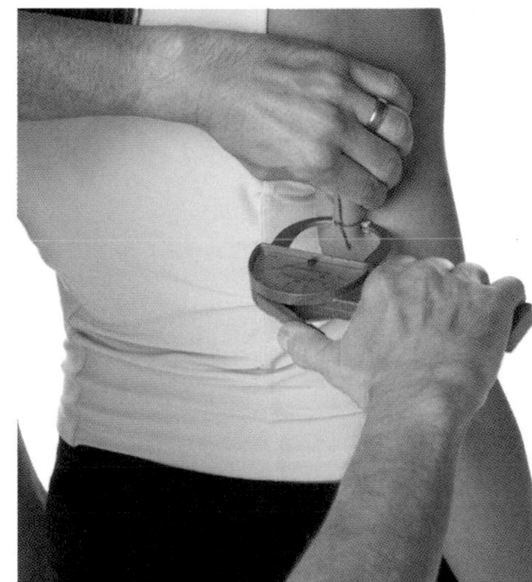

Figure 11-8
Triceps skinfold measurement for women

Locate the site midway between the acromion: (shoulder) and olecranon (elbow) processes.

Grasp a vertical fold on the posterior midline and pull it away from the muscle.

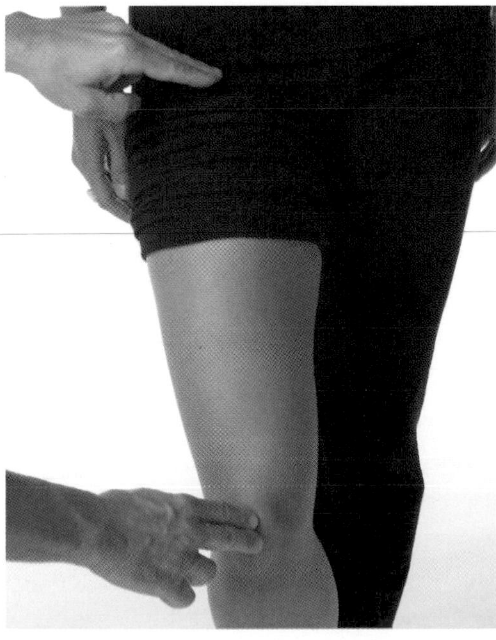

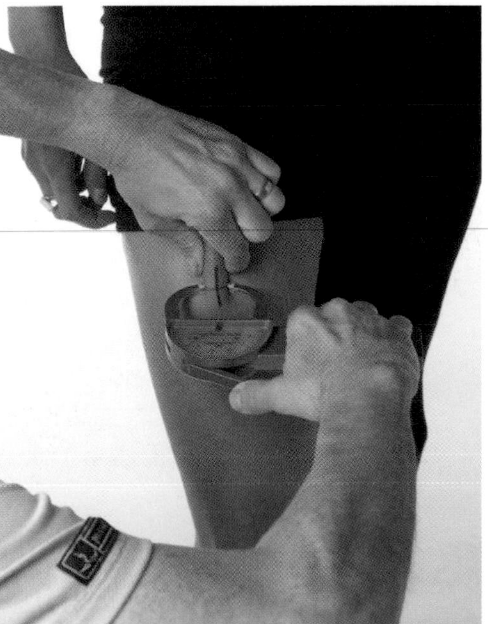

Figure 11-9
Thigh skinfold measurement for women

Locate the hip and the top of the patella and find the midpoint on the top of the thigh.

Grasp a vertical skinfold and pull it away from the muscle.

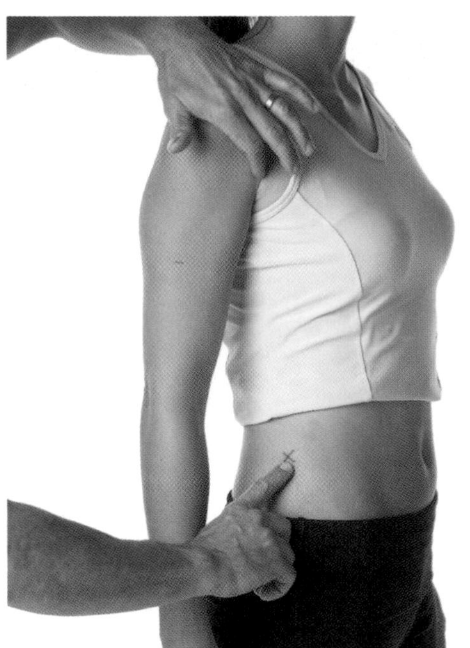

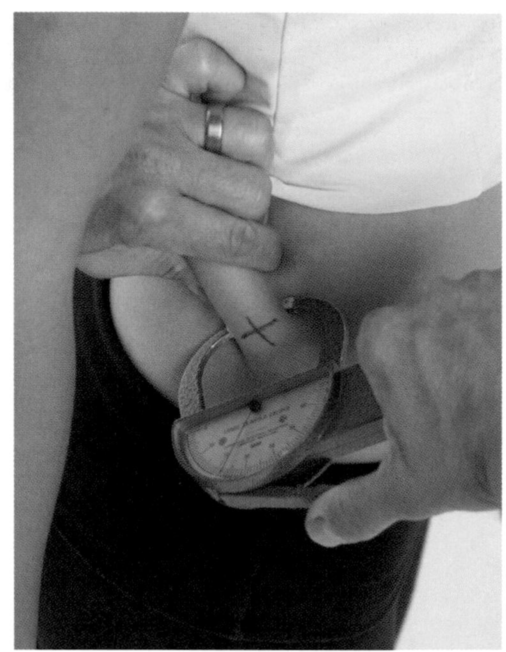

Figure 11-10
Suprailium skinfold measurement for women

Grasp a diagonal skinfold just above, and slightly forward of, the crest of the ilium.

After obtaining three satisfactory measurements, add them and refer to Table 11-9 for men and Table 11-10 for women. For example, a 47-year-old man has the following measurements: chest, 20; abdomen, 30; and thigh, 17, for a total measurement of 67. According to Table 11-9, at the intersection of the row corresponding to the sum of the skinfolds and the column corresponding to the age, his estimated body-fat percentage is 21.3%. This man's body-fat level falls within the acceptable range (see Table 11-3).

Bioelectrical Impedance

Bioelectrical impedance is a popular method for determining body composition. It is based on the principle that the conductivity of an electrical impulse is greater through lean tissue than through fatty tissue. An imperceptible electrical current is passed through two pairs of electrodes, which are placed on one hand and one foot. The analyzer, essentially an ohmmeter and a computer, measures the body's resistance to electrical flow and computes body density and body-fat percentage. The subject must lie still, with wrist and ankle electrodes accurately placed. The client should be well-hydrated and not have exercised in the past six hours or consumed any alcohol in the past 24 hours. Some research has shown the impedance method to be as accurate as the skinfold method, depending on the quality of the analyzer, the formula used to compute body density, and the adherence of the client to the aforementioned restrictions (Dehghan & Merchant, 2008). Assessing body composition via bioelectrical impedance is both fast and easy and requires minimal technical training. The cost of the analyzers ranges from $300 to $5,000, depending on design and report-generation capabilities (from simple digital readouts to elaborate multipage reports).

Body-fat scales and handheld devices are available for around $100 or less, though they are not accurate enough to be reliable measurement tools. The problem stems from the scales' inability to differentiate between body types and to provide consistent readings.

Table 11-9

Percent Body Fat Estimations for Men—Jackson and Pollock Formula

	Age Groups								
Sum of Skinfolds (mm)	Under 22	23-27	28-32	33-37	38-42	43-47	48-52	53-57	Over 57
8-10	1.3	1.8	2.3	2.9	3.4	3.9	4.5	5.0	5.5
11-13	2.2	2.8	3.3	3.9	4.4	4.9	5.5	6.0	6.5
14-16	3.2	3.8	4.3	4.8	5.4	5.9	6.4	7.0	7.5
17-19	4.2	4.7	5.3	5.8	6.3	6.9	7.4	8.0	8.5
20-22	5.1	5.7	6.2	6.8	7.3	7.9	8.4	8.9	9.5
23-25	6.1	6.6	7.2	7.7	8.3	8.8	9.4	9.9	10.5
26-28	7.0	7.6	8.1	8.7	9.2	9.8	10.3	10.9	11.4
29-31	8.0	8.5	9.1	9.6	10.2	10.7	11.3	11.8	12.4
32-34	8.9	9.4	10.0	10.5	11.1	11.6	12.2	12.8	13.3
35-37	9.8	10.4	10.9	11.5	12.0	12.6	13.1	13.7	14.3
38-40	10.7	11.3	11.8	12.4	12.9	13.5	14.1	14.6	15.2
41-43	11.6	12.2	12.7	13.3	13.8	14.4	15.0	15.5	16.1
44-46	12.5	13.1	13.6	14.2	14.7	15.3	15.9	16.4	17.0
47-49	13.4	13.9	14.5	15.1	15.6	16.2	16.8	17.3	17.9
50-52	14.3	14.8	15.4	15.9	16.5	17.1	17.6	18.2	18.8
53-55	15.1	15.7	16.2	16.8	17.4	17.9	18.5	19.1	19.7
56-58	16.0	16.5	17.1	17.7	18.2	18.8	19.4	20.0	20.5
59-61	16.9	17.4	17.9	18.5	19.1	19.7	20.2	20.8	21.4
62-64	17.6	18.2	18.8	19.4	19.9	20.5	21.1	21.7	22.2
65-67	18.5	19.0	19.6	20.2	20.8	21.3	21.9	22.5	23.1
68-70	19.3	19.9	20.4	21.0	21.6	22.2	22.7	23.3	23.9
71-73	20.1	20.7	21.2	21.8	22.4	23.0	23.6	24.1	24.7
74-76	20.9	21.5	22.0	22.6	23.2	23.8	24.4	25.0	25.5
77-79	21.7	22.2	22.8	23.4	24.0	24.6	25.2	25.8	26.3
80-82	22.4	23.0	23.6	24.2	24.8	25.4	25.9	26.5	27.1
83-85	23.2	23.8	24.4	25.0	25.5	26.1	26.7	27.3	27.9
86-88	24.0	24.5	25.1	25.7	26.3	26.9	27.5	28.1	28.7
89-91	24.7	25.3	25.9	26.5	27.1	27.6	28.2	28.8	29.4
92-94	25.4	26.0	26.6	27.2	27.8	28.4	29.0	29.6	30.2
95-97	26.1	26.7	27.3	27.9	28.5	29.1	29.7	30.3	30.9
98-100	26.9	27.4	28.0	28.6	29.2	29.8	30.4	31.0	31.6
101-103	27.5	28.1	28.7	29.3	29.9	30.5	31.1	31.7	32.3
104-106	28.2	28.8	29.4	30.0	30.6	31.2	31.8	32.4	33.0
107-109	28.9	29.5	30.1	30.7	31.3	31.9	32.5	33.1	33.7
110-112	29.6	30.2	30.8	31.4	32.0	32.6	33.2	33.8	34.4
113-115	30.2	30.8	31.4	32.0	32.6	33.2	33.8	34.5	35.1
116-118	30.9	31.5	32.1	32.7	33.3	33.9	34.5	35.1	35.7
119-121	31.5	32.1	32.7	33.3	33.9	34.5	35.1	35.7	36.4
122-124	32.1	32.7	33.3	33.9	34.5	35.1	35.8	36.4	37.0
125-127	32.7	33.3	33.9	34.5	35.1	35.8	36.4	37.0	37.6

Reprinted with permission from Jackson, A.S. & Pollock, M.L. (1985). Practical assessment of body composition. *Physician & Sports Medicine,* 13, 76–90.

Table 11-10

Percent Body Fat Estimations for Women—Jackson and Pollock Formula

	Age Groups								
Sum of Skinfolds (mm)	Under 22	23-27	28-32	33-37	38-42	43-47	48-52	53-57	Over 57
23-25	9.7	9.9	10.2	10.4	10.7	10.9	11.2	11.4	11.7
26-28	11.0	11.2	11.5	11.7	12.0	12.3	12.5	12.7	13.0
29-31	12.3	12.5	12.8	13.0	13.3	13.5	13.8	14.0	14.3
32-34	13.6	13.8	14.0	14.3	14.5	14.8	15.0	15.3	15.5
35-37	14.8	15.0	15.3	15.5	15.8	16.0	16.3	16.5	16.8
38-40	16.0	16.3	16.5	16.7	17.0	17.2	17.5	17.7	18.0
41-43	17.2	17.4	17.7	17.9	18.2	18.4	18.7	18.9	19.2
44-46	18.3	18.6	18.8	19.1	19.3	19.6	19.8	20.1	20.3
47-49	19.5	19.7	20.0	20.2	20.5	20.7	21.0	21.2	21.5
50-52	20.6	20.8	21.1	21.3	21.6	21.8	22.1	22.3	22.6
53-55	21.7	21.9	22.1	22.4	22.6	22.9	23.1	23.4	23.6
56-58	22.7	23.0	23.2	23.4	23.7	23.9	24.2	24.4	24.7
59-61	23.7	24.0	24.2	24.5	24.7	25.0	25.2	25.5	25.7
62-64	24.7	25.0	25.2	25.5	25.7	26.0	26.7	26.4	26.7
65-67	25.7	25.9	26.2	26.4	26.7	26.9	27.2	27.4	27.7
68-70	26.6	26.9	27.1	27.4	27.6	27.9	28.1	28.4	28.6
71-73	27.5	27.8	28.0	28.3	28.5	28.8	29.0	29.3	29.5
74-76	28.4	28.7	28.9	29.2	29.4	29.7	29.9	30.2	30.4
77-79	29.3	29.5	29.8	30.0	30.3	30.5	30.8	31.0	31.3
80-82	30.1	30.4	30.6	30.9	31.1	31.4	31.6	31.9	32.1
83-85	30.9	31.2	31.4	31.7	31.9	32.2	32.4	32.7	32.9
86-88	31.7	32.0	32.2	32.5	32.7	32.9	33.2	33.4	33.7
89-91	32.5	32.7	33.0	33.2	33.5	33.7	33.9	34.2	34.4
92-94	33.2	33.4	33.7	33.9	34.2	34.4	34.7	34.9	35.2
95-97	33.9	34.1	34.4	34.6	34.9	35.1	35.4	35.6	35.9
98-100	34.6	34.8	35.1	35.3	35.5	35.8	36.0	36.3	36.5
101-103	35.3	35.4	35.7	35.9	36.2	36.4	36.7	36.9	37.2
104-106	35.8	36.1	36.3	36.6	36.8	37.1	37.3	37.5	37.8
107-109	36.4	36.7	36.9	37.1	37.4	37.6	37.9	38.1	38.4
110-112	37.0	37.2	37.5	37.7	38.0	38.2	38.5	38.7	38.9
113-115	37.5	37.8	38.0	38.2	38.5	38.7	39.0	39.2	39.5
116-118	38.0	38.3	38.5	38.8	39.0	39.3	39.5	39.7	40.0
119-121	38.5	38.7	39.0	39.2	39.5	39.7	40.0	40.2	40.5
122-124	39.0	39.2	39.4	39.7	39.9	40.2	40.4	40.7	40.9
125-127	39.4	39.6	39.9	40.1	40.4	40.6	40.9	41.1	41.4
128-130	39.8	40.0	40.3	40.5	40.8	41.0	41.3	41.5	41.8

Reprinted with permission from Jackson, A.S. & Pollock, M.L. (1985). Practical assessment of body composition. *Physician & Sports Medicine,* 13, 76-90.

THINK IT THROUGH

After meeting your client for the first time, it is agreed that you will assess her body composition using the BIA device available in the fitness facility when you meet with her next week. A day later, you see your new client after she finishes taking a 60-minute high-intensity indoor cycling class. She asks you if you could assess her body composition now, before she leaves the gym for the day. How would you respond to this client?

Hydrostatic Weighing

Hydrostatic weighing, also known as underwater weighing, is considered the "gold standard" of body-composition assessment. The test involves suspending a client in a tank of water. Body density is calculated from the relationship of normal body weight to underwater weight. Body-fat percentage is calculated from body density. This method is most accurate when the client's residual volume (i.e., the amount of air left in the lungs after a complete expiration) is used in the calculation. When residual volume is estimated from a formula, the accuracy of the hydrostatic method can be significantly decreased. Though hydrostatic weighing is accurate, it is often impractical in terms of expense, time, and equipment.

Other Methods of Body-composition Assessment

The science of body-composition assessment is a relatively young discipline, but it is evolving rapidly due to the use of advanced technologies, such as **dual energy x-ray absorptiometry (DEXA), air displacement plethysmography (ADP),** and **near-infrared interactance (NIR).**

Dual Energy X-ray Absorptiometry

A relatively new technology that has been found to be very accurate and precise (an error rate of less than 1.5%), DEXA is based on a three-compartment model that divides the body into three components—total body mineral, fat-free soft (lean) mass, and fat tissue mass. This technique is based on the assumption that bone mineral content is directly proportional to the amount of photon energy absorbed by the bone being studied.

DEXA uses a whole-body scanner that has two low-dose x-rays at different sources that read bone and soft tissue mass simultaneously. The sources are mounted beneath a table with a detector overhead. The scanner passes across a person's reclining body with data collected at 0.5-cm intervals. A DEXA scan takes between three and five minutes, depending on the specific type of scanner used. This technique is safe and noninvasive, with little inconvenience to the individual (e.g., a person is not required to disrobe or monitor food or fluid consumption).

DEXA has become the "benchmark" for body-composition assessment techniques, because it has a higher degree of precision, while only involving one measurement, and has the ability to identify exactly where fat is distributed throughout the body (i.e., regional body-fat distribution). In fact, most clinical studies use DEXA to evaluate the accuracy of other body-composition assessment techniques. Research has shown DEXA to be a very reliable and useful tool for precisely measuring body-fat levels. Given its successful application in clinical settings and the increased awareness of the inherent dangers of excess body fat, the employment of DEXA in practical settings will undoubtedly become more commonplace in the future.

Air Displacement Plethysmography

Air displacement plethysmography (ADP) is another noninvasive and rapid way to assess body composition that predicts %BF within 1 to 3% of hydrostatic weighing results (Fields, Goran, & McCrory, 2002). ADP equipment, such as the BOD POD®, uses whole-body air displacement instead of water to measure body volume and density. The BOD POD determines body volume by measuring the volume of air in the chamber while empty and then with a person inside.

Near-infrared Interactance

Near-infrared interactance (NIR) technology was developed by the U.S. Department of Agriculture to measure the amount of fat contained in beef and pork carcasses following slaughter. NIR uses a small probe that emits an infrared light through the skin, fat, and lean tissues, and then records their optical densities (changes in color and tone) as the light is reflected off bone and back to the probe.

NIR equipment that has been adapted for use with humans, such as the Futrex® NIR model, is able to predict %BF based on the evidence that optical densities of FM and FFM are proportional to the amount of subcutaneous fat. By comparing known optical-density values for FM and FFM to the measured optical densities in subjects, one can estimate the amount of subcutaneous fat at the measured site. Most NIR equipment uses the anterior aspect of the biceps as the common NIR measurement site. Once the test is finished, NIR data is entered into a prediction equation based on the person's height, weight, frame size, and level of activity to estimate %BF.

Although NIR is an inexpensive and rapid way to measure %BF in humans, there has been significant debate over its reliability and validity. Factors such as probe pressure, skin color, and hydration status can affect results. At best, NIR provides a very general estimate of %BF, with an inherently high error rate.

APPLY WHAT YOU KNOW

Approaches to Discussing Results With Clients

Body-composition results should be used to help motivate clients and help them set realistic body-weight or fat-loss goals. They should never be used to humiliate, degrade, or categorize people. In addition, health coaches must always use positive and encouraging language. Never say, "Mr. Jones, your body-composition results indicate that your percent body fat is high, which means that you fall into the obese category. Boy, we sure have a lot of work ahead of us, don't we?" While this statement may be true, health coaches should be more encouraging: "Mr. Jones, your body-composition results indicate that you are above the range for good health, so I'm glad you made this appointment, and I'm excited to be working with you. I have set some very reasonable and attainable diet and exercise goals for you that I think will help bring your percent body fat down into a healthier range."

Health coaches must never focus on the numbers. Instead, they should consider the whole person when discussing the results of body-composition testing. When most people hear a number they think is too high, they tend to stop listening, because they have already made up their minds. For example, consider a client who is 5'7" and weighs 155 pounds (1.7 m; 70 kg), who tells you that he thinks he should weigh 135 pounds (61 kg) because he heard that a person can figure out his ideal weight by adding 5 pounds (2.3 kg) to a base of 100 for every inch of height over five feet. However, a body-composition test shows that 135 pounds (61 kg) would be unrealistic based on the client's amount of lean tissue (muscle). For example, if the client's body fat came out to 22%, then 78% of his weight, or 121 pounds (55 kg), is lean tissue. If he was to maintain that amount of lean tissue and lose 20 pounds (9.1 kg) of fat, he would weigh 135 pounds (61 kg), but his body composition would be down to 10% fat, which is an unrealistically low target for him.

Body-composition testing is only one tool to help guide a diet and exercise program. Body-composition results by themselves offer little value. In addition, body fat or weight is not the only measure of health. It is possible to be quite healthy by all other standards while exceeding a norm for body weight or body composition. Health coaches must discuss body-composition results by using phrases such as "within the desirable range," or "too high" or "too low," in addition to presenting the raw data. Saying that a body fat level is 28% likely means nothing to the client.

Summary

Body composition is an integral component of total health and physical fitness. Accordingly, fitness professionals have a responsibility to help educate those with whom they work and the general population regarding appropriate levels of body fat and how to safely and effectively achieve them. Not only can such an effort have a positive impact on the high prevalence of obesity in society, it can also help reduce the enormous healthcare costs that result from this very unhealthy condition. As such, a strong argument can be made that a body-composition evaluation should be included as an essential part of all health and fitness appraisals. The time for taking a more measured approached in the war on obesity and its related problems is now. Accurately assessing body composition and using that information to help design meaningful, personalized exercise programs should serve as the foundation for that approach.

References

Bray, G.A. & Gray, D.S. (1988). Obesity: Part I: Pathogenesis. *Western Journal of Medicine,* 149, 429–441.

Coppini, L.Z. et al. (2005). Limitations and validation of bioelectrical impedance analysis in morbidly obese patients. *Current Opinion in Clinical Nutrition and Metabolic Care,* 8, 3, 329–332.

Dehghan, M. & Merchant, A.T. (2008). Is bioelectrical impedance accurate for use in large epidemiological studies? *Nutrition Journal,* 7, 26–32.

Fields, D., Goran, M., & McCrory, M. (2002). Body-composition assessment via air-displacement plethysmography in adults and children: A review. *American Journal of Clinical Nutrition,* 75, 453–467.

Flegal, K.M. et al. (2010). Prevalence and trends in obesity among U.S. adults, 1999–2008. *Journal of the American Medical Association,* 303, 3, 235–241

Jackson, A.S. & Pollock, M.L. (1985). Practical assessment of body composition. *The Physician and Sportsmedicine,* 13, 76–90.

Klein, S. et al. (2007). Waist circumference and cardiometabolic risk. *Diabetes Care,* 30, 1647–1652.

Lohman, T.G., Roche, A. F., & Martorell, R. (Eds.). (1988). *Anthropometric Standardization Reference Manual.* Champaign, Ill.: Human Kinetics.

Metropolitan Life Insurance Company (1983). 1983 Metropolitan height and weight tables. *Statistics Bulletin Metropolitan Life Insurance Co.,* 64, 1–19.

Metropolitan Life Insurance Company (1959). New weight standards for men and women. *Statistics Bulletin Metropolitan Life Insurance Co.,* 40, 1–4.

National Heart, Lung, and Blood Institute (1998). Clinical guidelines on the identification, evaluation, and treatment of overweight and obesity in adults: The evidence report. *Obesity Research,* 6 (Suppl. 2), 51S–209S.

Ogden, C.L. et al. (2012). *Prevalence of Obesity in the United States 2009–2010.* NHCS Data Brief, No. 82. Washington, D.C.: Centers for Disease Control and Prevention.

Romero-Corral, A. et al. (2010). Normal weight obesity: A risk factor for cardiometabolic dysregulation and cardiovascular mortality. *European Heart Journal,* 31, 737–46.

Siri, W.E. (1961). Body composition from fluid space and density. In J. Brozek & A. Hanschel (Eds.) *Techniques for Measuring Body Composition* (p. 223–244). Washington, D.C.: National Academy of Science.

Tran, Z. & Weltman, A. (1989). Generalized equation for predicting body density of women from girth measurements. *Medicine & Science in Sports & Exercise,* 21, 101–104.

Tran, Z. Weltman, A., & Seip, R. (1988). Predicting body composition of men from girth measurements. *Human Biology,* 8, 60, 167–176.

Wolf, A.M. (2002). Economic outcomes of the obese patient. *Obesity Research,* 10, 58S–62S.

Suggested Reading

Brozek, J. et al. (1963). Densitometric analysis of body composition: Revision of some quantitative assumptions. *Annals of the New York Academy of Sciences,* 110, 113–140.

Chan J.M. et al. (1994). Obesity, fat distribution, and weight gain as risk factors for clinical diabetes in men. *Diabetes Care,* 17, 9, 961–969.

Finkelstein, E.A. et al. (2005). Economic causes and consequences of obesity. *Annual Review of Public Health,* April, 26, 239–257.

Heymsfield, S.B. et al. (2005). *Human Body Composition* (2nd ed.). Champaign, Ill.: Human Kinetics.

Heyward, V.H. & Wagner, D.R. (2004). *Applied Body Composition Assessment.* Champaign, Ill.: Human Kinetics.

Jackson, A.S. & Pollock, M.L. (1978). Generalized equations for predicting body density. *British Journal of Nutrition,* 40, 497–504.

National Institutes of Health (1998). *The Practical Guide on Identification, Evaluation, and Treatment of Overweight and Obesity in Adults.* Bethesda, Md.: National Institutes of Health.

Siri, W.E. (1961). Body composition from fluid space and density. In: Brozek, J. & Hanschel, A. (Eds.).

Techniques for Measuring Body Composition (pp. 223–244). Washington, D.C.: National Academy of Science.

Stunkard, A.J. & Wadden, T.A. (Eds.) (1993). *Obesity: Theory and Therapy* (2nd ed.). New York: Raven Press.

Thompson, D. et al. (1999). Lifetime health and economic consequences of obesity. *Archives of Internal Medicine*, 159, 2177–2183.

Wang, Y. et al. (2005). Comparison of abdominal adiposity and overall obesity in predicting risk of type 2 diabetes among men. *American Journal of Clinical Nutrition,* 81, 3, 555–563.

Yusuf, S. et al. on behalf of the INTERHEART Study (2005). Obesity and the risk of myocardial infarction in 27,000 participants from 52 countries: A case-control study. *The Lancet,* 366, 1640–1649.

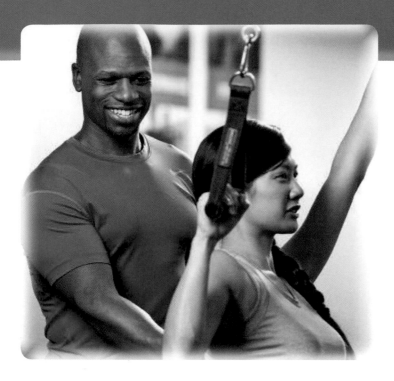

IN THIS CHAPTER:

Kelly Spivey, Ph.D., has a doctorate in Natural Health and a master's degree in Fitness Management. She has an extensive career in the health and fitness arena, ranging from cardiopulmonary rrehabilitation manager to owner/operator of three medically based fitness centers. Dr. Spivey is a Territory Manager for Freemotion Fitness, works with the University of Tampa in the Health Science & Human Performance Department, and serves as a subject matter expert for ACE. She has authored chapters in both the ACE Personal Trainer Manual *and the* ACE Advanced Health & Fitness Specialist Manual.

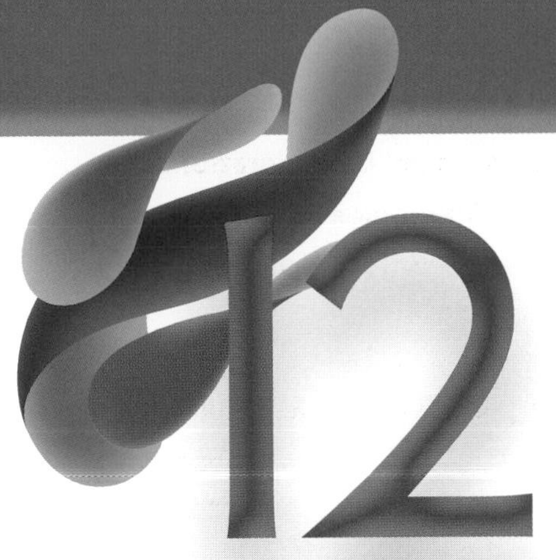

Physical-fitness Assessments

KELLY SPIVEY &
SABRENA JO

Sabrena Jo, M.S., has been actively involved in the fitness industry since 1987, successfully operating her own personal-training business and teaching group exercise classes. Jo is a former full-time faculty member in the Kinesiology and Physical Education Department at California State University, Long Beach. She has a bachelor's degree in exercise science as well as a master's degree in physical education/biomechanics from the University of Kansas. Jo, an ACE-certified Personal Trainer and Group Fitness Instructor, is an author, educator, and fitness consultant who remains very active within the industry.

The American Council on Exercise has created the ACE Integrated Fitness Training® (ACE IFT®) Model as a roadmap for the ACE-certified Health Coach and other health and fitness professionals to utilize in exercise programming and implementation. The ACE IFT Model provides a systematic progression, starting with assessment and risk stratification and continuing through exercise program design, implementation, and progression (see Chapters 16 and 17).

Phase 1 incorporates the components of health (**stability** and **mobility** training combined with aerobic-base training); phase 2 is fitness-related (movement training and aerobic-efficiency training); and phases 3 (load training and anaerobic-endurance training) and 4 (performance training and anaerobic-power training) are performance-related and incorporate sport-specific skills and movement patterns. Of course, each client may have a different starting point for each component, but it is up to the health coach to determine how and when to progress each individual based on his or her unique health needs and fitness goals. Figure 12-1 provides a sequential approach to conducting client assessments.

Pre-assessment Considerations

To enhance the evaluation experience, it is important for the client to feel at ease and have an idea of what to expect in the evaluation process. If possible, the health coach should provide a packet of paperwork prior to the initial meeting. The packet should include an overview of the evaluation process, including information on what to wear. Certain assessments also require avoidance of food, beverages, and/or prior exercise.

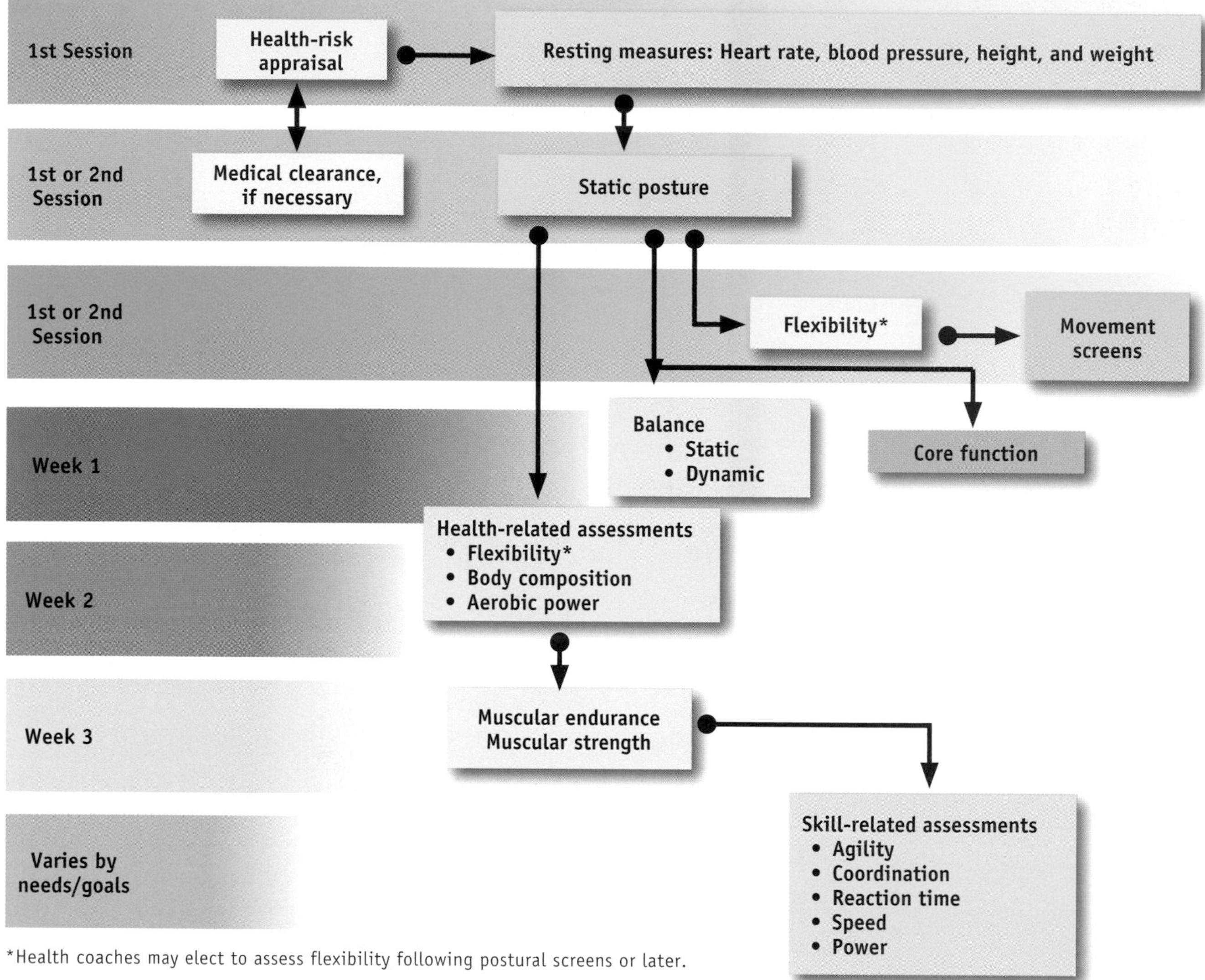

Figure 12-1
Sample assessment sequencing for the general client

Note: Refer to the *ACE Personal Trainer Manual* for information on those assessments not covered in this text.

To facilitate sharing of information, the evaluation setting should be private and free of distractions. All necessary assessment tools should be available and in good working order. When conducting physical assessments, the indoor temperature should be between 68 and 72° F (20–22° C). Health coaches should avoid outdoor testing in extreme environmental conditions. It is also important to ensure that emergency supplies are readily available.

General Assessment Guidelines

It is important for the health coach to consider the following guidelines for health screening and baseline data collection:

- Conduct a health-risk appraisal to identify any areas of concern or need for referral. For this reason, it is important to administer preliminary health-history questionnaires (see Figure 15-1, page 412) and resting measurements [i.e., **heart rate (HR)** and **blood pressure (BP)**] prior to beginning any fitness testing or supervised exercise program.
- Collect baseline data to use in exercise program design.
- Educate the client on his or her risk factors and areas of concern, especially those related to normative data for age and gender. For example, **cardiorespiratory fitness (CRF)**

scores are significant predictors of cardiac risk, as are abnormal BP responses to exercise.

- Motivate the client by establishing realistic goals and expectations. Injury and burnout are common side effects associated with starting an exercise program too aggressively. The health coach should remind clients that even small changes will positively impact their health.

Lastly, health coaches should be aware that not all clients desire or need a comprehensive fitness evaluation prior to engaging in an exercise program. In fact, physical-fitness assessments can be demotivating to some individuals, making them feel intimidated, embarrassed, or fearful of the exertion required and the results. Proper test selection can minimize these aspects. At the very least, it is prudent to conduct a health-risk appraisal for every client.

Baseline Resting Measurements

Heart Rate

The pulse rate (which in most people is identical to the HR) can be measured at any point on the body where an artery's pulsation is close to the surface. The following are some commonly palpated sites:

- *Radial artery:* The ventral aspect of the wrist on the side of the thumb, and less commonly, the ulnar artery on the pinky side, which is deeper and harder to palpate (Figure 12-2)
- *Carotid artery:* Located in the neck, lateral to the trachea; more easily palpated when the neck is slightly extended. When using the carotid artery for pulse detection, health coaches should instruct the client not to push too hard, as this may evoke a vagal response and actually slow down the HR (Figure 12-3).

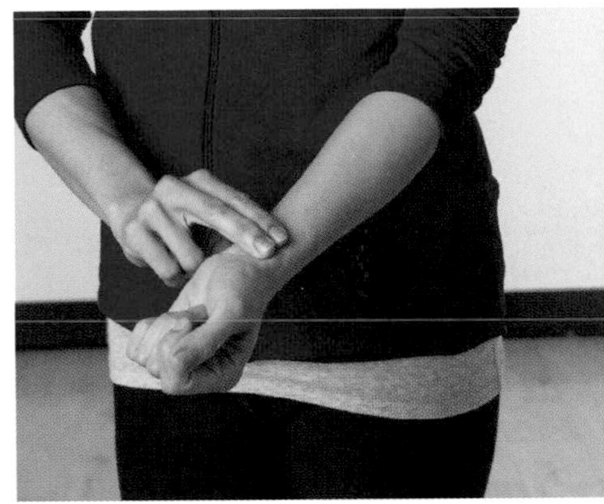

Figure 12-2
Taking the pulse at the radial artery

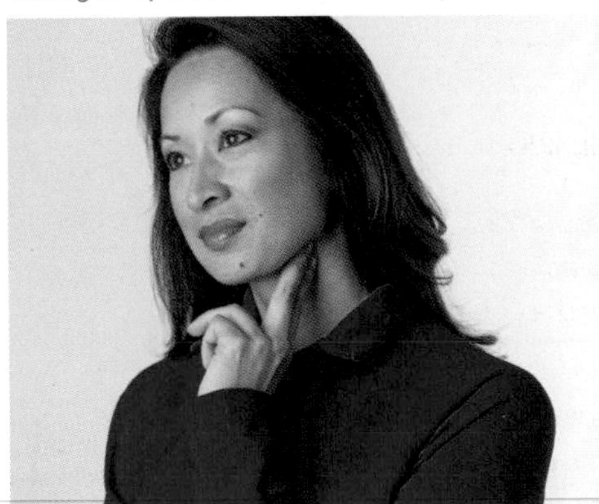

Figure 12-3
Taking the pulse at the carotid artery

It is also possible to auscultate the actual beat of the heart using a stethoscope placed over the chest. If when palpating the client's pulse, the health coach feels any irregularity in the rate or rhythm of the pulse, it is recommended that the client contact his or her personal physician.

Measurement of HR is a valid indicator of work intensity or stress on the body, both at rest and during exercise. Lower resting and submaximal HRs may indicate higher fitness levels, since cardiovascular adaptations to exercise increase **stroke volume (SV),** thereby reducing HR. Conversely, higher resting and submaximal HRs are often indicative of poor physical fitness. **Resting heart rate (RHR)** is influenced by fitness status, fatigue, body composition, drugs and medication, alcohol, caffeine, and stress, among other things. A traditional classification system exists to categorize RHRs:

- Sinus bradycardia, or slow HR: RHR <60 beats per minute (bpm)
- Normal sinus rhythm: RHR 60 to 100 bpm
- Sinus tachycardia, or fast HR: RHR >100 bpm

Average RHR is approximately 70 to 72 bpm, averaging 60 to 70 bpm in males and 72 to 80 bpm in females. The higher values found in the female RHR is attributed in part to:

- Smaller heart chamber size
- Lower blood volume circulating less oxygen throughout the body
- Lower hemoglobin levels in women

The following are some important notes about HR:

- Knowing a client's HR provides insight into the **overtraining syndrome,** as any elevation in RHR >5 bpm over the client's normal RHR that remains over a period of days is good reason to reduce or taper training intensities.
- Certain drugs, medications, and supplements can directly affect RHR. Individuals should abstain from consuming nonprescription stimulants or depressants for a minimum of 12 hours prior to measuring RHR.
- Body position affects RHR. Standing or sitting positions elevate HR more so than supine or prone positions due to the involvement of postural muscles and the effects of gravity.
- **Digestion** increases RHR, as the processes of **absorption** and digestion require energy, necessitating the delivery of nutrients and oxygen to the gastrointestinal tract.
- Environmental factors can affect RHR, as it is believed that noise, temperature, and sharing of personal information can place additional stress on the body, increasing HR as the body adjusts to the stressors.

During exercise, HR reflects exercise intensity. Because the heart plays a pivotal role in supplying oxygen and nutrients and removing waste products, HR is a valid indicator of the metabolic demands placed upon the body. Several methods are used to measure HR, both at rest and during exercise:

- 12-lead **electrocardiogram (ECG** or **EKG)**
- **Telemetry** (often two-lead, including commercial heart-rate monitors)
- **Palpation**
- **Auscultation** with stethoscope

Palpation and auscultation are each accurate within 95% of a heart-rate monitor.

Procedure for Measuring Resting Heart Rate

Keep in mind that true RHR is measured just before the client gets out of bed in the morning. Therefore, in most fitness environments, the health coach's assessment of RHR will not be reflective of true RHR. The pulsation heard through auscultation is generated by the expansion of the arteries as blood is pushed through after contraction of the left ventricle. This beat can be quite prominent in leaner individuals.

- The client should be resting comfortably for several minutes prior to obtaining RHR.
- The RHR may be measured indirectly by placing the fingertips on a pulse site (palpation), or directly by listening through a stethoscope (auscultation).
- Place the tips of the index and middle fingers (not the thumb, which has a pulse of its own) over the artery (typically, radial is used) and lightly apply pressure.
- To determine the RHR, count the number of beats for 30 or 60 seconds and then convert that value to beats/minute, if necessary.
    - ✓ It is important to remember that a health coach is counting cardiac cycles. Therefore, the first pulse measured should commence with "zero."
- When measuring by auscultation, place the bell of the stethoscope to the left of the client's sternum just above or below the nipple line. (It is important to be respectful of the client's personal space.)
- The client may also measure his or her own resting HR before rising from bed in the morning and report back.

Procedure for Measuring Exercise Heart Rate

- Measuring for 30 to 60 seconds is generally difficult during exercise. Therefore, exercise HRs are normally measured for shorter periods that are then converted to equal 60 seconds.
- Generally a 10- to 15-second count is recommended over a six-second count, given the larger potential for error with the shorter count.

Getting an Accurate Heart-rate Count

Conventional wisdom has long held that one should begin at "zero" when counting a client's pulse rate in order to accurately estimate the number of cardiac cycles. In fact, counting the first beat as zero will consistently underestimate exercise heart rate (Porcari, Robarge, & Veldhuis, 1993). If the pulse is counted for 10 seconds, the magnitude of the underestimation will be 6 bpm, since the 10-second count is multiplied by six. Starting at zero is only appropriate if the clock is started on a specific beat, but this method is very difficult in a fitness setting. Starting at "one" is particularly important in group settings, where exercisers will begin their counts at different points in the cardiac cycle.

Note: If the heart rhythm changes, or there are more than six skipped beats within a minute, exercise should immediately be terminated.

Determination of Exercise Target Heart Rate

Unless the client has had a recent **graded exercise test (GXT), maximal heart rate (MHR)** is not known at this point of the evaluation process. An exercise heart-rate range can be determined using the client's resting heart rate and an age-predicted maximal heart rate, which can be calculated by following equation (Tanaka, Monahan, & Seals, 2001):

MHR = 208 – (0.7 x Age)

A widely recognized formula for determining exercise heart-rate range is the Karvonen method:

Target HR (THR) = (HRR x % intensity) + RHR

Where: HRR = MHR – RHR

Note: HRR = Heart-rate reserve

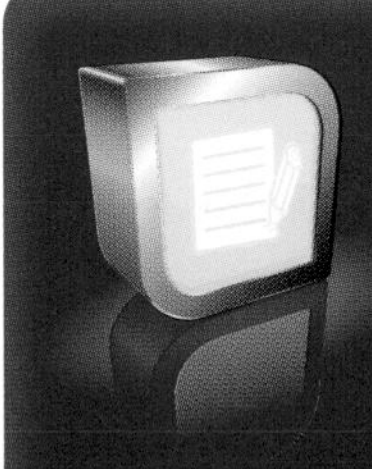

DO THE MATH

The initial evaluation with a deconditioned 50-year-old female client finds that her RHR is 90 bpm. What is her **target heart rate (THR)** range?

- MHR = 208 – (0.7 x Age)
- MHR = 208 – (0.7 x 50) = 173
- Since she is deconditioned, initial exercise intensity will be kept low to moderate, or 50–70% of **heart-rate reserve (HRR).**

Low-intensity, or 50% of HRR	Moderate-intensity, or 70% of HRR
HRR = 173 – 90 = 83 THR = (83 x 0.50) + 90 THR = 132	HRR = 173 – 90 = 83 THR = (83 x 0.70) + 90 THR = 148

As exercise duration increases, it is advisable to watch out for **cardiovascular drift.** Increases in heart rate often occur as exercise duration increases, even without an increase in intensity levels. This is likely due to gradual increases in core temperature, dehydration, and blood redistribution. It is also advisable to incorporate the use of **ratings of perceived exertion (RPE)** into each client's intensity regulation (see Table 12-3, page 324).

Blood Pressure

Blood pressure is defined as the outward force exerted by the blood on the vessel walls. It is generally recorded as two numbers. The higher number, the **systolic blood pressure (SBP),** represents the pressure created by the heart as it pumps blood into circulation via ventricular contraction. This represents the greatest pressure during one cardiac cycle. The lower number, the **diastolic blood pressure (DBP),** represents the pressure that is exerted on the artery walls as blood remains in the arteries during the filling phase of the cardiac cycle, or between beats when the heart relaxes. It is the minimum pressure that exists within one cardiac cycle. Blood pressure is measured within the arterial system. The standard site of measurement is the brachial artery, given its easy accessibility and the ability to hold it level to the heart position.

Blood pressure is measured indirectly by listening to the **Korotkoff sounds,** which are sounds made from vibrations as blood moves along the walls of the vessel. These sounds are only present when some degree of wall deformation exists. If the vessel has unimpeded blood flow, no vibrations are heard. However, under the pressure of a blood pressure cuff, vessel deformity facilitates hearing these sounds. This deformity is created as the air bladder within the cuff is inflated, restricting the flow of blood.

When inflated to pressures greater than the highest pressure that exists within a cardiac cycle, the brachial artery collapses, preventing blood flow. As the air is slowly released from the bladder, blood begins to flow past the compressed area, creating turbulent flow and vibration along the vascular wall. The first BP phase, signified by the onset of tapping Korotkoff sounds, corresponds with SBP. DBP is indicated by the fourth (significant muffling of sound) and fifth (disappearance of sound) phases (Figure 12-4). As the cuff is continuously

Figure 12-4
Korotkoff sounds and blood-pressure phases

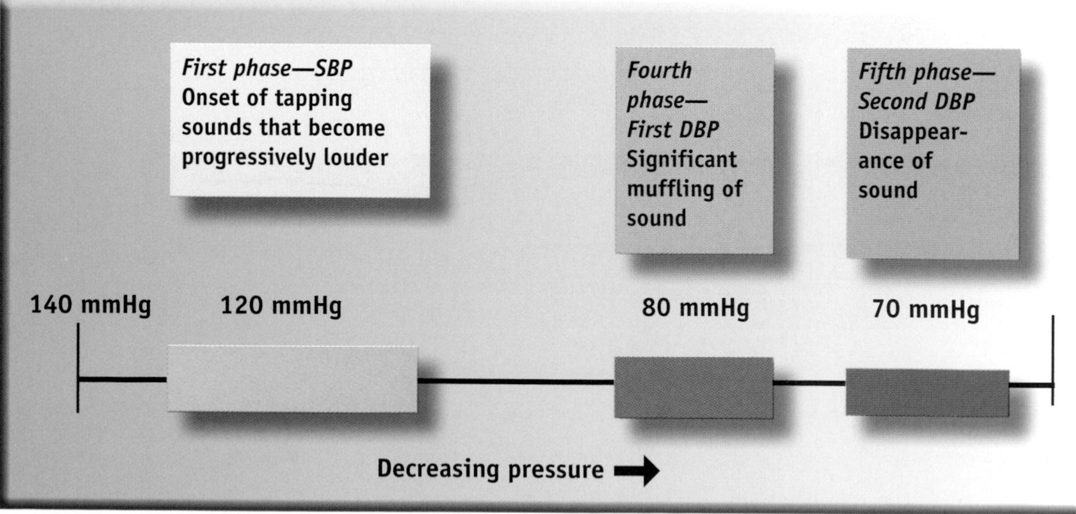

Note: SBP = Systolic blood pressure; DBP = Diastolic blood pressure

released, blood pressure within the vessel increases and eventually will exceed the pressure within the cuff. At this point, the blood pressure completely distends the vessel wall back to its original shape and the Korotkoff sounds will fade (fourth phase) and then disappear (fifth phase). Typically, in adults with normal blood pressure, the fifth phase is recorded as the DBP. However, in children and adults with a fifth phase below 40 mmHg, but who appear healthy, the fourth phase may be used.

Equipment:

- Sphygmomanometer (BP cuff)
- Stethoscope
- Chair

Procedure:

- Have the client sit with both feet flat on the floor for five minutes. *Note:* If the client is seated on an exam table as opposed to a chair, DBP may be increased by 6 mmHg. Crossing the legs or other changes in body position may affect SBP readings.
- Cuff placement:
  - ✓ While the right arm is considered standard, many individuals favor placing the cuff on the left arm due to the increased proximity to the heart, which amplifies the heart sounds. *Note:* Up to 20% of people will show a significant difference in BP readings between the right and left arms. Such a difference can be clinically significant and should be reported to the person's healthcare provider.
    - Smoothly and firmly wrap the blood pressure cuff around the arm with its lower margin about 1 inch (2.5 cm) above the antecubital space (i.e., the inside of the elbow). The tubes should cross the antecubital space. *Note:* In extremely obese individuals, a more accurate reading may be obtained by placing the cuff on the forearm and listening over the radial artery.
    - Since BP cuffs come in a variety of sizes (Table 12-1), it is important to ensure the correct size is used, as obese or muscular clients may have falsely elevated BP readings, while thin, small-framed individuals may have falsely low BP readings with a standard-sized cuff.
  - ✓ The client's arm should be supported either on an armchair or by the health coach at an angle of 0 to 45 degrees. *Note:* Positioning the arm above or below heart level can sway the reading by 2 mmHg. If the arm is elevated, BP readings may be reduced; if the arm is too low, BP readings may be increased.

Table 12-1

Blood-pressure Cuff Sizes Based on Arm Circumference

Arm Circumference	Size	Label
22 to 26 cm	12 × 22 cm	Small adult
27 to 34 cm	16 × 30 cm	Adult
35 to 44 cm	16 × 36 cm	Large adult

Source: Kaplan, N.M. & Victor, R.G. (2010). *Kaplan's Clinical Hypertension* (10th ed.). Baltimore, Md.: Wolters Kluwer/ Lippincott Williams & Wilkins.

Measuring procedure at rest:

- Turn the bulb knob to close the cuff valve (turning it all the way to the right, no more than finger tight) and rapidly inflate the cuff to 160 mmHg, or 20 to 30 mmHg above the point where the pulse can no longer be felt at the wrist.
- Place the stethoscope over the brachial artery using minimal pressure (do not distort the artery).
  - ✓ The stethoscope should lie flat against the skin and should not touch the cuff or the tubing.
  - ✓ The client's arm should be relaxed and straight at the elbow.
- Release the pressure at a rate of about 2 mmHg per second by slowly turning the knob to the left, listening for the Korotkoff sounds. *Note:* Deflation rates >2 mm per second can lead to a significant underestimation of SBP and overestimation of DBP.
  - ✓ SBP is determined by reading the dial at the first perception of sound (a faint tapping sound).
  - ✓ DBP is determined by reading the dial when the sounds cease to be heard or when they become muffled.
- If a BP reading needs to be repeated on the same arm, allow approximately five minutes between trials so that normal circulation can return to the area.
- Share measurements with the client, as well as the classification of values (Table 12-2).

Note: If abnormal readings result, repeat the measurement on the opposite arm. In fact, many within the medical community are recommending that BP measurements be taken in both arms. If there is a significant discrepancy (>10 mmHg) between readings from arm to arm, it could represent a circulatory problem, and the client should be referred to his or her physician for a medical evaluation (McManus & Mant, 2012).

Common errors in measuring blood pressure include:

- Cuff deflation that is too rapid
- Inexperience of the test administrator or inability of the test administrator to read pressure correctly
- Improper stethoscope placement and pressure
- Improper cuff size (see Table 12-1) or an inaccurate/uncalibrated sphygmomanometer
- Auditory acuity of the test administrator or excessive background noise

Measuring procedure during exercise:

- Blood pressure is very difficult to obtain during exercise due to the excessive amount of movement and noise, unless the person is riding a stationary bicycle.
- Traditionally, when exercise blood pressure measurements are justified, they are usually measured before and following exercise (to monitor against excessive **hypotension**).

Table 12-2

Classification of Blood Pressure for Adults Age 18 and Older*

Category	Systolic (mmHg)		Diastolic (mmHg)
Normal†	<120	and	<80
Prehypertension	120–139	or	80–89
Hypertension‡			
Stage 1	140–159	or	90–99
Stage 2	≥160	or	≥100

* Not taking antihypertensive drugs and not acutely ill. When systolic and diastolic blood pressures fall into different categories, the higher category should be selected to classify the individual's blood pressure status. For example, 140/82 mmHg should be classified as stage 1 hypertension, and 154/102 mmHg should be classified as stage 2 hypertension. In addition to classifying stages of hypertension on the basis of average blood pressure levels, clinicians should specify presence or absence of target organ disease and additional risk factors. This specificity is important for risk classification and treatment.

† Normal blood pressure with respect to cardiovascular risk is below 120/80 mmHg. However, unusually low readings should be evaluated for clinical significance.

‡ Based on the average of two or more readings taken at each of two or more visits after an initial screening.

Note: For individuals with diabetes or chronic kidney disease, HBP is defined as 130/80 mmHg or higher. HBP numbers also differ for children and teens.

Source: Chobanian, A.V. et al. (2003). *JNC 7 Express: The Seventh Report of the Joint National Committee on Prevention, Detection, Evaluation, and Treatment of High Blood Pressure.* NIH Publication No. 03-5233. Washington, D.C.: National Institutes of Health & National Heart, Lung, and Blood Institute.

- A sphygmomanometer with a stand and a hand-held gauge are better choices for measuring BP during exercise.
- If SBP drops during exercise, it should immediately be remeasured prior to terminating the session, just to ensure accuracy in measurement. If the client was anxious prior to the cardiorespiratory assessment, it is likely that the initial exercise SBP reading will drop.

Application:

The relationship between elevated blood pressure and cardiovascular events [e.g., **myocardial infarction** or **cerebrovascular accident (CVA)**] is unmistakable. For individuals 40 to 70 years old, each 20 mmHg increase in resting SBP or each 10 mmHg increase in resting DBP above normal *doubles* the risk of **cardiovascular disease** [American College of Sports Medicine (ACSM), 2014]. A difference of 15 mmHg or more between arms increases risk of **peripheral vascular disease** and **cerebral vascular disease** and is associated with a 70% risk of dying from heart disease (McManus & Mant, 2012). If the health coach discovers an abnormal BP reading, either at rest or during exercise, it is prudent to recommend that the client visit his or her personal physician.

Blood pressure can be reduced with medication or certain behavioral modifications (i.e., exercise, weight loss, sodium restriction, smoking cessation, and stress management). For those with **prehypertension**, BP can realistically be reduced with lifestyle interventions; for those with true clinical **hypertension** (see Table 12-2), it is likely that their personal physicians will want to treat the hypertension with medication *and* lifestyle interventions. The health coach can provide guidance and motivation on appropriate lifestyle-modification practices.

EXPAND YOUR KNOWLEDGE

Understanding Hypertension

Hypertension, also known as high blood pressure, is a significant risk factor for heart disease and stroke and can damage other organs such as the kidneys and eyes. According to the National Heart, Lung, and Blood Institute (NHLBI), one in three Americans has hypertension (Chobanian et al., 2003). Hypertension can go unnoticed for years because, for many people, there are no discernible warning signs. Once detected, hypertension is a very treatable condition, so it is very important for the health coach to assess blood pressure on every new client and report any abnormal findings to his or her personal physician. The health coach may discover fluctuations in blood pressure. Approximately 15 to 20% of people with stage 1 hypertension may exhibit "white coat syndrome," where blood pressure may only be elevated in the presence of a healthcare worker, particularly a physician. In these cases, individuals are recommended to monitor blood pressure at home, with regular recordings throughout the day (Pickering et al., 2005).

Blood pressure is the actual force exerted by the blood on the vessel walls. Blood pressure needs to be sufficient to perfuse blood to all the vital organs. High blood pressure can be dangerous and contributes to many health problems ranging from heart attack to stroke. Low BP, or hypotension, may be normal for many people. Low BP readings are usually only significant when accompanied by other symptoms like dizziness, faintness when changing positions, pale skin color, or chest pain.

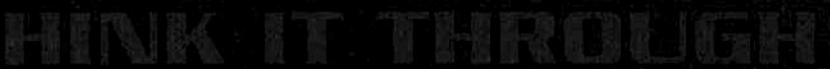

At the beginning of an initial assessment, you take your client's resting HR and blood pressure. After repeatedly measuring your new client's resting blood pressure, you determine that his results fall into the "hypertension" category. How would you handle this situation? What would your next steps be within that initial assessment session?

Ratings of Perceived Exertion

Ratings of perceived exertion are used to subjectively quantify a participant's overall feelings and sensations during the stress of physical activity. Subjective measures of exertion are useful since they can be compared with previous sessions and have been validated against the physiological measure of HR. RPE can be used to complement or replace HRs in providing feedback on exercise intensity (e.g., when the client is taking certain drugs that may blunt the heart-rate response to exercise, such as **beta blockers**). Two standardized ratings exist: the Borg 15-point scale (6 to 20 scale) and a modified 0 to 10 category ratio scale, which is a revision of the original Borg scale (Table 12-3). On the original 6 to 20 Borg scale, each value closely corresponds to a HR. For example:

- Borg score: 6 = corresponding HR of 60 bpm
- Borg score: 12 = corresponding HR of 120 bpm
- Borg score: 20 = corresponding HR of 200 bpm

Common trends:

- Men tend to underestimate exertion, while women tend to overestimate exertion.
- The use of RPE has a significant learning curve that demonstrates deviation toward the mean as the client becomes more familiar with the scale.
- Initially, very **sedentary** individuals may find it difficult to use RPE charts, as they often find any level of exercise fairly hard.
- Conditioned individuals may under-rate their exercise intensity if they focus on the muscular tension requirement of the exercise rather than cardiorespiratory effort.

Recommendations for usage:

- The 6 to 20 scale is difficult to use and should only be utilized if HR equivalents are needed and the actual exercise HR is not a reliable indicator of exertion (e.g., when a client is taking medications that affect HR responses, such as beta blockers).
- The 0 to 10 scale should be used to gauge intensity when the health coach does not need to measure HR via the RPE.

Table 12-3

Ratings of Perceived Exertion (RPE)

RPE	Category Ratio Scale
6	0 Nothing at all
7 Very, very light	0.5 Very, very weak
8	1 Very weak
9 Very light	2 Weak
10	3 Moderate
11 Fairly light	4 Somewhat strong
12	5 Strong
13 Somewhat hard	6
14	7 Very strong
15 Hard	8
16	9
17 Very hard	10 Very, very strong
18	* Maximal
19 Very, very hard	
20	

Data from: Borg, G. (1998). *Borg's Perceived Exertion and Pain Scales*. Champaign, Ill.: Human Kinetics.

Cardiorespiratory Fitness Testing

Each new client will have a unique point of entry into the ACE IFT Model. Therefore, it is up to the health coach to identify the most appropriate assessments. The initial focus for a beginning client is to provide positive experiences and encourage exercise participation; therefore, intensive fitness testing is discouraged. Further fitness testing will likely be conducted as the client progresses.

It is important to note that the physiological demands of exercise can uncover underlying disease or dysfunction that may not be revealed while a person is sedentary. During the administration of any exercise test involving exertion (e.g., a CRF test), health coaches must always be aware of signs or symptoms they can identify that merit immediate test termination and referral to a more qualified healthcare professional. These symptoms include:

- Onset of **angina pectoris** or angina-like symptoms that center around the chest
- Significant drop (>10 mmHg) in SBP despite an increase in exercise intensity
- Excessive rise in blood pressure: SBP >250 mmHg or DBP >115 mmHg
- Fatigue, shortness of breath, difficult or labored breathing, or wheezing (does not include heavy breathing due to intense exercise)
- Signs of poor perfusion: lightheadedness, pallor (pale skin), **cyanosis**, nausea, or cold and clammy skin
- Increased nervous system symptoms (e.g., **ataxia,** dizziness, confusion, and syncope)
- Leg cramping or **claudication**
- Physical or verbal manifestations of severe fatigue

The test should also be terminated if the client requests to stop or the testing equipment fails.

CRF is an indication of how well the body can perform dynamic activity using large muscle groups at a moderate to high intensity for extended periods of time. CRF depends on the efficiency and interrelationship of the cardiovascular, respiratory, and skeletal muscle systems.

CRF assessments are also valuable mechanisms in assessing the overall health of an individual. Exercise testing for cardiorespiratory fitness is useful to:

- Determine **functional capacity,** using predetermined formulas based on age, gender, and in some cases, body weight
- Determine a level of cardiorespiratory function [commonly defined as either **maximal oxygen uptake ($\dot{V}O_2$max)** or **metabolic equivalent (MET)** level] that serves as a starting point for developing goals for aerobic conditioning
- Determine any underlying cardiorespiratory abnormalities that signify progressive stages of cardiovascular disease
- Periodically reassess progress following a structured fitness program

The risk of heart attack and sudden cardiac death during exercise among fitness facility members, though very low, still exists. The risk can be further reduced with appropriate pre-exercise screening and careful observation of clients during and following exercise.

$\dot{V}O_2$max, an excellent measure of cardiorespiratory efficiency, is an estimation of the body's ability to use oxygen for energy, and is closely related to the functional capacity of the heart and circulatory system. Measuring $\dot{V}O_2$max in a laboratory involves the collection and analysis of exhaled air during maximal exercise. Conducting a cardiorespiratory assessment at maximal effort is not always feasible and can actually place certain populations at risk. Therefore, it is recommended that submaximal tests be used in the fitness setting.

Submaximal cardiorespiratory assessments will provide accurate values that can be extrapolated to determine expected maximal efforts. In exercising individuals, as workload increases, so do HR and **oxygen uptake.** In fact, HR and oxygen uptake exhibit a fairly linear relationship to workload. This relationship allows the health coach to accurately estimate $\dot{V}O_2$max from the heart-rate response to exercise with fairly good accuracy. The lack of accuracy related to estimated maximal oxygen uptake is influenced by two key variables:

- Most estimations of $\dot{V}O_2$max are based on the calculation of "220 – Age" for estimating MHR (Fox, Naughton, & Haskell, 1971). This formula is subject to a standard deviation of approximately ±12 beats per minute (bpm). This means that in a room of 100 40-year-old individuals (for whom this standard MHR calculation would yield an MHR of 180 bpm), the actual MHR for 68% of them would range between 168 and 192 bpm, while the remaining 32% would fall further outside that range.
- Maximal oxygen uptake is determined by estimating MHR at submaximal workloads. The charts and equations that are used to determine maximal oxygen uptake are based on the assumption that everyone expends exactly the same amount of energy and uses the same amount of oxygen at any given work rate (remember, $\dot{V}O_2$max is calculated from equations devised after repeated tests that actually measured oxygen uptake). For this reason, a submaximal test is likely to *underestimate* the true maximum for an individual who is very deconditioned and *overestimate* $\dot{V}O_2$max for a very fit individual. The true value of submaximal cardiorespiratory testing is seen when the client can repeat the same test a few months later and then compare his or her individual test results.

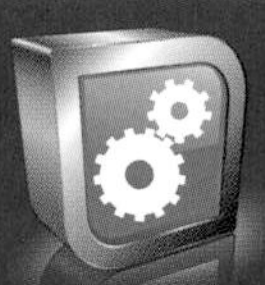

EXPAND YOUR KNOWLEDGE

Maximal Heart Rate: How Useful Is the Prediction Equation?

Two methods exist for determining maximal heart rate (MHR). The most accurate way is to directly measure the MHR with an EKG monitoring device during a graded exercise test. The other way is to estimate MHR by using a simple prediction equation or formula. In 1971, the formula "220 – Age" was introduced and was widely accepted by the health and fitness community (Fox, Naughton, & Haskell, 1971). However, the validity of the formula has come under attack for several reasons. The subjects used in the study to determine the formula were not representative of the general population. In addition, even if the prediction equation did represent a reasonable average, a significant percentage of individuals will not fit the average. In fact, standard deviations of plus or minus 10 to 20 beats per minute have been observed. Consequently, basing a client's exercise intensity (i.e., training HR) on a potentially flawed estimation of MHR is somewhat dubious. Using a submaximal fitness test will provide a more reliable MHR value. When the training HR is based on an estimated MHR, it should be used in combination with the ratings of perceived exertion scale. Health coaches should modify the intensity of the workout if a client reports a high level of perceived exertion, even if his or her training HR has not been achieved.

Cardiorespiratory Assessments for the Lab or Fitness Center

Cardiorespiratory testing in a laboratory or fitness center provides a controlled environment in which the setting is generally more private, the temperature is usually constant, and all of the equipment is centrally located for easy test administration.

GXTs conducted in laboratory and fitness settings typically use a treadmill, cycle ergometer, arm ergometer, or aerobic step to measure cardiorespiratory fitness, though cycle ergometer, arm ergometer, and step tests are not the most suitable for the obese populations and are not presented in this manual. Some of the tests are administered in stages that incorporate gradual increases in exercise intensity, while others measure the heart-rate response to a single-stage bout of exercise. On a treadmill, the intensity is raised by increasing the speed and/or incline.

GXTs are used extensively in both clinical and fitness settings. In the clinical setting, a GXT is typically performed to maximal exertion, which means that the test is terminated when the client can no longer tolerate the activity, when signs or symptoms arise that warrant test termination, or when the client has achieved a predetermined age-predicted MHR. There are certain risks associated with maximal GXTs, the most severe being cardiac arrest. For this reason, maximal exercise tests are not typically administered in fitness centers or other nonclinical settings.

Submaximal exercise testing is safer and, in many cases, provides a reliable indicator of maximal effort. The information obtained from a submaximal exercise test can be used to determine $\dot{V}O_2$max. Table 12-4 defines the norms for maximal oxygen uptake, or "aerobic fitness."

The workload can also be measured in METs. Workload is a reflection of oxygen uptake and, hence, energy use (i.e., 1 MET is the equivalent of oxygen uptake at rest, or approximately 3.5 mL/kg/min). For example, most **activities of daily living (ADL)** require a functional capacity of 5 METs.

In addition to measuring cardiorespiratory fitness, a GXT is also a valuable tool in identifying those who are at risk of a coronary event. The major indicators include the following (ACSM, 2014; Miller, 2008):

- *A decrease—or a significant increase—in blood pressure with exercise:* SBP that is lower during exercise compared to SBP taken immediately

Table 12-4

Percentile Values for Maximal Oxygen Uptake (mL/kg/min)

	Age				
Percentile*	20-29	30-39	40-49	50-59	60-69
Men					
90	54.0	52.5	51.1	46.8	43.2
80	51.1	48.9	46.8	43.3	39.5
70	48.2	46.8	44.2	41.0	36.7
60	45.7	44.4	42.4	38.3	35.0
50	43.9	42.4	40.4	36.7	33.1
40	42.2	41.0	38.4	35.2	31.4
30	40.3	38.5	36.7	33.2	29.4
20	39.5	36.7	34.6	31.1	27.4
10	35.2	33.8	31.8	28.4	24.1
Women					
90	47.5	44.7	42.4	38.1	34.6
80	44.0	41.0	38.9	35.2	32.3
70	41.1	38.8	36.7	32.9	30.2
60	39.5	36.7	35.1	31.4	29.1
50	37.4	35.2	33.3	30.2	27.5
40	35.5	33.8	31.6	28.7	26.6
30	33.8	32.3	29.7	27.3	24.9
20	31.6	29.9	28.0	25.5	23.7
10	29.4	27.4	25.6	23.7	21.7

*To realize the health benefits of aerobic conditioning, clients should aim to achieve >30th percentile.

Note: $\dot{V}O_2$max below the 20th percentile is associated with an increased risk of death from all causes (Blair et al., 1995).

Study population for the data set was predominately white and college educated. A modified Balke treadmill test was used with $\dot{V}O_2$max estimated from the last grade/speed achieved. The following may be used as descriptors for the percentile rankings: well above average (90), above average (70), average (50), below average (30), and well below average (10).

Reprinted with permission from The Cooper Institute, Dallas, Texas from *Physical Fitness Assessments And Norms For Adults And Law Enforcement*. Available online at www.cooperinstitute.org.

prior to the test in the same posture as the test is being performed (i.e., baseline measurement); SBP that rises above 250 mmHg during exercise; or SBP that increases during immediate post-exercise recovery

- *An inadequate HR response to exercise:* An increase in HR of <80% of age-predicted value or <62% for clients on beta blocker medication during exercise
- *Exercise duration:* Stated simply, the longer the individual can tolerate the treadmill test, the less likely he or she is to die soon of CAD—or of any cause.
- *Heart-rate recovery:* An individual standing in an upright position should show a reduction of 12 bpm at one minute post-exercise, and an individual in a sitting position should show a reduction of 22 bpm two minutes post-exercise.

Visit www.ACEfitness.org/HealthCoachResources to download a free PDF of a physical-fitness assessment form that you can use to record the results of all assessments introduced in this chapter, as well as other forms and assessment tools that you can use throughout your career as a health coach.

The health coach should clarify important information from the client's health-history questionnaire and review a few key procedural issues prior to any cardiorespiratory assessment:

- Medication/supplement usage. If the client is on a beta blocker (atenolol, metropolol, or propranalol), the test will be invalid due to a blunted HR response. Use of stimulants may exaggerate the HR response.
- Recent musculoskeletal injury or limiting orthopedic problem(s)
- Any sickness or illness (cold, flu, or infection)
- Time of last meal or snack (especially important to avoid **hypoglycemia**)
- It is the client's responsibility to perform the test as advised, as the validity of fitness testing is based on precise protocols being followed.
- Clients should provide RPE when requested, as well as information on personal signs and symptoms.
- The health coach will assess HR and BP at specific intervals throughout the test. The test may be terminated if there is an inappropriate HR or BP response to exercise, even without complaints from the client.
- The health coach should remind the client that the test will immediately cease if the client reports any significant discomfort at any point during the test. The client is free to stop the test at any time, for any reason.

The following variables should be constantly assessed and recorded during an exercise test:

- *Heart rate:* Monitor continuously and record during the last 15 seconds of each minute
- *Blood pressure:* Measure and record during the last 45 seconds of each stage
- *Ratings of perceived exertion (RPE):* Record during the last five seconds of each minute (see Table 12-3)
- *Signs and symptoms (S/S):* Monitor continuously and record both personal observations and subjective comments from the client

Again, aerobic testing can be initiated during the second week of training, if deemed appropriate by the health coach. The following three tests are described in this section:

- Ventilatory threshold testing (**talk test**) using a treadmill
- Treadmill test: Balke & Ware treadmill exercise test
- Field test: Rockport fitness walking test (1 mile)

If any negative signs or symptoms arise during exercise testing, the client's personal physician should be notified immediately. Emergency medical services (EMS) should be called when severe signs or symptoms arise, including the following:

- Unconsciousness
- Chest pain or other signs or symptoms of heart attack or cardiac distress
- Extreme difficulty in breathing that cannot be controlled with discontinuing exercise and several minutes of rest

Ventilatory Threshold Testing/Talk Test

Ventilatory threshold testing is based on the physiological principle of ventilation. As exercise intensity increases, ventilation increases in a somewhat linear manner. The deflection points seen in Figure 12-5 are associated with metabolic changes within the body. The first notable point is called the "crossover" point and represents a level of intensity where blood **lactate** begins to accumulate. This marks the **first ventilatory threshold (VT1).** At lower intensities, fats are the major fuel and only small amounts of lactic acid are being produced. The need for oxygen is met primarily through an increase in **tidal volume** as breathing deepens. Therefore, the ability to talk should not be compromised and should not appear challenging or uncomfortable. Past the crossover point, ventilation rates begin to increase, as a quickened expiration rate helps to blow off more carbon dioxide in an effort to buffer blood lactate, a by-product of burning predominantly carbohydrate. The **second ventilatory threshold (VT2)** is marked by an exaggerated increase in respiratory rate (RR) and associated with a rapid increase in blood lactate (>4.0 mmol). Talking at this point becomes difficult and labored.

Figure 12-5
Ventilatory response to increasing exercise intensity

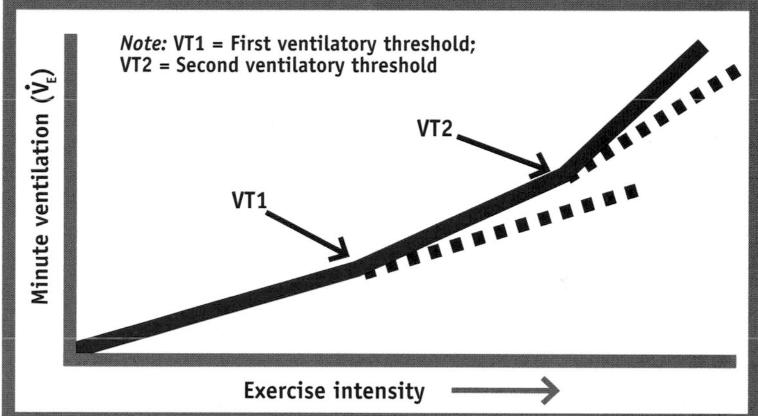

EXPAND YOUR KNOWLEDGE

Understanding the Ventilatory Response to Exercise

During exercise, higher intensities increase respiratory rates, moving larger volumes of air into and out of the lungs. This volume of air, called minute ventilation (V_E), reflects the body's metabolism and defines the volume of air moved through the lungs on a minute-by-minute basis. As exercise intensity progressively increases, the air moving into and out of the respiratory tract increases linearly, or similarly. As the intensity of exercise continues to increase, there is a point at which ventilation starts to increase in a non-linear fashion (i.e., VT1). This point where ventilation deviates from the progressive linear increase corresponds (but is not identical) with the development of muscle and blood acidosis. Blood buffers, which are compounds that help to neutralize acidosis, work to reduce the muscle fiber acidosis. As exercise intensity increases, and the predominant fuel changes from fats to carbohydrates, carbon dioxide increases. The body responds by increasing the ventilatory rate in an effort to expel the excess CO_2.

Some facilities may have metabolic analyzers that can identify VT1 and VT2, but since the majority of health and wellness facilities do not have access to this sort of equipment, field testing can be used to identify these markers. This section reviews field tests for measuring HR at VT1 and VT2. This type of testing is also useful for athletes interested in estimating their lactate threshold.

Since target heart-rate range calculations based on an age-predicted maximum have a significant margin of error, the ventilatory threshold test offers a viable solution for determining exercise training range. The objective of the test is to determine the HR at which talking becomes uncomfortable-to-challenging, but not difficult. This is defined as the intensity where the individual can continue to talk while breathing with minimal discomfort, reflecting an increase in tidal volume. It is before the point where respiratory rate increases significantly, which makes continuous talking difficult.

There are two different assessments for ventilatory threshold testing. Assessing VT1 is important for the deconditioned exerciser and those with certain health risks. With an advanced client, VT2 testing becomes appropriate since higher levels of exercise intensity are required. The end-point of the test is not a predetermined HR, but is based on monitoring changes in metabolism that are determined by the client's ability to talk during exercise (specifically, reciting the Pledge of Allegiance or a similar combination of phrases from memory or reading from text.) *Note:* Reading as opposed to reciting from memory may not be advised if it compromises focus and balance on a treadmill. Conversations with questions and answers are also not suggested, as the test needs to evaluate the challenge of talking continuously, not in brief bursts as in conversation.

Contraindications

This type of testing is not recommended for:

- Individuals with certain breathing problems [**asthma** or other **chronic obstructive pulmonary disease (COPD)**]
- Individuals prone to panic/anxiety attacks, as the labored breathing may create discomfort or spawn an attack

It is important to note that progressing past the point where breathing rate increases significantly and continuous talking becomes difficult is not necessary and will render the test inaccurate.

Equipment:

- Treadmill
- Stopwatch
- HR monitor with chest strap (optional)
- Cue cards (if not using the Pledge of Allegiance); any 30- to 50-word paragraph will do

Pretest procedure:

- As this test involves small, incremental increases in intensity specific to each individual, the testing stages need to be predetermined. The goal is to incrementally increase the workload in small quantities to determine VT1. Large incremental increases may result in the individual passing through VT1, thereby invalidating the test:

- ✓ The recommended workload increases are approximately 0.5 mph, 1% grade, or 15 to 20 watts.
- ✓ The objective is to increase **steady state heart rate (HRss)** at each stage by approximately 5 bpm.
- ✓ Plan to complete this test within eight to 16 minutes to ensure HRss is achieved at each stage. Localized muscle fatigue from longer durations of exercise should not be an influencing factor.
- ✓ Any strength training conducted prior to testing can cause a noticeably higher exercise HR. Thus, clients should be tested before performing any resistance-training exercises or assessments.

- Measure pre-exercise HR and BP (if necessary), both sitting and standing, and then record the values on the testing form.
- Describe the purpose of this graded exercise test. Each stage of the test lasts one to two minutes to achieve a HRss at each workload.
- Toward the latter part of each state (i.e., last 20 to 30 seconds), measure the HR and then ask the client to recite the Pledge of Allegiance or another predetermined text. The client's ability to talk without difficulty will be evaluated. A HRss must be achieved prior to moving to the next stage (within 2 or 3 bpm).
- Conversations with the client during testing are discouraged, as the test needs to evaluate the challenge of talking continuously, not in brief conversational bursts.
- Allow the client to walk on the treadmill to warm up and get used to the apparatus. A three- to five-minute warm-up at an RPE of 2 to 3 is recommended. The HR should be kept below 120 bpm.
- Clients should avoid holding the handrails on the treadmill. If the client is too unstable without holding onto the rails, consider using another testing modality, as the results of a treadmill test will not be accurate if the client must hold on to the handrails the entire time.

Test protocol and administration:

- Once the client has warmed up, adjust the workload intensity so the client's HRss is approximately 120 bpm, or a 3- to 4-out-of-10 effort.
- Each stage should be one to two minutes in length, allowing enough time to achieve HRss. During the last 20 to 30 seconds of each stage, ask the client to recite the predetermined text. At the completion of this task, ask the client to identify whether he or she felt this task was easy, uncomfortable-to-challenging, or difficult.
- Record the client's response.
- If VT1 is not achieved, eliciting a response of "uncomfortable-to-challenging," progress through the successive stages, repeating the protocol at each stage until breathing is labored and VT1 is reached.
- At the end of this stage, increase the intensity until the client's HR achieves steady state at the new intensity. Record HRss, repeat the test, and evaluate the breathing discomfort.
- Once the client's response is "uncomfortable," or the health coach notices that

breathing has become difficult (associated with a significant increase in breathing rate), note the client's HR, terminate the test, and begin the three- to five-minute cool-down process.

- Continue to observe the client, as negative symptoms can arise immediately post-exercise.
- The final exercise HR that corresponds to an "uncomfortable" response is recorded on the testing form as the VT1 HR.
- Ideally, the test should be conducted on two separate occasions with the same exercise modality to determine an average VT1 HR. *Note:* HR varies between treadmills, bikes, etc., so it is important to conduct the tests with the exercise modality that the client uses most frequently.

The HR at VT1 can now be used as an objective target for determining an appropriate exercise intensity. Those interested in sports conditioning and/or competition would benefit from training at higher intensities, but those interested in general health and fitness are well served to stay at, or slightly below, this exercise intensity. Periodic reassessments can be performed to evaluate changes in metabolic functioning and fitness level.

Second Ventilatory Threshold

Another important metabolic marker is the determination of a client's lactate threshold, the point at which lactic acid accumulates at rates faster than the body can buffer and remove it. This marker represents an exponential increase in the concentration of blood lactate, indicating an exercise intensity that can no longer be sustained. This is an important marker, as it represents the highest sustainable level of exercise intensity, a strong indicator of exercise performance. Continually measuring blood lactate is an accurate method to determine VT2. However, the cost of lactate analyzers and handling of biohazardous materials make it improbable for most fitness facilities. Consequently, field tests have been created to challenge an individual's ability to sustain high intensities of exercise for a predetermined duration to estimate VT2. This entails sustaining the highest intensity during a single bout of steady-state exercise, which mandates high levels of conditioning and experience in pacing. Consequently, VT2 testing is only recommended for well-conditioned individuals with performance-oriented goals. Refer to the *ACE Personal Trainer Manual* for more information on VT2 testing.

Treadmill Exercise Testing

The type of test chosen to assess cardiorespiratory fitness should be individualized and based on the client's capabilities. Walking on a treadmill may make some clients uneasy. In such cases, a field walking test could be used. Ideally, a submaximal graded fitness test should take between eight and 12 minutes (ACSM, 2014), allowing ample time in each stage to allow the client's HR to reach HRss.

Treadmill tests are a simple and reliable means of assessing cardiorespiratory fitness. The type of treadmill test used will also depend on the client. While there are several treadmill tests used in fitness settings, the Balke & Ware treadmill test is preferred for older and deconditioned clients, because the progressive increases in workload are more modest, making it the best option for most overweight clients.

Contraindications

Treadmill exercise testing should be avoided in a client with:

- Visual or balance problems, or who cannot walk on a treadmill without using the handrails
- Orthopedic problems that create pain with prolonged walking. Low-back pain (LBP) can be aggravated at inclines exceeding 3 to 5%. As obese individuals may suffer from both balance and orthopedic issues, treadmill testing may not be an appropriate modality for them.
- Foot neuropathy

Balke & Ware Treadmill Exercise Test

The Balke & Ware treadmill test is a common treadmill test used in both clinical and fitness settings to assess cardiorespiratory fitness. The test is administered in one- to three-minute stages until the desired HR is achieved or symptoms limit test completion. In a clinical setting, the test is typically performed to maximal effort to evaluate cardiac function in addition to fitness. When performed in a fitness setting, this test should be terminated when the client achieves 85% of his or her age-predicted MHR. Since speed is held constant, this test is more appropriate for deconditioned individuals, the elderly, and those with a history of cardiovascular disease.

Equipment:

- Commercial treadmill
- Stopwatch
- Stethoscope and sphygmomanometer
- RPE scale
- HR monitor (optional)

Pretest procedures:

- Measure pre-exercise HR, sitting and standing, and record the values on a testing form or data sheet.
- Estimate the submaximal target exercise HR (MHR x 0.85). Record the value on a testing form.
- Discuss RPE and remind the client that he or she will be asked for RPE levels throughout the test.
- Describe the purpose of the treadmill test. The protocols for men and women are different, as illustrated in Table 12-5:
  - ✓ For men, the treadmill speed is set at 3.3 mph, with the incline starting at 0%. After 1 minute the incline is raised to 2% and increased by 1% each minute thereafter until any test termination criteria is achieved (i.e., signs, symptoms, or 85% of MHR).
  - ✓ For women, the treadmill speed is set at 3.0 mph, with the incline starting at 0%. After three minutes the incline is raised to 2.5% and increased by 2.5% every three minutes thereafter until any test termination criteria is achieved (i.e., signs, symptoms, or 85% MHR).
- Secure the BP cuff on the client's arm (tape the cuff in place with medical tape to avoid slippage). Check the accuracy of the HR monitor if one is being used.
- Allow the client to walk on the treadmill for three to five minutes to warm up and get used to the apparatus. He or she should avoid holding the handrails. If the client is too

Table 12-5

Balke & Ware Treadmill Exercise Test Protocol

Minute	Incline (Males)	Incline Females)
1	0	0
2	2	
3	3	
4	4	2.5
5	5	
6	6	
7	7	5.0
8	8	
9	9	
10	10	7.5
11	11	
12	12	
13	13	10
14	14	
15	15	
16	16	12.5

Note: This test utilizes a constant speed of 3.3 mph for men and 3.0 mph for women.

unstable without holding onto the rails, consider using another testing modality, as test results will not be accurate.

Test protocol and administration:

- This treadmill test begins at 3.0 mph for a female client or 3.3 mph for a male client with a 0% incline.
- Assess and record exercise HR and RPE at each minute; assess and record exercise BP with 30 seconds to go in each stage.
- The stages progress as shown in Table 12-5.
- The test should be performed until 85% maximal effort is achieved or until symptoms develop that warrant test termination.
- Upon completion of the test, allow the client to cool down on the treadmill by walking at a moderate speed until breathing returns to normal and HR drops below 100 bpm.
- Estimate $\dot{V}O_2$max and maximal MET level using the following conversion formulas (Pollock et al., 1982; 1976).
  ✓ Men: $\dot{V}O_2$max = 1.444 (time in minutes) + 14.99
  ✓ Women: $\dot{V}O_2$max = 1.38 (time in minutes) + 5.22
  ✓ To calculate METs, divide the $\dot{V}O_2$max by 3.5 mL/kg/min
- Record all values on the testing form.
- Continue to observe the client as he or she cools down, as negative symptoms can arise immediately post-exercise.
- Using Table 12-4, rank the client's maximal oxygen uptake.

Field Testing

Most field tests are simple to administer, involve very little expense, and can even be used for testing multiple clients. Many of the field tests described in this section can also be self-administered, allowing clients to periodically reassess their own progress.

Since many of the field tests can be performed outside, it is important to be mindful of extreme weather conditions and avoid exercise testing during extreme heat and humidity or when the weather turns cold.

Contraindications

Outdoor walk/run testing would not be appropriate:

- In extreme weather conditions
- For individuals with health challenges that would preclude continuous walking (e.g., extreme obesity, intermittent leg claudication, or **osteoarthritis** of the lower extremity)
- For individuals with breathing difficulties exacerbated by pollution or outdoor allergens

Running tests are not recommended for those who are deconditioned.

Rockport Fitness Walking Test (1 Mile)

The purpose of the Rockport fitness walking test is to estimate $\dot{V}O_2$max from a client's HRss response. This test involves the completion of a 1-mile course as fast as possible, with $\dot{V}O_2$max being calculated using the client's HRss or immediate post-exercise HR and his or her 1-mile walk time. This test is suitable for many individuals, easy to administer, and inexpensive to conduct. However, considering that walking may not elicit much of a cardiorespiratory challenge to conditioned individuals, this test will generally under-predict $\dot{V}O_2$max in fit individuals and is therefore not appropriate for that population group. A running track is the preferred testing surface. Most running tracks are a quarter-mile in distance, which means that walking four times around on the innermost lane will equal 1 mile. This test is also suitable for testing large groups of people, and clients can periodically reassess their own fitness levels by self-administering this test. This method of testing would also be preferred for a client who intends to walk/run outdoors as his or her primary mode of fitness training.

Research has shown that clients using a treadmill and walking on a track achieved similar $\dot{V}O_2$max results. When the weather is inclement and/or a track is not available, a treadmill test can be administered (Nieman, 2010).

Equipment:

- Quarter-mile track or suitable alternative (e.g., treadmill)
- Stopwatch
- RPE chart
- HR monitor with chest strap (optional)

Pretest procedure:

- After explaining the purpose of the 1-mile Rockport fitness walking test, define the 1-mile course.
- The goal of the test is to walk as fast as possible for 1 mile. Running is not permitted for this test. Pacing is strongly recommended throughout the test.
- Discuss RPE and remind the client that he or she will be asked for perceived exertion levels throughout the test.

Test protocol and administration:

- On the health coach's "go," the stopwatch is started and the client begins.
- The client's 1-mile time, RPE, and HRss, or immediate post-exercise HR, are recorded on the testing form. If a HR monitor is not being used, a manual pulse count should be done for 15 seconds and then multiplied by four to determine an accurate HR immediately post-exercise.
- Encourage a three- to five-minute cool-down, followed by stretching of the lower extremities.

Evaluation of performance:

- The client's information is plugged into one of the following formulas (ACSM, 2008):
  - ✓ *Females:* $\dot{V}O_2$ (mL/kg/min) = 132.853 – (0.1692 x Weight in kg) – (0.3877 x Age) – (3.265 x Walk time in minutes to the nearest 100th) – (0.1565 x HR)
  - ✓ *Males:* $\dot{V}O_2$ (mL/kg/min) = 139.168 – (0.1692 x Weight in kg) – (0.3877 x Age) – (3.265 x Walk time, expressed in minutes to the nearest 100th) – (0.1565 x HR)
- Record the values on the testing form. It is also important to include weather, surface conditions, or any other variables that may have impacted overall time.
- Continue to observe the client, as negative symptoms can arise immediately post-exercise.
- Evaluate the client's score using Table 12-4 , or use Table 12-6 to classify performance using normative data.

Table 12-6		
Normative Values for the Rockport Walking Test		
Rating	Males (Age 30–69)	Females (Age 30–69)
	Time (minutes : seconds)	Time (minutes : seconds)
Excellent	<10:12	<11:40
Good	10:13–11:42	11:41–13:08
High average	11:43–13:13	13:09–14:36
Low average	13:14–14:44	14:37–16:04
Fair	14:45–16:23	16:05–17:31
Poor	>16:24	>17:32
Percentile	Males (Age 18–30)	Females (Age 18–30)
90%	11:08	11:45
75%	11:42	12:49
50%	12:38	13:15
25%	13:38	14:12
10%	14:37	15:03

Adapted with permission from Morrow, J.R. et al. (2011). *Measurement and Evaluation in Human Performance* (4th ed.). Champaign, Ill.: Human Kinetics.

DO THE MATH

Jessica, a 26-year-old client weighing 125 lb (56.8 kg), completes the 1-mile walk in 16:40 with a HRss of 132 bpm. Calculate her $\dot{V}O_2max$.

$\dot{V}O_2max$ = 132.853 – (0.1692 x Weight in kg) – (0.3877 x Age) – (3.265 x Walk time, expressed in minutes to the nearest 100th) – (0.1565 x HR)

= 132.853 – (0.1692 x 56.8) – (0.3877 x 26) – (3.265 x 16.67) – (0.1565 x 132)

= 132.853 – 9.61 – 10.08 – 54.43 – 20.66 = 38.07 mL/kg/min

Application of Information From Cardiorespiratory Fitness Testing

Cardiorespiratory fitness is a strong predictor of **morbidity** and **mortality.** Low levels of cardiorespiratory fitness have been linked to increased risk of premature death from all causes, especially from cardiovascular disease. High levels of cardiorespiratory fitness are associated with increased levels of regular physical activity, which translates to numerous health benefits.

Once a client's cardiorespiratory fitness level has been established, and any cardiovascular health risks have been ruled out, it is important to understand how to safely and efficiently improve upon his or her results. Health coaches should keep in mind that physical fitness exists in a continuum, ranging from basic function and health to peak sports performance. The time and energy commitments required to improve sport performance are obviously much more involved than the requirements for improving overall health.

The *2008 Physical Activity Guidelines for Americans* suggest that adults should participate in structured cardiorespiratory-related physical activity at a moderate intensity for at least 150 minutes per week or a vigorous intensity for at least 75 minutes per week to experience the health benefits of exercise. In addition, it is recommended that most adults incorporate muscle-strengthening activities at least two days a week (U.S. Department of Health and Human Services, 2008).

For clients who are not capable of achieving these recommendations at the outset, reaching this level of activity should be the primary goal during the initial conditioning stage. It is prudent for the health coach to encourage regular participation in cardiorespiratory-endurance activities. Chapter 16 provides guidelines for developing safe and effective cardiorespiratory-endurance exercise plans.

Initially, intensity of exercise is not important. For beginning exercisers, or those who are returning after a significant break, intensity should be kept low in order to promote positive experiences and exercise **adherence.**

If the cardiorespiratory testing was unremarkable, an appropriate fitness program can be initiated. For novice exercisers and those who score in the lowest percentiles, improving on cardiovascular fitness should be addressed in a twofold manner. The first goal is to establish an aerobic base by gradually increasing exercise duration. This allows the body to adapt to the new demands of exercise and respond accordingly (e.g., increase in capillary density, increase in mitochondrial size/number, and enhanced ability to remove lactic acid). Initially, training volume can be increased by 10 to 20% per week until the desired training volume is achieved.

For those who already have a solid cardiorespiratory training base, the second phase of training focuses on increasing aerobic efficiency in an effort to increase $\dot{V}O_2$max. As long as there are no contraindications to higher-intensity training, it is then appropriate to move into the anaerobic-endurance phase, which incorporates higher-intensity steady-state training as well as interval training. The anaerobic-power phase is typically reserved for athletes and those who aim to achieve peak performance levels.

Assessment of Stability Through Static Posture Observation

New clients often enter a supervised fitness and nutrition program with a desire to lose weight, increase energy levels, tone their muscles, or even reduce certain health risks such as hypertension or cancer. Exercise is an integral component in achieving any of these goals. Nonetheless, both cardiorespiratory-endurance and resistance-training activities place extra stress upon the body. For this reason, it is important to assess potential areas of cardiorespiratory or musculoskeletal weakness so as not to exacerbate any underlying conditions.

The initial physical assessments should begin with a basic assessment of standing posture and muscular fitness. When clients have adequate movement efficiency, which is positively influenced by proper posture and good muscular balance and control, the performance of ADL as well as sports and fitness activities requires less energy and poses a reduced risk for musculoskeletal injury. Functional imbalances, such as those that can be detected through basic posture and muscular fitness assessments, should be addressed prior to initiating any physical activities. The following list presents three examples of how functional imbalances can lead to musculoskeletal problems.

- If a client has excessive ankle **pronation,** continuous treadmill walking may reinforce these structural deficiencies and place undue stress on the knee joint.
- If a client comes into the program with weak core muscles, many movement patterns

may be altered under physical stress. For example, a weak core can cause the lower back to arch excessively when performing an overhead shoulder press, placing undue stress on the lumbar spine.

- Posture can be compromised when the body's frame is carrying excessive amounts of body weight. Excessive abdominal fat can contribute to **lordosis** of the lower back that may lead to back pain and dysfunction over time.

Information gained from a thorough postural and muscular fitness assessment can be used to improve musculoskeletal dysfunction and areas of instability, thus improving movement efficiency and overall stability. Figure 12-6 outlines the components included in the basic assessment of posture and muscular fitness.

Figure 12-6
A chronological plan for conducting postural assessments and movement screens

Note: Refer to the *ACE Personal Trainer Manual* for information on muscle length testing and the phases of training.

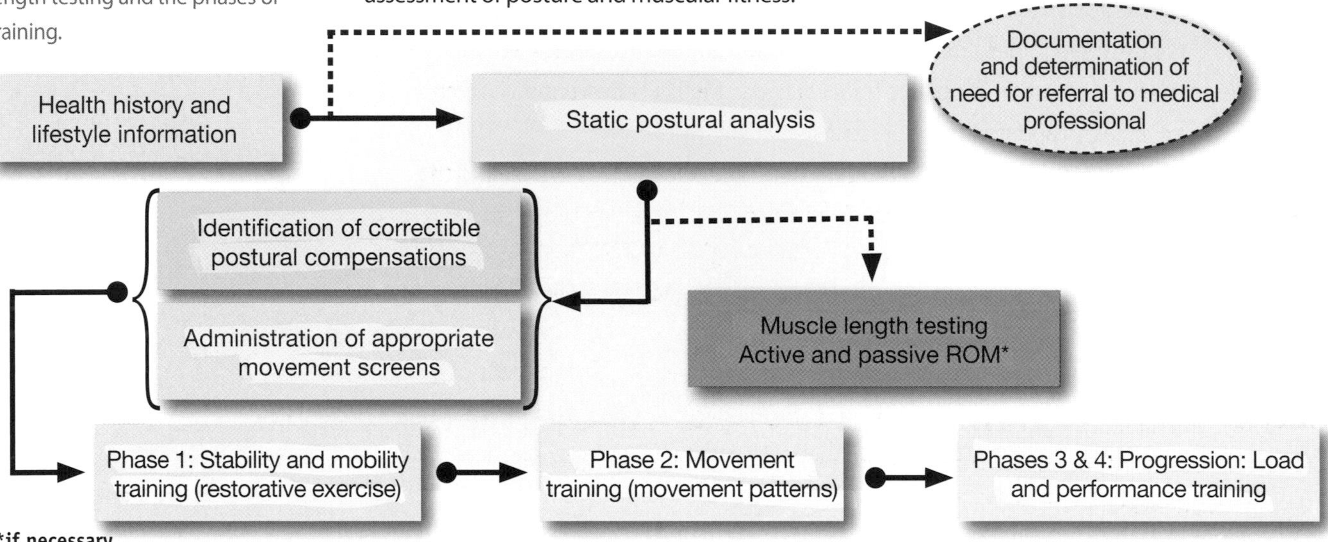

Static Posture

Good posture occurs when bodily parts are symmetrically balanced in all planes. Ideal postural alignment allows the body's muscles, joints, and nerves to function efficiently and effectively. Even digestion and breathing are enhanced by good posture. The structural integrity of the body relies mostly on the deeper, stabilizing muscles of the core that are capable of holding **isometric** contractions for extended periods of time. Improper training techniques, poor body mechanics, or prolonged periods of inactivity (such as sitting at a desk) can create muscle imbalances throughout the body. Muscular imbalance often contributes to a decreased **range of motion (ROM)** at the joints, dysfunctional movement patterns, joint instability, and eventually pain.

Muscle imbalances and postural deviations are often correctable, especially if these are due to certain lifestyle factors and behaviors. Correctable factors include the following:

- Muscular pattern overload, often from repetitive movements (e.g., long-distance running)
- Ungainly positions or movements (e.g., slouching)
- Side dominance (as in tennis players or golfers)
- Lack of joint stability
- Lack of joint mobility
- Imbalanced strength-training program

Non-correctable factors include congenital conditions like **scoliosis**, extreme trauma, skeletal structural deviations, and certain diseases or dysfunctions, like **rheumatoid arthritis.**

Posture and Good Health

With chronic poor posture, the supporting musculature eventually adapts by either shortening or lengthening. Prolonged misalignment adversely affects the structure and function of nerve tissue as well. The resulting muscular imbalances can lead to a number of health issues.

Postural issues tend to vary by population and age of onset. For adolescents, upright posture is important for overall growth and development. Environmental factors (such as overloaded bags and backpacks and poorly designed school desks) and sitting for extended hours in front of a video game or computer can negatively affect posture. Growth spurts and increased self-awareness of body image (which can lead to slouching to hide one's body) can also lead to postural misalignment. Scoliosis, which is more common in adolescent females than males, is the most common idiopathic spinal disorder. Medical intervention is often required in the evaluation and treatment of scoliosis.

Occupational and sports-related activities often contribute to postural deviations in the adult. Prolonged sitting or standing can certainly cause muscle imbalance. Repetitive motions and heavy manual labor can also be harmful, especially if proper body mechanics are not employed. Wearing high heels and restrictive clothing, as well as sleeping on nonsupportive mattresses, can also lead to postural problems.

In older adults, postural changes can occur from a general weakening of the musculoskeletal system that is associated with a decline in physical activity. Age-related limitations caused by poor posture include difficulty with the following actions:

- Walking or standing for prolonged periods
- Stooping, crouching, or kneeling
- Getting in and out of a car
- Reaching or extending the arms overhead

Postural limitations also include pushing and pulling large objects, such as a heavy trashcan. Osteoporosis is also a concern in the aging population and can certainly lead to postural changes such as **kyphosis** and related compensations [including a shift in **center of gravity (COG),** shortening of stride length in gait, and reduction in physical activity].

Assessments are a necessary component of uncovering postural changes. Health and fitness professionals need to develop interventions to minimize both postural deviations and limitations. If not addressed, joint misalignments and muscular weaknesses can become more pronounced.

Static Postural Assessment

A basic postural assessment provides a good starting point to determine muscular imbalances. Figure 12-7 demonstrates proper alignment and anatomical positioning in all three planes:

- **Sagittal plane:** A longitudinal line that divides the body or any of its parts into right and left sections
- **Frontal plane:** A longitudinal line dividing the body into anterior and posterior parts
- **Transverse plane:** A horizontal line that divides the body or any of its parts into superior and inferior sections

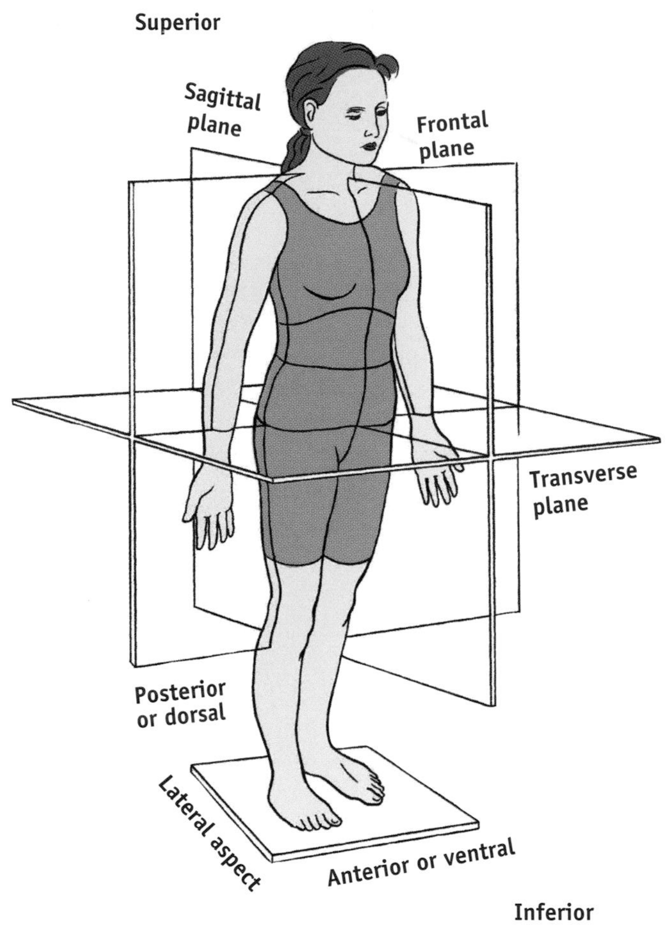

Figure 12-7
Anatomical position and planes of motion

Since all movement is based on a person's posture, a health coach should be able to recognize the important characteristics associated with proper spinal alignment and good overall posture. The following points represent what a health coach should look for when assessing a client's standing posture.

- Lateral view (Figure 12-8a)
  The head should be suspended (not pushed back or dropped forward) with the ears in line with the shoulders, shoulders over hips, hips over knees, and knees over ankles. An imaginary plumb line dropped from overhead should pass through the cervical and lumbar vertebrae, hips, knees, and ankles.
  Clients should maintain the three natural curves of the spine. A decrease or increase in the spinal curvature changes the amount of compression the spine can withstand. The hips can be tucked slightly, particularly for individuals with exaggerated lumbar lordosis, pregnant women, and clients with a large, protruding abdominal area. The knees should be unlocked or soft. Hyperextended knees shift the pelvis, contributing to an increased low-back curve and back strain, along with decreased blood flow to and from the legs.
- Anterior and posterior views (Figures 12-8b and 12-8c)
  The feet should be shoulder-width apart with the weight evenly distributed. Excessive pronation or **supination** could lead to musculoskeletal injuries if a client performs high volumes of exercise with poor foot mechanics. Any individual who complains of joint pain in the ankles, knees, hips, or back should consult his or her healthcare provider, especially if he or she exhibits high arches (excessive supination) or flat feet (excessive pronation). There should be overall symmetry between the two sides of the body with no visible lateral shifting or leaning to one side.
- Anterior view (Figure 12-8b)
  The arms should hang with equal spaces between the arm and the torso, and the hands should hang such that only the thumbs and index fingers are visible (i.e., no knuckles should be visible from the anterior view). A one-sided, asymmetrical space between the arm and the torso indicates a muscular imbalance at the trunk or shoulder girdle complex. Hands that hang with the knuckles facing forward indicate an imbalance of the muscles of the shoulder and/or forearm.
  The kneecaps (patellae) should be oriented forward without deviation into internal or external rotation. A patella that appears rotated inward or outward is an indication of a potential muscular imbalance or structural deviation of the hips and/or foot/ankle complex.

The health coach should keep in mind that the body is rarely symmetrical. Therefore, it is important to focus on areas of obvious muscle imbalance and gross deviations that differ from ideal alignment by more than 1/4 inch (0.6 cm). Client health history will provide

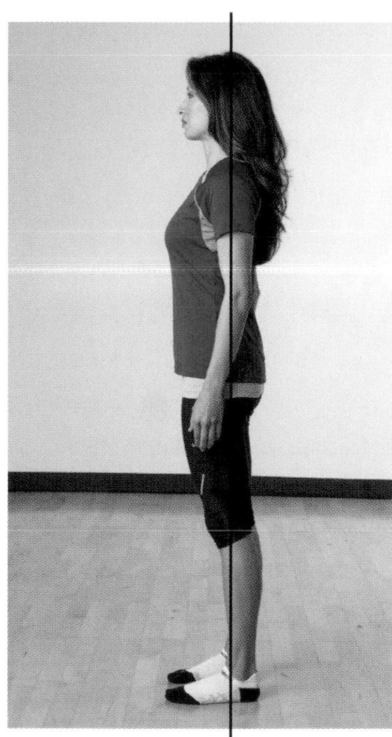
a. Lateral view

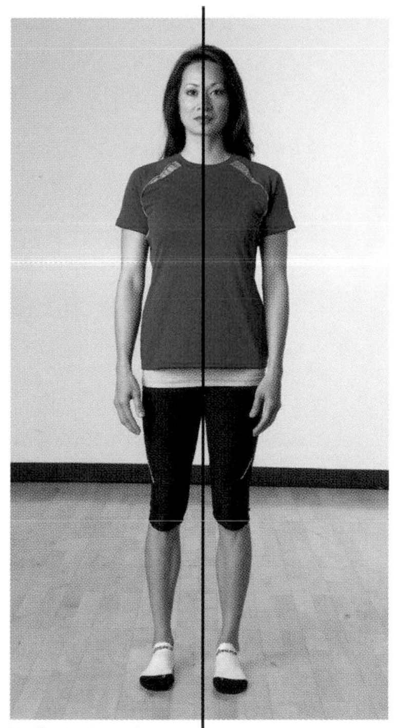
b. Anterior view

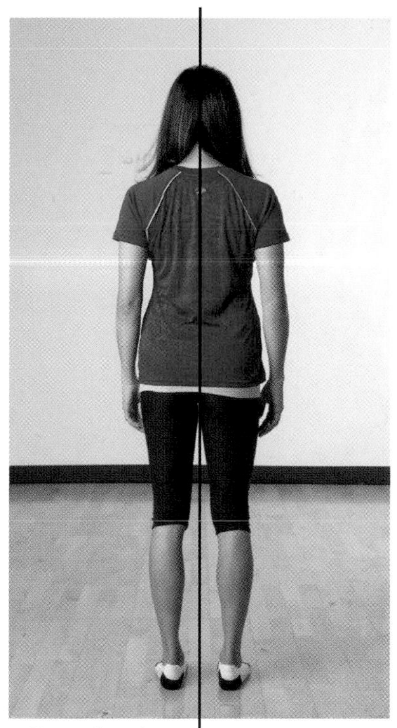
c. Posterior view

Figure 12-8
Assessing a participant's posture

valuable information on past injuries and/or musculoskeletal problems. The visual and manual observations from the postural assessment will enable a targeted focus on any problematic areas. It is important to maintain professional courtesy and respect personal boundaries and **scope of practice.** A health coach is not qualified to diagnose any condition and should be vigilant in referring to a healthcare professional when necessary. If a client reports persistent musculoskeletal pain (i.e., lasting longer than two weeks), or if a structural or congenital condition (e.g., scoliosis) is suspected, the client should be referred to his or her primary healthcare professional and receive medical clearance prior to engaging in a new exercise program.

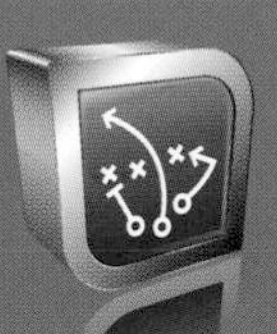

APPLY WHAT YOU KNOW

Familiarize Yourself With Postural Alignment

It is important to be familiar with anatomical landmarks and human anatomy prior to undertaking a comprehensive postural assessment. It is also helpful to maneuver your own body through many of the postural deviations to learn the impact on the kinetic chain. For example, notice how ankle pronation/supination affects the movement of the femur: Stand barefoot on a firm surface while placing your hands on your upper thighs. Standing in front of a full-length mirror is also helpful for visual observation. Notice what happens to the alignment of the knees and the orientation of the thighs when moving between ankle pronation and supination. Also, observe how the calcaneus everts as the ankle moves into pronation. Some of these positions may seem unnatural—but notice which muscles are activated, and thus can become overworked.

There are a number of quality workshops that focus entirely on postural assessments and exercise programming. Visit the ACE website for a comprehensive listing of continuing education courses—www.ACEfitness.org/continuingeducation.

THINK IT THROUGH

Upon visiting with a client during the initial interview process, you observe that she has noticeable kyphosis while she is completing the health-history questionnaire. During the interview she confides that she does not want to undergo any formal physical-fitness testing because it makes her uncomfortable to be scrutinized and compared to norms. What would you do in this situation? How would you handle the topic of postural assessment with this client? How would you approach her training program if she refuses to participate in a baseline postural assessment?

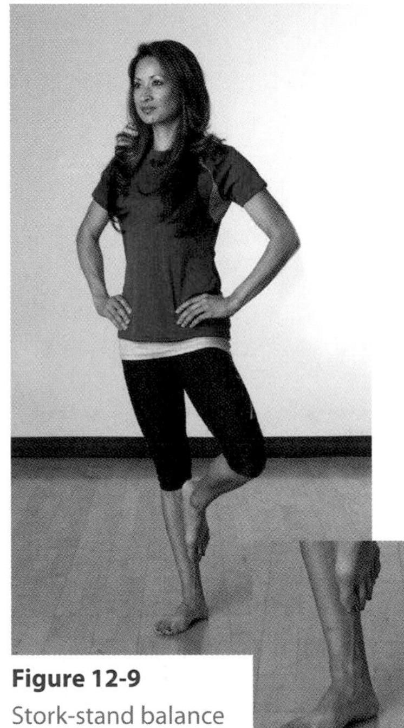

Figure 12-9
Stork-stand balance test: Starting position

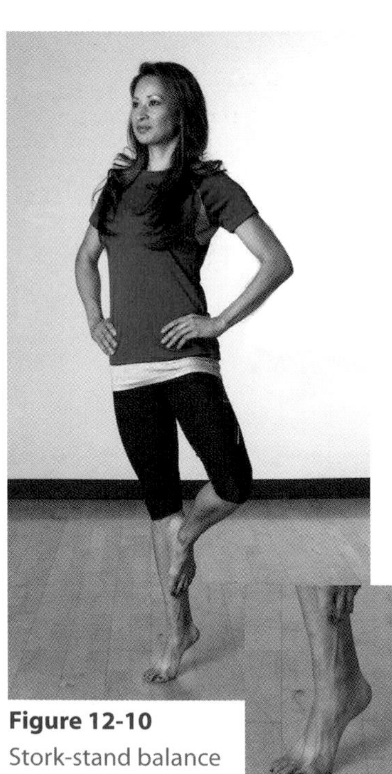

Figure 12-10
Stork-stand balance test: Test position

Balance and the Core

Baseline assessments of balance are important to evaluate the need for comprehensive balance training and core conditioning during the early stages of an exercise program. Often, abdominal obesity shifts the center of gravity anteriorly. This can lead to instability and balance problems. The following two tests measure a client's basic level of static balance.

Stork-stand Balance Test

Source: Johnson & Nelson, 1986

Objective: To assess static balance by standing on one foot in a modified stork-stand position

Equipment:

- Firm, non-slip surface
- Stopwatch

Test protocol and administration:

- Explain the purpose of the test.
- Ask the client to remove his or her shoes and stand with feet together, hands on the hips.
- Instruct the client to raise one foot off the ground and bring that foot to lightly touch the inside of the stance leg, just below the knee (Figure 12-9).
  - ✓ The client must raise the heel of the stance foot off the floor and balance on the ball of the foot (Figure 12-10).
  - ✓ Stand behind the client for support if needed.
  - ✓ Allow 1 minute of practice trials.
  - ✓ After the practice trial, perform the test, starting the stopwatch as the heel lifts off the floor.
- Repeat with the opposite leg.
- Allow up to three trials per leg position and record the best performance on each side.

Observations:

- Timing stops when any of the following occurs:
  - ✓ The hand(s) come off the hips.
  - ✓ The stance or supporting foot inverts, everts, or moves in any direction.
  - ✓ Any part of the elevated foot loses contact with the stance leg.
  - ✓ The heel of the stance leg touches the floor.
  - ✓ The client loses balance.

General interpretation:

- Use the information provided in Table 12-7 to categorize the client's performance.

Table 12-7					
The Stork-stand Balance Test					
Rating	Excellent	Good	Average	Fair	Poor
Males	>50 seconds	41–50 seconds	31–40 seconds	20–30 seconds	<20 seconds
Females	>30 seconds	25–30 seconds	16–24 seconds	10–15 seconds	<10 seconds

Source: Johnson B.L. & Nelson, J.K. (1986). *Practical Measurements for Evaluation in Physical Education* (4th ed.). Minneapolis, Minn.: Burgess.

Sharpened Romberg Test

Sources: Black et al. 1982; Newton, 1989

Objective: To assess static balance and postural control while standing on a reduced base of support while removing visual sensory perception

Equipment:

- Firm, flat, non-slip surface
- Stopwatch

Test protocol and administration:

- Explain the purpose of the test.
- Instruct the client to remove his or her shoes and stand with one foot directly in front of the other (tandem or heel-to-toe position), with the eyes open.
- Ask the client to fold his or her arms across the chest, touching each hand to the opposite shoulder (Figure 12-11).
- Allow sufficient practice trials. Once the client feels stable, instruct the client to close his or her eyes. Start the stopwatch to begin the test.
- Always stand in close proximity as a precaution to prevent falling.
- Continue the test for 60 seconds or until the client exhibits any test-termination cue, as listed in the "Observations" section below.
- Allow up to two trials per leg position and record the best performance on each side.

Observations:

- Continue to time the client's performance until one of the following occurs:
  - ✓ The client loses postural control and balance.
  - ✓ The client's feet move on the floor.
  - ✓ The client's eyes open.
  - ✓ The client's arms move from the folded position.
  - ✓ The client exceeds 60 seconds with good postural control.

General interpretations:

- The client needs to maintain his or her balance with good postural control (without excessive swaying) and not exhibit any of the test-termination criteria for 30 or more seconds.
- The inability to reach 30 seconds is indicative of inadequate static balance and postural control.

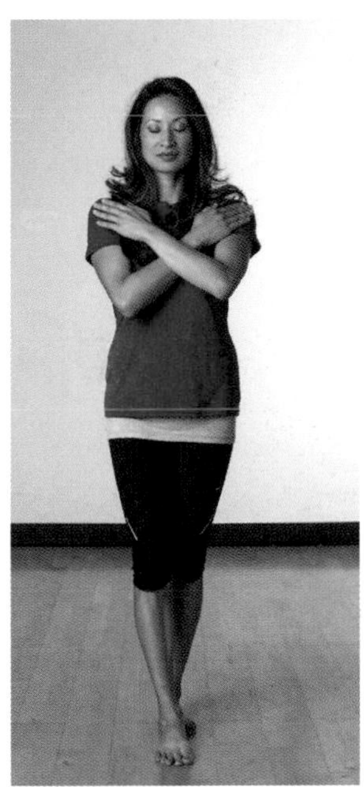

Figure 12-11
Sharpened Romberg test

McGill's Torso Muscular Endurance Test Battery

There is more to core stability than showing off a "six pack." Possessing a strong core is important for the performance of simple ADL, from lifting a heavy laundry basket to swinging a golf club. Core stability involves complex movement patterns that continually change as a function of the three-dimensional torque needed to support the various positions of the body. Dr. Stuart McGill (2007) states that back problems can often be alleviated by improving and then grooving the motor patterns of the abdominal musculature. To determine balanced core strength and stability, it is important to assess all sides of the torso. The benefit of each one of these tests is to assess the interrelationships among the three torso tests. The tests are evaluated collectively. Poor endurance capacity of the torso muscles or an imbalance between these three muscle groups is believed to contribute to low-back dysfunction and core instability.

Trunk Flexor Endurance Test

The flexor endurance test is the first in the battery of three tests that assesses **muscular endurance** of the deep core muscles (i.e., transverse abdominis, quadratus lumborum, and erector spinae). It is a timed test involving a static, isometric contraction of the anterior muscles, stabilizing the spine until the individual exhibits fatigue and can no longer hold the assumed position. As clients move through this battery of tests, make sure they are not holding their breath.

Contraindications

This test may not be suitable for individuals who suffer from low-back pain, have had recent back surgery, and/or are in the midst of an acute low-back flare-up.

Equipment:

- Stopwatch
- Board (or step)

Pretest procedure:

- After explaining the purpose of the flexor endurance test, describe the proper body position.
  - ✓ The starting position requires the client to be seated, with the hips and knees bent to 90 degrees, aligning the hips, knees, and second toe.
  - ✓ Instruct the client to fold his or her arms across the chest, touching each hand to the opposite shoulder, lean against a board positioned at a 60-degree incline, and keep the head in a neutral position (Figure 12-12).
  - ✓ It is important to ask the client to press the shoulders into the board and maintain this position throughout the test.
  - ✓ Instruct the client to engage the abdominals to maintain a flat-to-neutral spine. The back should never be allowed to arch during the test.
  - ✓ The health coach can anchor the toes under a strap or manually stabilize the feet if necessary.
- The goal of the test is to remove the back support and ask the client to hold this 60-degree position for as long as possible.
- Encourage the client to practice this position prior to attempting the test.

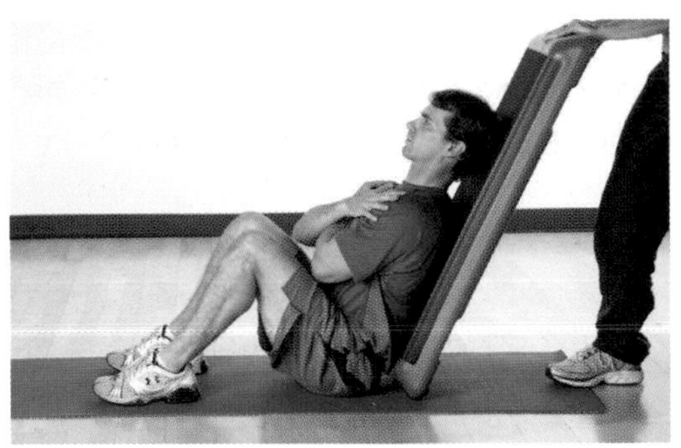
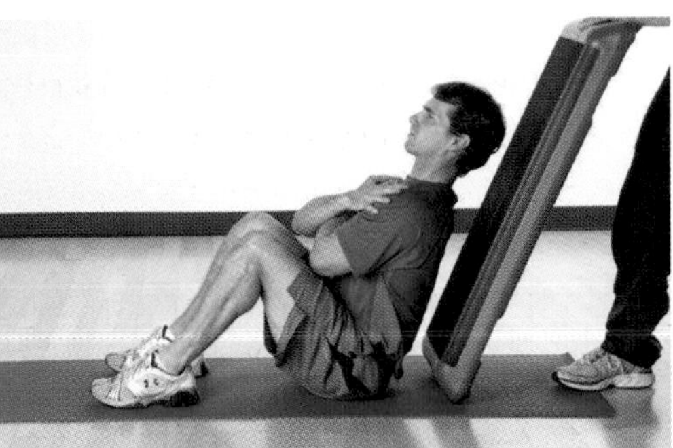

Figure 12-12
Trunk flexor endurance test

Test protocol and administration:

- The health coach starts the stopwatch as he or she moves the board about 4 inches (10 cm) back, while the client maintains the 60-degree, suspended position.
- Terminate the test when there is a noticeable change in the trunk position:
  - ✓ Watch for a deviation from the neutral spine (i.e., the shoulders rounding forward) or an increase in the low-back arch.
  - ✓ No part of the back should touch the back rest.
- Record the client's time on the testing form.

Trunk Lateral Endurance Test

The trunk lateral endurance test, also called the side-bridge test, assesses muscular endurance of the lateral core muscles (i.e., transverse abdominis, obliques, quadratus lumborum, and erector spinae). Similar to the trunk flexor endurance test, this is a set of timed tests involving isometric contractions of the lateral muscles on each side of the trunk that stabilize the spine.

Contraindications

This test may not be suitable for individuals:

- With shoulder pain or weakness
- Who suffer from low-back pain, have had recent back surgery, and/or are in the midst of an acute low-back flare-up

Equipment:

- Stopwatch
- Mat (optional)

Pretest procedure:

- After explaining the purpose of this test, describe the proper body position.
  - ✓ The starting position requires the client to be on his or her side with extended legs, aligning the feet on top of each other or in a tandem position (heel-to-toe).
  - ✓ Have the client place the lower arm under the body and the upper arm on the side of the body.
  - ✓ When the client is ready, instruct him or her to assume a full side-bridge position, keeping both legs extended and the sides of the feet on the floor. The elbow of the lower arm should be positioned directly under the shoulder with the forearm facing out (the forearm can be placed palm down for balance and support), and the upper

arm should be resting along the side or across the chest to the opposite shoulder.

✓ The hips should be elevated off the mat and the body should be in straight alignment (i.e., head, neck, torso, hips, and legs). The torso should only be supported by the client's foot/feet and the forearm (Figure 12-13).

- The goal of the test is to hold this position for as long as possible. Once the client breaks the position, the test is terminated.
- Encourage the client to practice this position prior to attempting the test.

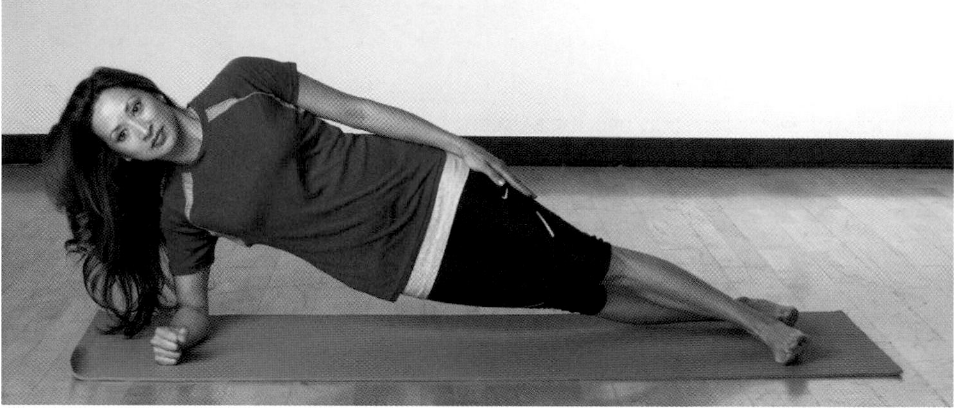

Figure 12-13
Trunk lateral endurance test

Test protocol and administration:

- The health coach starts the stopwatch as the client moves into the side-bridge position.
- Terminate the test when there is a noticeable change in the trunk position.
  - ✓ A deviation from the neutral spine (e.g., the hips dropping downward)
  - ✓ The hips shifting forward or backward in an effort to maintain balance and stability
- Record the client's time on the testing form.
- Repeat the test on the opposite side and record this value on the testing form.

Trunk Extensor Endurance Test

The trunk extensor endurance test is generally used to assess muscular endurance of the torso extensor muscles (i.e., erector spinae, longissimus, ilicostalis, and multifidi). This is a timed test involving an isometric contraction of the trunk extensor muscles that stabilize the spine.

Contraindications

This test may not be suitable for:

- A client with major strength deficiencies, where the subject cannot even lift the torso from a forward flexed position to a neutral position
- A client with a high body mass, in which case it would be difficult for the health coach to support the client's suspended upper-body weight
- Individuals who suffer from low-back pain, have had recent back surgery, and/or are in the midst of an acute low-back flare-up

Equipment:

- Elevated, sturdy exam table
- Nylon strap
- Stopwatch

Pretest procedure:

- After explaining the purpose of the test, explain the proper body position.
  - ✓ The starting position requires the client to be prone, positioning the iliac crests at the table edge while supporting the upper extremity on the arms, which are placed on the floor or on a riser.
  - ✓ Secure the lower extremity with the legs supported on a table while the torso, or upper body, is suspended over the ground.
  - ✓ While the client is supporting the weight of his or her upper body, anchor the client's lower legs to the table using a strap. If a strap is not used, the health coach will have to use his or her own body weight to stabilize the client's legs. Client body size in relation to the health coach may become a limiting factor in this particular test.
- The goal of the test is to hold this position for as long as possible. Once the client falls below horizontal, the test is terminated.
- Encourage the client to practice this position prior to attempting the test.

Test protocol and administration:

- When ready, the client lifts/extends the torso until it is parallel to the floor with his or her arms crossed over the chest (Figure 12-14). This position requires activation of the torso extensor muscles (i.e., erector spinae, longissimus, iliocostalis, and multifidi).
- Start the stopwatch has soon as the client assumes this position.
- Terminate the test when the client can no longer maintain the position.
- Record the client's time on the testing form.

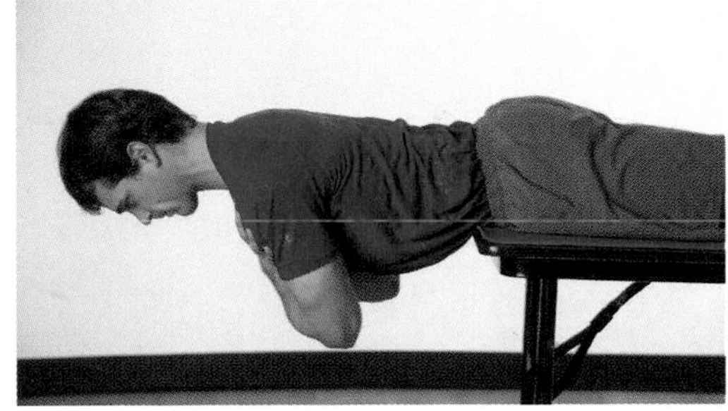

Figure 12-14
Trunk extensor endurance test

Evaluation and Application of Performance for McGill's Torso Muscular Endurance Test Battery

Each individual test in this testing battery is not a primary indicator of current or future back problems. McGill (2007) has proven that the *relationships* among the tests are important indicators of muscle imbalances that can lead to back pain. In fact, even in a person with little or no back pain, the ratios can still be off, suggesting that low-back pain may eventually occur without diligent attention to a solid core-conditioning program. McGill (2007) suggests that the following ratios indicate balanced endurance among the muscle groups:

- Flexion/extension ratio should be less than 1.0.
  - ✓ For example, a flexion score of 120 seconds and an extension score of 150 seconds generate a ratio score of 0.80.
- Right-side bridge (RSB):left-side bridge (LSB) scores should be no greater than 0.05 from a balanced score of 1.0 (i.e., 0.95 to 1.05).
  - ✓ For example, an RSB score of 88 seconds and an LSB score of 92 seconds generate a ratio score of 0.96, which is within the 0.05 range from 1.0.
- Side bridge (either side): extension ratio should be less than 0.75.
  - ✓ For example, an RSB score of 88 seconds and an extension score of 150 seconds generate a ratio score of 0.59.

Demonstrated deficiencies in these core functional assessments should be addressed during exercise programming as part of the foundational exercises for a client. The goal is to create ratios consistent with McGill's recommendations. Muscular endurance, more so than

muscular strength or even ROM, has been shown to be an accurate predictor of back health (McGill, 2007). Low-back stabilization exercises have the most benefit when performed daily. When working with clients with low-back dysfunction, it is prudent to include daily stabilization exercises in their home exercise plans.

Basic Assessment of Mobility

Muscular fitness encompasses both muscular endurance and muscular strength. Muscular endurance represents a muscle's ability to resist fatigue and perform sustained work for many successive repetitions, while muscular strength defines a muscle's ability to overcome external resistance. Both are essential health-related fitness components. The following list describes the many benefits of muscular fitness:

- Enhances the ability to carry out activities of daily living, which can increase self-esteem and foster a sense of independence
- Provides for musculoskeletal integrity, which can decrease the occurrence of common musculoskeletal injuries
- Enhances or maintains fat-free mass and ultimately increases **resting metabolic rate (RMR),** which is an important aspect of weight management
- Enhances glucose tolerance, which can protect against **type 2 diabetes**

Muscular strength assessments typically involve a client performing few repetitions with a very heavy load. For example, in **one-repetition maximum (1 RM)** testing, individuals lift a weight load that is so heavy it can only be lifted one time. Because the risk for injury is higher with muscular strength testing, and because assessing muscular strength is not necessary—especially for clients new to exercise or those who are deconditioned or obese—muscular-strength testing is not addressed in this text. Muscular-endurance testing assesses the ability of a specific muscle group to perform repeated contractions to sufficiently invoke muscular fatigue. Assessment criteria are typically based on the number of repetitions that can be performed with correct form or the length of time a muscle contraction can be held while keeping the body in correct postural alignment (e.g., McGill's torso endurance battery described in the previous section). The muscular assessments in this section focus on tests that can be easily administered and are only moderately challenging for most deconditioned individuals. One of the most important things to observe during any muscular fitness test is that the client is maintaining the integrity of joint movement during each repetition and/or the recommended posture for the specific exercise movement. In this respect, the following muscular fitness tests can also act as assessments of appropriate joint mobility and overall movement patterns. In essence, these assessments can be thought of as movement screens.

Modified Body-weight Squat Test

The modified body-weight squat test assesses muscular fitness of the lower extremity when performing repetitions of a squat-to-stand movement. It also allows the health coach to observe a client's movement pattern while he or she performs a squat, which is an essential movement required in many ADL. This test can be used to effectively gauge relative improvements in a client's lower-extremity muscular fitness.

Equipment:

- None needed

Pretest procedure:

- After explaining the purpose of the modified body-weight squat test, explain and demonstrate the proper technique.
- Allow for adequate warm-up and stretching if needed.

Test protocol and administration:

- Instruct the client to perform six to 10 repetitions of a squat at a depth that is tolerable to his or her lower-extremity joints.
- Evaluate the depth of the squat using the following criteria (Figure 12-15a):
  - ✓ Knees flex between 0 and 45 degrees (poor)
  - ✓ Knees flex between 45 and 90 degrees (good)
- To enhance balance and stability, the client may extend his or her arms to the sides or front for balance.
- The goal of the test is to complete as many controlled and proper repetitions (up to 10) as possible. Once the client exhibits muscular fatigue (e.g., shakiness) or needs a pause to rest, terminate the test.

Test evaluation:

- After the repetitions are complete, ask the client where he or she felt the muscles working the most. That is, did the client feel the movement mainly in the lower back and upper area of the posterior hips, the front of the thighs and knees, or the lower area of the posterior hips and back of the thighs?
  - ✓ If the client felt it mainly in the lower back and/or upper portion of the posterior hips, he or she is likely performing a lumbar-dominant squat.
  - ✓ If the client felt it mainly in the front of the thighs and/or knees, he or she is likely performing a quadriceps-dominant squat.
  - ✓ If the client felt it mainly in the lower portion of the posterior hips and/or the back of the thighs, he or she is likely performing a glute-dominant squat.
- The depth of the squat is also important in that it shows the client's tolerance for loading the lower-extremity joints in a flexed position and the client's ability to balance while lowering and raising his or her center of gravity in a squat movement pattern.
  - ✓ The lower the client can squat while maintaining proper form, the better he or she is able to tolerate the squat movement pattern and to maintain balance while performing it.
  - ✓ Use the depth of squat information to compare to the client's follow-up assessment to gauge relative improvement.
- Lastly, when viewed from the front, the alignment of the knees, ankles and feet during the squatting movement can indicate the amount of **valgus** or **varus** strain—if any—in the client's lower extremities (Figure 12-15b).
- Varus strain (i.e., femoral abduction and tibial adduction) is associated with knee pain and instability and excessive supination at the feet.
  - ✓ Valgus strain (i.e., femoral adduction and tibial abduction) is also associated with knee pain and instability, but it is more correlated with excessive pronation at the feet. Clients will most likely present with a valgus misalignment rather than a varus deviation, as valgus strain is more common in the general population.

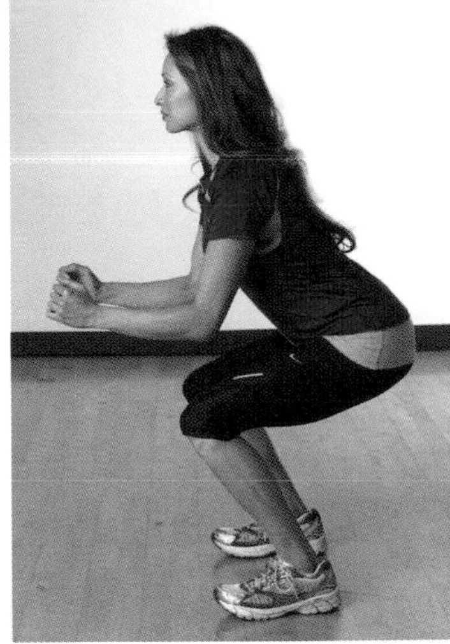

Figure 12-15
a. Body-weight squat test—adequate depth

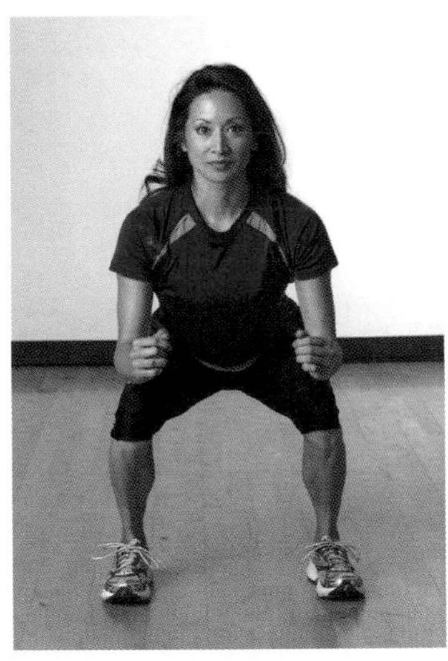

b. Anterior view

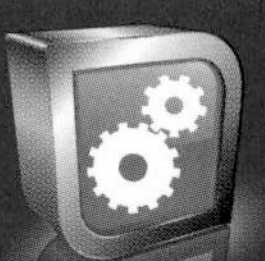

EXPAND YOUR KNOWLEDGE

Movement Patterns During a Squat

The gluteals and core musculature play an important role in the squat movement, during which individuals can exhibit "lumbar dominance," "quadriceps dominance," or "glute dominance."

- *Lumbar dominance:* This implies a lack of core abdominal and gluteal muscle strength to counteract the force of the hip flexors and erector spinae as they pull the pelvis forward during a squat movement. In this scenario, the individual experiences excessive loads within the lumbar spine as it moves into extension during the squat. The muscles of the abdominal wall and gluteal complex do not contribute enough in this situation to spare the back and foster proper execution of the squat (McGill, 2006). Chronically tight hip flexors, such as those experienced by individuals who sit for prolonged periods throughout the day, may also contribute to the this problem.
- *Quadriceps dominance:* This implies reliance on loading the quadriceps group during a squat movement. The first 10 to 15 degrees of the downward phase are initiated by driving the tibia forward, creating shearing forces across the knee as the femur slides over the tibia. In this lowered position, the gluteus maximus does not eccentrically load and cannot generate much force during the upward phase. Quadriceps-dominant squatting transfers more pressure into the knees, placing greater loads on the anterior cruciate ligament (ACL) (Wilthrow et al., 2005).
- *Glute dominance:* This implies reliance on eccentrically loading the gluteus maximus during a squat movement. The first 10 to 15 degrees of the downward phase are initiated by pushing the hips backward, creating a hip-hinge movement. In the lowered position, this maximizes the eccentric loading on the gluteus maximus to generate significant force during the upward, concentric phase. The glute-dominant squat pattern is the preferred method of squatting, as it spares the lumbar spine and relieves undue stress on the knees.

Front Plank

The front plank test assesses the core musculature's ability hold the spine in neutral alignment when the body is in a forearm plank position. To perform the assessment, the client adopts a prone plank position in which the forearms and toes are in contact with the floor. The elbows should be aligned directly underneath the shoulders and the body should maintain a straight line from shoulders to heels (i.e., the hips should not rise above or fall below shoulder level). Clients can also be given the option of supporting the lower body using the knees instead of the toes if they feel that attempting to hold the position on the toes will be too challenging.

Equipment:

- Stopwatch
- Exercise mat

Pretest procedure:

- After explaining the purpose of the front plank test, explain and demonstrate the proper technique.
- Allow for adequate warm-up and stretching if needed.

Test protocol and administration:

- Instruct the client to adopt the forearm plank position. As soon as the client is in the position and exhibiting proper alignment, start the stopwatch and cue the client to hold the position for 30 seconds (or as long as possible) (Figure 12-16).

- The goal of the test is to hold the forearm plank position with the body in proper alignment for as long as possible, up to 30 seconds. If the client breaks form and comes out of proper position, terminate the test and record the number of seconds attained.

Test evaluation:

- After the test is complete, ask the client where he or she felt the muscles working the most. That is, did the client feel the work mainly in the lower back or the abdomen?
  - ✓ If the client felt it mainly in the lower back, it is an indication that he or she lacks appropriate core stability.
  - ✓ If the client reports feeling it mainly in the abdominal muscles, it is an indication that he or she is recruiting the appropriate musculature to support the spine in the forearm plank position.
- If the client is able to hold proper alignment throughout the duration of the test, it is an indication that his or her core muscles are able to effectively stabilize the spine. Evaluate the muscular fitness of the core using the following criteria:
  - ✓ Unable to hold proper alignment for 30 seconds (poor)
  - ✓ Able to hold proper alignment for 30 seconds (good)

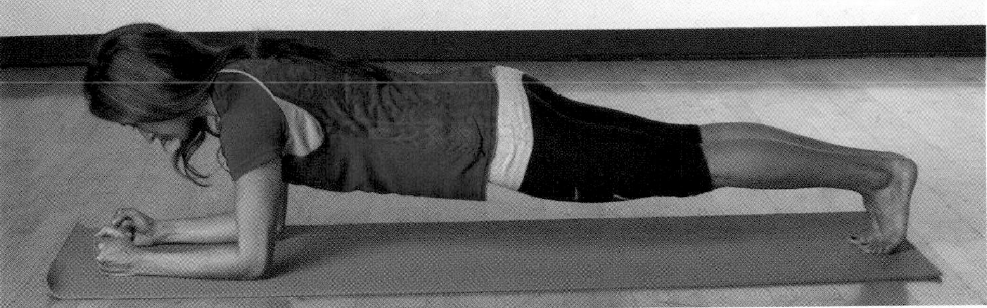

Figure 12-16
Front plank with good alignment

Overhead Reach

The overhead reach test assesses the mobility of the shoulder joints in external rotation. Limited mobility in the shoulder is a common problem in individuals who execute daily tasks with poor posture and/or dysfunctional biomechanical movement patterns. For example, clients who work for extended periods in a slouched position with the arms in front of the body, such as those who sit at a desk working on a computer throughout the day, may present with limited external rotation of the shoulder because their arms are positioned in habitual internal rotation.

Equipment:

- Exercise mat

Pretest procedure:

- After explaining the purpose of the overhead reach test, explain and demonstrate the proper technique.
- Allow for adequate warm-up and stretching if needed.

Test protocol and administration:

- Instruct the client to lie in the supine position with the knees bent and the feet flat on the floor about 18 inches in front of, and in line with, the hips. The hands should be placed on the mat alongside the body with the thumbs pointed up toward the ceiling. Cue the client to keep the arms straight (i.e., elbows fully extended) and the lower back pressed into the mat as he or she reaches the arms as far as possible overhead (Figure 12-17).

- The goal of the test is to see how far the client can reach his or arms overhead in a position of external rotation at the shoulder joint. If the client cannot touch the thumbs to the floor, it indicates limited ROM at the shoulder joint. Inadequate shoulder flexibility is also indicated if the client allows the back to arch upward off the floor while reaching overhead, thus effectively furthering his or her reach by repositioning the spine instead of moving through the shoulder joints.

Test evaluation:

- After the test is complete, ask the client where he or she felt the stretch the most. That is, did the client feel the work mainly in the shoulders or the back?
  - ✓ If the client felt it mainly in the back and the back arched upward off the floor, it is an indication that he or she lacks appropriate shoulder mobility and core stability.
  - ✓ If the client felt it mainly in the shoulders, was able to keep the back flat on the mat, yet could not touch the thumbs to the floor, it indicates a lack of adequate shoulder mobility.
  - ✓ If the client felt it mainly in the shoulders, was able to keep the back relatively flat on the mat, and could touch the thumbs to the floor, it indicates good shoulder mobility.

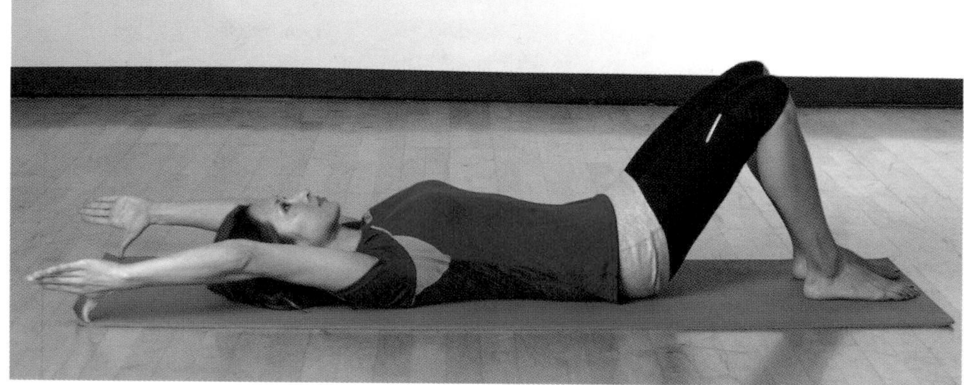

Figure 12-17
Overhead reach with adequate ROM

The Next Step After Postural Assessment and Muscular Fitness Testing

It is important for the health coach to initially assess and identify any postural problems or deviations and/or accompanying pain. The next step is to discuss these specific deficiencies and educate the client on the long-term ramifications. Using the guidelines presented in this chapter, or guidance from the client's rehabilitation professional, health coaches should develop and implement a restorative exercise program to strengthen and lengthen appropriate muscle groups. Keen observation and feedback will facilitate client awareness on key postural issues. Health coaches should monitor body mechanics throughout each training session. The goal is to foster new healthier habits that will not only improve the body's structure and function, but also reduce the likelihood of pain, injury, and dysfunction.

Additional assessments of joint ROM may be conducted. For further information on techniques and acceptable parameters, refer to the *ACE Personal Trainer Manual*.

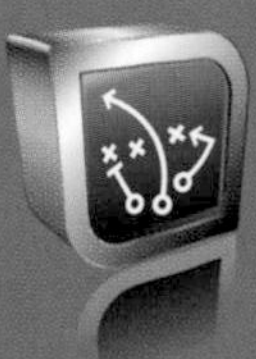

APPLY WHAT YOU KNOW

Discussing Physical Fitness Assessment Results With Clients

Collecting assessment information through conducting physical fitness tests can be an important step in exercise program development for clients. The baseline data, as well as follow-up data, can be invaluable in guiding clients through the journey of improving health and fitness that ultimately helps them achieve their goals. For this information to be meaningful and motivating to the client, the health coach must present assessment results in a way that is easily understood and relevant to the client's goals. The following example illustrates how a health coach can effectively communicate a client's physical-fitness assessment data in a clear manner that teaches the client how the results apply to his or her personal situation.

Jennifer, a busy health coach who works in a fitness facility, has just retained Ben as a client. Ben is a 65-year-old retiree who is interested in improving lower-body strength because he has noticed that rising up out of a chair is becoming more challenging the older he gets. Ben has just completed the modified body-weight squat test (see page 348) and reports that he felt the work mainly in the "tops of his thighs." Additionally, Jennifer observed the following characteristics during Ben's test:

- Completed 10 repetitions at a depth of 30 degrees of knee flexion
- Valgus tendencies with both knees

To help Ben understand the assessment results and make them relevant to his personal goals, Jennifer explained the data in the following way:

"Ben, you completed all 10 repetitions, which is very good. This indicates that your muscular endurance—or the ability to sustain exercise without becoming too fatigued—is at the right level. I also noticed that the depth of your squat was less than 90 degrees and that your knees had a tendency to drop inward during the movement. This lets me know that we need to work on improving muscular strength in your legs as well as on increasing your ability to maintain knee alignment during squat-type movements. Working on alignment is important so that as you gain strength you also move properly, protecting the joints from unnecessary wear and tear. I have some very effective exercises and stretches in mind to address these issues, which will also help you with your goal of standing up from a seated position more easily."

While the scenario described above portrays just one component of a client's overall conditioning program, it gives an example of how technical assessment data can be delivered in a meaningful way. The health coach can take this approach with all assessment-result information to facilitate the client's understanding of why the assessments were performed and how they apply directly to the client.

For clients who have a good understanding of physiology and kinesiology, it may be more appropriate to communicate test results using more technical language. In these situations, it is up to the health coach to gauge the knowledge level and interest of the client in using exercise science–related terminology. If, through the initial interview process and the course of conversation, it is discovered that a client possesses advanced knowledge of anatomical and health-related topics, it would be prudent to speak to the level of understanding of the client. Communicating in such a manner adds to the professionalism of the health coach and lets the client know that the health coach is not attempting to "speak down" to him or her.

Fitness Testing Accuracy

There are many causes of inaccuracy in fitness testing, ranging from equipment failure to human error (Table 12-8). Most clients are motivated by improvements in their fitness assessments. Clients like to see that the hard work and dedication to their fitness programs have paid off. There may be test inaccuracies, but repeating the same test, in the same environment, and at the same time of day, will ensure test reliability when compared to earlier test outcomes. For example, even if optimal results are not always attainable, a client who sees his or her performance assessment move from "below average" to "average" will likely be thrilled with the results and motivated to continue with a regular program of exercise.

Table 12-8

Causes of Fitness Test Inaccuracy

CLIENT	HEALTH COACH OR TEST TECHNICIAN
Fatigue, lack of sleep Motivation, lack of conviction Excess activity prior to test Food intake prior to test Hydration level Chronic health condition(s) Medications or supplements	Inexperience with testing protocol Poor application of testing protocol Partiality; trying to affect results Level of encouragement
EQUIPMENT	**ENVIRONMENT**
Improper calibration Mismatched to subject Failure, out of order	Distractions Privacy Temperature Weather conditions

Summary

The role of a health coach is multifaceted. A comprehensive evaluation can help determine the type of support that is needed to assist in meeting health and fitness goals. To enhance the evaluation experience, it is important for the client to feel at ease and have an idea of what to expect in the evaluation process. To facilitate sharing of information, the evaluation setting should be private and free of distractions.

Conducting assessments to determine clients' cardiorespiratory fitness, balance, core function, and muscular fitness is a valuable practice for health coaches to guide initial exercise programming and continued progression. Once the tests are administered and evaluated, effectively communicating a client's physical-fitness assessment data in a clear manner that translates to the client how the results apply to his or her personal situation (without negatively labeling the client) enhances the rapport between the health coach and the client. This approach facilitates the client's understanding of why the assessments were performed and how they apply directly to the client, thus increasing motivation and ultimately adherence to the program.

References

American College of Sports Medicine (2014). *ACSM's Guidelines for Exercise Testing and Prescription* (9th ed.). Philadelphia: Wolters Kluwer/ Lippincott Williams & Wilkins.

American College of Sports Medicine (2008). *ACSM's Health-Related Physical Fitness Assessment Manual* (3rd ed.). Philadelphia: Lippincott Williams & Wilkins.

Black, F.O. et al. (1982). Normal subject postural sway during the Romberg test. *American Journal of Otolaryngology*, 3, 309–318.

Blair, S.N. et al. (1995). Changes in physical fitness and all-cause mortality: A prospective study of healthy and unhealthy men. *Journal of the American Medical Association*, 273, 14, 1093–1098.

Borg, G. (1998). *Borg's Perceived Exertion and Pain Scales*. Champaign, Ill.: Human Kinetics.

Chobanian, A.V. et al. (2003). *JNC 7 Express: The Seventh Report of the Joint National Committee on Prevention, Detection, Evaluation, and Treatment of High Blood Pressure. NIH Publication No. 03-5233.* Washington D.C.: National Institutes of Health and National Heart, Lung, and Blood Institute.

Fox III, S.M., Naughton, J.P., & Haskell, W.L. (1971). Physical activity and the prevention of coronary heart disease. *Annuals of Clinical Research*, 3, 404–432.

Kaplan, N.M. & Victor, R.G. (2010). *Kaplan's Clinical Hypertension* (10th ed.). Baltimore, Md.: Wolters Kluwer/Lippicott Williams & Wilkins.

Johnson B.L. & Nelson, J.K. (1986). *Practical Measurements for Evaluation in Physical Education* (4th ed.). Minneapolis, Minn.: Burgess.

McGill, S. (2007). *Low Back Disorders: Evidence Based Prevention and Rehabilitation* (2nd ed.). Champaign, Ill.: Human Kinetics.

McGill, S.M. (2006). *Ultimate Back Fitness and Performance* (4th ed.). Waterloo, Canada: Backfitpro.com

McManus, R.J. & Mant, J. (2012). Do differences in blood pressure between arms matter? *The Lancet*, 379, 9819, 872–873.

Miller, T.D. (2008). The exercise treadmill test: Estimating cardiovascular prognosis. *Cleveland Clinic Journal of Medicine*, 75, 6.

Morrow, J.R. et al. (2011). *Measurement and Evaluation in Human Performance* (4th ed.). Champaign, Ill.: Human Kinetics.

Newton, R. (1989). Review of tests of standing balance abilities. *Brain Injury*, 3, 4, 335–343.

Nieman, D.C. (2010). *Exercise Testing and Prescription: A Health-Related Approach* (7th ed.). New York: McGraw-Hill.

Pickering, T.G. et al. (2005). AHA Scientific Statement: Recommendations for blood pressure measurement in humans and experimental animals. *Circulation*, 11, 697–716.

Pollock, M.L. et al. (1982). Comparative analysis of physiologic responses to three different maximal graded exercise test protocols in healthy women. *American Heart Journal*, 103, 363–373.

Pollock, M.L. et al. (1976). A comparative analysis of four protocols for maximal treadmill stress testing. *American Heart Journal*, 92, 39–46.

Porcari, J.P., Robarge, M., & Veldhuis, R. (1993). Counting heart rate right. *Fitness Management*, August.

Tanaka, H., Monahan, K.D., & Seals, D.R. (2001). Age-predicted maximal heart revisited. *Journal of the American College of Cardiology*, 37, 153–156.

U.S. Department of Health & Human Services (2008). *2008 Physical Activity Guidelines for Americans: Be Active, Healthy and Happy*. www.health.gov/paguidelines/pdf/paguide.pdf

Wilthrow, T.J. et al. (2005). The relationship between quadriceps muscle force, knee flexion and anterior cruciate ligament strain in an *in vitro* simulated jump landing. *American Journal of Sports Medicine*, 34, 2, 269–274.

Suggested Reading

American College of Sports Medicine (2009). *ACSM's Exercise Management for Persons with Chronic Disease and Disabilities* (3rd ed.). Champaign, Ill.: Human Kinetics.

American College of Sports Medicine (2007). *ACSM's Health/Fitness Facility Standards and Guidelines* (3rd ed.). Champaign, Ill.: Human Kinetics.

American Council on Exercise (2014). *ACE Personal Trainer Manual* (5th ed.). San Diego, Calif.: American Council on Exercise.

Baechle, T.R. & Earle, R.W. (2008). *Essentials of Strength Training and Conditioning* (3rd ed.). Champaign, Ill.: Human Kinetics.

Bassett D.R. & Howley, E.T. (2000). Limiting factors for maximum oxygen uptake and determinants of endurance performance. *Medicine & Science in Sports & Exercise,* 32, 70–84.

Block, P. & Kravitz, L. (2005). The "talk test." *IDEA Fitness Journal,* 2, 2, 22–23.

Cooper Institute of Aerobic Research (2009). *Physical Fitness Assessments and Norms for Adults and Law Enforcement.* Dallas, Tex.: Cooper Institute.

Flávio, O. et al. (2008). Ventilation behavior in trained and untrained men during incremental test: Evidence of one metabolic transition point. *Journal of Sports Science and Medicine,* 7, 335–343.

Golding, L.A., Clayton, R.M., & Sinning, W.E. (1989). *Y's Way to Physical Fitness* (3rd ed.). Champaign, Ill.: Human Kinetics.

Heyward, V. (2010). *Advanced Fitness Assessments and Exercise Prescription* (6th ed.). Champaign, Ill.: Human Kinetics.

Londeree, B.R. (1997). Effect of training on lactate/ventilatory thresholds: A meta-analysis. *Medicine & Science in Sports & Exercise,* 29, 6, 837–843.

Maud, P.J. & Foster, C. (2006). *Physiological Assessment of Human Fitness.* Champaign, Ill.: Human Kinetics.

McArdle, W., Katch, F., & Katch, V. (2010). *Exercise Physiology: Energy, Nutrition, and Human Performance* (7th ed.). Philadelphia: Wolters Kluwer/Lippincott Williams & Wilkins.

Neder, J.A. & Stein, R. (2006). A simplified strategy for the estimation of the exercise ventilatory thresholds. *Medicine & Science in Sports & Exercise,* 38, 5, 1007–1013.

Pierce, A. (1999). *The American Pharmaceutical Association Practical Guide to Natural Medicines.* New York: Stonesong Press.

Pressman, A. & Shelley, D. (2000). *Integrative Medicine.* New York: St. Martin's Press.

Riegelman, R.K. (2012). *Studying a Study and Testing a Test: How to Read the Medical Evidence* (6th ed.). Philadelphia: Wolters Kluwer/Lippincott Williams & Wilkins.

U.S. Department of Health & Human Services (1996). *Physical Activity and Health: A Report of the Surgeon General.* Atlanta, Ga.: U.S. Department of Health & Human Services, Centers for Disease Control and Prevention, National Center for Chronic Disease Prevention and Health Promotion.

SECTION V

PROGRAM DESIGN AND IMPLEMENTATION

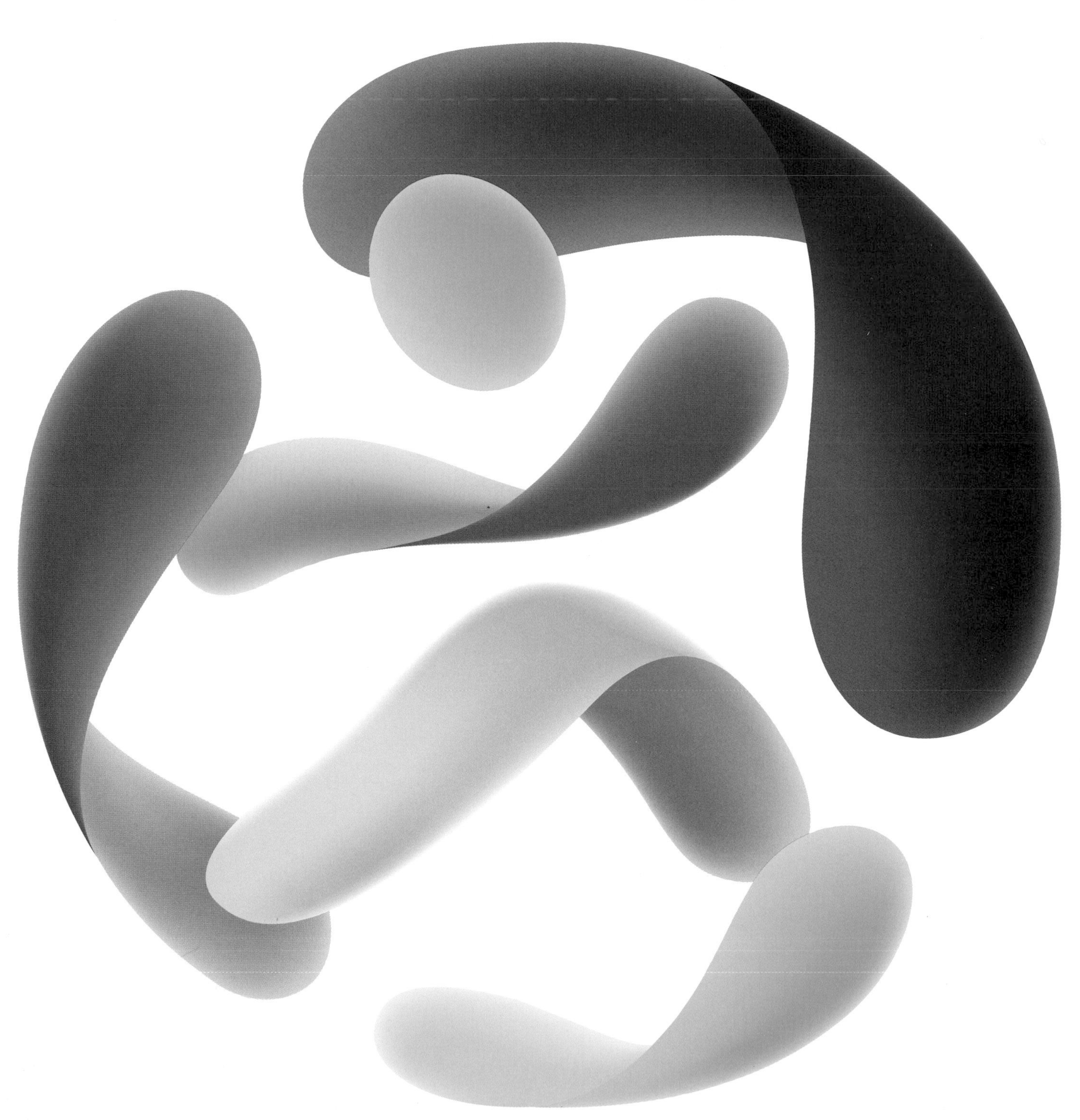

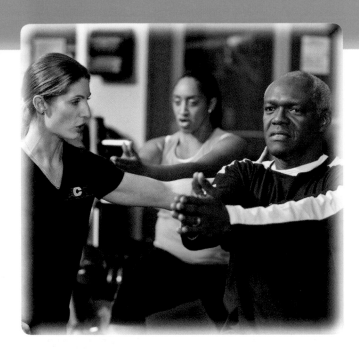

IN THIS CHAPTER:

13

A Realistic Approach to Goal-setting

JONATHAN ROSS

Jonathan Ross' "800 pounds of parents" directly inspired his prolific fitness career. He lost his father to obesity at over 400 pounds, then helped his mother lose 170 pounds. This ability to bring fitness to those who need it the most has made Ross a two-time Personal Trainer of the Year Award Winner (ACE and IDEA), fitness expert for Discovery Fit *and* Health, *and a fitness industry thought leader. An ACE-certified Personal Trainer and a prolific author and speaker, Ross shares compelling fitness information through live appearances, his book,* Abs Revealed, *and numerous articles and blogs.*

Realistic goals benefit both the ACE-certified Health Coach and the client, as they ensure that the client's energy and effort are appropriately placed and the instruction and coaching from the health coach are effectively tailored to the individual needs of the client.

Realistic goals are easier to achieve because they provide a level of detail and relevance to the client that connects the goals to what the client values in life. Goals can be focused on past, present, or future accomplishments exclusively, or on some combination of the three. Health coaches who ask the right questions will gain a detailed understanding of the motivations of the client that is indispensable when developing recommendations for lifestyle change. Well-chosen questions provide the health coach with absolute clarity on client goals and on the obstacles to achieving those goals—a terrific aid to adherence.

SMART Goals

Clients often express fairly general training goals, such as wanting to "tone muscles" or "lose some weight." The health coach should help clients define goals in more specific and measurable terms so that progress can be evaluated. Effective goals are commonly said to be **SMART goals,** which means they are:

Specific: Goals must be clear and unambiguous, stating specifically what should be accomplished.

Measurable: Goals must be measurable so that clients can see whether they are making progress. Examples of measurable goals include performing a given workout two times a week or losing 5 pounds (2.3 kg).

Attainable: Goals should be realistically attainable by the individual client. The achievement of attaining a goal reinforces commitment to the program and encourages the client to continue exercising.

Relevant: Goals must be relevant to the particular interest, needs, and abilities of the individual client.

Time-bound: Goals must contain estimated timelines for completion. Clients should be evaluated regularly to monitor progress toward goals.

The SMART goal concept is ubiquitous in training manuals and articles on goal-setting. While this should form the foundation for the health coach's goal-setting process with clients, the health coach does not need to consciously "tick off the boxes" when helping clients establish their program goals. In other words, the health coach does not need to ask if each goal is "SMART." Instead, the client and health coach should work together to develop long- and short-term objectives that work within this framework as a natural part of the process. Eventually, a health coach will be able to easily recognize a well-constructed goal when he or she hears one. This chapter employs real-world, practical applications and implications of using the SMART goal-setting approach with clients.

Why Goals Are Essential

How does a goal turn into real and lasting change in someone's life? More importantly, how can health coaches properly and effectively facilitate the process of goal-setting at the beginning of the professional relationship with a new client?

Goals benefit both the client and the health coach, as they have the power to motivate clients during the entire process of change. They provide clarity that aids the client in directing action on a daily basis to make steady progress toward goals. Perhaps most importantly, goals may help reduce **relapse** and enhance program adherence, especially in adults and adolescents who engage in dietary and physical-activity behavioral change practices (Shilts, Horowitz, & Townsend, 2009; 2004). Being mindful of goals can help clients overcome the obstacles that will inevitably arise during any process of lifestyle change.

For the health coach, personal client goals provide insights that are useful in developing specific recommendations on lifestyle modification, designing exercise programs, and providing nutritional education, and then developing coaching strategies to successfully deliver this information to the client. Figure 13-1 presents a list of questions that can be used either in written form or asked in person during the initial stages of the client–health coach relationship to provide realistic goal-setting opportunities. This gives the health coach an opportunity to identify areas for follow-up questioning that require a higher level of detail than the client provided initially. This serves two important purposes: (1) it demonstrates to the client that the health coach will be circumspect in examining all potential opportunities for success and obstacles to that success, and (2) it reminds the client that he or she will need to go beyond the customary simple answers to goal-setting and provide thoughtful responses to the questions to help the health coach provide relevant guidance.

Asking the right questions has the power to bring clients back to a more thoughtful approach to lifestyle change, as opposed to a more reactive approach. This helps clients proceed at their own pace with help from the health coach to organize the steps into an action plan.

Figure 13-1
Client goal questionnaire

Client goal questionnaire

- What are your short-term goals (three to six months) and long-term goals (beyond six months)?
- What could hinder your fitness program (e.g., work schedules, commute times, and child care/activities)?
- What motivates you?
- What things are most important to you? How will a healthy lifestyle complement or support this?
- What kinds of exercise programs have you tried in the past?
- What did you like most and least about your previous exercise programs?
- What types of exercise or activities do you currently enjoy?
- What is your favorite exercise or activity?
- How will you integrate exercise into your life?
- How much time do you have to commit to exercise?
- What kind of support (e.g., family and friends) do you have to help you change your lifestyle?
- What is something you are good at now? Did you know you were good at it before you did it or the first time you did it?
- When was the last time you exercised regularly (at least three times per week) and how long did it last? Why did you stop?

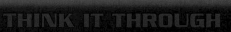

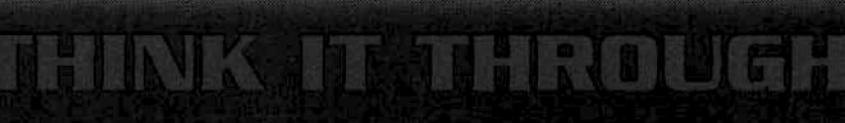

Practice using the questionnaire presented in Figure 13-1 with a friend or family member. Were you able to draw out any unexpected details from him or her? How would this discussion help you develop a comprehensive weight-management plan?

Developing Meaningful Goals

Imagine someone planning a vacation. If he or she says, "I want to go on vacation," and never provides any additional details, it is very unlikely that he or she will ever get anywhere. Without sufficient details of where to go, how long to stay, and how to travel, the vacation will not happen.

Yet this is the exactly the same approach that many clients take when stating goals to a health coach. Clients will often state goals such as "be healthier," "feel better," "have more energy," "lose weight," or "get in shape." Failing to ask for additional details at this critical stage can greatly diminish the chances of success with the program.

There is a difference between knowing *how* to act, and being *motivated* to act. However, when leading a client to behavioral change, the first instinct is often to teach and advise. It is the motivational aspect of change that is most important, as it has the power to enhance a client's desire to adopt healthy behaviors, and perhaps more importantly, provide the confidence and will to overcome obstacles and setbacks when they arise.

When the health coach discovers the specific, highly personal goals of a client, they reflect a level of detail that provides an obvious connection to what the client values in life and cares about most. Knowing why the goal matters to a client is essential information for the health coach, as this information is not only useful at the beginning when developing a plan, but also during the course of the client–health coach relationship when challenges arise. If the health coach can successfully and continuously remind the client of the connection between specific day-to-day behaviors and the larger goal by linking the behaviors to the goal through what the client values, the client will more effectively overcome obstacles.

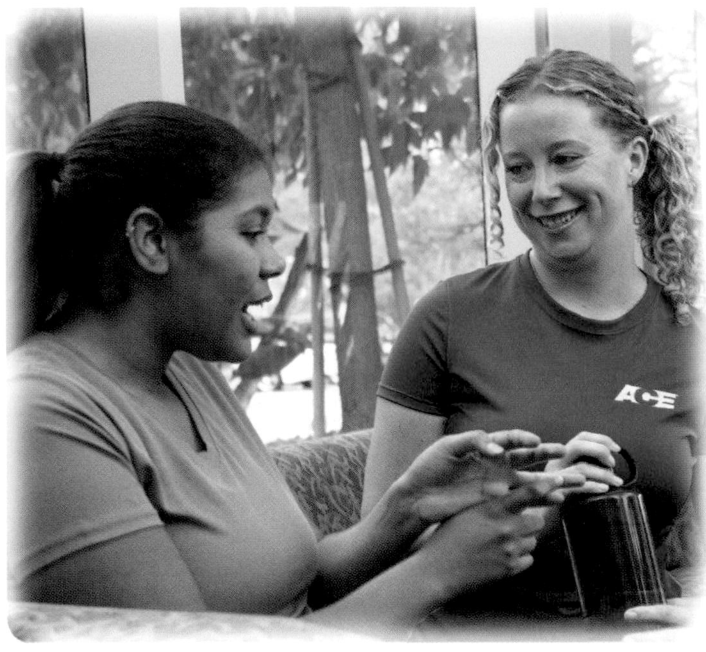

When a client and health coach collaborate to develop realistic goals, an essential component of this process is to identify common obstacles for the client. These can be either external factors, such as pressure at work, at home, or from a family member, or internal factors, such as a client's previous failed attempts at health improvement and a resulting lack of confidence or negative mindset. Once common obstacles are identified, the client and health coach can work to develop solutions before those challenges arise. The stress of facing a challenge often leads clients away from healthy behaviors and impairs their decision-making ability. As a result, it is essential to plan a strategy for how to react to common obstacles and challenges before a client is actually faced with them by always linking specific behaviors to the goals. This teaches a client to focus on his or her goals rather than on the obstacle itself. The result is that the client can direct his or her energy to finding a way around the obstacle rather than on the frustration or stress of the obstacle itself.

APPLY WHAT YOU KNOW

Preparing for Obstacles

A client that came to you initially with a goal of weight loss is three weeks into her program. The client is now dealing with major pressures at work and at home and, as a result, is beginning to have trouble following the exercise and healthy eating plan the two of you created together. She arrives for a session 10 minutes late and says to you, "I'm so sorry. I'm just overwhelmed at work and at home and haven't worked out the past few days and I'm upset because I haven't lost much weight yet." Your response in this situation will often determine whether the client overcomes the obstacles and continues progressing or continues to struggle.

From your early sessions with this client, you know that she is motivated by a desire to be fit enough to play with her kids and enjoy recreational activities with the family, even though the initial goals were simply stated as "weight loss." You also discovered that the client has a history of stopping and starting exercise programs because, invariably, situations just like the current one arise and the circumstances force her to miss a few workouts. She gets very upset and discouraged with herself, which only adds to the stress of dealing with the work and home pressures. When the additional disappointment of not seeing much progress with her weight-loss efforts is added to the mix, it all feels like too much. This client is on the brink of losing her commitment, so your response is critical. In this situation, by knowing the history of this tendency in the client and her usual all-or-nothing response, you can work with the client to develop a different strategy.

Health coach: "It sounds like you have a lot going on and I can see how it's tough for you to get your workouts in. Would you like it if we came up with a shorter workout you could do on the days that get out of control and don't leave you with enough time to perform your full workout?"

It is very likely that the client will appreciate this approach, since it gives her an opportunity to feel successful in the face of challenges. As for the disappointment expressed regarding the client's goals, it is important to relay to her that her feelings are valid.

Health coach: "I understand that you're frustrated right now with the lack of progress. Have you had a chance to do something active with your kids recently?"

Client: "It's funny you should ask. Last weekend, we had a family gathering and my son wanted me to play tag with him and the other kids. I did so for several minutes and had a great time. It was only after I stopped that I realized that I wasn't nearly as tired as I normally would be after doing that."

Health coach: "That's terrific. You had mentioned that along with weight loss, one of your goals was to have more energy to play with your kids, and that is already happening. That is a clear sign that your body is changing and getting fitter. If you can find a way to keep this good momentum going, you'll notice that additional results will soon follow."

Client: "You know, I guess I've gotten so used to looking at the scale as a way to measure progress that I'd forgotten about the other significant and meaningful goals I had mentioned."

Health coach: "I'd imagine that it's quite a great feeling to be able to play with your kids."

Client: "Yes, and I know I have a lot going on right now, but I can find a way to still get my workouts in.

Health coach: "The exercise will actually help you deal with the stress you're experiencing and keep you on track for reaching your goals."

This exchange is impossible unless the health coach takes the time to ask the right questions, and most importantly, helps the client arrive at her own solutions by validating the feelings of frustration, disappointment, and stress, while at the same time guiding the client to tap into positive emotions that can be drawn on for strength to overcome the current obstacle.

Realistic Goals Begin With a Past, Present, or Future Emphasis

Helping a client achieve health goals ultimately involves creating a better version of who the client already is. As such, the goals should have an emphasis on the past, present, or future—or some combination of all three. A simple way to remember these categories is to realize that most goals can be categorized by a desire to:

- Be all you used to be (past)
- Be better now (present)
- Be all you can be (future)

Past Goals

A client who focuses on past goals typically wants to resume participation in a cherished sport or recreational activity, or perhaps lose weight to return to a period of life when he or she felt better and more energetic. Often, when stating a weight-loss goal of a specific number of pounds, a client may say something like, "When I weighed 'x' number of pounds, I felt better, enjoyed being active, and liked how my clothes fit." It is important when encountering this type of goal to note the significance the client places on getting back to a feeling. In this example, there is nothing transformative about the client achieving the target weight. It is the behaviors that might lead to weight loss that will create the feeling the client is seeking. In most cases, if a client is feeling the way he or she wants to feel, the weight will matter less. Thus, it is essential to simply state the importance of the positive feelings associated with behavioral change and perhaps introduce the idea of a lowered emphasis on weight without making too much of an issue about it. In this case, it is better to ask for additional details and information about how he or she felt "back then." The more detail the health coach can get from the client about the positive feelings associated with behavioral change for weight loss, the more the health coach can connect those feelings with current behaviors.

Other clients may desire to participate in a sport they used to play. This typically means they are trying to recapture a feeling of competition or camaraderie. Some important considerations here are the practicality of returning to the sport and any necessary modifications to the intensity of the sport given the client's current conditioning levels. For example, a client who used to play rugby or American football may find it impractical to do so as an adult. In this case, it may be best to discuss other opportunities for expressing this goal that might be more appropriate, as the level of organization and equipment needs may prohibit pursuit of the original sport. In another case, the health coach may have a client who was previously a competitive singles tennis player and, given the need to respect current conditioning levels, it may be prudent to recommend resuming tennis through doubles play while following an exercise program geared toward preparing the client for a possible return to singles tennis.

For those who have never played sports (and have no desire to do so), there may be a desire to return to a cherished recreational activity such as hiking, skiing, gardening, or any number of other possibilities. The same considerations would apply in terms of practicality for the return to the activity in the event it requires a period for the body to readjust to the stresses placed on it.

In all of the above scenarios, setting appropriate goals is achieved by the health coach questioning or probing to find out details about why the client is looking back to capture a feeling or experience from his or her past.

There is one major caveat with recurring goals that were first created in the past: The health coach should be vigilant for old goals that are no longer appropriate, relevant, or motivating, yet are still expressed by the client. For example, a woman in her fifties may state a target weight that she maintained in her thirties. She may have been stating the goal for so long that it has become automatic to do so without examining the current strength of the desire for this goal. Often, fitness goals will naturally evolve or shift steadily and in subtle ways over the years. Sometimes the shift can happen so gradually that clients do not realize that their goals have changed. When working with this type of individual, there may be a high risk of frustration for the health coach, as recommended actions and behaviors are not adopted, results are less than expected for the client, and compliance becomes a continual struggle. It is best to avoid this situation when possible by learning as much as possible about the client's motivations for achieving a goal. The danger is that sometimes these goals appear very reasonable and realistic, but just not for the client at this time in his or her life. As a result, it may not be immediately apparent to the health coach that seemingly reasonable goals are not realistic for a particular individual. This is another reason why it is advisable to gather as much additional information as possible about a client's goals before recommending a course of action.

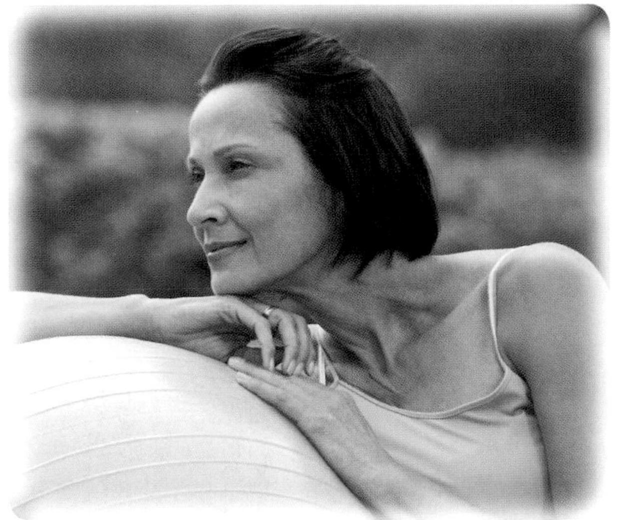

Present Goals

Many clients will obtain the services of a health coach for help with something that has motivated them to take action now. It may be medical or experiential in nature. A client may want to improve health and fitness measures now (e.g., lower **blood pressure,** lower **body fat,** increase muscle mass, or increase bone density), or may have a desire for a greater ability to physically perform in an area that is more immediate (e.g., playing with grandchildren, getting in shape for a short-term upcoming event such as a vacation or wedding, or perhaps being a short-term caregiver for an aging parent.)

A client may have had a recent doctor's appointment and received news of high blood pressure, high **cholesterol,** low bone density, high **triglycerides,** or some other indicator of less-than-optimal health. If this is the main motivation for someone, it will likely not be enough on its own to provide the drive for long-term success. The health coach must find out what elements of the client's life will be made better by improvement in these measures, as these health measures are typically rather abstract in nature, in that most people feel no symptomatic effects of the imbalance. In this case, it may shift the goal to more of a future perspective. For example, upon further investigation, a parent struggling with **obesity,** with test results showing elevated blood pressure and high blood sugar, may be motivated by a desire to live long enough to see his or her child get married or graduate college. As a result, the health coach can frame the present goal in terms of enjoyment of future experiences.

Other clients have a looming event such as a class reunion, wedding, vacation, or "active vacation" where they may be attempting a long and challenging hike, for example, which directs all effort and action in the short-term toward achieving the goal. In this case, setting realistic goals is often fairly straightforward, as the timeline and nature of the event dictate most of the program variables.

Better health often expands the physical sense of self. In other words, through the process of achieving one goal, new abilities and a sense of physical competency may give birth to new goals that neither the client nor the health coach could have envisioned at the outset. It is wise for the health coach to look for opportunities during the process of achieving the current goal to actively encourage the client to consider any new goals that might develop. This provides the health coach with a natural and seamless way to promote the adoption of healthy behaviors beyond the current goals.

For example, a health coach may have a client who is preparing for a vacation and simply wants to feel good about how she looks in a bathing suit. This concern may occupy her focus at the outset. However, as she is progressing, a focus on psychological and physical function may emerge as she experiences better reactions to stressful situations and more stamina during recreational activity. The health coach will want to connect these improvements with the healthy behaviors the client has adopted, as many clients will often be unaware of the cause-and-effect nature of global improvements to many areas of life when better health is attained. Identifying these unintended consequences of better health is essential for converting someone who has a singular, immediate goal into someone who finds ongoing reasons to pursue a healthy lifestyle that makes everyday living better.

Future Goals

A client may want to prepare for a long-term upcoming event (e.g., extended travel with a lot of walking) or may have a fitness goal such as participating in a charity event or other endurance race after a long layoff from exercise. The main differences between a "present" goal and a "future" goal are the timeline and focus. A present goal has a relatively short timeline and the goal itself captures the client's imagination and energy. With a future goal, the timeline is generally longer and, while the client is of course focused on the goal, he or she typically is aware of, and often directly seeking, many of the secondary benefits associated with the goal.

For example, a client may say, "I'd like to do a triathlon, as a few of my friends have started doing them and it will give me something to shoot for. But right now I just want to exercise consistently and feel better on a day-to-day basis." In this case, many of the same healthy behaviors that will move the client toward the future goal of completing a triathlon will also address the more immediate goal of having more energy now.

Future goals can be inspirational in terms of the client seeking to achieve something new and challenging that will require a lifestyle effort in a number of areas. Future goals can also be related to the pursuit of a new experience. This new experience might allow the client to have a great experience with a loved one, reclaim a sense of physical mastery, or travel to a destination best experienced and enjoyed through better fitness. Future goals are often broader in scope, which can be an aid to the health coach in that the client will already realize that there will be physical, mental, and lifestyle aspects of achieving the goal.

With these goals, it is helpful for the health coach to prioritize the smaller goals and behaviors that are necessary to achieve the larger ones, as it is often difficult for clients to easily organize a future goal into smaller actions.

For example, a health coach may have a client who has been **sedentary** for years and has decided he wants to complete a marathon. To achieve this goal, the health coach will want to collaborate with the client to lay out a schedule of actions. This might start with setting a more short-term, realistic goal of the client completing a 5K or "fun run" and beginning the exercise programming, nutrition education, and recovery strategies with that smaller goal in mind.

Another good example includes a health coach who has a client who is the less-fit half of a couple that is planning a backpacking trip. In this case, the client may have a number of goals, all relating to the main goal of being able to physically perform in a way that allows him or her to enjoy the trip. The client may want to be able to keep up with his or her partner and avoid the embarrassment of having to stop often, to be comfortable enough to actually enjoy the surroundings without exhaustion dampening the experience, and may have some joint concerns that reflect a need to develop the ability to handle the repetitive nature of the activity.

An important realization for the health coach in situations like this is that the goals themselves are actually secondary to the *feelings* associated with the goal. It is unlikely in this scenario that the exercise program itself and the feeling of greater hiking ability will be adequate to sustain motivation. To some extent, the goals are motivated by the emotions of the client surrounding the upcoming experience rather than the physical performance he or she can expect. Therefore, it is imperative for the health coach to appropriately frame the goals and program. For example, it may be wise to schedule an occasional outdoor workout session during which the health coach asks the client to notice or identify various things about the surroundings. Similarly, the health coach should gather information on the current conditioning level of the client's partner, so standards of physical performance can be used that will be most meaningful for the client.

Why Do Clients' Goals Matter?

Health coaches often have expertise in the "how" of lifestyle change. That is, programming exercise and providing healthy eating education are common actions taken by competent health coaches to help their clients effectively lead healthier lives. However, the "why" behind the client's desire to change is often the hardest information to come by, but is essential when making lifestyle changes, as it provides ample motivation for a client to successfully navigate the ups and downs of the process of change.

Connecting Goals With Values

It is imperative for the health coach to discover why the client's goals matter and how the client's health efforts will connect to what the client values in life. This information will help the health coach provide guidance for the client to overcome obstacles and challenges. By knowing what the client values in life, the health coach can help ensure that goals are real and relevant for the client by framing the lifestyle behaviors in terms of those values.

As discussed previously, many clients will initially provide generic, vague, and ambiguous goals. By putting the goals in context of what the client values, the health coach can facilitate the process of transforming the goals from abstract ideas into a specific and realistic plan of action that the client is motivated to begin. This is done by continuously and repeatedly asking "why?" with open-ended questions until the reasons for why the goal matters to the client are uncovered. See Chapter 5 for more information on how to properly use open-ended questions.

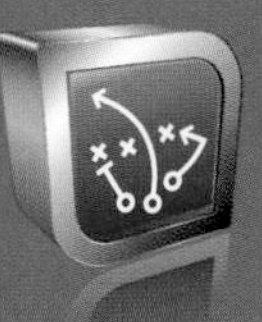

APPLY WHAT YOU KNOW

Client–Health Coach Role Play

Health coach: "Please tell me your health and fitness goals."

Client: "I'd like to lose weight—about 50 pounds."

Health coach: "What will be different in your life if you achieve that goal?"

Client: "I want my clothes to fit better and feel like I have more energy."

Health coach: "And why is this important to you?"

Client: "I just want to feel better. I sometimes get so tired that I have little energy left and snap at my kids and husband at the end of a long day."

Health coach: "How do you see your weight-loss goal having a connection to this?"

Client: "I don't know."

Health coach: "Do your responsibilities at home and work leave you feeling like you have no time for yourself and that you are doing for others all day?"

Client (begins to get emotional): "Now that you mention it, I often think to myself that I just would like some 'me' time. And I get down on myself, as I want to set a good example for healthy living to my kids, but I just feel like I can't get started when I have to keep handling everything that comes my way each day."

Health coach: "Could it be that you've never really progressed in your weight-loss goal because weight loss, in and of itself, isn't really your most important goal? It seems to me that having some time for yourself so you can give to others without losing yourself and setting a good example for your kids so they grow up with healthy behaviors is very important to you. Does that sound accurate?"

Client: "You know, I've never really thought of it that way, but you're right. I've always put my own goals on hold when life gets busy and I just feel so drained inside because I can't escape the things I do for others."

Health coach: "Have you considered that by carving out some time for exercise, getting proper rest, and having better nutrition, you might be more efficient and effective in your other roles, while also setting a good example for your kids on how to manage their lives when they become adults? If they see you reacting to the stresses of the day and ignoring your own needs, they might wind up following the same pattern when they are older."

Client: "Wow. That sure gives me a lot to think about. Fitness has always been something I've felt like I was supposed to do, but also felt guilty about taking the time to pursue."

In this example, the same behaviors that might achieve weight loss are put in the context of the client having some time for herself, becoming more efficient, and setting a good example for her kids. By attaching the goals to the client's values, they take on new relevance.

Lasting Motivation Comes From Within

A crucial aspect in connecting goals to what a client values involves determining if his or her health goals are originating from a desire for personal fulfillment (**intrinsic motivation**), from direct environmental input such as the praise and support from family members or a physician (**extrinsic motivation**), or some combination of the two (a blend of intrinsic and extrinsic motivation).

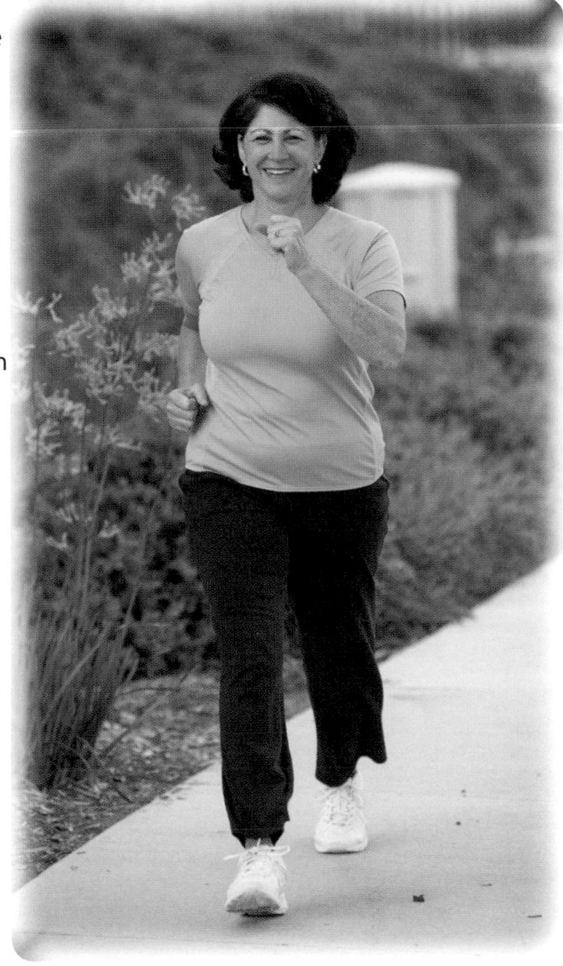

Intrinsically motivated behaviors are engaged in for their own sake and for the pleasure and satisfaction derived from the process of engaging in the activity. Intrinsically motivated behaviors are associated with psychological well-being, interest, enjoyment, fun, and persistence (Ryan & Deci, 2000). Ultimately, the objective is to develop some amount of intrinsic motivation in all clients, as the pursuit of health goals for primarily extrinsically motivated factors is rarely adequate to sustain motivation to progress, especially in the case of adherence to physical activity or exercise (Buckworth et al., 2007).

A common statement among many people struggling to achieve health goals is that they are "always doing for others," so it may appear that extrinsic motivation is a significant source of motivation. However, even those who do a lot for others do so because it provides them with a pleasant emotional response. Further, the immediate satisfaction of doing for others can allow someone to put off the harder job of focusing on self-improvement. Ultimately, everyone is, to a significant degree, self-motivated, which is perfectly normal, though many people are taught to eschew self-motivation for self-sacrifice. The health coach's ability to facilitate a client's reframing of extrinsic motivations as internal ones will enhance the likelihood of success.

Intrinsic Motivation

Some clients will naturally begin with health goals for their own personal achievement and thus are intrinsically motivated at the outset. A client may want to get back in shape after childbirth, reverse poor posture from a sedentary lifestyle, feel more confident about his or her body, enjoy more effortless movement during an activity, or increase performance in some physical pursuit. The main role of the health coach with these types of goals is to ensure that the goals are realistic given the client's current physical abilities and ability to commit to the changes necessary given time demands.

One area to investigate with any client—but especially so with clients with primarily self-interested goals—is the level of support the client has at home, and perhaps at work. Often, if someone is pursuing a change for his or her own benefit and the change is significant enough to affect food choices and leisure-time choices, there can be passive resistance from the client's family and/or coworkers. If a client is seeking significant health improvement, he or she may no longer be curling up on the sofa to watch television in the evening and may begin to skip going out to lunch with coworkers. This can result in subtle resistance from any individual whose preferences are challenged and negatively impacted by the behaviors of the client.

For example, a new client who has signed up for a 5K run and begun resistance training and improving nutrition habits in an effort to reduce body fat might get complaints about the different foods and meals at home and the time spent performing evening workouts that used to be spent watching favorite television shows. At work, the client may have coworkers who dislike the fact that the client no longer joins them to eat out at restaurants with poor quality food, or a client may work in an office that insists on having pastries available every morning or having a cake for everyone's birthday in the office. In isolation, any one of these challenges to a client's resolve in making a change could potentially be handled well. But the cumulative effect of "getting it from all sides" (i.e., overload of environmental stimuli) can leave the client exhausted mentally and prone to slipping back into familiar behavioral patterns from the subtle pull of the people in his or her life. In this case, it is essential for the health coach to be the client's partner in identifying these potential interpersonal challenges and discussing strategies for working around them to equip the client to successfully navigate future obstacles.

APPLY WHAT YOU KNOW

Overcoming Environmental Stimuli Obstacles

A new client works in an office where someone always brings in doughnuts to the weekly staff meeting. In addition, there are a large number of people on staff and the office manager insists on having a cake or cupcakes for everyone's birthday. The client finds it hard to resist these constant temptations. It is absolutely essential at this time to avoid reminding the client of the physical impact of consuming such foods. Instead, the health coach can help the client find a way around this common obstacle.

Client: "I can usually resist the sweets once or twice, but I have a sweet tooth, so when my coworkers start hassling me to just relax and tell me that one cupcake won't kill me, I eventually cave."

Health coach: "If I was your client and you were the coach, how would you tell me to solve this problem?"

Client: I don't know... maybe make sure you're really full from a healthy lunch before the birthday party or something like that."

Health coach: "That's a great idea! If you know in advance of when this occurs, you can plan accordingly by making sure you've eaten just before. Can I try to expand this concept for you?"

Client: "Please do. I feel like I need help with this."

Health coach: "Sometimes you might not be full enough after eating or you might not know exactly when the sweets will be served. Can you keep a toothbrush and toothpaste in your desk? Right before an office gathering where sweets are going to be served, go brush your teeth in the washroom. This might make it easier to say no, since it will affect the taste. What do you think of that idea? Does it sound like a good solution to you?"

Client: "That's great! I'll either make sure I eat a proper meal or brush my teeth right before the office party."

Health coach: "And once you've done this enough times that you've broken the behavioral pattern, you will likely be able to decline the sweets even when you aren't full or haven't just brushed your teeth. We're just using those methods to disrupt the automatic reaction you have to the sweets right now to give you a chance to build your confidence and the ability to make better choices."

In this scenario, the client and health coach strategize short-term solutions to give the client a feeling of success and a break from the stress of having to exhaust willpower fighting to decline sweets. The client either chooses the behavior herself or agrees to suggestions (not directives) from the health coach. This gives the client a chance to experience some "wins," which builds confidence and reinforces the ability to make the desired choice when necessary.

Extrinsic Motivation

Some clients will begin with health goals established mostly as a result of direct input from social contacts or other environmental stimuli, and are therefore primarily extrinsically motivated at the outset. This may derive from the need to be a caregiver for an aging parent, the need to physically keep up with grandchildren as a part-time babysitter, the result of a stern warning from the doctor after some test results, or a spouse or partner who is pressuring the client to get back in shape to maintain physical attraction.

It is essential to realize that while the health goals may have an external origin, the client is ultimately seeking the internal satisfaction of pleasing the other party, so the motivations are simply not yet connected to the behaviors and actions necessary to get results. The external factors are less likely to provide long-term motivation, so the health coach should look for opportunities to reframe the goals in terms of the internal satisfaction that the client receives.

For example, a health coach may have a client whose children have gone off to college, and the client's spouse wants to take the opportunity to travel and explore places best seen on foot with a lot of walking. If the client is not as interested in this goal, but is pursuing better fitness to participate with his or her spouse, it is likely that the client will have adherence problems should any challenges arise in pursuit of the goal. The health coach can make the goal more meaningful by finding out what the client is interested in and seek ways to make the goal more relevant to those deeper, more personal desires while still steering the eventual programming in the direction of the initially stated goal. This uncovers both the internal and external motivators and provides the health coach the opportunity to instill the notion in the client that it is acceptable to focus on one's own goals.

The health coach will find it helpful to use some of the questions identified in Figure 13-1, such as "What things are most important to you? How will a healthy lifestyle complement or support this?" The health coach could also ask, "What do you hope to get out of this experience of getting fit enough to travel and being able to walk comfortably for longer distances?" This helps the health coach dig a little deeper to reveal the intrinsic motivators for this client, even though the main reasons for getting started are extrinsic. Most clients will have a combination of intrinsic and extrinsic goals at the outset.

Combined Intrinsic and Extrinsic Motivation

It is common for clients to present with goals that are initially a combination of intrinsic and extrinsic factors, as both motivations exist within individuals to different degrees (Vallerand, 1997). In many ways, this can be helpful, since the goals will originate from many aspects of the client's life, so there are more opportunities to reinforce the goals. However, the majority of a client's motivation should become intrinsic for long-term success to become more likely. This ensures that there is enough internal drive to overcome obstacles and enjoy successes while staying focused on the daily tasks required for health-behavior change. For example, a client may present with a directive from his or her doctor to exercise because of some health concerns such as high blood pressure, high cholesterol, or **anxiety** from stress. This directive may have triggered the client to recall that he or she used to enjoy a variety of activities before the career and raising a family took over. He or she may have been into hiking and played tennis once a week. The "need" to get back in shape coming from the doctor (extrinsic motivator) has stimulated the desire to return to these two cherished activities (intrinsic motivators). When putting together the recommendations for this client, the health coach will be able to achieve both goals by focusing efforts primarily on the intrinsic motivators, as those will be more relevant for the client and most likely generate better program adherence.

THINK IT THROUGH

If a health coach can uncover the "why" of a client's motivation toward a goal, the client and health coach can use this information to support his or her intentions to stick with the program to reach the goal. What techniques would you use to help clients discover why they have decided to pursue a particular goal?

Big Changes Come From Small Goals

When the goal is better health and fitness, it is often a "big" goal for the client and, as great as it would feel to achieve the goal, it can paradoxically be discouraging and make consistent progress harder if the goal is not shaped and made smaller and more realistic.

There are three key reasons to transform large goals into smaller, more realistic goals:

- Overly general or unrealistic goals demotivate and overwhelm people.
- Small goals direct energy to manageable actions and tasks.
- Transforming larger aspirations into a series of smaller goals provides a clearer picture, or roadmap, for success.

General or Unrealistic Goals Demotivate and Overwhelm

If a client is seeking a return to health and fitness after many years of ignoring it and has "let him- or herself go," there may be a large difference between his or her ultimate vision of fitness compared with the current situation. This discrepancy can easily discourage a client the moment a challenge or obstacle appears. The health coach can help make the goals more realistic by having the client clearly define them. This involves having the client imagine what life would be like if the goal was reached, and imagine, in very small and simple ways, what life would be like if the client were living in a more fit and capable body. A health coach can ask the following questions to help facilitate discovering the specific vision that a client has for his or her health goals:

- What would be the first thing you would do in the morning if you were more fit?
- What activities would you engage in?
- With whom would you engage in these activities?
- How would you spend your free time?

Smaller Goals Direct Energy to Actions and Tasks

Vague intentions to increase fitness are not as useful as clearly defined goals. Even if action is taken, if the goal is unclear, the slightest obstacle or challenge can lead the client to abandon the goal for more immediate concerns. The health coach can help clients discover what fitness means to them by getting clients to provide their own definitions in clear, specific terms relating to the *experience* of living in a healthy body. This helps make fitness more personal and meaningful. If a client develops a series of smaller goals that are within immediate reach, it is easy to generate a feeling of real possibility and hope about achieving goals in general. This positive emotional response is essential, as it has the power to broaden the client's sense of his or her ability to achieve goals. Small goals must have two main characteristics: (1) They must be meaningful to the client and (2) be within immediate reach (i.e., they should have a relatively short timeline, such as a daily or weekly task).

For example, if a client has a goal to "eat healthier," it is very unlikely that this will translate into specific behaviors. What does "eat healthier" mean when the client arrives home after sitting in traffic, is already hungry, and has nothing planned for dinner? The client's immediate needs will outweigh any general sense of eating healthier. When challenged or under pressure, the most familiar path is always the first option. If that means ordering a pizza, this behavior is exactly what will continue to happen. The goal to eat healthier needs to be made clearer by defining specific actions for the client. For example, the client might agree to schedule a time on the weekends to write out a plan for dinners for every weeknight, go shopping to buy the necessary foods for those meals, and always carry a bottle of water to sip on throughout the day. These actions should be chosen by the client, with the health coach making recommendations about which behaviors may need to change and the client making the choices from a list of actions related to how to make the change.

Persevere With Small Goals

Successful behavioral change is almost always the result of small achievements accumulated over time. It is worth pointing out to clients that the opposite is also true—the cumulative effect of repeatedly engaging in a series of small behaviors (e.g., getting a little less physical activity, eating a few "treats" every day, or skipping a meal or two every few days) can have a big impact over time. These are the ways people make physical changes—for better or for worse. A decade of small, poor choices and unhealthy behaviors may lead someone to a decision to get back in shape and hire a health coach for guidance. Often, once the decision is made to get in shape, a client will expect to see results very rapidly. The client may even say something like, "I need to make big changes." In reality, the client needs to make a series of small behavioral changes in a number of areas that will create the big change. The typical client's focus on big changes means he or she will often be very intense at the outset and think that the necessary changes will take a big effort and vast willpower. Clients may even appear very committed when sitting in front of the health coach discussing the goals.

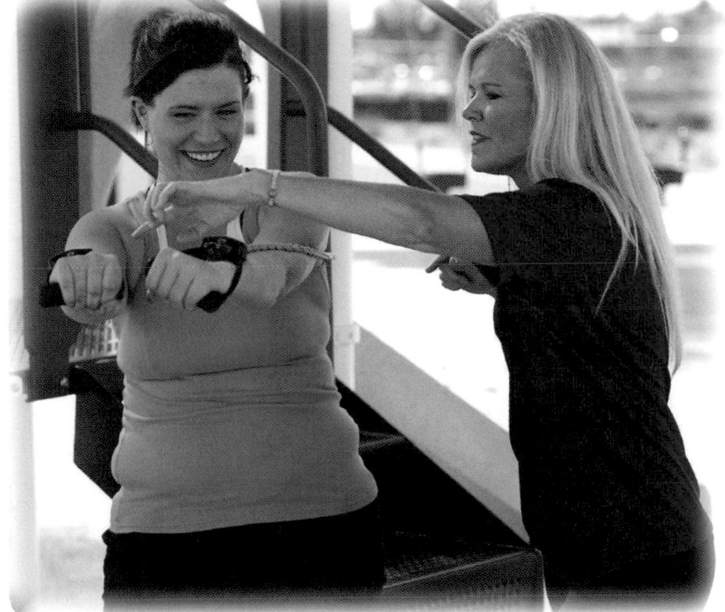

However, when daily life takes over and they are behind on errands, work projects, and home or family demands, the continued effort to change will seem like too much and will be pushed aside for more immediate concerns.

EXPAND YOUR KNOWLEDGE

Willpower

Willpower is the ability to ignore temporary pleasure or discomfort to pursue a longer-term goal, and it is a biological function. It is a mind-body response, not a virtue. Anyone using willpower for long periods or for multiple tasks will have less resolve to make better choices. A review of the literature on self-control and decision-making abilities has shown that willpower is inherently limited (Baumeister, 2003). That is, self-control depletes willpower in much the same way that exercise temporarily depletes physical power. Researchers have found that in experiments where people exert their willpower on one occasion, they have difficulty doing so a second time (Baumeister, 2003). This effect was discovered with all sorts of self-control tasks, such as avoiding tempting foods, suppressing emotions, and sticking with challenging problems.

Using willpower is, in essence, using one's rational side to control or dictate what the emotional side wants—and it is not really a fair fight, as emotions are a more powerful driver of decisions than reason. If clients set too many goals or have goals that are too large and imposing, they can, by force of will, maintain things for a short period. At the first sign of trouble, however—when they get stuck in traffic on the way home from work or have extra responsibilities in dealing with family matters—their resolve crumbles, and they get too worn out to maintain the new, difficult behaviors.

Given that willpower is inherently limited, clients should have strategies to conserve it. Planning in advance for moments of weak self-control reinforces willpower when it is needed most. For example, when a client makes food choices when he or she is hungry or tired, the choices made are often of poor nutritional quality. A better strategy is to organize meals for the day in advance when the client has moments of greatest strength. Another effective strategy for conserving willpower is to think in advance about how to deal with specific obstacles as they arise. In a study on exercise and self-regulation, investigators found that people who wrote in a journal about how they would handle barriers to exercise were more likely to stick with an exercise program (Sniehotta et al., 2005). Another study found that journaling in advance about overcoming barriers helped people succeed at a challenging self-control task, even after a previous task had depleted their willpower (Webb & Sheeran, 2003).

Realistic Goals, Realistic Obstacles

Realistic goals can only come from a realistic examination of the obstacles to health-behavior change. Many clients will have a history of starting and failing, often repeating the same patterns. The specific circumstances may change, but the client's challenges—and reactions to those challenges—can provide insights for the health coach into the obstacles to success that need to be discussed early on. There are two main steps to this process:

- Discover the potential obstacles to achieving the client's goals.
- Help the client find solutions to navigate the obstacles before he or she faces them.

Identify Potential Obstacles

The pattern of starting a fitness program and then stopping the effort is familiar to many people. Often, at the start of a program, the client will be more focused and motivated because it is the beginning of a new endeavor. But there may be significant reasons why the client never enjoys real and lasting change. Uncovering these reasons is valuable information to the health coach when developing a program. Furthermore, it is essential to reexamine the goals in light of any obstacles and discuss potential changes that may be warranted.

Common obstacles to health-behavior change—just like the motivations for health-behavior change—can be either internal or external. Internal obstacles relate to a client's attitudes, opinions, thoughts, feelings, and self-talk about health, fitness, exercise, or nutrition. External obstacles can include time, family, and work responsibilities.

Internal Obstacles

Even though someone may have secured the services of a health coach to provide guidance to make change, there is often an unhealthy mindset in the client that can adversely affect his or her attitudes, thoughts, and feelings toward change. This type of individual has often tried several times to change and failed each time. There is also frequently a sense of loss of control of one's own choices. People often feel overwhelmed by daily demands, and their significant unhappiness with how they feel or look has eroded hope that change is possible. What develops from this are statements like "Exercise does not work for me," or "I have tried everything and nothing works." Statements such as these reflect a mindset of inability to change. Psychologist Carol Dweck (2008) refers to this as a fixed mindset, which is characterized by a deterministic view of the world, or in the language of fitness, a belief that health and fitness are determined by one's genes. As a result, they avoid challenges, give up easily, see effort as fruitless, and feel threatened by the success of others. It should be apparent that in this case, it is imperative for the health coach to steer the client toward a growth mindset, which is characterized by a desire to learn and grow, embrace challenges, persist in the face of setbacks, view effort as the path to improvement, and find lessons and inspiration in the success of others. To facilitate this change, the health coach can simply begin to examine the potential challenges a client faces now and has faced previously in pursuit of health improvement. An important part of this is interviewing the client about what he or she feels could have been done to cope with challenges more effectively in the past and how he or she plans on coping with current challenges. This process helps the health coach avoid the common practice of telling clients what to do and instead treat them like they possess the ability to find the best way around their own obstacles by facilitating the development of their own solutions.

For example, a client has admitted that he or she needs to drink more water. Instead of telling the client how much water to drink, the health coach can ask more questions such as, "How will you ensure that you begin to drink more water?" and wait for the client's response. The client might have an idea about how best to achieve this goal. If the client needs help, then the health coach can offer suggestions, while still allowing the client to choose which of the offered suggestions seems to be the most practical and suitable. For example, the health coach may offer the following options to help the client achieve the goal of drinking more water:

- Always carry water in the car, at work, and throughout the daily routine.
- Link the behavior to something commonly done throughout the day, such as taking a sip of water every time the client sends a text message or email.
- When eating, the client can take a sip of water every three bites.

The client gets to choose which of these might work. If none of them are agreeable to the client, they still may inspire a new solution from the client. Either way, the client chooses which behavior(s) to use to achieve the goal, not the health coach.

External Obstacles

Frequently, when discussing goals and the available time for commitment to the exercise and nutrition changes necessary, a client will provide the health coach with best-case scenario answers. It is important for the health coach to gain an understanding of the realistic time available and motivation level of the client. This aids the health coach in developing recommendations that will truly fit a client's life and avoid setting up a situation where the lifestyle changes are in direct competition with other priorities and commitments. A realistic examination of the opportunities for change remaining in a client's life, after including all the daily work and family responsibilities, is the first step in identifying external obstacles.

For example, a client may state that he or she has five days per week available to exercise, with 90 minutes per session. Upon further investigation, this might only be true if there are no traffic problems to and from work, if there are no major deadlines requiring extra work, and there are no school events that require getting the children to and from practices, games, or performances. It might also be true that the 90 minutes includes travel time to and from the gym, and time to park, get into the club, and change clothes. The client may have significantly less actual exercise time available given these considerations. If these factors are not uncovered initially and the health coach simply proceeds with the program, the client will eventually feel the stress and pressure of the competing demands and the health program will often be what is compromised.

APPLY WHAT YOU KNOW

Everyone Has Time for Results

Many people cite a lack of results as the reason they cease fitness programs, while a perceived lack of time is the most commonly cited reason why people do not begin exercising in the first place. It is important to note how one often leads to the other. With full-time careers, children to raise, long commutes with long workdays (which often do not stop once people are home), there are many demands on people's time and energy. These significant time, family, and work commitments can overwhelm anyone's efforts to change, but are less likely to do so if clients are getting results or if they truly believe they will get meaningful results.

Typically, when someone begins to feel better, move more fluidly, or has clothes that fit better, the enthusiasm that ensues enables the person to overcome most obstacles to continued participation in a fitness program. Conversely, after the initial rush of enthusiasm passes, if someone is not getting results, the time and energy he or she devotes to the fitness program will seem less worthwhile and a few missed workouts may lead to complete relapse. Stated simply, people do not typically choose to continually devote time and energy to something that is providing no discernable positive benefit in return. If there is effort without reward, motivation wanes and the effort will soon disappear.

Consider the client from the "Preparing for Obstacles" sidebar (see page 364). In this scenario, the client was guided to focus on what has improved—the increased ability to play with her kids—and reminded of the importance of this goal. Whenever someone is engaging in the right behaviors, there will be positive changes to discuss. Often, the client will focus on only the bigger parts of the goal and may need to be reminded of smaller goals that he or she has already expressed. The client may need to be encouraged to consider other signs of progress that he or she may not be aware of yet because of the focus on the larger goals.

Develop Solutions Before Problems Appear

It is best to have a client develop his or her own solutions to common obstacles so he or she develops improved reactions to challenges that are more in line with health goals. Another reason this is essential in the initial stages of a client–health coach relationship is that this provides the client the opportunity to think of solutions when not actually facing an obstacle. When facing an obstacle that has historically thrown the client off course from his or her health goals, the most familiar path will be the one that is taken unless a different response has been planned.

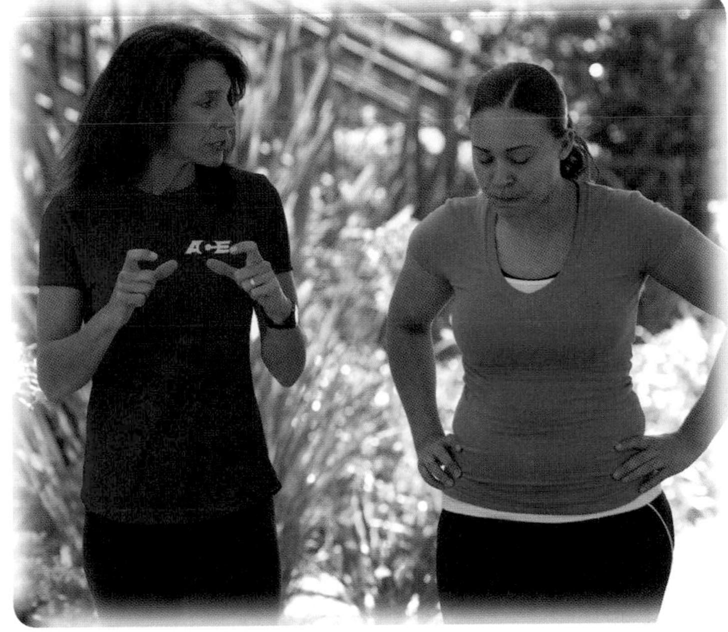

Through facilitation by the health coach, the client can gain confidence from the knowledge that there has been a different solution created in collaboration with a competent, caring fitness professional, and often the boost to morale that comes from this is enough to provide the client with the motivation to successfully work through an obstacle. Simply altering the familiar path of facing obstacles alone without effective coping strategies is enough to enhance clients' abilities to successfully navigate challenges that had previously derailed their efforts. For example, a client may have a history of missing a workout or two, and then getting discouraged and engaging in negative self-talk. The powerful negative emotions take control and overshadow her desire to follow through on her efforts. After discussing this with the health coach, the client has realized that she will not get in great shape from one or two workouts and, similarly, she will not get out of shape from missing one or two workouts. This has helped her keep a more long-term perspective on things.

Everyone Is Good at Something

The widespread difficulty experienced by people from all walks of life in pursuit of health and fitness has created an interesting situation for fitness professionals. It is common to encounter people who are successful in their careers and in organizing home and family, and are very confident when performing tasks in those areas. Yet, when the topic turns to exercise, nutrition, or other health-related behaviors, many people lack confidence in their own abilities, are susceptible to the latest fads, and have difficulty keeping their goals in focus.

Everyone has an area where they are confident, capable, and in control, either professionally or at home. For example, a project manager can smoothly organize many people and tasks to achieve a larger objective. A parent might successfully manage multiple family schedules and get everyone where they need to be on time and well-fed. Some people may do both. If the health coach reframes a health goal as a goal or project in areas where the client is already confident, the client can bring the same skills that he or she already possesses to bear on health goals. This helps the client uncover unrecognized strength.

People often compartmentalize their skills and abilities. For example, a client might describe herself as an excellent accountant, but have terrible nutrition and exercise habits.

The attention to detail and organizational skills required to be a successful accountant are not that different from those required to successfully follow through on lifestyle change. The same could be said of any worthwhile pursuit of a professional or personal nature. The health coach can present to clients the idea that they already possess the skills necessary for successful lifestyle change by pointing out the areas in which the client is already confident and capable. Many people will appreciate—and perhaps even be a bit surprised by—this fresh take on their abilities to succeed.

A simple way to introduce this concept is to ask clients what they are good at now. Then ask them if they were good at it the first time they did it or before they were experienced or practiced? *Everything in life is hard before it is easy*. From learning the alphabet to mastering calculus, anything new is hard until it has been done often enough for the person to get better at it. This is a simple but important lesson for many clients.

Decisional Balance Worksheet

Visit www.ACEfitness.org/HealthCoachResources to download a free PDF of the decisional balance worksheet, as well as other forms and assessment tools that you can use throughout your career as a health coach.

Even though the benefits of making positive lifestyle changes are readily apparent, it would surprise some health coaches to know that in the minds of many individuals, there are also benefits to *not* making those changes. During the assessment process, it can be useful for the health coach to use a decisional balance worksheet with clients (Figure 13-2). This classic concept was developed by psychologists Janis and Mann in the 1960s and used as a way to look at decision-making (Janis & Mann, 1977). The balance sheet recognizes that both gains and losses can be consequences of a single decision. The balance sheet is a place to record the advantages and disadvantages of different options facing an individual. Clients can use this tool to detail everything that could affect their decision to make changes. The client writes down all of his or her positive and negative perceptions about exercise (or any other health-related behavioral change), which helps him or her connect with the benefits of change and remove barriers to change.

Any behavioral change will have pros and cons—even behaviors that are unequivocally positive. Clients can sometimes experience a sense of ambivalence, wherein they sometimes

Figure 13-2
Sample decisional balance worksheet

Behavior	Disadvantages	Advantages
Continue to *not* exercise	Cannot play with kids Have to buy new clothes Depression Low energy	More free time Easier
Begin to exercise	Requires a lot of effort Takes up time More laundry from workouts	More confidence Better mood Better problem-solving skills Feel better in clothes Less back pain Feel more attractive

see a real need for change, but sometimes feel it is simply not worth the effort. The decisional balance worksheet helps the health coach and the client ensure that there is motivation toward the desired changes for health improvement. The health coach can give the client a blank worksheet with instructions to either complete it in advance of the first session or together with the health coach—whichever is most relevant and convenient for the client.

Summary

A realistic approach to goal-setting involves going beyond the first answer to the question, "What are your health and fitness goals?" Gathering additional details surrounding a client's goals will enable the health coach to understand the motivations for the goals, their relevance to the client, and the potential obstacles the client faces. It is imperative for the health coach to discover why the client's goals matter and how the client's health efforts will connect to what the client values in life. This information will help the health coach provide guidance for the client to overcome obstacles and challenges. By knowing what the client values, the health coach can help ensure that goals are relevant for the client by framing the lifestyle behaviors in terms of those values. This understanding will greatly amplify the quality of the experience the client has with the health coach and allow the achievement of results that are perhaps even better than the client expects.

References

Baumeister, R.F. (2003). Ego depletion and self-regulation failure: A resource model of self-control. *Alcoholism: Clinical and Experimental Research*, 27, 281–284.

Buckworth, J. et al. (2007). Decomposing intrinsic and extrinsic motivation for exercise: Application to stages of motivational readiness. *Psychology of Sport and Exercise*, 8, 441–461.

Dweck, C. (2008). *Mindset: The New Psychology of Success.* New York: Ballantine Books.

Janis, I.L. & Mann, L. (1977). *Decision Making: A Psychological Analysis of Conflict, Choice, and Commitment.* New York, Free Press.

Ryan, M.R. & Deci, L.E. (2000). Self-determination and the facilitation of intrinsic motivation, social development, and well-being. *American Psychologist*, 55, 68–78.

Shilts, M.K., Horowitz, M., & Townsend, M.S. (2009). Guided goal setting: Effectiveness in a dietary and physical activity intervention with low-income adolescents. *International Journal of Adolescent Medicine and Health*, 21, 111–122.

Shilts, M.K., Horowitz, M., & Townsend, M.S. (2004). Goal setting as a strategy for dietary and physical activity behavior change: A review of the literature. *American Journal of Health Promotion*, 19, 81–93.

Sniehotta, F.F. et al. (2005). Long-term effects of two psychological interventions on physical exercise and self-regulation following coronary rehabilitation. *International Journal of Behavioral Medicine*, 12, 244–255.

Webb, T.L. & Sheeran, P. (2003). Can implementation intentions help to overcome ego-depletion? *Journal of Experimental Psychology*, 39, 279–286.

Vallerand, R.J. (1997). Toward a hierarchical model of intrinsic and extrinsic motivation. In: Zanna, M.P. (Ed.) *Advances in Experimental Social Psychology* (pp. 271–360). New York: Academic Press.

Suggested Reading

DiSalvo, D. (2011). *What Makes Your Brain Happy and Why You Should Do the Opposite.* Amherst, N.Y.: Prometheus Books.

Heath, C. & Heath, D. (2010). *Switch: How to Change Things When Change is Hard.* New York: Crown Business.

McGonigal, K. (2012). *The Willpower Instinct.* New York: Penguin Group.

Medina, J. (2009). *Brain Rules: 12 Principles for Surviving and Thriving at Work, Home, and School.* Seattle, Wash.: Pear Press.

Miller, W. & Rollnick, S. (2012). *Motivational Interviewing: Preparing People for Change* (2nd ed.). New York: Guilford Press.

Patterson, K. et al. (2011). *Crucial Conversations: Tools for Talking When Stakes Are High.* Columbus, Ohio: Mc-Graw-Hill.

Ratey, J. (2008). *Spark: The Revolutionary New Science of Exercise and the Brain.* New York: Little, Brown, and Company.

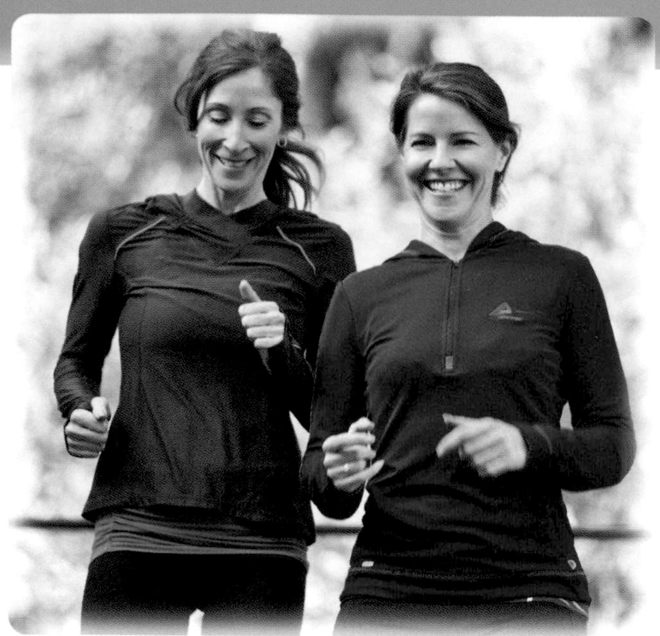

IN THIS CHAPTER:

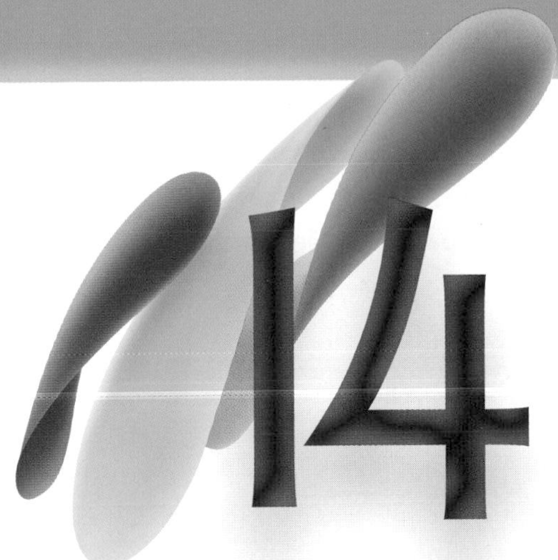

14 Lifestyle Modification and Behavioral Change

BARBARA A. BREHM

Barbara A. Brehm, Ed.D., is professor of exercise and sport studies at Smith College, Northampton, Mass., where she teaches courses in nutrition, health behavior, and stress management. She is also director of the Smith Fitness Program for Faculty and Staff. Dr. Brehm is the author of several books, including Successful Fitness Motivation Strategies.

Most clients will likely tell their ACE-certified Health Coach that starting a weight-loss plan is easy; sticking to the plan is the hard part. Clients often say, "I know what I am supposed to do. I just can't seem to get myself to do it."

For many health and fitness professionals, mastering the basics of exercise science and nutrition is fairly straightforward. Soon after developing this foundation, they become comfortable with recommending exercise programs, giving advice on preventing injury, and guiding clients on how to make healthier nutrition choices. Helping clients stick with their plans, however, is often the biggest challenge.

Lifestyle modification and behavioral change are simple in theory. First, health coaches help clients figure out what lifestyle habits and daily behaviors are problem areas. Then, they help clients come up with plans to replace problematic habits with behaviors that promote a healthier weight. Clients modify their lifestyles as planned, and they lose weight—simple!

Of course, if losing weight was really that easy, much of the world would not be facing an **obesity** crisis. In reality, changing one's lifestyle is a complicated and difficult challenge. Lifestyles evolve for various reasons over many years, and people behave the way they do because their behaviors "work" for them. Clients' eating and activity patterns have adapted over the years, and have been influenced by such factors as friends, family, culture, financial constraints, current health status, and work. Some clients may use eating and other behaviors to cope with negative moods, connect with family and friends, celebrate triumphs, and soothe jangled nerves.

While working with clients to implement lifestyle-modification and behavior-change programs, a health coach must transition from being an expert to acting as a cheerleader and guide. While fitness professionals may know more about exercise and nutritional science than their clients, it is the clients who are ultimately in control of choosing a healthier lifestyle.

When studying lifestyle modification and behavioral change, it is important to keep in mind the material presented in Chapter 5 on the importance of good communication. Good listening skills are essential. A health coach must listen with **empathy** and keep an open mind when talking to clients about their weight-control issues and other challenges.

What Determines Behavior?

Several theories attempt to explain health behaviors. Keep in mind that theories are approximations that can help health coaches better understand their clients. Theories will not, however, always apply to every individual. Nevertheless, they give health coaches a starting point for their work, from which they can make adjustments as they get to know their clients better.

Socio-ecological Model

People are social creatures, so their eating and physical-activity habits, as well as their stress and coping patterns, are greatly influenced by the social and physical environments in which they live. Ecological perspectives, which are sometimes referred to as the **socio-ecological model (SEM),** can help the health coach better understand the health behaviors of their clients and more effectively structure behavior-change programs. Ecological perspectives look at the interrelationships between individuals and the environments in which they live and work, and examine the many levels at which individuals are influenced, both in terms of support for healthy behaviors and barriers to improving health behavior (Fisher, 2008) (Figure 14-1).

Figure 14-1
Ecological perspective

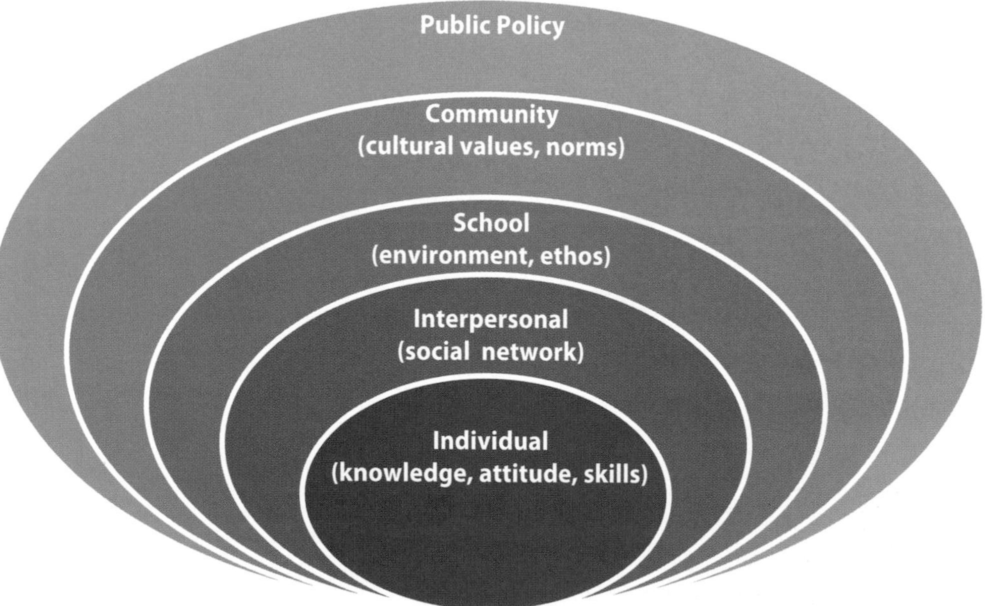

Much behavior-change research has focused on individual decision-making and health outcomes. But the individual decisions that deal with engaging in physical activity and making wise food choices are influenced by the various levels depicted in Figure 14-1. For example, on an individual level, a person's prior experiences with physical activity influence his or her current attitudes regarding what types of activities are appealing. Family influences can provide much-needed support for change, as when a helpful older child watches the younger children while a parent goes for a walk. Of course, families can also create strong barriers to change. Family responsibilities, such as needing to care for a disabled family member, can create high levels of stress or limit the time available to the caretaker for exercise. Close friends, neighborhoods, and social networks tend to support certain lifestyle habits, both good and bad. Clients may be encouraged to walk to the store because safe sidewalks promote walking to neighborhood destinations, or to go out for ice cream every Sunday afternoon with friends. Norms regarding body size, physical activity, and diet influence what clients see as acceptable and desirable. When friends and family members gain weight, obesity may become more acceptable to an individual. An interesting study examining weight changes in 12,067 participants in the renowned Framingham Heart Study found that the risk of weight gain increases when a person's close friends and family members gain weight (Christakis & Fowler, 2007). Subjects in this study experienced a 57% increase in risk of gaining weight (above what would normally be predicted to occur over time) if a close friend gained weight. Risk increased by 40% if a sibling gained weight and by 37% if one's spouse gained weight. While researchers could not pinpoint any particular causes for these associations, they ruled out shared environment as the strongest influence, since the effect of close friends did not vary with proximity to the test subject. In other words, whether best friends lived thousands of miles apart or in the same town, the effect was the same. Instead, the researchers proposed that friends and family affect each other's *perception* of fatness, and change each other's ideas of what kind of body size is acceptable.

Other levels in the ecological perspective also influence health behaviors. Workplaces and community organizations may enlarge or restrict options for exercise and choices of meal options. Yet other influences, such as public health policies and economic structures, influence important factors such as local food availability and healthcare opportunities.

A health coach must try to understand the clients who come to him or her for help. If a client's cultural background differs from that of the health coach, it is the health coach's responsibility to learn about the client's diet, traditions, belief system, and family structure. Advice on behavior change will not be relevant without an understanding of a client's lifestyle and the various ecological levels in which the client operates.

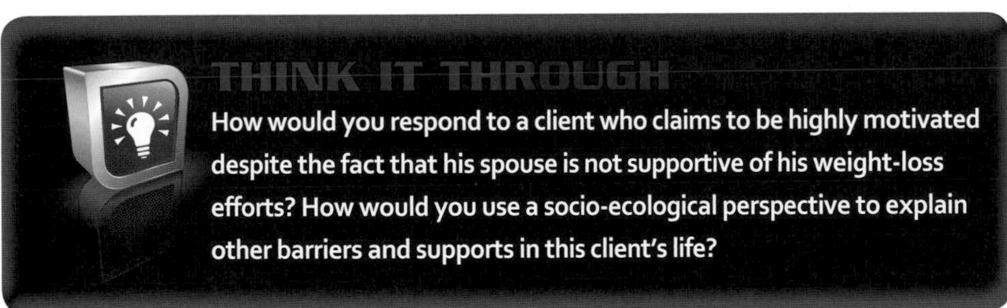

THINK IT THROUGH
How would you respond to a client who claims to be highly motivated despite the fact that his spouse is not supportive of his weight-loss efforts? How would you use a socio-ecological perspective to explain other barriers and supports in this client's life?

Stages of Change

The **transtheoretical model of behavioral change (TTM)** emphasizes the importance of determining a client's readiness for change (see Chapter 3). According to this model, which is also called the **stages-of-change model,** people who change their behavior go through several stages, from **precontemplation** (not thinking about changing), to **contemplation** (weighing the pros and cons of changing), **preparation** (getting ready to make a change), **action** (practicing the new behavior), and finally to **maintenance** (incorporating the new behavior into one's lifestyle). Refer to Table 3-1 on page 60 for a summary of the stages of change for exercise and a list of effective intervention approaches for clients in each stage.

For effective weight-loss intervention, it is essential that health coaches determine where a new client is in the behavior-change process. Fitness professionals often assume that people who come to them for exercise advice are eager to begin an exercise program. While this is often the case, many times these people are still weighing the pros and cons of starting an exercise program and have not yet formed a strong intention to commit to the group exercise class or regularly visit the fitness center. Yet fitness professionals plow ahead in designing a delightfully complicated exercise program for their clients—and then wonder why they stop attending after a few weeks.

Moreover, applying the stages-of-change model in a weight-management program requires addressing different behaviors simultaneously. Some changes come more easily than others, and clients may be ready to change some behaviors, but not others. For example, a client might already be entering the action stage in terms of reducing empty-calorie foods, but have doubts about his or her ability to stick to an exercise program. This scenario is not uncommon for people with a history of obesity. They may have avoided exercise in the past because physical activity was embarrassing or difficult for them, but may have had plenty of experience with various diet programs. Health coaches should assess stages of exercise and diet readiness separately, and use appropriate intervention strategies according to each client's readiness for change.

Health Belief Model

The **health belief model** suggests that a person's health beliefs influence decisions about behavioral change (see Chapter 3). According to this model, it is best if clients perceive obesity as a potential health problem that has serious consequences, so they become motivated to do something about it. Addressing health beliefs with **overweight** clients is especially important in the early stages of behavioral change.

Health coaches should discuss clients' beliefs about obesity, weight loss, nutrition, and physical activity, and correct misperceptions with accurate information from handouts, pamphlets, websites, and other reputable sources, such as www.ACEfitness.org/getfit/default.aspx. Useful information and tools will help clients weigh the pros and cons of behavioral change and may create an incentive to modify their current lifestyles.

Health coaches should help clients understand that lifestyle modification is the best option for addressing obesity. Perceiving obesity as a health threat can motivate behavior change, as long as the change is perceived as feasible by the client. Health coaches should also build clients' **self-efficacy** so that they feel empowered to modify their lifestyles to reduce health risks (see Chapter 3 for more information on how to enhance self-efficacy).

Principles of Lifestyle Modification

Health psychology research has clarified many helpful principles of lifestyle modification for health coaches. While some of these principles may have intimidating names and terminology, they are congruent with common sense and should be remembered while working with clients to evaluate and guide their lifestyle-modification efforts.

Motivation for Change: Self-determination Theory

People generally do not like to be told what to do, especially by someone younger and less experienced than themselves. For health coaches who have never had a weight problem, identifying with overweight or obese clients may be difficult. Clients do not want to be judged or criticized, especially by someone who "just doesn't understand." Health coaches must examine and correct their own prejudices regarding obese clients (Teachman & Brownell, 2001). Health coaches can use the suggested readings at the end of this chapter to learn more about the experiences of overweight people.

After extensive research into the motivation behind behavioral change, psychologists Edward Deci and Richard Ryan (2008) believe that people are naturally motivated to pursue activities and goals in which they are interested, and from which they feel they derive benefit. Deci and Ryan point out that people also act in response to external forces that pressure them into behaving in certain ways. These researchers have described different types of motivation in their **self-determination theory (SDT).** Autonomous motivation occurs when people feel like they are acting as a result of their own free will and doing something because they want to. Controlled motivation means people are doing something because they feel pushed by external forces. People prefer to change their lifestyles because of autonomous motivation rather than controlled motivation.

Deci and Ryan (2008) break motivation down into five categories:

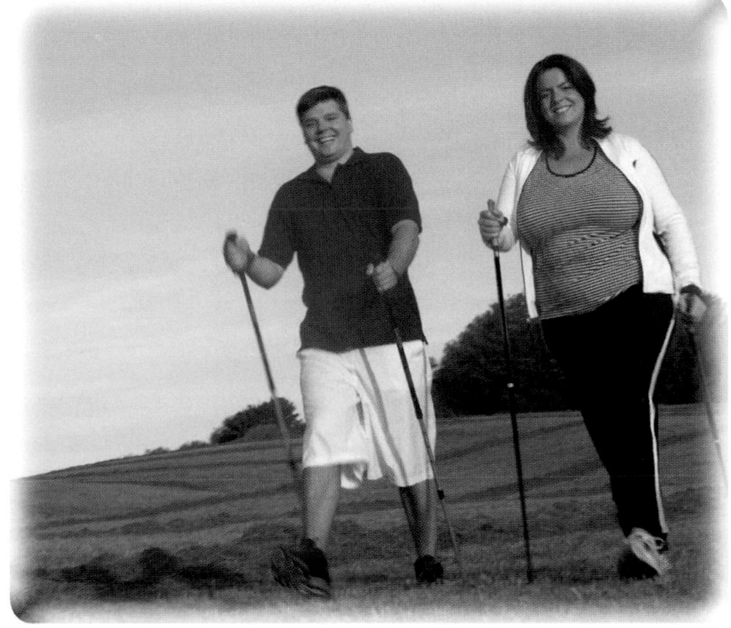

- *Intrinsic motivation:* People engage in an activity because it is inherently interesting or enjoyable. For example, people may go hiking because they enjoy it, or drink tomato juice because they like the taste. Intrinsic motivation is a form of autonomous motivation and is the most effective type of motivation for behavior change.
- *Integrated regulation:* The behavior and its goals have become integrated into a person's self-concept. People with integrated regulation see themselves as cyclists, runners, or weight-room regulars.
- *Identified regulation:* People engage in an activity because it helps them reach a personally meaningful goal, even though they may not actually enjoy the activity very much. For example, people may go for a hike because they know it will help them control their blood pressure, or drink tomato juice because they think it will benefit their health. People have integrated the goal of the activity into their personal values, and their behavior feels autonomous.
- *Introjected regulation:* People engage in an activity because they think they should, even though they really do not want to. Individuals motivated by introjected regulation act to avoid feeling guilty or obtain contingent self-worth. For example, people may join an exercise class because a spouse bullied them into it. They may join the class to appease the spouse, but they do not feel good about joining. Introjected regulation feels more like

controlled regulation, and people generally do not enjoy feeling like they are being forced to do something they do not want to do.

- *External regulation:* People engage in an activity solely from external pressure to avoid punishment or gain rewards. For example, children may participate in physical education activities only because they must, simply to avoid punishment. External regulation is a form of controlled motivation. People trying to change behavior for this reason are rarely committed to long-term behavioral change.

Deci and Ryan (2008) have also described three factors that guide human development and influence lifestyle change:

- *Autonomy* refers to the fact that people like to feel they have choices and are acting in accordance with their own values and wishes.
- *Competence* refers to the fact that people like to feel that they have some skill in the activities in which they engage. They like to feel competent, or at least like they are improving and doing fairly well in a given activity. When people feel incompetent, they lose motivation to continue trying.
- *Connection* means that people feel a bond to others. As social creatures, humans have a basic drive to connect with others. These positive connections are motivational, and they help people continue working toward their goals, even in the face of adversity.

As health coaches work with clients, they should use their good communication skills to establish a feeling of connection with clients. They should help clients be as successful as possible in their lifestyle-modification programs in order to build feelings of competence. To maximize client motivation, health coaches must encourage clients take the lead in designing their own lifestyle-modification and behavior-change programs. Every person is different, and each client's life circumstances must be regarded with dignity and respect. Health coaches must combine their knowledge of behavior-change research with the emotional intelligence needed to respond with their hearts and minds to the unique experiences of every client.

Self-efficacy

Self-efficacy refers to a person's belief that he or she can perform a given task (Bandura, 1997). While self-efficacy is similar to self-confidence, it is always situation- or behavior-specific. For example, a client may be very confident in his ability to reduce calorie intake, but have low self-efficacy in terms of sticking to an exercise program. Self-efficacy is synonymous with feelings of competence as described in the SDT.

Self-efficacy predicts how much effort clients will exert in sticking to their lifestyle-modification programs. Self-efficacy also predicts how hard clients will persist in their behavior-change efforts when facing difficulties (Bandura, 1997).

Strengthening self-efficacy is important at all stages of behavioral change. That said, precontemplators and contemplators tend to have especially low self-efficacy in the realm of weight-control behaviors (see Chapter 3). Much of a health coach's work with clients in these stages will be focused on helping them believe that they can modify their lifestyles and change problematic behaviors.

Operant Conditioning

Operant conditioning examines the relationships between behaviors and their

consequences (see Chapter 3). Behaviors followed by a reward are likely to be repeated, whereas behaviors followed by a punishment are less likely to be repeated. Of course, for humans, eating behavior is usually wrapped up with a complex system of punishments (feeling guilty for overeating) and reward (enjoyment of eating, feeling nourished and satisfied). For the purpose of weight control, health coaches should focus on factors that reward exercise and healthful eating behaviors, keeping in mind the SDT principle stating that autonomous motivations are best. For example, clients who choose to walk with a good friend might find the experience enjoyable. In this case, the enjoyment of being with the friend is a reward, reinforcing the walking behavior. Through the pleasant experience, the client not only feels rewarded, but he or she may also develop more autonomous motivation to exercise.

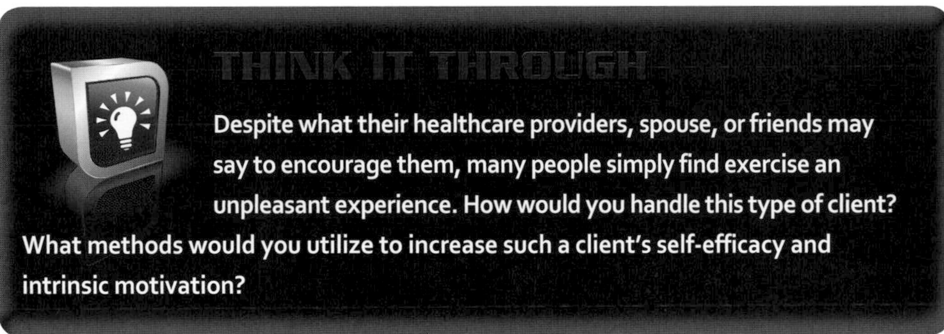

Despite what their healthcare providers, spouse, or friends may say to encourage them, many people simply find exercise an unpleasant experience. How would you handle this type of client? What methods would you utilize to increase such a client's self-efficacy and intrinsic motivation?

Principle of Limited Self-control

Clients will often say, "If only I had more willpower, I would…" It takes effort to change one's lifestyle, exercise regularly, and change one's eating habits. Psychologists who study willpower refer to this concept as **self-regulation** or **self-control.** Their research has several applications for health coaches.

First, psychologists believe that for each person, self-control is a limited resource (Muraven & Baumeister, 2000). While some clients have more self-control than others, no one has a limitless supply. The more health coaches and clients can minimize the amount of self-control needed to maintain lifestyle modifications, the more successful they will be. For example, clients who "clean up" their eating environments at home by eliminating foods they are trying to avoid will not have to exert self-control to avoid eating foods that are sitting in plain sight on the kitchen counter.

Second, habits are comfortable and require little self-control. The more quickly lifestyle modifications can become habits, the happier and more successful a client will be. People are creatures of habit and tend to settle into daily routines. Researchers who study self-control believe that most people are able to tolerate only a relatively small disruption in their daily routines before experiencing stress (Vohs & Heatherton, 2000).

Third, coping with stress requires a certain level of self-control. This observation helps explain why it is more difficult to change a habit when under a lot of stress. The emotional energy that would otherwise be used to exert self-control in a particular situation gets used up when a person is dealing with stress. Encourage clients to begin a lifestyle-modification program when stress levels are relatively low, such as after (rather than during) the holidays. Managing stress and negative emotions must be an integral part of every lifestyle-modification program.

Lastly, self-control appears to be renewed daily. It is highest in the mornings, and then gradually diminishes as the day goes on. This observation helps explain why people who exercise in the morning tend to be most successful in sticking to their exercise programs. It also explains why dieters are more able to follow their plans in the early part of the day, but often give in to temptation in the late afternoon and evening.

Contrary to popular belief, many overweight people actually have a great deal of self-control, even though they often do not think so. A failure to lose weight is often attributed to a failure of willpower rather than to the fact that (1) their diets were impossible to follow, or (2) that people often establish totally unrealistic weight-loss goals. Health coaches should help clients design lifestyle-modification strategies that call for realistic levels of self-control, and help clients understand that changing behaviors becomes easier as those behaviors develop into lifelong habits.

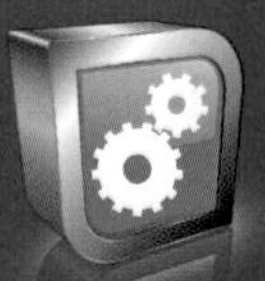

EXPAND YOUR KNOWLEDGE

The Force of Habit

Research on people who have successfully lost weight supports the idea that modifying lifestyle is a crucial component of successful weight-management efforts. Some of the most interesting data on successful lifestyle-modification practices come from research work done by Rena Wing, James O. Hill, and colleagues at the National Weight Control Registry (NWCR). The NWCR was created in 1994, and follows individuals who have lost at least 30 pounds (13.6 kg) and maintained the weight loss for one year or more.

Data from the NWCR have found the following lifestyle-modification strategies to be most commonly used among people who have been successful in their weight-management efforts (Wing & Phelan, 2005):

- Engaging in high levels of physical activity, at least one hour each day
- Eating a low-calorie, low-fat diet
- Eating breakfast daily
- Self-monitoring body weight regularly
- Maintaining a consistent eating pattern every day, on both weekdays and weekends

Participants in the NWCR who maintained their weight loss for more than two years had greater long-term success rates, suggesting that lifestyles had become modified, with the force of habit supporting weight maintenance. Data from this study also support the health belief model, in that a medical incentive for weight loss (e.g., treatment of hypertension) was associated with long-term success.

The False-hope Syndrome and the Planning Fallacy

As Alexander Pope wrote, "Hope springs eternal in the human breast." While this idea can be helpful during a weight-management effort, psychologists have observed that hope can be problematic when it leads to unrealistic goals. People's tendency to set unrealistic goals is called the **false-hope syndrome** (Polivy & Herman, 2000). Setting ambitious goals makes people feel good. Their self-image improves, and they feel optimistic and in control. "I will lose 20 pounds in the next five weeks." But what happens as time goes by and goals are not reached? Clients are disappointed in themselves, feel bad, and ultimately discontinue their behavior-change programs.

The **planning fallacy** states that people consistently underestimate the time, energy, and other resources required to complete a given task (Buehler, Griffin, & Ross, 1994). Whether someone is building a space shuttle, remodeling the kitchen, starting an exercise program, or changing eating habits, most projects end up taking more money, time, and effort than anticipated. Clients often say that they will spend more time exercising than they really can, or that they will change their eating habits more drastically than they can really tolerate.

Therefore, health coaches must keep the false-hope syndrome and planning fallacy in mind when helping clients design lifestyle-modification programs. Health coaches must encourage clients to get positive results, but explain that changing habits takes a great deal of time and effort. It is important to help clients set modest goals and take small, manageable steps that reinforce feelings of self-efficacy and the belief that they can stick with the program.

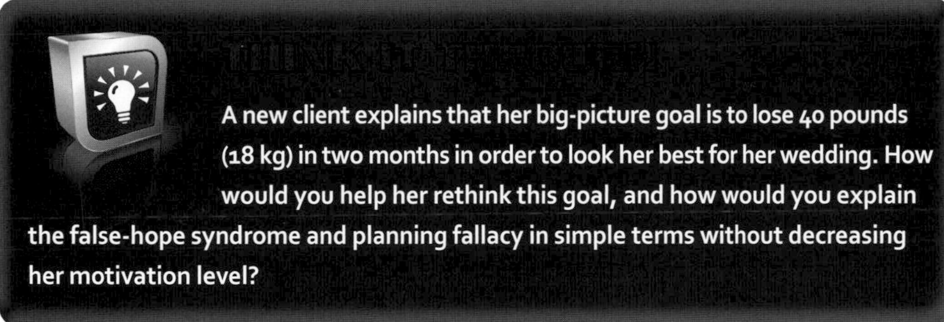

A new client explains that her big-picture goal is to lose 40 pounds (18 kg) in two months in order to look her best for her wedding. How would you help her rethink this goal, and how would you explain the false-hope syndrome and planning fallacy in simple terms without decreasing her motivation level?

Stress Management and Negative Mood

Stress is the most common reason that people abandon their plans to change behavior. Stress depletes self-control, lowers feelings of self-efficacy, and decreases energy and motivation. Too much stress triggers negative emotions such as **anxiety,** anger, and sadness. When people feel bad, they look for ways to feel better. Coping with negative emotions is more important for most people than sticking to a lifestyle-modification program. The perceived future benefits of lifestyle modification can be overwhelmed by feelings of deprivation at the present time (Tice, Bratslavsky, & Baumeister, 2001).

Some people respond to feelings of stress and to extreme emotional states (both negative and positive) by eating, even when they are not hungry. Eating triggered by emotional states is referred to as **emotional eating.** This response is fairly widespread in the general population, not just among those who are overweight (Geliebter & Aversa, 2003). Emotional eating becomes a problem when people are trying to reduce food intake. The stress associated with lifestyle modification can compound the problem of emotional eating. In other words, eating less than normal causes stress, which can lead, paradoxically, to overeating.

Guiding clients to monitor and manage stress levels must be an integral and continuing component of all lifestyle-modification and behavior-change recommendations. Lifestyle modifications should create as little stress as possible, and clients, especially emotional eaters, must learn new ways of coping with stress and negative moods, instead of simply reaching for their favorite comfort foods.

Lifelong Sustainability and Relapse Prevention

A sobering principle that all clients must face is that obesity is a chronic disease with no quick fix. The lifestyle modifications and behavioral changes that lead to weight loss must be maintained to prevent weight regain. People who succeed in maintaining weight loss continue to exercise and watch their eating habits for a lifetime (Wing & Phelan, 2005). Successful weight control requires lifelong lifestyle modifications.

A hectic lifestyle offers many opportunities for disruption to lifestyle-modification programs, even for people with the best of intentions. Clients must understand that achieving perfection is impossible, and that they may occasionally overeat or skip exercise sessions. The goal of relapse-prevention work is to prevent a lapse (i.e., a short-term disruption in a lifestyle-modification program) from turning into relapse (i.e., a return to one's former behaviors and the act of "giving up" on the lifestyle-modification program) (Hendershot, Marlatt, & George, 2009).

Relapse-prevention discussions with clients can encourage them to anticipate and visualize occasions during which they may experience lapses in their behavior-change programs. Health coaches can help clients understand that lapses are normal and should be accepted and taken in stride. While feelings of disappointment may arise when lapses occur, it is important for clients to avoid feelings of failure and guilt, as these negative thoughts and emotions can deplete self-control and energy, increase feelings of stress, and lead to total relapse and motivational collapse. Lapses are a fact of life. Clients should use their behavior-change skills to avoid them as much as possible, but should also know that they can get back on track if disruptions occur.

Lifestyle-modification Strategies

Successful lifestyle-modification strategies derive from an understanding of the principles presented earlier in this chapter. The following strategies may be incorporated into either individual or group formats.

Strengthen Autonomous Motivation to Change

Use good listening and coaching skills to encourage clients to take responsibility for their own lifestyle-modification programs. While the health coach should be ready with simple, helpful advice, this advice should only be offered when clients are ready to consider it. The health coach should learn about clients' hopes and dreams, and try to connect lifestyle modification with goals that sincerely matter to clients, so that motivation will be as self-directed as possible.

Increase Readiness to Change

When clients are in the contemplation or preparation stages, the health coach can shape discussions to help them weigh the pros and cons of change and make a decision to engage in a lifestyle-modification program. Discussions can occur either in a group or one-on-one format. Weight-control groups usually meet weekly and follow a curriculum that includes educational discussions that address topics of interest to participants. Health coaches can also engage in educational discussions with individual clients. These discussions should be informational and motivational. The goal of the health coach is to strengthen the reasons for changing, while helping clients make plans for overcoming barriers to change.

Health coaches should assess clients' readiness to change eating habits and engage in physical activity early on. Educational discussions should be designed to help clients form and strengthen their intentions to change behavior (Armitage, 2006). Clients in the earlier stages of behavior change, who are still weighing the pros and cons, should be given information on the dangers of obesity and the benefits of exercise and proper nutrition, as well as concrete ideas for implementing a lifestyle-modification program that will lead to weight loss. If health coaches are leading group discussions, the group members will speak up and add to those discussions. It is the health coach's role to correct misinformation and give clients the take-home message that, while lifestyle modification does take effort, it is the only way to achieve healthy, lifelong weight control.

As health coaches discuss lifestyle-modification issues and assess clients, it is important to find out if clients are ready to make a change. Be sure that clients are at least in the preparation stage for lifestyle modification before asking too much of them.

Help Clients Set Realistic Goals

Health coaches should help clients set both weight-loss and lifestyle-modification/behavior-change goals. Remembering that clients will tend to be overly ambitious, health coaches should help clients set realistic goals.

While most clients will want to focus on weight loss, health coaches should help them focus more on behavior. After all, they will have more control over their behavior than their weight. Simply adhering to their exercise and nutrition plans each day should be seen as reaching a goal. Health coaches can explain to clients that the behavior is the means by which the weight-loss goal will be accomplished.

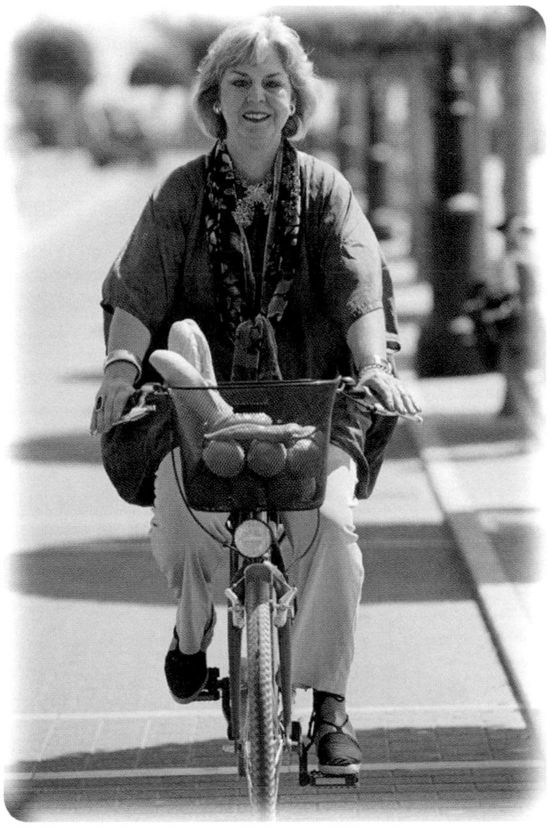

When working with clients to develop healthy exercise and diet guidelines, health coaches should focus on adherence. Health coaches should ask themselves, "Is this advice something the client can really follow long-term?" Remember that the new behaviors the clients are adopting should require as little self-control as possible so that they can become habits as quickly as possible.

Advice on behavior change should include a great deal of structure for meals (Berkel et al., 2005). Meal structure decreases the effort required for meal planning and decision making, and reduces temptation and guesswork. Clients who quickly develop a daily routine for eating will be most successful in modifying their lifestyles. To avoid **scope of practice** concerns, health coaches should be sure to use resources such as the USDA's *Dietary Guidelines for Americans* and the MyPlate Food Guidance System (www.ChooseMyPlate.com) when making nutrition recommendations.

Exercise recommendations can be somewhat more flexible, with some built-in choices to accommodate each client's schedule. Exercise recommendations that are too structured may make adherence difficult, and some researchers suggest encouraging people who are overweight to engage in more lifestyle activity, such as walking, doing yard work, and taking stairs (Andersen et al., 1999). See Chapter15 for specific information about exercise programming.

Encourage Clients to Modify Environmental Cues

Obesity has been called an environmental issue (Carlos Poston & Foreyt, 1999). Environmental cues encourage excessive calorie intake and low levels of physical activity. Clients will probably have a lot to say about how their environment encourages overeating and prevents them from exercising.

Health coaches should encourage clients to become aware of environmental cues that trigger food intake and physical activity. Many environmental factors will be out of a client's control. For example, a client will not be able to change the price of fresh fruits and vegetables, decrease restaurant portion sizes, or move to a new apartment to avoid living next door to a fast-food restaurant.

As clients prepare to improve their eating habits, one of the first steps many of them take is to clean up their immediate environments at home and at work. They can give away (or stop purchasing) high-calorie, nutrient-poor foods. They can keep food out of view, in cupboards or containers. These preparations help reduce cues for eating foods of limited nutritional value or eating when not hungry. Similarly, clients may prepare to become more active by buying exercise videos or exercise clothes, or seeking out exercise opportunities near home or work.

Look for Ways to Increase Self-efficacy

Self-efficacy helps clients stick to their lifestyle-modification programs. Research suggests that fitness professionals can help clients build self-efficacy in several ways (McAuley & Blissmer, 2000).

As the old adage states, success breeds even more success. Health coaches can help clients achieve success early in their lifestyle-modification programs by setting realistic goals that they can reasonably accomplish. Health coaches must provide continued positive reinforcement, as this will help clients feel like they are being successful. Health coaches should help clients find concrete evidence of success, such as their diet records or exercise log. In the early stages of a lifestyle-modification program, the focus should remain on consistent participation and successful adherence.

Clients should be exposed to a variety of role models. People of a similar size, age, gender, and ethnic background who exercise regularly and have lost weight and maintained it encourage the belief that, "If they can do it, so can I." If a client feels "different" from everyone else in the group or at the fitness center, self-efficacy may decline. The key to enhancing self-efficacy is to uncover the defining variables that make the client feel "different." For example, if a client is older than most other gym members, he may lack self-efficacy because he thinks he is too old. Therefore, his role models should be old as well, at least in his eyes.

Where are role models found? Real people are best. Perhaps the health coach can invite former clients, friends, or acquaintances who could serve as role models to talk to the client or group. Role models might be willing to exercise with the client or perform their own workouts at the same time as the client. This will give the client the opportunity to observe and ultimately model effective behavior first-hand. The health coach might be able to recommend an exercise class or group that includes people with whom the client identifies, or start a group for this particular demographic. If role models are difficult to find, the health coach can direct clients to videos, articles, books, and websites featuring people similar to the client.

Health coaches should help clients feel comfortable in the exercise environment by advising them on what to wear, where to go, and how to act. They should also help clients find exercise opportunities that are not embarrassing for them and environments where they feel comfortable.

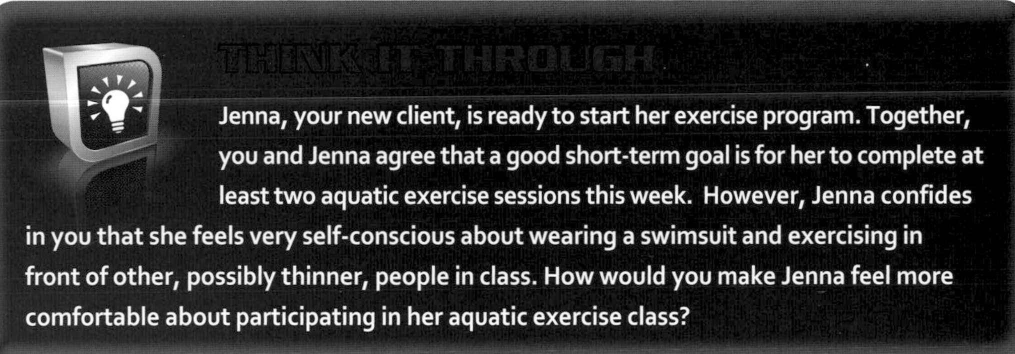

Jenna, your new client, is ready to start her exercise program. Together, you and Jenna agree that a good short-term goal is for her to complete at least two aquatic exercise sessions this week. However, Jenna confides in you that she feels very self-conscious about wearing a swimsuit and exercising in front of other, possibly thinner, people in class. How would you make Jenna feel more comfortable about participating in her aquatic exercise class?

Encourage Clients to Build Social Support

Positive social support enhances feelings of self-efficacy, as well as the likelihood that clients will be successful in their lifestyle-modification efforts. Social support can reinforce positive behavioral change in several ways. Friends and family may provide encouragement and praise, which help clients continue their efforts. Sometimes social support comes in the form of logistical support. For example, a client may be able to work out in the morning because her husband takes the children to school. Another client may be able to exercise during his lunch hour because a coworker is available to take calls while he is away.

Many clients find that a workout partner helps them stick to their behavior-change programs. A partner may "force" other partners to show up, even though they may not feel like it. Workout partners may make exercise more fun (or at least less boring) for people who do not enjoy exercise very much.

Clients can also be encouraged to join a lifestyle and weight management program with a friend. That way, they can exercise together and boost each other's self-confidence. If a friend is not available to join the program, perhaps clients can find others who will support them in their efforts to change eating behaviors. Friends can agree to not give the client foods he or she is trying to avoid, or help the client stay busy and away from situations that might lead to overeating. The health coach should encourage clients to think of ways in which friends and family members can help them succeed in their behavior-change efforts.

Help Clients Manage Stress and Negative Mood

Most clients already have many stress-management strategies in place, as well as ways to cope with negative moods. In a group situation, clients can share the things they do to make themselves feel better when they are feeling bad. In one-on-one sessions, clients can brainstorm a list of things that they enjoy, such as listening to music, enjoying a cup of tea, reading a good book, talking to a friend, or watching a funny movie.

It is the health coach's responsibility to reinforce the pleasures and psychological benefits of physical activity. Research shows that regular physical activity can reduce feelings of **depression,** stress, and anxiety, and improve mood and energy levels (Brehm, 2000). Help clients identify enjoyable activities, and encourage them to tune into the positive effects of exercise. If clients get "hooked" on exercise, they achieve three rewards: They perform the physical activity that is part of their weight-control programs; they reduce stress; and, by reducing stress, they increase the energy available for self-control.

Some clients find relaxation techniques, such as meditation and breathing exercises, helpful in reducing stress levels. Many techniques are simple to teach and learn (Brehm, 1998). Relaxation techniques can teach clients to be more mindful of their eating habits, slow down and enjoy their food more, and reduce emotional eating during stress. Clients who disclose that stress and negative moods are especially disruptive to their eating habits should be referred to a mental-health specialist, such as a psychotherapist or other licensed counseling professional (See "Knowing When to Refer," page 404).

Create Self-monitoring Systems

It is important to set up systems for self-monitoring of food intake and physical activity early in the working relationship with each client. Health coaches may ask clients to monitor themselves even *before* making diet and exercise recommendations to determine a baseline for behaviors. Continuing to refine self-monitoring systems will help clients evaluate their lifestyle-modification plans and make appropriate adjustments as needed.

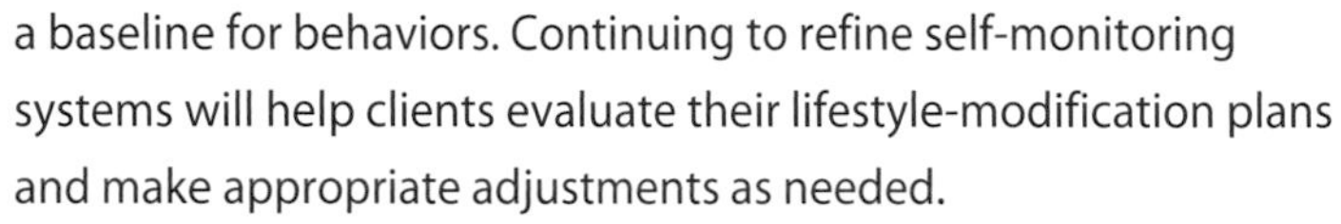

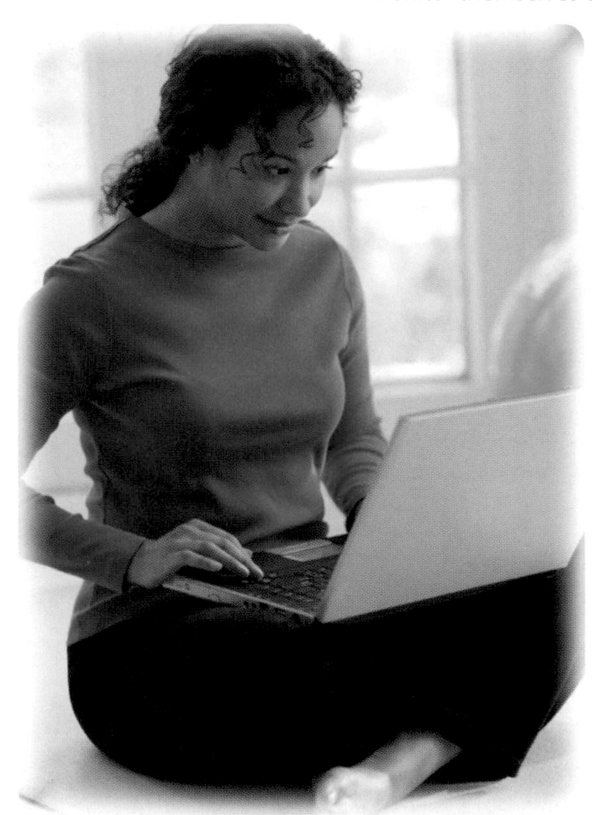

Self-monitoring systems usually consist of written or computer forms in which clients record the behaviors they are working to change. Clients will need ways to record both food intake and physical activity. Clients may also want to record body weight daily or weekly. Once clients get used to record keeping, it is also useful to ask them to observe thoughts and feelings, both helpful and unhelpful, that precede eating and exercise behaviors.

Research has consistently shown that self-monitoring is one of the most important components of successful weight-control and weight-maintenance programs (Boutelle & Kirschenbaum, 1998). Self-monitoring systems help in several ways. First, they increase people's self-awareness. For example, clients may not realize how many extra calories they consume while nibbling as they prepare dinner or snacking as they watch television. Self-monitoring acts as a mirror, giving clients a more objective view of their behavior.

Second, self-monitoring systems forge a link between the health coach and the client outside of sessions. Clients will anticipate careful surveillance of their records. Hopefully, they will stick to their lifestyle-modification and behavior-change programs and be proud of their accomplishments when the health coach next reviews their records.

Third, self-monitoring systems will serve as an important tool for evaluating clients' lifestyle-modification and behavior-change successes and challenges. While reviewing clients' records each week, the health coach can note occasions where challenges arose. Why did this occasion of overeating occur? What triggered this response? Clients and health coaches can then brainstorm ways to eliminate negative **triggers** when possible and identify better responses to those situations to prevent relapses. Self-monitoring systems will reveal times when lifestyle-modification efforts are working. Health coaches should help clients analyze what works and what does not.

Lastly, self-monitoring records can serve as a form of positive reinforcement and increase self-efficacy. A completed exercise log or a chart showing a good daily intake of vegetables, for instance, shows clients that they are being successful in their lifestyle-modification and behavior-change programs.

Guide Clients in Problem-solving and Cognitive Restructuring

Problem-solving often evolves naturally from self-monitoring, as clients become aware of the situations in which they overeat, eat the wrong things, or skip their exercise sessions. While it may be tempting for the health coach to solve the problems themselves, problem-solving must be client-driven, so that solutions are more congruent with clients' needs and lifestyles.

Consciously changing the way one perceives or thinks about something is called **cognitive restructuring.** Cognitive restructuring requires developing a mindful awareness of one's automatic thoughts, or self-talk, and consciously changing counterproductive thoughts. Over time, and with practice, clients can learn to change the way they think, and thus, the ways they feel and behave. Thinking is intimately tied to behavior, so it is important for clients to be aware of their thought patterns as they work on changing specific behaviors (Fabricatore, 2007).

Health coaches can help clients apply cognitive restructuring when weighing the pros and cons of starting a weight-control program. As health coaches educate clients about the benefits of exercise, the goal should be to make physical exercise appealing to them. This will be a continued effort while working with clients. For example, clients who say they "hate" exercise should try to see physical activity in a more positive light. Cognitive restructuring may make them more aware of the things they say to themselves about exercise. This can be part of their self-monitoring routine. For example, they can make a note of the thoughts and feelings that occur as they get ready to participate in physical activity.

To continue this example, suppose a client who was overweight as a child associates exercise with being teased in school. The health coach should explore this association and help the client understand that there are ways to be active that do not involve teasing. Health coaches should strive to help clients adopt new ways of thinking and create more positive feelings about physical activity. This means steering them away from any negative automatic thoughts relating to exercise, and then creating more positive associations.

Clients may uncover other automatic thoughts that produce feelings of stress and weaken self-efficacy. For example, many clients feel that if they are not perfect, they are failures. They may judge themselves as always falling short or discount positive results because they have not reached unrealistic expectations. When automatic thoughts are brought into the light of day, they often sound silly. "I must be perfect in my weight-control behaviors," will sound unreasonable for most clients. The health coach can guide clients to rephrase such thoughts to be more supportive and realistic. "Nobody is perfect. I am making improvements in several areas (list) and I am getting healthier and stronger every day."

Especially harmful is all-or-nothing thinking. Many clients develop the attitude that they are either "on" or "off" the diet. "On" means being perfect; "off" can mean destructive behaviors such as overeating and not exercising. The beauty of lifestyle-modification programs is that they help clients learn to think about lifelong behavior change, rather than being on or off diets.

Hopefully, as clients become aware of counterproductive thinking, they can learn to replace negative thoughts with more positive and realistic ones.

Cognitive restructuring requires a great deal of practice and self-monitoring. It also requires the ability to observe one's own thinking, and to not accept one's immediate thoughts as "reality." Positive thinking alone is not enough; clients must restructure thoughts in ways that are believable, as well as positive. "I love exercise," may not ring true to a client, but "I don't mind walking on the treadmill while I watch TV," might *become* true.

Implementing a Lifestyle-modification Program

The specifics of implementing a lifestyle-modification program will vary depending upon the environment in which the health coach works. Health coaches may lead lifestyle- and weight-management groups or work more as personal trainers with certain clients. The following suggestions may be incorporated into either individual or group work. Specific suggestions for group programs are included at the end of this section.

Many health coaches ask clients to commit to a minimum timeframe for lifestyle- and weight-management programs. Research suggests that programs should last at least 16 to 26 weeks to foster success (Renjilian et al., 2001). Health coaches must plan a general progression to the program that accommodates the timeframe in which they work, but allows for flexibility depending upon client needs and interests.

Health coaches should remain positive in all aspects of their work. Working with a health coach must be a positive experience for clients, or they will go elsewhere. It is important to always be understanding and supportive of clients, even when questioning their behaviors. Remember that while the behavior may be a problem, these clients are doing the best they can. Therefore, health coaches need to express confidence in every client's ability to change.

Lifestyle Assessment and Overview of the Program

Before diving into assessment procedures, health coaches need to obtain health histories and medical-clearance forms (when necessary) from their clients, and make sure that they are qualified to work with clients who have certain health conditions. They should also discuss the forms with clients to ensure that all health information is complete and accurate.

Most lifestyle-modification programs include exercise, nutrition, and behavior-change components. Advice in all of these areas will begin with the initial client assessment. Looking at current lifestyle behaviors is a key to ensuring long-term success. Exercise, diet, and weight history reveal a lot about a client's lifestyle and the various factors that account for the client's weight problems. Health coaches must be sure to discuss clients' past successes with diet, exercise, and weight loss. What worked in the past may work again, and discussing successful experiences will enhance clients' self-efficacy.

The big question that the health coach and the client are trying to answer is "Why is the client overweight?" Health coaches must consider biological and environmental influences, including exercise, diet, and weight-loss history. Health coaches should also ask clients about social-support networks, stress levels, and stress-management techniques (Fabricatore & Wadden, 2005).

During the initial assessment, health coaches should analyze the client's stage of change for physical activity and diet. Simply by coming to a health coach, clients indicate that they are probably preparing to make changes in their behavior, either in diet or physical activity, or both. Keep in mind, however, that the stage of change may differ for exercise and diet. Health coaches can assess the stage of change by asking clients questions about their readiness, or by using a questionnaire (Brehm, 2004). If a health coach senses that a client is not yet in the preparation stage for exercise or diet, he or she can spend more time on discussion and education to help the client develop the intention to change.

Health coaches should initially ask clients to keep a daily food and activity log for one week. In addition to helping the health coach gain a better understanding of their clients' current lifestyle habits, this log will also help clients set lifestyle-modification goals. Be sure that the format of this log matches each client's specific interests and abilities. Keep logs simple at first to get clients into the self-monitoring habit. Record keeping can become more complex over time if necessary. Difficult logs should not be allowed to form a barrier to action. Computerized logs are fine, but only if a client uses a computer on a daily basis and finds computer use easy and convenient.

Health coaches should provide an overview of the program early in the relationship with each client. Health coaches should tailor programs to accommodate each client's needs and explain that losing weight and changing one's lifestyle take commitment, time, and effort.

Establish Goals for Interventions

After completing the initial exercise, diet, and lifestyle assessments, health coaches should work with the client to establish program goals, including weight-loss and behavioral goals. Use the information from Chapters 15 and 16 to establish goals for physical activity and diet. Remember that goals must be specific, measurable, attainable, relevant, and time-bound (i.e., **SMART goals**). If the health coach and client are meeting regularly, the health coach can help the client create a specific guide to what should be accomplished during the week.

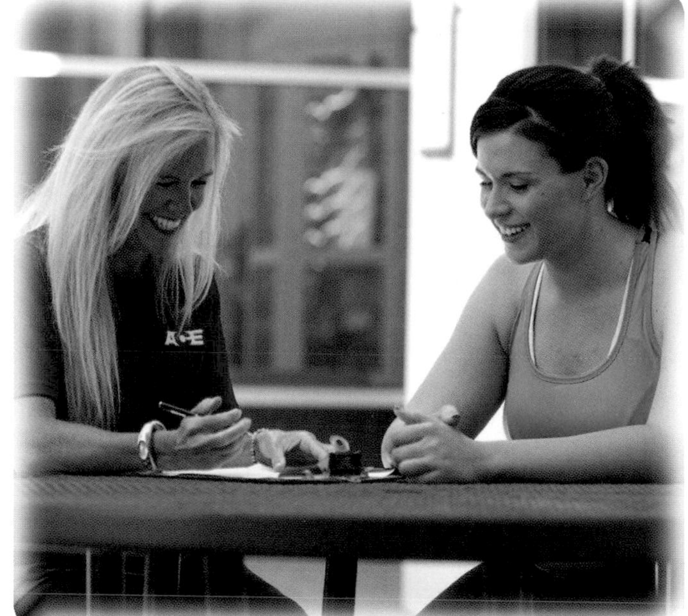

How elaborate should the goal-setting process be? It is easy to overwhelm clients with information and motivational suggestions during the first few weeks of a new program. Clients often come in very ambitious and willing to take it all on at once. Health coaches should err on the side of caution to be sure that clients are successful in meeting their lifestyle-modification goals early in the program. Suggest behavioral changes that clients have successfully accomplished in the past and are willing to try again. Early weight-loss success is associated with adherence and long-term weight control (Renjilian et al., 2001). Refer to Chapter 13 for a realistic approach to goal-setting.

Self-monitoring and Problem-solving: The Heart of Lifestyle Modification

At subsequent meetings, health coaches should review clients' lifestyle-modification records. Did they meet their behavioral goals? Why or why not? Discuss both helping and hindering factors. Let the clients do most of the talking in problem-solving situations. Listen and ask questions, but try not to make suggestions right away. Remember that each client is the expert on his or her lifestyle.

In many cases, clients will indicate specific triggers that make them eat too much, or eat the wrong things. They may describe situations that cause them to skip an exercise session. Health coaches should take detailed notes, as this is the critical information that will enable health coaches to help their clients make plans that will result in lifestyle modification.

In other cases, clients may overlook, or be in denial about, the factors and situations that trigger negative eating and exercise behaviors. Keeping a record of food intake that includes notes on reasons for eating and situations that trigger eating helps both the health coach and the client take an objective look at a client's behavior and evaluate how it is influenced both positively and negatively by **antecedents** and consequences.

Consider a client who is struggling with evening snacking. The health coach must first understand what is causing the behavior. Is the client actually hungry? If so, he or she may need to increase daily caloric intake. Is he or she eating for other reasons (e.g., boredom, stress, or habit)? If the client does not know why he or she eats in the evening, ask the client to note the factors that seem to precede and follow the evening snacking during the coming week. Ask the client to record his or her observations of thoughts and feelings in the self-monitoring work. The client's work in the program will hopefully help him or her uncover the antecedents and reinforcements to the problematic snacking behavior.

Once the client understands some of the factors that contribute to the evening snacking, he or she can try to design some ways to support a change in this behavior. Can he or she eliminate any of the factors that trigger the snacking? If the client finds that he or she eats out of boredom, can he or she get out of the house, or stay busy and away from snacks? Can he or she get rid of the snack foods at home? If the client cannot stop snacking, can he or she snack on healthier foods? How can friends and family help?

Problem-solving is about defining the problem, then brainstorming possible solutions. Clients should weigh the pros and cons of solutions, decide which ones to implement, and then evaluate their success during the next meeting. Health coaches and clients should revise tactics until they find workable solutions. Theoretically, this process should lead to behavioral changes, which become habits, and then result in a new, healthier lifestyle.

As clients weigh the pros and cons of possible solutions, health coaches need to stay supportive, but also evaluate the likelihood that clients will adopt the new behaviors. Asking clients if these new behaviors could really work for them, and defining strategies to achieve them, will be critical to the long-term success of the program.

Health coaches should ask clients if self-talk has affected their eating and exercise behaviors, and whether they have become more aware of thoughts and feelings that lead to overeating and negative self-talk. Health coaches can have clients keep track of the negative thoughts and feelings and then help them substitute a positive version of each. For example, if a client writes, "I blew my diet and gained 2 pounds," the health coach can suggest replacing this negative thought with, "I slipped on my diet and gained 2 pounds, but tomorrow is a new day and I will get right back on track." They can then work together to list action steps to help the client achieve this immediate goal.

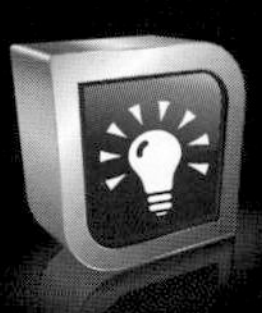

THINK IT THROUGH

Imagine that you are working with an overweight client who wants to lose 20 pounds (9 kg) to help control her newly diagnosed diabetes. She loves to cook and bake, and while she admits that she eats more when she has just baked cookies and other treats, she would hate to quit making desserts entirely since her family enjoys them so much. What are some ways your client can continue to prepare food for her family that will be more supportive of the client's weight-loss efforts? What questions might you ask the client to guide her to discover more healthful ways of preparing food for her family? What kinds of skills might she need to learn to move in this direction?

Continue Education and Self-monitoring

Continue to review and discuss clients' lifestyle-modification records throughout the program's duration. Give clients educational material that addresses their questions and specific behavior-change issues. Most clients appreciate motivational reading and want to learn about physical activity, nutrition, and weight control. Topics typically included in weight-management curricula include eating out, managing the holidays, traveling, cooking, grocery shopping, reading food labels, managing stress, avoiding emotional eating, and preventing relapses.

Between sessions, the health coach should think about each client and develop strategies that might be used to promote self-efficacy and behavior-change success. Review the material in this chapter on lifestyle-modification principles and strategies. While clients will take the lead, be prepared to make helpful suggestions, or ask new questions, at each session. Would a client like to try a new exercise class at the fitness center and ask a friend to join him? How will his exercise program change now that it is getting dark earlier in the day? How will he eat during the holidays? The health coach should help clients anticipate and plan for challenges before they arise.

Relapse Prevention

People are creatures of habit, and most find it difficult to change their daily routines. For this reason, most people experience lapses during their behavior-change efforts. Lifestyle-modification programs for weight loss can be especially difficult to maintain long-term, as they involve modification of many different behaviors and habits. Helping clients accept the difficulty of this process and anticipate factors that contribute to both success and relapse may help them stick to their weight-loss programs.

Most clients can identify high-risk situations and anticipate ways in which they might abandon their behavior-change programs. The health coach's goal in discussing these situations is to help clients understand that it is human to make mistakes, and that self-forgiveness is the correct response, followed by continued efforts to resume a healthful lifestyle. A *lapse* need not be interpreted as a *relapse.*

High-risk situations are typically accompanied by feelings of stress and negative moods. Lapses are often preceded by such thoughts as, "It's been a tough day. I deserve a mocha frappuccino."

Health coaches should continue to encourage clients to monitor their thoughts and feelings, and to develop effective ways to cope with stressful situations.

Some people relapse because of the mistaken belief that behavior-change programs are "all-or-nothing" efforts. Consequently, when these clients "break their rules" about eating or exercise (for example, overeating one evening), they blame themselves, feel a loss of control, and fall into relapse. This tendency is called the **abstinence violation effect,** a term borrowed from addiction treatment programs to describe the behavior of people who resume alcohol or drug abuse after a period of abstinence (Witkiewitz & Marlatt, 2004). Dieting can be the same way. Once people "break" their diet, they often continue to overeat and lose all motivation to stick to a lifestyle-modification program. Health coaches need to step in and help clients break that vicious cycle. Health coaches can help clients see that lapses are solvable problems, not indicators of failure. Clients must avoid all-or-nothing thinking when it comes to making lifelong behavior change.

Lifestyle and Weight-management Groups

Research suggests that lifestyle- and weight-management groups tend to be more effective than individual consultations, regardless of whether individuals say they prefer group or individual counseling (Renjilian et al., 2001). When it comes to working with groups, experienced health coaches have often found that group members provide valuable support, motivation, and information to one another.

Group members generally follow the same progression outlined earlier in this chapter, from assessment and goal-setting to self-monitoring and problem-solving. Most group programs follow a set curriculum that includes weekly readings and "homework"—self-monitoring assignments that focus on a particular behavior-change topic.

Health coaches with teaching experience may feel more confident leading group discussions, as groups require good listening and observation skills. The role of a group leader is to ensure that discussions are not dominated by a few individuals, that individuals listen respectfully to each other, and that each member feels comfortable. Before leading a lifestyle- and weight-management group, health coaches should participate or assist in a group led by an experienced leader. See Chapter 3 for more information on working with groups.

Weight-loss maintenance is enhanced when people have ongoing contact with their health coaches and fellow group members (Renjilian et al., 2001). Consider offering ways to keep in touch with participants once the program has ended.

Knowing When to Refer

In general, if a health coach has concerns about a particular client and wonders about whether to refer that client to another qualified healthcare professional, then he or she should do so. Health coaches may find themselves referring clients for many reasons.

Sometimes a health coach will want to refer a client back to his or her primary healthcare provider because the health coach cannot figure out why the client is overweight. If the client already has a healthy lifestyle, exercises daily, and eats healthfully, health coaches have little more to offer. If the client's behaviors are not the problem, then the health coach does not have the solution. Perhaps the obesity has additional causes that other providers can address.

Obese clients often have other health conditions such as **diabetes** and **hypertension.** If their primary healthcare providers "clear" them to exercise and work with a health coach, then the health coach should still proceed with caution. If clients complain of health symptoms that may indicate poor control of their medical conditions, the health coach should refer them back to their healthcare providers. Such symptoms include chest pain, dizziness, and any new health symptoms that develop during the program. Orthopedic problems, such as knee or foot pain, might also develop. If chronic orthopedic pain is not relieved by appropriate exercise program modifications (e.g., reduced duration and/or intensity, **RICE,** increased stretching, and cross training) and persists for several weeks, the client should be referred as well.

Health coaches should immediately refer clients to the appropriate healthcare provider if there is any suspicion of an eating disorder. Excessive calorie restriction (dieting), bingeing, and purging all indicate psychological problems that are outside the health coach's scope of practice. Review the warning signs of eating disorders presented in Chapter 9. People with **binge eating disorder** may continue to work with health coaches to modify their behavior with their therapist's consent, since research shows that lifestyle modification is helpful for binge eaters (Gladis et al., 1998).

Sometimes clients struggle with addictions, which also necessitate a referral. The underlying issue with a weight problem can be an alcohol or drug problem. Lifestyle modification can support recovery for certain addictions, but clients also need to be in therapy.

Mood disorders such as depression and anxiety also require the appropriate referral. Obesity may be associated with a higher severity of negative thoughts and feelings about oneself, at least among those obese individuals who have sought treatment (Anderson, Reiger, & Caterson, 2006). Research comparing obese individuals who sought treatment in a professional hospital-based program to obese people who did not seek treatment suggests that obese people seeking treatment report greater rates of mood disturbances than obese people who do not seek treatment (Fitzgibbon, Stolley, & Kirschenbaum, 1993). While everyone feels sad and anxious at times, clients who report ongoing negative feelings or symptoms that interfere with daily living need to be referred to a qualified healthcare provider.

Health coaches need to establish a referral network early on in their careers (see Chapter 2). Health coaches who make sound decisions regarding referrals will earn the respect of clients and other allied healthcare professionals, and lift the reputation of fitness professionals to a higher level.

THINK IT THROUGH

Ben has worked with you for the past six months on improving his eating habits and incorporating more physical activity into his daily routine so that he can lose about 20 pounds (9.1 kg). Even though Ben has never skipped an exercise session with you, his progress toward his weight-loss goal has been minimal. Upon your request, Ben keeps a food diary for one week. Even though it appears to show an appropriate balanced diet to meet his needs and transition his body toward weight loss, you have a feeling that Ben is not being completely honest about his daily calories. When you ask Ben if he might be forgetting to log a specific food or beverage, he responds by admitting that he never writes down the alcohol he drinks with his nightly meal. Upon further discussion, Ben looks very concerned and admits to you that he cannot give up drinking and thinks that he might have a problem with alcohol. As a health coach, what would you do in this situation?

Summary

Behavioral change is essential for lifelong weight management. Health coaches should teach lifestyle-modification strategies throughout their work with weight-control clients, in addition to helping clients discover and address the specific causes of their obesity. Health coaches should understand the theories and principles that help explain health behavior, as well as the many variables that affect motivation and weight-loss success. Lifestyle-modification strategies built on self-monitoring can help health coaches work with clients to address readiness to change, goal-setting, environmental cues, self-efficacy, stress management, cognitive restructuring, and problem-solving.

References

Andersen, R.E. et al. (1999). Effect of lifestyle activity vs. structured aerobic exercise in obese women. *Journal of the American Medical Association,* 281, 335–340.

Anderson, K., Reiger, E., & Caterson, I. (2006). A comparison of maladaptive schemata in treatment-seeking obese adults and normal-weight control subjects. *Journal of Psychosomatic Research*, 60, 245–252.

Armitage, C.J. (2006). Evidence that implementation intentions promote transitions between the stages of change. *Journal of Consulting and Clinical Psychology,* 74, 1, 141–151.

Bandura, A. (1997). *Self-efficacy: The Exercise of Control.* New York: Freeman.

Berkel, L.A. et al. (2005). Behavioral interventions for obesity. *Journal of the American Dietetic Association,* 105, 5, Suppl. 1, 35–43.

Boutelle, K.N. & Kirschenbaum, D.S. (1998). Further support for consistent self-monitoring as a vital component of successful weight control. *Obesity Research,* 6, 219–224.

Brehm, B.A. (2004). *Successful Fitness Motivation Strategies*. Champaign, Ill.: Human Kinetics.

Brehm, B.A. (2000). Maximizing the psychological benefits of physical activity. *ACSM's Health & Fitness Journal,* 4, 6, 7–11, 26.

Brehm, B.A. (1998). *Stress Management: Increasing Your Stress Resistance.* New York: Addison, Wesley, Longman.

Buehler, R., Griffin, D., & Ross, M. (1994). Exploring the "planning fallacy": Why people underestimate their task completion times. *Journal of Personality and Social Psychology,* 67, 366–381.

Carlos Poston, W.S., II, & Foreyt, J.P. (1999). Obesity is an environmental issue. *Athlerosclerosis,* 146, 2, 201–209.

Christakis, N.A. & Fowler, J.H. (2007). The spread of obesity in a large social network over 32 years. *New England Journal of Medicine*, 357, 4, 370–379.

Deci, E.L. & Ryan, R.M. (2008). Facilitating optimal motivation and psychological well-being across life's domains. *Canadian Psychology,* 49, 1, 14–23.

Fabricatore, A.N. (2007). Behavior therapy and cognitive-behavior therapy of obesity: Is there a difference? *Journal of the American Dietetic Association,* 107, 92–99.

Fabricatore, A.N. & Wadden, T.A. (2005). Lifestyle modification in the treatment of obesity. In: Goldstein, D.J. (Ed.). *The Management of Eating Disorders and Obesity* (2nd ed.). (pp 209–229). Totowa, N.J.: Humana Press.

Fisher, E.B. (2008). The importance of context in understanding behavior and promoting health. *Annals of Behavioral Medicine,* 35, 3–18.

Fitzgibbon, M.L., Stolley, M.R., & Kirschenbaum, D.S. (1993). Obese people who seek treatment have different characteristics than those who do not seek treatment. *Health Psychology,* 12, 342–345.

Geliebter, A. & Aversa, A. (2003). Emotional eating in overweight, normal weight, and underweight individuals. *Eating Behavior,* 3, 4, 341–347.

Gladis, M.M. et al. (1998). A comparison of two approaches to the assessment of binge eating in obesity. *International Journal of Eating Disorders,* 23, 17–26.

Hendershot, C.S., Marlatt, G.A., & George, W.H. (2009). Relapse prevention and the maintenance of optimal health. In: Shumaker, S.A. et al. (Eds.) *The Handbook of Health Behavior Change.* New York: Springer.

McAuley, E. & Blissmer, B. (2000). Self-efficacy determinants and consequences of physical activity. *Exercise and Sport Sciences Reviews,* 28, 2, 85–88.

Muraven, M. & Baumeister, R.F. (2000). Self-regulation and depletion of limited resources: Does self-control resemble a muscle? *Psychological Bulletin,* 126, 2, 247–259.

Polivy, J. & Herman, C.P. (2000). The false-hope syndrome: Unfulfilled expectations of self-change. *Current Directions in Psychological Science,* 9, 4, 128–131.

Renjilian, D.A. et al. (2001). Individual vs. group therapy for obesity: Effects of matching participants to their treatment preference. *Journal of Consulting and Clinical Psychology,* 69, 717–721.

Teachman, B.A. & Brownell, K.D. (2001). Implicit

anti-fat bias among health professionals: Is anyone immune? *International Journal of Obesity,* 25, 1525–1531.

Tice, D.M., Bratslavsky, E., & Baumeister, R.F. (2001). Emotional distress regulation takes precedence over impulse control: If you feel bad, do it! *Journal of Personality and Social Psychology,* 80, 1, 53–67.

Vohs, K.D. & Heatherton, T.F. (2000). Self-regulatory failure: A resource-depletion approach. *Psychological Science,* 11, 3, 249–254.

Wing, R.R. & Phelan, S. (2005). Long-term weight loss maintenance. *American Journal of Clinical Nutrition,* 82, 1, 222S–225S.

Witkiewitz, K. & Marlatt, G.A. (2004). Relapse prevention for alcohol and drug problems: That was Zen, this is Tao. *American Psychologist,* 59, 4, 224–235.

Suggested Reading

Annesi, J.J. (2002).The exercise support process: Facilitating members' self-management skills. *Fitness Management,* 18, 10 (Suppl), 24–25.

Baumeister, R.F. & Tierney, J. (2011). *Willpower: Rediscovering the Greatest Human Strength.* New York: Penguin Press.

Brehm, B.A. (2004). *Successful Fitness Motivation Strategies.* Champaign, Ill.: Human Kinetics.

Brehm, B.A. (2000). Maximizing the psychological benefits of physical activity. *ACSM's Health & Fitness Journal,* 4, 6, 7–11, 26.

Carlos Poston, W.S., II, & Foreyt, J.P. (2000). Successful management of the obese patient *American Family Physician,* 61, 3615–3622.

McKay, M., Davis, M., & Fanning, P. (2011). *Thoughts and Feelings: Taking Control of Your Moods and Your Life.* Oakland, Calif.: New Harbinger Publications.

Miller-Kovach, K. (2006). *Weight Watchers Family Power: 5 Simple Rules for a Healthy-Weight Home.* Hoboken, N.J.: John Wiley & Sons.

Rippe, J.M. and Weight Watchers (2005). *Weight Loss That Lasts: Break Through the 10 Big Diet Myths.* Hoboken, N.J.: John Wiley & Sons.

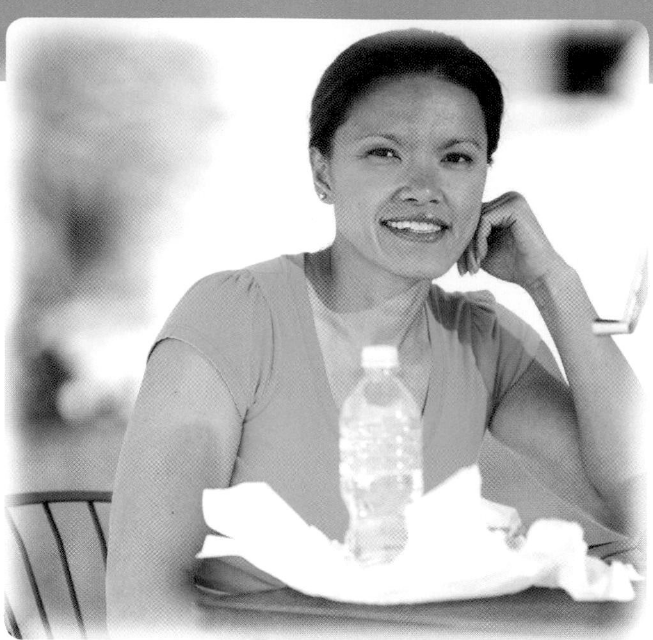

IN THIS CHAPTER:

*Debra Wein, M.S., R.D., L.D.N., C.S.S.D., NSCA-CPT*D, is on the faculty at the University of Massachusetts Boston and the Massachusetts General Hospital (MGH) Institute for Health Professions, where she teaches courses in nutrition, sport nutrition, and worksite wellness, and is the president of Wellness Workdays. She has worked with the United States of America Track and Field Association, U.S. Navy Seals, The Boston Ballet, and numerous marathon training teams. Wein is also certified as a personal trainer by the American College of Sports Medicine (ACSM-HFI) and the National Strength and Conditioning Association (NSCA-CPT*D). Wein holds undergraduate and graduate degrees in nutritional sciences from Cornell and Columbia Universities.*

15 Nutritional Programming

DEBRA WEIN

& MEGAN MIRAGLIA

Megan Miraglia, M.S., R.D., L.D.N., is a nutritionist with Wellness Workdays and Sensible Nutrition. She is a noted author and has published works in the American Journal of Lifestyle Medicine *and the* International Journal of Cancer, *and has also contributed articles to LIVESTRONG.com. Miraglia is a certified Freshstart facilitator for the American Cancer Society's Freshstart tobacco cessation program. She received her master of science degree in nutrition from Tufts University Friedman School of Nutrition and completed her dietetic internship at the Frances Stern Nutrition Center, affiliated with Tufts Medical Center. Miraglia completed her undergraduate degree at the State University of New York College at Oneonta, graduating Magna Cum Laude and earning the Outstanding Dietetics Student award.*

Clients will often describe schedules that barely allow them enough time to sleep, let alone eat healthy meals and exercise regularly. Grocery shopping and preparing meals are often out of the question. Even though clients may be well aware that fueling their bodies with healthy foods is important, "life" often gets in the way.

It is important to help clients understand that they will not *find* the time to exercise and eat right—they must *make* the time. Contrary to popular belief (or popular excuses), eating a healthy diet is not impossible. Like anything else, it takes knowledge, practice, and planning to set goals and overcome barriers. (For more information on assessing a client's readiness for change, see Chapter 3.)

Eating behaviors, which are among the most complex of human behaviors, are learned habits that are deeply entrenched and strongly influenced by religious, ethnic, and family customs. Emotional influences also play an important role in why, when, and what people eat. Despite the many factors involved, it is possible for people to "relearn" how to eat more healthfully. The processes of eating, cooking, and choosing foods are shaped by one's past, but these behaviors can be modified. Behavioral modification, however, takes time. When working with clients, the focus should remain on gradually modifying eating and exercise behaviors, both of which are necessary for sustainable weight loss. ACE-certified Health Coaches should remind clients that small, permanent changes in both behavior and weight loss are better than large, temporary ones.

Behavioral modification involves the following:

- Modifying old ways of eating and developing healthier eating habits
- Taking small steps in a consistent direction
- Focusing on environmental or situational control of eating in a program that is designed to reduce the exposure, susceptibility, and response to environmental situations that result in high calorie intake and/or low energy expenditure
- Self-monitoring and self-management

The Nutrition Interview

Understanding a Client's Current Dietary Habits

An effective way to learn about a client's current dietary habits is to administer a lifestyle and health-history questionnaire (Figure 15-1), which may be used to identify clients' areas of concern as well as identify clients whose needs fall outside the **scope of practice** of a health coach. Alternatively, this questionnaire can be administered by the health coach in an interview format, which might stimulate greater conversation, insight, and connection.

Figure 15-1
Sample lifestyle and health-history questionnaire

Medical Information

1. How would you describe your present state of health? ❑ very well ❑ healthy ❑ unhealthy ❑ ill ❑ other:__________
2. Are you taking any prescription medication? ❑ Yes ❑ No
   If yes, what medications and why?__________
   Do these interact with foods or weight loss in any way?__________
3. Do you take any over-the-counter medication? ❑ Yes ❑ No
   If yes, what medications and why?__________
4. When was the last time you visited your physician?__________
5. Have you ever had your cholesterol checked? ❑ Yes ❑ No
   Date of test:__________ What were the results?
   Total Cholesterol:__________ HDL:__________ LDL:__________ TG:__________
6. Have you ever had your blood sugar checked? ❑ Yes ❑ No
   What were the results?__________
7. Please check any that apply to you and list any important information about your condition:

❑ Allergies (Specify:__________)
❑ Amenorrhea
❑ Anemia
❑ Anxiety
❑ Arthritis
❑ Asthma
❑ Celiac disease
❑ Chronic sinus condition
❑ Constipation
❑ Crohn's disease
❑ Depression
❑ Diabetes
❑ Diarrhea
❑ Disordered eating
❑ Gastroesophageal reflux disease (GERD)
❑ High blood pressure
❑ Hypoglycemia
❑ Hypo/hyperthyroidism
❑ Insomnia
❑ Intestinal problems
❑ Irritability
❑ Irritable bowel syndrome (IBS)
❑ Menopausal symptoms
❑ Osteoporosis
❑ Premenstrual syndrome (PMS)
❑ Polycystic ovary syndrome (PCOS)
❑ Pregnant
❑ Ulcer
❑ Skin problems
❑ Major surgeries: __________
❑ Past injuries: __________
❑ Describe any other health conditions that you have:__________
____
____
____
____

Family History

8. Has anyone in your immediate family been diagnosed with the following?

❑ Heart disease If yes, what is the relation: __________ Age of diagnosis: __________
❑ High cholesterol If yes, what is the relation: __________ Age of diagnosis: __________
❑ High blood pressure If yes, what is the relation: __________ Age of diagnosis: __________
❑ Cancer If yes, what is the relation: __________ Age of diagnosis: __________
❑ Diabetes If yes, what is the relation: __________ Age of diagnosis: __________
❑ Osteoporosis If yes, what is the relation: __________ Age of diagnosis: __________

9. What are your dietary goals?____________________

10. Have you ever followed a modified diet? ❑ Yes ❑ No
If so, describe:____________________

11. Are you currently following a specialized diet (e.g., low-sodium or low-fat)? ❑ Yes ❑ No
If so, what type of diet?____________________

12. Why did you choose this diet?____________________
Was the diet prescribed by a physician? ❑ Yes ❑ No
How long have you been on the diet?____________________

13. Have you ever met with a registered dietitian? ❑ Yes ❑ No
Are you interested in meeting with one? ❑ Yes ❑ No

14. What do you consider to be the major issues in your diet and eating plan? (e.g., eating late at night, snacking on high fat foods, skipping meals, or lack of variety)____________________

15. How many glasses of water do you drink per day? ________ 8-ounce glasses

16. Do you have any food allergies or intolerance? ❑ Yes ❑ No
If so, what?____________________

17. Who prepares your food?
❑ Self ❑ Spouse ❑ Parent ❑ Minimal preparation

18. How often do you dine out? ________ times per week

19. Please specify the type of restaurants for each meal:
Breakfast:____________________ Lunch: ____________________
Dinner:____________________ Snacks:____________________

Habits

20. Do you crave any foods? ❑ Yes ❑ No
If so, please specify:____________________

21. How is your appetite affected by stress? ❑ increased ❑ not affected ❑ decreased

22. Do you drink alcohol? ❑ Yes ❑ No
How often? ________times per week Average amount? ______glasses

23. Do you drink caffeinated beverages? ❑ Yes ❑ No
Average number per day:____________

24. Do you use tobacco? ❑ Yes ❑ No
How much (cigarettes, cigars, or chewing tobacco per day)?____________________

25. Do you take any vitamin, mineral, or herbal supplements? ❑ Yes ❑ No
Please list type and amount per day:____________________

26. Do you currently participate in any structured physical activity? ❑ Yes ❑ No
If so, please describe: ____minutes of cardiovascular activity, ____times per week
____strength-training sessions, ____times per week
____minutes of flexibility training, ____times per week
____minutes of sports per week
List sports:____________________
Do you engage in any other forms of regular physical activity?____________________
Please describe your activity level during the work day:____________________

27. Have you experienced any injuries that may limit your physical activity?
If so, please describe:____

28. On a scale of 1–10, how ready are you to adopt a healthier lifestyle?
1 = very unlikely 10 = very likely __________

Weight History

29. What would you like to do with your weight?
❑ lose weight ❑ gain weight ❑ maintain weight

30. What was your lowest weight within the past 5 years? ____lb

31. What was your highest weight within the past 5 years? ____lb

32. What do you consider to be your ideal weight (the weight at which you feel best)? ____lb ❑ don't know

33. What is your present weight? ____lb

34. What are your current waist and hip circumferences? ________waist ________hip ❑ don't know

35. What is your present body composition? ____% body fat ❑ don't know

Note: HDL = High-density lipoprotein; LDL = Low-density lipoprotein; TG = Triglycerides

Figure 15-1
Continued

Visit www.ACEfitness.org/HealthCoachResources to download a free PDF of the lifestyle and health-history questionnaire and food diary/food record, as well as other forms and assessment tools that you can use throughout your career as a health coach.

Several methods can be used to learn more about a client's eating and lifestyle patterns, including food diaries/food records, 24-hour recall, and food-frequency questionnaires. With practice, a health coach may find that certain clients may be very likely to complete food records, while others may only be willing or able to give a 24-hour diet recall. Regardless of which method is used, the information gleaned from these tools will be invaluable in helping clients meet their goals.

Food Diary/Food Record

Keeping a food diary involves having clients describe a "typical" eating day, including all foods and beverages. Clients should be urged to be specific and estimate amounts as best they can. Be sure to discuss weekends versus weekdays. Space is provided in the food diary for the client to note how hungry he or she is when the food is consumed. Additional space could be added to include information on mood, location, and time of day for more detailed intake information.

One thing to consider is that people generally underestimate or under-report their caloric intake and tend to eat more salads, vegetables, and lower-calorie foods when using a food diary than their weight might suggest. Experience with probing the client, asking nonjudgmental questions, and offering a supportive environment is likely to reveal a more truthful picture of a client's eating pattern.

Proper instruction on how to keep food records will often yield better results than just handing a client a sheet of paper and instructing him or her to "write down what you eat." Health coaches should adhere to the following guidelines to help clients more accurately report their food intakes (Figure 15-2):

- Have clients keep a record for three consecutive days, including one weekend day (i.e., Thursday-Friday-Saturday or Sunday-Monday-Tuesday). Advise them to choose three days that would be typical of their usual intake (to obtain the most accurate picture of each client's diet).

Meal/Snack Time		Food/Beverage & Amount	Food Group Servings	Hunger Level	Mood/ Thoughts	Location	Challenges
BREAKFAST							
SNACK							
LUNCH							
SNACK							
DINNER							

Figure 15-2
Sample food diary/record

- Have clients record everything they eat or drink during those days, including water, any added salt, candies, gum, condiments, **vitamin**/**mineral** supplements, sports drinks, coffee, tea, medications, and alcoholic beverages.
- Clients should use a separate sheet of paper for each day and create columns with the following titles: Meal/Snack Time, Food/Beverage & Amount, Food Group Servings, Hunger Level, Mood/Thoughts, Location, and Challenges.

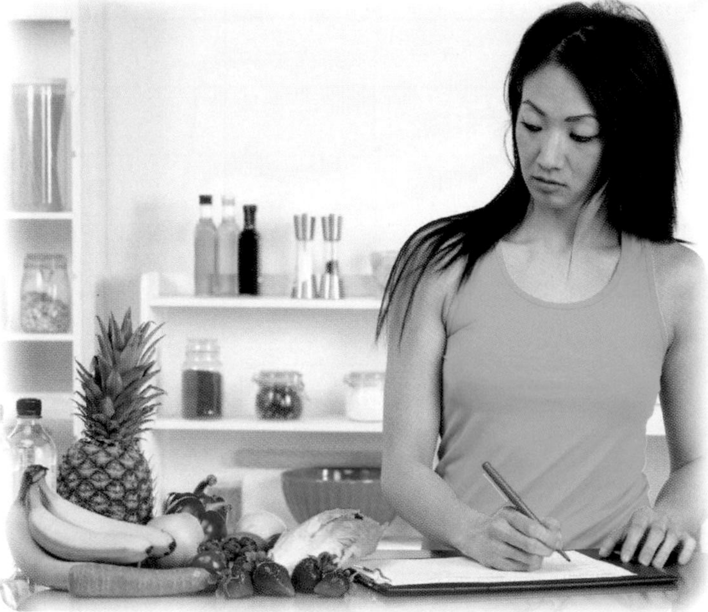

- In the first column, clients record whether the foods and/or beverages were part of a meal (and which one) or consumed as part of a snack, as well as the time when all foods and beverages were consumed. It is also important to record everything immediately after each meal or snack so that they do not forget what was eaten.
- In the second column, clients should give as much specific information as possible:
  - ✓ Method of cooking (e.g., baked, broiled, fried, boiled, or toasted)
  - ✓ Brand names of commercial products
  - ✓ Descriptive words on the packaging such as low-fat or low-sodium
  - ✓ Specific foods and drinks
    - Bread (whole wheat, white, rye; number of slices per loaf)
    - Milk (whole, low-fat, skim, **protein**-enriched)
    - Margarine (stick, tub, diet)
    - Vegetables (canned, fresh, frozen)
    - Meats (fat trimmed, weighed with bone, skinned)
    - Drinks (light, low-calorie, diet, low-fat), including additions such as cream and sugar
    - Snacks (pretzels, chips, dry roasted or raw nuts)
    - Size of fruits or vegetables (small, medium, large, extra large)
    - Ingredients/condiments used in salads, sandwiches, or on food items (e.g., mayonnaise, ketchup, mustard, gravy, sauce, grated cheese, salad dressing, lettuce, and tomato)
- Clients should also list the amount of food or beverage consumed, measured by a scale (for weight in ounces or grams), a ruler (for height, length, and width), or via a household measure (for volume: cups, tablespoons, or teaspoons). If possible, clients should weigh and measure foods after preparation and indicate when it was done. They can use package-label information on commercially made products.
- Clients should also record any significant feelings or emotions they were experiencing before and after eating, their hunger level, where the food was eaten, and any obstacles that were faced when making decisions and choices.

There are also a number of websites and phone applications now available that enable users to track their daily food intake in a convenient fashion via the phone, tablet device, or computer. These websites and "apps" provide a database of foods to choose from, as well as detailed nutrient information for all foods entered. Users can then track their daily calorie, protein, **fat,** and **carbohydrate** intake along with **micronutrients.** Many of these resources also provide an exercise diary that allows individuals to view their calorie expenditure and/or workout history.

Description and Procedure

Sources: Bountziouka et al., 2010; Nataranjan et al., 2010; Svendsen et al., 2006

- The client records intake throughout the day, including water and beverages. The client also records daily physical activity. The client is solely responsible for the foods and beverages consumed throughout the day, as well as for recording them.
- By reviewing food intake along with the calories and fat consumed, the health coach can easily pinpoint any trouble spots with food (e.g., late-night eating or meal skipping).
- The client must be very specific. Instead of writing "ham sandwich," he or she should write down how much ham was actually on the sandwich. Was it 3 ounces (88 mL) or 8 ounces (237 mL)? It is important to include what types of condiments were used as well.

Necessary Components

- The client only needs to record his or her food intake in a food diary booklet, in a notebook, or on pieces of paper. Health coaches should teach clients that it is best to record food intake immediately after consumption, instead of writing it down at the end of the day when it is easy to forget foods consumed.

Pros

- Easy to administer
- Economical
- Increased awareness of habits and foods consumed

Cons

- Dependent on the literacy of the client
- Respondent burden
- Recall bias: Records may not reflect "typical" intakes because interest in "pleasing" the health coach may alter consumption or tracking
- Lack of knowledge on estimating **portion** sizes, calories, and fat content of foods consumed

24-hour Recall

The same tools used for the food diary can be used when administering the 24-hour recall (see Figure 15-2). Obviously, a major limitation of the 24-hour recall is that "yesterday" may not truly reflect the scope of a person's typical eating patterns. In addition, this tool relies heavily on memory.

Description and Procedure

Sources: Takachi et al., 2011; Schatzkin et al., 2003

- Obtain information on food and fluid intake for the previous day or previous 24 hours.
- The 24-hour recall is based on the assumption that the intake described is typical of daily intake.
- A five-pass method can be used that includes the following:
  - ✓ A "quick list" pass in which the respondent is asked to list everything consumed in the previous day
  - ✓ A "forgotten foods" pass in which a standard list of foods and beverages that are often forgotten is read to prompt recall
  - ✓ A "time and occasion" pass in which the time and name for each eating occasion is collected
  - ✓ A "detailed" pass in which the detailed descriptions and portion sizes are collected and the time interval between meals is reviewed to check for additional foods
  - ✓ The "final" pass: one last opportunity to recall the foods consumed

Necessary Components

- Time that the food or beverage was consumed
- The food or beverage item
- **Serving** size of the food or beverage item
- How the food was prepared
- Where the client consumed the food or beverage item
- Any relevant notes regarding the meal or food item

Pros

- Easy to administer
- Not dependent on the literacy of the respondent
- Precision and, when multiple days are assessed, reliability
- Low administration costs

Cons

- The need to obtain multiple recalls to reliably estimate usual intake
- Participant burden
- Difficulty of the estimation of portion sizes
- Recall bias: Records may not reflect "typical" intakes because interest in "pleasing" the health coach may alter consumption or tracking

Visit www.ACEfitness.org/HealthCoachResources to download a free PDF of the food-frequency questionnaire, as well as other forms and assessment tools that you can use throughout your career as a health coach.

Food-frequency Questionnaire

Food-frequency questionnaires (FFQ) may be challenging for clients, as it can be difficult to truly estimate the number of times an individual food is eaten. However, the benefit of this tool is that the client is less likely to forget foods, because they are listed on the chart. It is also easy to identify the type of diet the client typically follows (e.g., low-fat/high-fiber or high-protein/high-fat). Figure 15-3 presents a portion of a sample food-frequency questionnaire.

Figure 15-3
Sample food-frequency questionnaire

Food	Every Day (Always)	3 or 4 Times/Week (Often)	Every 2 or 3 Weeks (Sometimes)	Don't Eat (Never)
Dairy Products				
Milk, whole				
Milk, reduced fat				
Milk, nonfat				
Cottage cheese				
Cream cheese				
Other cheeses				
Yogurt				
Ice cream				
Sherbet				
Puddings				
Margarine				
Butter				
Other				
Meats				
Beef, hamburger				
Poultry				
Pork, ham				
Bacon, sausage				
Cold cuts, hot dogs				
Other				
Fish and Other Protein Sources				
Canned tuna				
Breaded fish				
Fresh or frozen fish				
Eggs				
Peanut butter				
Grain products				
Bread, white				
Bread, whole wheat				
Rolls, muffins				
Pancakes, waffles				
Bagels				
Pasta, spaghetti				
Pasta, macaroni and cheese				
Rice				
Crackers				
Other				

Figure 15-3
Continued

Food	Every Day (Always)	3 or 4 Times/Week (Often)	Every 2 or 3 Weeks (Sometimes)	Don't Eat (Never)
Cereals				
Sugar-coated				
High-fiber (bran)				
Natural (granola)				
Plain (e.g., Cheerios®)				
Fortified				
Other				
Fruits				
Oranges, orange juice				
Tomatoes, tomato juice				
Grapefruit, grapefruit juice				
Strawberries				
Cranberry juice				
Apples, apple juice				
Grapes, grape juice				
Fruit drink				
Peaches				
Bananas				
Other				
Vegetables				
Peppers				
Potatoes				
Lettuce				
Broccoli				
Spinach				
Carrots				
Corn				
Squash				
Peas				
Green beans				
Beets				
Other				
Snacks and Sweets				
Chips (potato, corn)				
Pretzels				
Popcorn				
French fries				
Cookies				
Pastries				
Candy				
Sugar, honey, jelly				
Soda, regular				
Soda, diet				
Cocoa				
Other				

Description and Procedure

Sources: Takachi et al., 2011; Bountziouka et al., 2010; Svendsen et al., 2006; Schatzkin et al., 2003; Willett, 2001

- The FFQ identifies foods that the client most commonly eats.
- The client indicates, on average, how much and how often he or she consumes different foods.
- Analysis of the FFQ data provides information about the daily intake of many nutrients.

Necessary Components

- Vary among FFQs, but typically include a large list of foods with their corresponding frequency of consumption

Pros

- Relatively low administrative costs
- Ability to assess usual and longer-term intake

Cons

- Inaccuracy of absolute nutrient values
- Fluctuation of nutrient values depending on instrument length and structure
- Lack of detail regarding specific foods
- General imprecision
- Recall bias: Records may not reflect "typical" intakes because interest in "pleasing" the health coach may alter consumption or tracking
- Seasonal variability
- Cultural/diet variability (e.g., vegetarians or individuals on therapeutic diets)

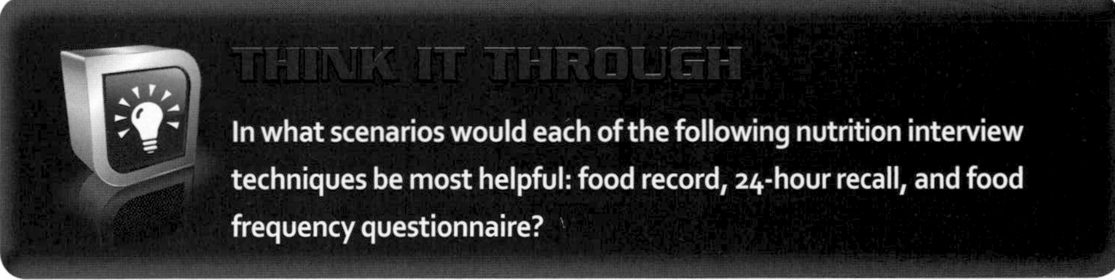

THINK IT THROUGH
In what scenarios would each of the following nutrition interview techniques be most helpful: food record, 24-hour recall, and food frequency questionnaire?

Food Models and Portion Estimates

A portion is the amount of food a person chooses to eat, while a serving is a standardized amount of a food used to estimate and/or evaluate one's intake. Increases in portion sizes have been frequently cited as an important contributing factor to the growing rates in obesity seen over the past several decades (Figure 15-4). Portions are very difficult for some to estimate, and correct estimates could mean the difference between a 1,400-calorie diet and a 2,200-calorie diet.

Health coaches can assist clients in a number of ways when estimating their portions. The guidelines presented in Table 15-1 can be used to help clients more accurately determine the amount of food that they are consuming.

In addition, there are a number of tools that can be purchased to help clients better understand their portion sizes. For example, the National Dairy Council sells paper cutouts of various foods with detailed nutrition information on the back. Also, various companies sell plastic food models that demonstrate average and large sizes. Food models range from

Figure 15-4
Increases in portion sizes

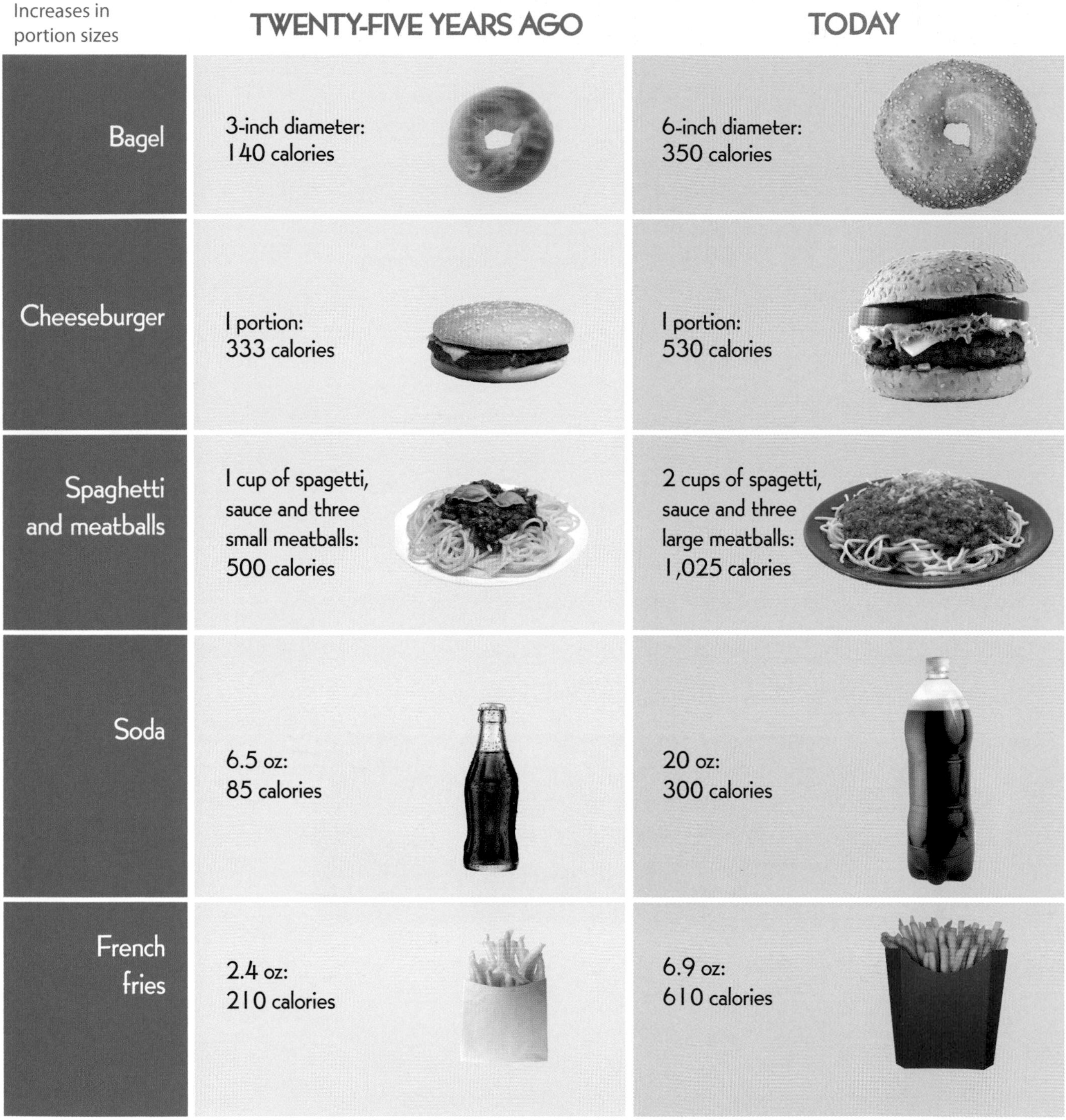

	TWENTY-FIVE YEARS AGO	TODAY
Bagel	3-inch diameter: 140 calories	6-inch diameter: 350 calories
Cheeseburger	1 portion: 333 calories	1 portion: 530 calories
Spaghetti and meatballs	1 cup of spagetti, sauce and three small meatballs: 500 calories	2 cups of spagetti, sauce and three large meatballs: 1,025 calories
Soda	6.5 oz: 85 calories	20 oz: 300 calories
French fries	2.4 oz: 210 calories	6.9 oz: 610 calories

$2 for a single food to $125 for an extensive package. Some of these companies also sell index cards with pictures of foods in specific serving sizes. The sizes range from 1-ounce servings to "supersize" servings, so clients can visualize the difference and understand how portion-size choices impact their diets.

Comparing food portion sizes to common items is also a helpful way for clients to visualize the foods they eat, adopt better habits, and eat more appropriate foods amounts. For example, in Table 15-1, servings are compared to common household items for reference.

Table 15-1

Estimating Portion Size

Food Group	Key Message	What Counts?	Looks Like ...
Grains	Make half your grains whole.	1 oz equivalent =	
		1 slice of bread	CD cover
		1 cup of ready-to-eat cereal	A baseball
		½ cup cooked rice, pasta, or cooked cereal	½ a baseball
		5 whole-wheat crackers	
Vegetables	Vary your veggies. Make half your plate fruits and vegetables.	1 cup =	
		1 cup of raw or cooked vegetable	Baseball
		2 cups of raw leafy salad greens	Softball
		1 cup of vegetable juice	
Fruits	Make half your plate fruits and vegetables.	1 cup =	
		1 cup raw fruit	Tennis ball
		½ cup dried fruit	2 golf balls
		1 cup 100% fruit juice	
Milk	Switch to fat-free or low-fat (1%) milk.	1 cup =	
		1 cup of milk, yogurt, or soy milk	Baseball
		1.5 ounces of natural cheese or	1½ 9-volt batteries
		2 ounces of processed cheese	
Protein Foods	Choose lean proteins.	1 ounce =	
		1 oz of meat, poultry, or fish	Deck of cards (3 oz) for lean meats; checkbook = 3 oz fish
		¼ cup cooked dry beans	½ golf ball
		1 egg	½ of a Post-it® note
		1 Tbsp peanut butter	Golf ball
		½ oz nuts or seeds	
		2 Tbsp hummus	
Oils	Choose liquid oils and avoid solid fats.	3 tsp =	
		1 Tbsp vegetable oils	Tip of thumb
		½ medium avocado	
		1 oz peanuts, mixed nuts, cashews, almonds, or sunflower seeds	

For more specific amounts, please visit www.ChooseMyPlate.gov.

Using the 2015-2020 Dietary Guidelines for Americans *and MyPlate*

The *2015-2020 Dietary Guidelines for Americans* provide science-based advice aimed at promoting health and reducing the risk for major chronic diseases through diet and physical activity [United States Department of Agriculture (USDA), 2015]. The intent of the *Dietary Guidelines* is to summarize and synthesize knowledge regarding individual nutrients and food components into recommendations for a healthy eating pattern that focuses on nutrient-dense foods and beverages that help the public achieve and maintain a healthy weight.

The *Guidelines* encourage most Americans to eat fewer calories, be more active, and make informed food choices. A basic premise of the *Dietary Guidelines* is that nutrient needs should be met primarily through consuming foods. Foods provide an array of nutrients and other compounds that may have beneficial effects on health. In certain cases, fortified foods and dietary supplements may be useful sources of one or more nutrients that otherwise might be consumed in less than recommended amounts. Dietary supplements, while recommended in some cases, cannot replace a healthful diet. The complete guidelines can be found at www.health.gov/dietaryguidelines.

With the release of the *2010 Dietary Guidelines for Americans,* the USDA took the old Food Guide Pyramid, which recommends a number of food groups and serving sizes to consume on a daily basis, one step further with the unveiling of www.ChooseMyPlate.gov. This new, simplified approach to nutrition and food group recommendations breaks down food groups by balancing the correct portions of each food group on a plate for an easy visual (Figure 15-5). Fruits and vegetables make up one half of the plate, grains take up one quarter, and the final quarter of the plate is protein. Additionally, there is a glass of milk (or any dairy item) paired with the plate of food groups. Unlike the old Food Guide Pyramid, new recommendations are now offered in a measureable quantity (ounces or cups) rather than servings to help individuals put recommendations into action. By logging on to www.ChooseMyPlate.gov. individuals can receive personalized nutrition recommendations in their "Daily Food Plan" based on age, gender, weight, height, and physical-activity level. To appreciate the role of the personalized "Daily Food Plan" in helping an overweight client

Figure 15-5
MyPlate

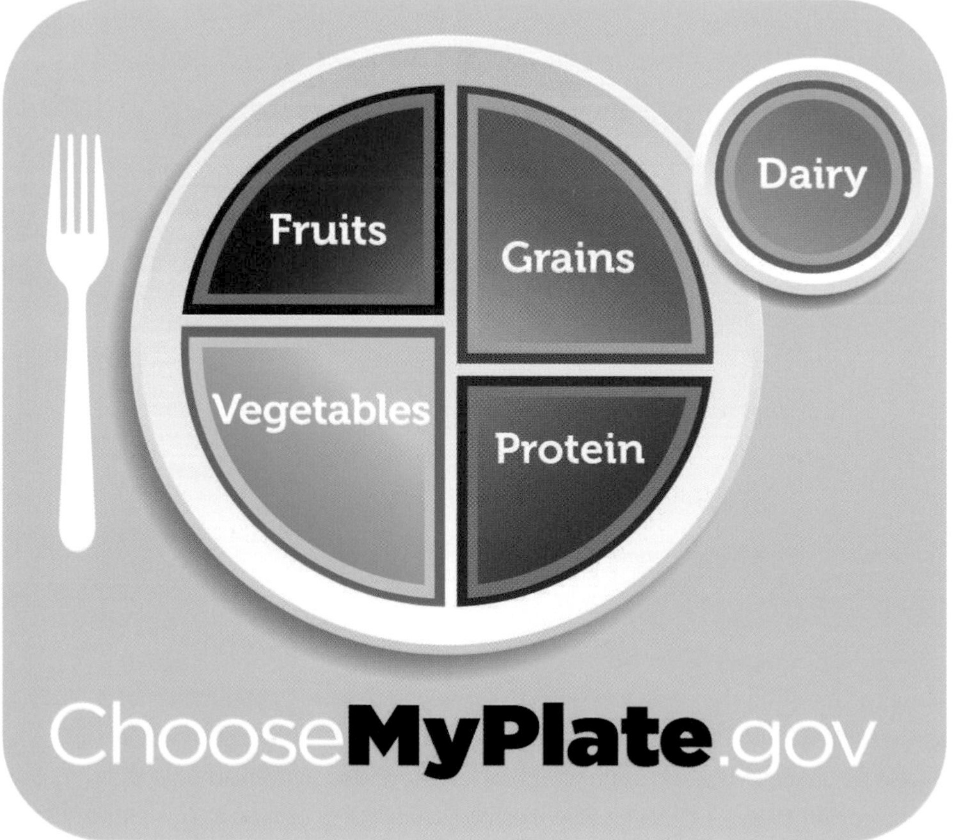

plan his or her daily intake of food, an 1,800-calorie diet is described below. In this example, the personalized "Daily Food Plan" is designed for a 45-year-old female who is 5'4" (1.6 m), 185 pounds (84 kg), and sedentary. To move toward a healthier weight, this individual should consume the following amount of food from each food group for her 1,800-calorie food plan:

- 6 ounces of grains
- 2.5 cups of vegetables
- 1.5 cups of fruits
- 3 cups of milk and dairy
- 5 ounces of protein foods

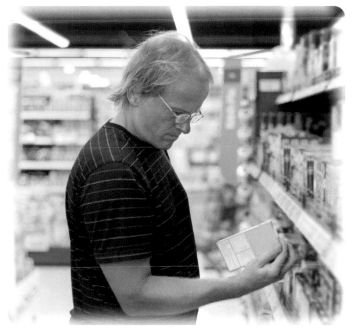

ChooseMyPlate aims to simplify servings. Serving sizes are not designed to portray how much a person should consume at a meal or a snack, but rather to serve as a pattern with which to compare his or her intake throughout the day. To clear up any confusion, it is important to outline the appropriate food group serving sizes and tips as described in Table 15-1. Food intake patterns that outline the breakdown of foods groups by calorie recommendations can be found at www.choosemyplate.gov/professionals/pdf_food_intake.html.

The *2015-2020 Dietary Guidelines for Americans* offer five big-picture recommendations that are key to good nutrition. An overview of these five key recommendations, how they pertain to health and fitness professionals, and how you can best use this information to support clients in achieving their nutrition goals are provided here. In addition, readers are referred to www.health.gov/dietaryguidelines for a full review of the report.

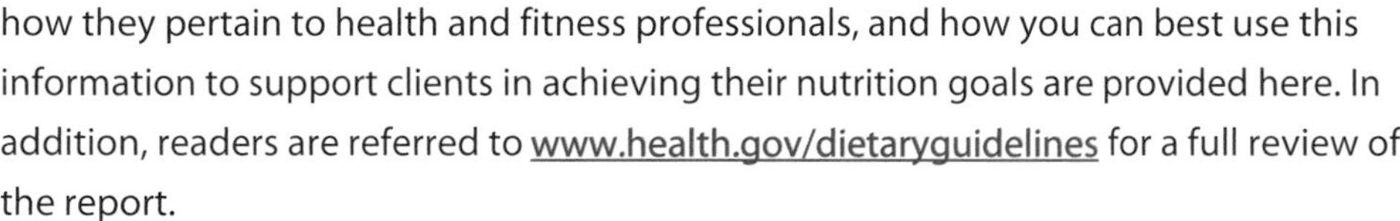

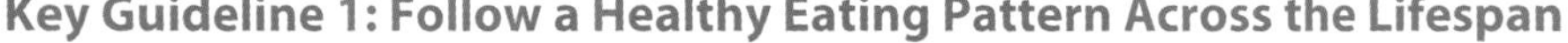

Key Guideline 1: Follow a Healthy Eating Pattern Across the Lifespan

All food and beverage choices matter. Choose a healthy eating pattern at an appropriate calorie level to help achieve and maintain a healthy body weight, support nutrient adequacy, and reduce the risk of chronic disease.

The *2015-2020 Dietary Guidelines for Americans* make a point to emphasize overall eating patterns more so than individual nutrients, recognizing that the overall nutritional value of a person's diet is more than "the sum of its parts."

The main components of a healthy eating pattern include:

- A variety of vegetables from five different groups—dark green, red and orange, legumes (beans and peas), starchy, and other
- Fruit
- Grains, primarily whole grains
- Fat-free or low-fat dairy, including milk yogurt, cheese, and/or fortified soy products
- A variety of foods rich in protein, including seafood, lean meats and poultry, eggs, legumes (beans and peas), nuts, seeds, and soy products
- Limited amounts of saturated fats and trans fats (less than 10% of calories), added sugars (less than 10% of calories), and sodium (less than 2,300 mg per day). If alcohol is

consumed, it should be consumed in moderation, defined as up to one drink per day for women and two drinks per day for men.

The three types of healthy eating patterns discussed at most length in the *Dietary Guidelines* are the **Healthy U.S.-Style Eating Pattern,** the **Healthy Mediterranean-Style Eating Pattern,** and the **Healthy Vegetarian Eating Pattern**. The Healthy U.S.-Style Eating Pattern is based on the types and proportions of foods Americans typically consume, but in nutrient-dense forms and appropriate amounts. It is designed to meet nutrient needs while not exceeding calorie requirements and while staying within limits for overconsumed dietary components. The Healthy Mediterranean-Style Eating Pattern contains more fruits and seafood and less dairy, meats, and poultry than does the Healthy U.S.-Style Eating Pattern. The pattern is similar to the Healthy U.S.-Style Eating Pattern in nutrient content, with the exception of providing less calcium and vitamin D. The Healthy Vegetarian Eating Pattern is adapted from the Healthy U.S.-Style Pattern, modifying amounts recommended from some food groups to more closely reflect eating patterns reported by self-identified **vegetarians.** This pattern is similar in meeting nutrient standards to the Healthy U.S.-Style Eating Pattern, but somewhat higher in calcium and **fiber** and lower in vitamin D.

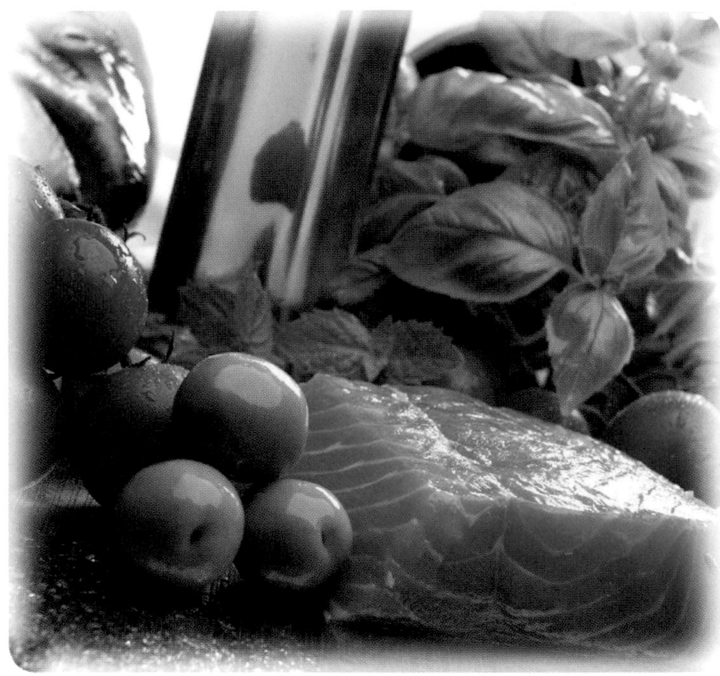

Key Guideline 2: Focus on Variety, Nutrient Density, and Amount

To meet nutrient needs within calorie limits, choose a variety of nutrient-dense foods across and within all food groups in recommended amounts.

The *Dietary Guidelines* suggest that Americans are most likely to meet nutrient needs and manage weight by choosing nutrient-dense foods, which provide high levels of vitamins, minerals, and other nutrients that may have health benefits relative to caloric content. Categories of nutrient-dense foods include vegetables, fruits, grains, dairy, protein foods, and oils.

- *Vegetables:* Vegetables are an important contributor to a healthy eating pattern. Vegetables are classified into five subgroups—dark green, red and orange, legumes (beans and peas), starchy, and other.
- *Fruits:* Whole fruits, including fresh, frozen, canned, and dried forms, provide key nutrients, including dietary fiber, potassium, and vitamin C.
- *Grains:* Grains include foods such as rice, oatmeal, and popcorn, as well as products that contain grains like bread, cereals, crackers, and pasta. Whole grains contain the entire grain kernel and provide health and nutritional value, including fiber, iron, zinc, manganese, folate, magnesium, copper, thiamin, niacin, vitamin B6, phosphorus, selenium, riboflavin, and vitamin A. Whole grains include foods such as brown rice, quinoa, and oats.

- *Dairy:* The dairy group includes milk, yogurt, cheese, and fortified soy beverages. Dairy products are high in calcium, phosphorus, vitamin A, vitamin D (usually through fortification), riboflavin, vitamin B12, protein, potassium, zinc, choline, magnesium, and selenium.
- *Protein foods:* Protein foods include a diversity of foods from plant and animal sources, including the following subgroups: seafood; meats, poultry, and eggs; and nuts, seeds, and soy products. Protein foods are high in nutrients, such as niacin, vitamin B12, vitamin B6, riboflavin, selenium, choline, phosphorus, zinc, copper, vitamin D, and vitamin E.
- *Oils:* Oils are fats that contain a percentage of monounsaturated fats and polyunsaturated fats and are liquid at room temperature. Oils are not a food group; however, the *Dietary Guidelines* recognizes them as an important part of a healthy eating pattern because they contain essential fatty acids and vitamin E.

Key Guideline 3: Limit Calories from Added Sugars and Saturated Fats and Reduce Sodium Intake

Consume an eating pattern low in added sugars, saturated fats, and sodium. Cut back on foods and beverages higher in these components to amounts that fit within healthy eating patterns.

The *Dietary Guidelines* urge Americans to pay attention to—and limit—consumption of foods with low to no nutritional value, especially those that are, or may be, harmful to health such as added sugars, saturated fat, and sodium. New to the *2015-2020 Dietary Guidelines* compared to previous editions, dietary cholesterol is no longer noted as a nutrient to limit, as it is likely not harmful to health for most people.

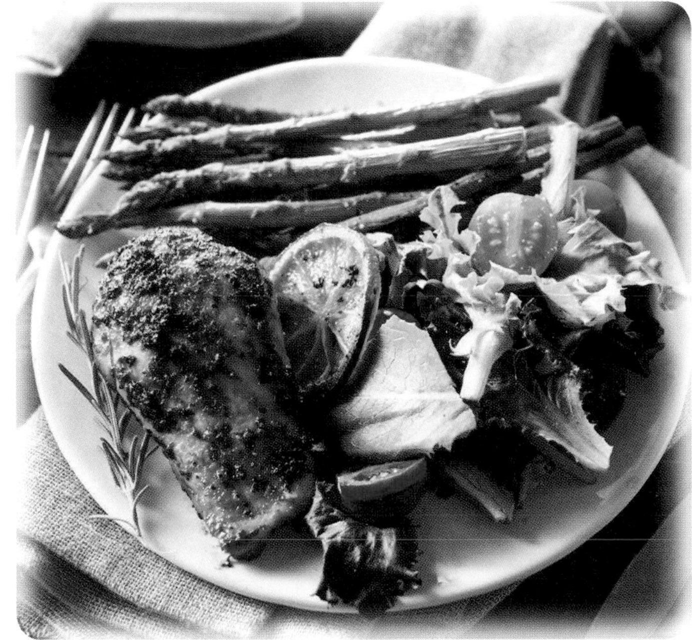

- *Added sugars:* Natural sugars include fruit sugar (fructose) and milk sugar (lactose). However, most sugars in the typical American diet are added sugars. The *Dietary Guidelines* recommend that Americans consume no more than 10% of calories from added sugars, while staying within calorie limits.
- *Saturated fats:* The *Dietary Guidelines* recommend a diet containing <10% of total calories from saturated fat. Major sources of saturated fat for Americans include full-fat cheese, pizza, grain-based desserts, dairy-based desserts, fried foods, sausage, franks, bacon, and ribs.
- *Trans fats:* Trans fats are found naturally in some foods ("ruminant trans fats"), but the majority of intake comes from processed foods ("artificial trans fats"). Americans should consume as little artificial trans fats as possible.
- *Sodium and the Dietary Approaches to Stop Hypertension Eating Plan:* The health and fitness professional can help clients decrease sodium intake with the following advice:
  - ✓ Read nutrition labels and pay attention to sodium content
  - ✓ Consume more fresh foods and fewer processed foods

- ✓ Eat more home-prepared meals and add little table salt or sodium-containing seasonings
- ✓ When eating out, ask that salt not be added
- ✓ Reduce calorie intake (since most foods also contain sodium)

In addition, individuals with hypertension are advised to follow the low-sodium Dietary Approaches to Stop Hypertension (DASH) eating plan to optimize health and decrease blood pressure.

Key Guideline 4: Shift to Healthier Food and Beverage Choices

Choose nutrient-dense foods and beverages across and within all food groups in place of less healthy choices. Consider cultural and personal preferences to make these shifts easier to accomplish and maintain.

While the *Dietary Guidelines* advocate an overall healthy and balanced nutrition pattern that is low in added sugars and sodium, the reality is that most Americans eat nothing like the eating patterns recommended by the *Dietary Guidelines.* By making shifts in dietary patterns, Americans can achieve and maintain a healthy body weight, meet nutrient needs, and decrease the risk of chronic disease.

Overall, the *Dietary Guidelines* advise that Americans shift their eating patterns to:

- Consume more vegetables
- Consume more fruits
- Consume more whole grains, and fewer refined grains
- Consume more dairy products
- Increase variety in protein food choices and choose more nutrient-dense foods. That is, eat more seafood in place of meat, poultry, or eggs and use legumes or nuts and seeds in mixed dishes instead of some meat or poultry.

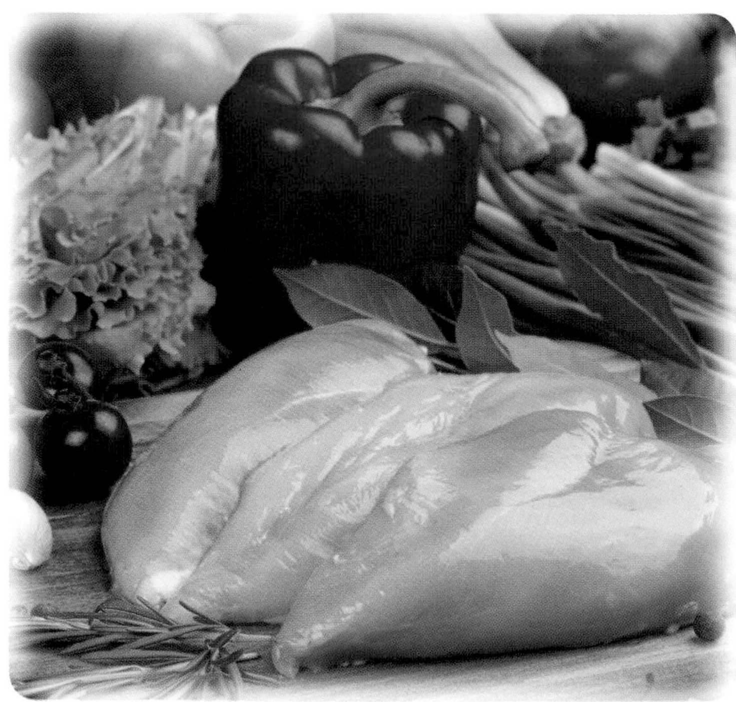

- Men and teenage boys should consume less protein, especially meat, poultry, and eggs
- Exchange solid fats for oils
- Reduce added sugar consumption to less than 10% of calories per day
- Reduce saturated fat

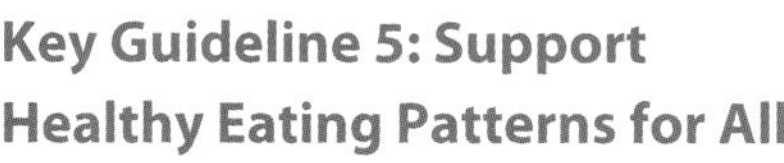

Key Guideline 5: Support Healthy Eating Patterns for All

Everyone has a role in helping create and support healthy eating patterns in multiple settings nationwide, from home to school to work to communities.

The *Guidelines* charge all sectors of society to play an active role in the movement to make the United States healthier by developing coordinated partnerships, programs, and policies to support healthy eating,

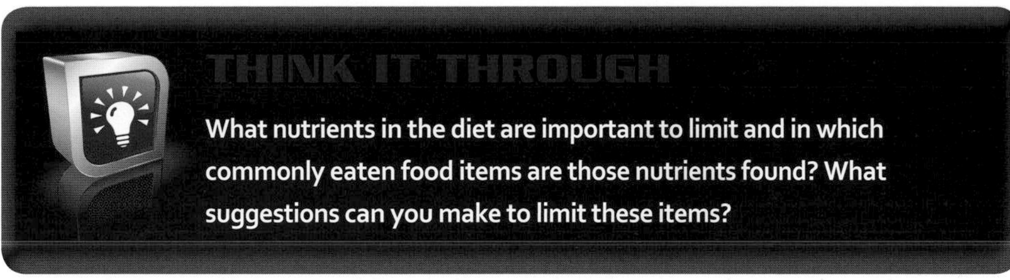
THINK IT THROUGH
What nutrients in the diet are important to limit and in which commonly eaten food items are those nutrients found? What suggestions can you make to limit these items?

Addressing a Client's Nutritional Needs While Staying Within the Health Coach's Scope of Practice

Making specific nutrition/nutrient recommendations and developing meal plans are beyond the scope of practice of a health coach. However, providing general information on nutrition and weight management can be helpful and useful for clients. A health coach must know when to tackle and when to refer nutrition issues, as doing so will help maintain professionalism as well as decrease the risk of liability (see Chapters 2 and 20 and Appendix A).

Table 15-2 features a list of issues that a health coach might discuss with clients, as well as issues that are more appropriate for referral. Every health coach must ultimately determine what topics are appropriate to discuss with the client based upon his or her level of education and expertise. A health coach should not hesitate to refer a client to a **registered dietitian (R.D.)** or more qualified professional if the client's needs exceed the health coach's training and level of expertise. Refer to Chapter 2 for more information on making appropriate referrals.

Table 15-2

Scope of Practice Guidelines for Nutrition

Appropriate Nutrition Topics for a Health Coach	
• MyPlate Guidelines • Suggestions for weight loss • Pre-evaluations and use of food diary • Lifestyle changes	• Hydration • Recipes • Support • Basic pre- and post-exercise nutrition • Weight-loss physiology
Nutrition Areas That Should Be Referred	

• Specific meal plans
• Tailored plans
• Medications
• Diseases
  ◦ Cardiovascular disease
  ◦ Hypertension
  ◦ Hyperlipidemia
  ◦ Diabetes
  ◦ Eating disorders
  ◦ AIDS
	• Medical diagnoses
	  ◦ Anemia
	  ◦ Osteoporosis
	  ◦ Polycystic ovary disease
	• Post-op
	• Yo-yo dieting
	• Supplements
	• Large weight loss or morbid obesity

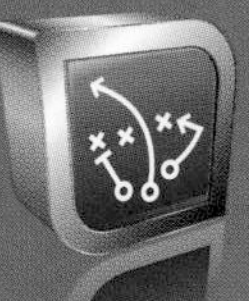

APPLY WHAT YOU KNOW

Qualified registered dietitians can be located through the following organizations and channels:

- The Academy of Nutrition and Dietetics (formerly the American Dietetic Association, www.eatright.org)
- Sports, Cardiovascular, and Wellness Nutritionists (www.scandpg.org)
- Professional meetings
- Local fitness centers
- Medical professionals
- Professional networking

Questions the registered dietitian should be asked:

- How does he or she stay up-to-date on the latest research?
- To which organizations does he or she belong ? With what hospital or medical group is he or she affiliated?
- What journals or research does he or she read?
- What are the fees? What is included in the appointment?
- What is his or her area of specialty or expertise (e.g., age groups or certain populations)?
- Does he or she sell vitamins, supplements, or foods?

In addition, the health coach can discuss a current client situation (while maintaining client confidentiality) with the registered dietitian to get a better idea of his or her approach or philosophy on nutrition.

THINK IT THROUGH

Based on your personal knowledge, what nutrition topics do you feel you can appropriately and professionally handle and what areas would be best to refer to an R.D. for optimal care of your clients?

Nutritional Program Planning for the Weight-loss Client

Estimating Caloric Needs

There are a variety of methods that can be used to estimate a client's daily calorie needs. Daily energy needs (caloric requirement) are determined by three factors:

- **Resting metabolic rate (RMR)**
- **Thermogenesis** (calories required for heat production)
- Physical activity

Resting metabolic rate is the amount of energy (measured in calories) expended by the body during quiet rest. RMR makes up between 60 and 75% of the total calories used daily (see Chapter 8). Physical activity is the second largest factor contributing to daily energy expenditure or calorie requirements. This is the most variable component of 24-hour energy expenditure, as this number changes based on the frequency, intensity, and duration of an individual's workouts. Thermogenesis, also referred to as the **thermic effect of food,** is the smallest component. This is the amount of calories needed to digest and absorb the foods that are consumed. While certain diets claim to enhance this component (e.g., food-combining programs), no research exists to support that concept. The bottom line is that regular physical activity is the most effective way to increase total caloric expenditure.

The following section reviews methods for determining a client's energy needs. This information does not, however, take into account a client's disease risk in relation to his or her weight or nutritional habits. For more information on how to use tools such as **waist-to-hip ratio** and **body mass index (BMI),** see Chapter 11.

Calculating Energy Needs

There are numerous ways to calculate a client's daily caloric needs. The simplest method is to multiply the client's weight (in pounds) by the appropriate conversion factor (Table 15-3). This calculation will yield an approximation of how many calories the individual needs to maintain his or her current weight, based on activity level and gender.

The Harris-Benedict equation for **basal metabolic rate (BMR)** takes into account the individual's weight, height, age, and gender. However, it has been shown to slightly underestimate BMR in females and slightly overestimate BMR in males (Harris & Benedict, 1919).

Table 15-3

Conversion Factors for Estimating Daily Caloric Requirements Based on Gender and Activity Level

	Activity Level		
	Light	Moderate	Heavy
Male	17	19	23
Female	16	17	20

Light activity level: Walking (level surface, 2.5–3.0 mph), housecleaning, child care, golf

Moderate activity level: Walking (3.5–4.0 mph), cycling, skiing, tennis, dancing

Heavy activity level: Walking with a load uphill, basketball, climbing, football, soccer

Harris-Benedict Equation

For men: BMR = [13.75 x weight (kg)] + [5.003 x height (cm)] – [6.775 x age] + 66.5

For women: BMR = [9.563 x weight (kg)] + [1.850 x height (cm)] – [4.676 x age] + 655.1

Note: To determine weight in kg, divide weight in pounds by 2.2. To determine height in cm, multiply height in inches by 2.54. Incorporate an activity correction factor between 1.2 and 1.5 to account for the individual's average amount of physical activity.

Table 15-4 includes several RMR prediction equations that can be used to help clients understand how many calories they burn throughout the day while at rest. Some of these equations provide more accurate results for certain populations than others, so health coaches must be sure to choose the most appropriate equation for each client.

In addition to the estimation equations presented in Table 15-4, another method called **indirect calorimetry** is used to predict resting metabolic rate. Since oxygen is used in

Table 15-4

RMR Prediction Equations (kcal/day)

Mifflin-St. Jeor Equations
(Frankenfield, Roth-Yousey, & Compher, 2005; Frankenfield et al., 2003; Mifflin et al., 1990)

Men: RMR = (9.99 x weight) + (6.25 x height) – (4.92 x age) + 5
Women: RMR = (9.99 x weight)+ (6.25 x height) – (4.92 x age) – 161

Multiply the RMR value derived from the prediction equation by the appropriate activity correction factor:

1.200 = sedentary (little or no exercise)
1.375 = lightly active (light exercise/sports one to three days per week)
1.550 = moderately active (moderate exercise/sports three to five days per week)
1.725 = very active (hard exercise/sports six to seven days per week)
1.900 = extra active (very hard exercise/sports and a physical job)

Note: This equation is more accurate for obese than non-obese individuals.

Schofield Equation
(Tverskaya et al., 1998; Schofield, 1985; Harris & Benedict, 1919)

Age	Males	Females
15–18	BMR = 17.6 x weight + 656	BMR = 13.3 x weight + 690
18–30	BMR = 15.0 x weight + 690	BMR = 14.8 x weight + 485
30–60	BMR = 11.4 x weight + 870	BMR = 8.1 x weight + 842
>60	BMR = 11.7 x weight + 585	BMR = 9.0 x weight + 656

Note: This equation slightly underestimates for women and slightly overestimates for men.

Owen Equation
(Owen et al., 1987; 1986)

Males: RMR = (10.2 x weight) + 879
Females: RMR = (7.18 x weight) + 795

Cunningham Equation
(Cunningham, 1991)

All subjects: REE (kcal/day) = (21.6 x FFM) + 370

Note: This is considered one of the better prediction equations for athletes because it takes into account fat-free mass.

Wang Equation
(Bauer, Reeves, & Capra, 2004)

All subjects: REE (kcal/day) = (21.5 x FFM) + 407

Note: This equation is potentially better for athletes because it takes into account fat-free mass.

Note: All methods of determining RMR are estimates only; Equations use weight in kilograms (kg) and height in centimeters (cm); REE = Resting energy expenditure; FFM = Fat-free mass; RMR = Resting metabolic rate; BMR = Basal metabolic rate; Note that RMR and BMR are sometimes used interchangeably.

the metabolic process to create energy, a person's metabolic rate can be determined by measuring how much oxygen he or she consumes when breathing. There is a relationship between the body's use of oxygen and the energy it expends, so scientists use formulas to convert gas usage into energy (calories) used.

Historically, oxygen-uptake measurements were only performed with a medical device called a metabolic cart, which can cost between $20,000 and $50,000. Newer technology has made it possible to measure oxygen uptake using hand-held devices, making the analysis more accessible and affordable.

Using Caloric Information to Affect Weight

Once the client's daily caloric needs have been estimated, this information can be used to help the client lose, gain, or maintain weight. To change weight by 1 pound (0.45 kg), caloric intake must be decreased or increased by 3,500 calories. For weight loss, it is advisable to reduce daily caloric intake by 250 calories per day and to increase daily expenditure (through physical activity) by 250 calories. This 500-calorie difference, when multiplied by seven, creates a weekly negative caloric balance that results in a loss of 1 pound (0.45 kg). These numbers may be doubled to achieve a loss of 2 pounds (0.91 kg) per week, but that may be too great a goal for some clients. Most health organizations recommend a weight-loss rate of 1 to 2 pounds (0.45 kg to 0.91 kg) per week.

To gain approximately one-half pound (0.23 kg) of weight per week, clients can add 300 to 500 calories to their daily intake. It is crucial that the exercise routine be maintained so that additional calories are used to fuel muscles, rather than to simply store additional fat. Advise clients to follow this new calorie plan for a few months and make changes as needed (American College of Sports Medicine, 2010; Baechle & Earle, 2008).

THINK IT THROUGH

If a client is aiming to gain weight, what recommendations would you make to safely and effectively help him or her gain lean body mass? What recommendations would you make to help your client lose weight while preserving lean body mass?

APPLY WHAT YOU KNOW

Weight Loss and Fatigue in the Adolescent Athlete

Anna is a 15-year-old classical ballet dancer studying for an Intermediate Level Ballet Examination. She is about 5'7" (1.7 m) and 150 pounds (68 kg). She attends a 90-minute classical ballet class four times per week and completes one class of repertoire, contemporary, and jazz ballet each Saturday. Anna has recently moved from her local suburban dancing school to one that provides a highly regarded but rigorous dance training program.

Anna's ballet teachers are concerned about her increasing weight, which is 15 pounds (6.8 kg) higher than when she first started at their school nine months earlier. In addition to the weight concern, Anna has recently become moody, tired, and less motivated.

Anna has been dieting in an attempt to reduce weight with little success since her menstrual cycle began 18 months previously. She tried almost every diet given to her by other ballet students, but any weight loss achieved seemed to rapidly reappear. The experience of "nothing seeming to work" left Anna convinced that her metabolism was slow and that she would never be able to lose weight.

Given Anna's height, weight, and activity level, her calorie needs are approximately 2,800 calories per day. To lose about 1 pound (0.45 kg) a week she aims to consume about 500 fewer calories per day. According to the *2015-2020 Dietary Guidelines*, this calorie level (the closest plan is 2,400 kcal) calls for 2 cups of fruits, 3 cups of vegetables, 8 oz-equivalents of grains, 6.5 oz-equivalents of protein (meat, beans, nuts, seeds, seafood, etc.), 3 cups of milk, and 31 g of oils, with an allowance of about 350 discretionary calories. Below is the 24-hour recall representative of Anna's current diet.

Anna's Current Diet

Meal	Anna's 24-hour Recall
Breakfast	Nothing or one slice whole-meal toast with jam (no butter) 1 cup unsweetened tea
Lunch	Green salad One apple Diet soda
Dinner	Steamed chicken or fish with steamed vegetables 1 cup tea
Snacks	Diet soda and, if feeling really low before class, a chocolate bar or two

After evaluating Anna's 24-hour recall, a few key concerns arise that a health coach should address. The following suggestions can be made to improve calcium, iron, and fiber intake, boost nutrient-dense food intake, facilitate weight loss, control cravings, and improve satiety and hydration. Making these small changes in Anna's diet will help her reach her goals of regulating her metabolism to lose weight and alleviate her moodiness, fatigue, and lack of motivation.

- Consume a balanced diet that includes three meals a day and nutrient-dense snacks between meals such as fresh fruit, reduced-fat milk or yogurt, whole-grain crackers, or vegetables and hummus.
- Incorporate balance at every meal by including a fruit and/or vegetable, whole grain, and lean protein to boost satiety, energy levels, and fiber intake. Complex carbohydrates help maintain blood glucose levels and glycogen stores to power through exercise sessions. Examples include:
  - ✓ Breakfast: Whole-grain cereal or oatmeal with non-fat milk, an orange (to boost iron absorption), and a glass of milk or water instead of tea. Tea can inhibit iron absorption.
  - ✓ Lunch: Whole-grain wrap filled with salad greens, mixed veggies and beans, cheese, or poultry for added protein and staying power. Include a glass of milk or yogurt for extra calcium intake.
  - ✓ Dinner: Salmon with mango salsa, grilled asparagus, and wild rice.
- Increase fruit and vegetable intake by incorporating more fresh fruit for snacks, on salads, on cereal, or as dessert. Include more vegetables as snacks, and in soups, stews, casseroles, or sandwiches.
- Substitute water for diet soda. Adequate water intake is important for many biological processes and will help to prevent muscle fatigue. Aim for about half the body weight (in pounds) in ounces per day.
- Use a food diary to monitor food intake, cravings, and feelings. Allow chocolate or another treat once or twice a week to help prevent binge eating.
- Consider adding low-impact aerobic training (e.g., walking, cycling, swimming, or deep-water running) to help with weight loss via increasing energy expenditure and strength training to preserve lean tissue.

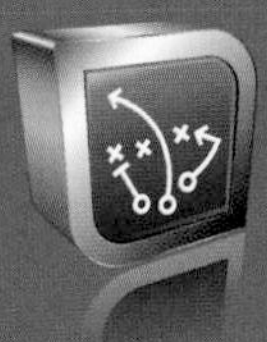

APPLY WHAT YOU KNOW

Eating to Recover After Training

Henry is an 20-year-old male college quarterback competing to be the team's starting quarterback in the upcoming season. Henry is 6'1" (1.9 m) and weighs 192 pounds (87 kg). In preparation for the new season, Henry undertook a program of 90 minutes per day of weight training five times a week, and about one hour playing a game of pick-up basketball most days of the week.

Within the first month of spring practice Henry had lost 7 pounds (3.2 kg) despite reporting eating "all of the time." He is fatigued and starving by the end of the workouts and is frustrated with his weight loss. He feels that lack of recovery between training sessions is preventing him from making the desired weight and performance gains.

Henry ate the bulk of his energy in the afternoon and evening. He grabs a sports bar and Gatorade in the morning before weight training around 10:30 a.m. and typically goes without breakfast during the week. He eats his lunch out every day, usually a burrito or sub sandwich. Henry avoids soda, but drinks lemonade with meals, and water before and after practice. Sometimes between afternoon practice and pick-up basketball Henry grabs another sports bar, but his main energy intake comes at dinner time. On the drive home, he often stops and gets a medium pizza with sausage and a glass of lemonade. Before bed, he always has a protein shake made with 1% milk.

Given Henry's height, weight, and athletic training, his daily energy needs are 4,650 calories to maintain his current weight. To gain 0.50 pounds (0.2 kg) per week, he needs 1,750 more calories per week or 250 more calories per day (4,650 calories + 250 calories = 4,900 calories). To follow the balance recommended by the *Dietary Guidelines*, he would need to consume 4 cups of fruits, 6 cups of vegetables, 15 oz-equivalents of grains, 12-oz equivalents of meat and beans, 6 cups of milk, and 15 tsp of oils, with an allowance of about 800 discretionary calories.

Considering his weight-loss concerns and his desire to enhance his energy and performance, what types of nutrient intervention would you recommend?

Henry's 24-hour Recall				
Morning Snack	Lunch	Afternoon Snack	Dinner	Evening Snack
Sports bar Gatorade®	Large chicken burrito Mexican rice Lemonade	Sports bar Water	Medium sausage pizza Lemonade	16-oz 1% milk and a scoop of protein powder

Goals are set to increase Henry's daily energy and carbohydrate intake, obtain the recommended fiber and micronutrients, fruit, and vegetable intake, and moderate his sodium intake. To achieve these changes, the following recommendations may be made:

- Start the day off with complex carbohydrates, protein, and fruit, such as a whole-wheat bagel, peanut butter, and banana before the morning weight-training session.
- Eat a high-carbohydrate snack with a high glycemic index within 30 minutes of all training sessions—fruit, bagel, or sports bar and Gatorade.
- For lunch, look for healthier options on the menu, such as a grilled chicken sandwich with lettuce and tomato on a whole-wheat roll. Pair a sweet potato or brown rice with a large vegetable salad to help reduce sodium and increase intake of vegetables.
- Replace high-fat dinner choices with a meal that is rich in complex carbohydrates, has adequate protein, and is low in fat. For example, replace the whole sausage pizza with half of a medium whole-wheat thin crust

vegetarian pizza, a garden salad, a piece of fruit, and water. Better yet, skip pizza and choose a dinner rich in lean protein, complex carbohydrates, and vegetables, such as salmon, wild rice, and asparagus.

- Replace the sports bar with whole foods such as a piece of fruit with low-fat cottage cheese/yogurt or almonds; whole-wheat crackers and almonds; or whole-grain breakfast cereal and low-fat milk.
- Encourage fluid intake throughout the day and during training sessions, especially water. Sports drinks may be used during workouts or mixed with water.
- Add a scoop of peanut butter or low-fat yogurt to the protein shake to increase energy content.
- Avoid sugar-sweetened beverages, like lemonade. Filling up on high-sugar beverages depletes the body of needed nutrients such as calcium.

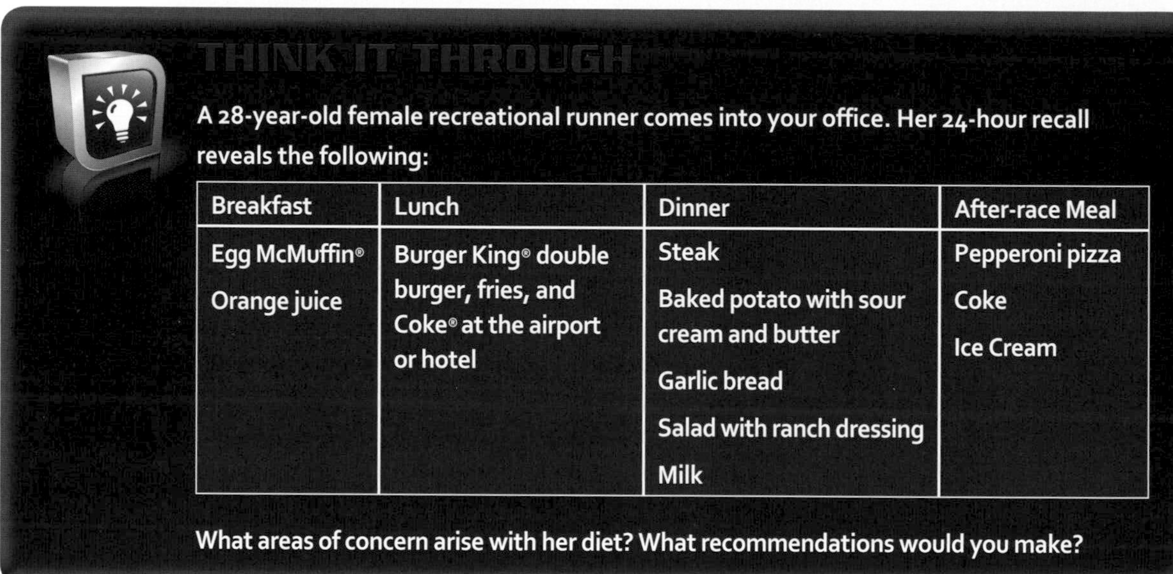

THINK IT THROUGH

A 28-year-old female recreational runner comes into your office. Her 24-hour recall reveals the following:

Breakfast	Lunch	Dinner	After-race Meal
Egg McMuffin® Orange juice	Burger King® double burger, fries, and Coke® at the airport or hotel	Steak Baked potato with sour cream and butter Garlic bread Salad with ranch dressing Milk	Pepperoni pizza Coke Ice Cream

What areas of concern arise with her diet? What recommendations would you make?

Summary

The client interview is a time not only to assess a client's current dietary habits and readiness for change, but also develop **rapport** and build a foundation for the client–health coach relationship. Health coaches should understand which programming tools to use with each client, as well as how to modify those tools as needed. Finally, it is essential for the health coach to stay within his or her scope of practice when it comes to nutritional programming.

References

American College of Sports Medicine (2010). *ACSM's Resource Manual for Guidelines for Exercise Testing and Prescription* (6th ed.). Philadelphia, Pa.: Lippincott Williams & Wilkins.

Baechle, T.R. & Earle, R.W. (2008). *Essentials of Strength Training and Conditioning* (3rd ed.). Champaign, Ill.: Human Kinetics.

Bauer, J., Reeves, M.M., & Capra, S. (2004). The agreement between measured and predicted resting energy expenditure in patients with pancreatic cancer: A pilot study. *Journal of the Pancreas*, 5, 1, 32–40.

Bountziouka, V. et al. (2010). Statistical methods used for the evaluation of reliability and validity of nutrition assessment tools used in medical research. *Journal of Current Pharmaceutical Design*, 34, 3770–3775.

Cunningham, J.D. (1991). Body composition as a determinate of energy expenditure: A synthetic review and a proposed general prediction equation. *American Journal of Clinical Nutrition*, 54, 963–969.

Frankenfield, D., Roth-Yousey, L., & Compher, C. (2005). Comparison of predictive equations for resting metabolic rate in healthy nonobese and obese adults: A systematic review. *Journal of the American Dietetic Association*, 105, 5, 775–789.

Frankenfeld, D. et al. (2003). Validation of several established equations for resting metabolic rate in obese and nonobese people. *Journal of the American Dietetic Association*, 103, 9, 1152–1159.

Harris, J. & Benedict, F. (1919). A biometric study of basal metabolism in man. *Key Facts in Clinical Nutrition*. Washington, D.C.: Carnegie Institute of Washington.

Mifflin, M.D. et al. (1990). A new predictive equation for resting energy expenditure in healthy individuals. *American Journal of Clinical Nutrition*, 51, 241–247.

Miraglia, M. et al. (2011). Dietary recommendations for primary prevention: An update. *The American Journal of Lifestyle Medicine*, 5, 144–155.

Nataranjan, L. et al. (2010). Measurement error of dietary self-report in intervention trials. *American Journal of Epidemiology*, 172, 819–827.

Owen, C.E. et al. (1987). A reappraisal of caloric requirements of men. *American Journal of Clinical Nutrition*, 46, 75–85.

Owen, C.E. et al. (1986). A reappraisal of caloric requirements in healthy women. *American Journal of Clinical Nutrition*, 44, 1–19.

Schatzkin, A. et al. (2003). A comparison of a food-frequency questionnaire with a 24-hour recall for use in an epidemiological cohort study: Results from the biomarker-based Observing Protein and Energy Nutrition (OPEN) study. *International Journal of Epidemiology*, 32, 1054–1062.

Schofield, R. (1985). Equations for estimating basal metabolic rate (BMR). *Human Nutrition: Clinical Nutrition*, 39C, 5–41.

Svendsen, M. et al. (2006). Accuracy of food intake reporting in obese subjects with metabolic risk factors. *British Journal of Nutrition*, 95, 640–649.

Takachi, R. et al. (2011). Validity of a self-administered Food Frequency Questionnaire for middle-aged urban cancer screenees: Comparison with 4-day weighed dietary records. *Journal of Epidemiology*, 1–12.

Tverskaya, R. et al. (1998). Comparison of several equations and derivation of a new equation for calculating basal metabolic rate in obese children. *Journal of the American College of Nutrition*, 17, 4, 333–336.

U.S. Department of Agriculture (2015). *2015-2020 Dietary Guidelines for Americans* (8th ed.). www.health.gov/dietaryguidelines

Willett, W. (2001). Commentary: Dietary diaries versus food frequency questionnaires—A case of undigestible data. *International Journal of Epidemiology*, 30, 317–319.

Suggested Reading

Ainsworth, B.E. et al. (2011). 2011 compendium of physical activities: A second update of codes and MET values. *Medicine & Science in Sports & Exercise,* 8, 1575–1581.

Anderson, J.W. et al. (2001). Long-term weight-loss maintenance: A meta-analysis of US studies. *American Journal of Clinical Nutrition,* 74, 579–584.

Lazzer, S. et al. (2009). Relationship between basal metabolic rate, gender, age, and body composition in 8,780 white obese subjects. *Obesity,* 18, 71–78.

Mahabir, S. (2006). Calorie intake misreporting by diet record and food frequency questionnaire compared to doubly labeled water among postmenopausal women. *European Journal of Clinical Nutrition,* 60, 561–565.

Ohsiek, S. et al. (2011). Psychological factors influencing weight loss maintenance: An integrative literature review. *Journal of American Academy of Nurse Practitioners,* 11, 592–601.

Prado de Oliveira, E. (2011). Comparison of predictive equations for resting energy expenditure in overweight and obese adults. *Journal of Obesity,* 1–5.

Wadden, T.A. et al. (2005). Randomized trial of lifestyle modification and pharmacotherapy for obesity. *New England Journal of Medicine,* 353, 2111–2120.

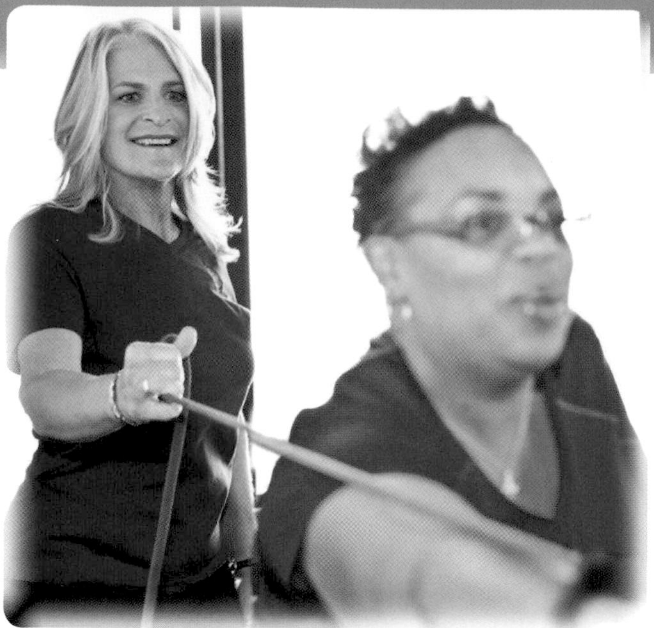

IN THIS CHAPTER:

Todd Galati, M.A., is the director of credentialing for the American Council on Exercise. He holds a bachelor's degree in athletic training, a master's degree in kinesiology, and four ACE certifications [Personal Trainer, Advanced Health & Fitness Specialist, Group Fitness Instructor, and Health Coach (formerly Lifestyle & Weight Management Coach)]. Prior to joining ACE, Galati was a program director with the University of California, San Diego School of Medicine, where he researched the effectiveness of youth fitness programs in reducing risk for cardiovascular disease, obesity, and type 2 diabetes. Galati's experience includes teaching biomechanics and applied kinesiology classes at Cal State San Marcos, working as a research physiologist with the U.S. Navy, personal training in medical fitness facilities, and coaching endurance athletes.

Sabrena Jo, M.S., has been actively involved in the fitness industry since 1987, successfully operating her own personal-training business and teaching group exercise classes. Jo is a former full-time faculty member in the Kinesiology and Physical Education Department at California State University, Long Beach. She has a bachelor's degree in exercise science as well as a master's degree in physical education/biomechanics from the University of Kansas. Jo, an ACE-certified Personal Trainer and Group Fitness Instructor, is an author, educator, and fitness consultant who remains very active within the industry.

16

Exercise Programming Considerations and Guidelines

TODD GALATI,
SABRENA JO, &
FABIO COMANA

Fabio Comana, M.A., M.S., is the director of continuing education for the National Academy of Sports Medicine (NASM) and a faculty member in Exercise Science and Nutrition at San Diego State University and UC San Diego. Comana holds numerous fitness certifications from ACE, NASM, the American College of Sports Medicine, and the International Society of Sports Nutrition. Previously, he was an exercise physiologist and certification manager for the American Council on Exercise (ACE) where he played a key role in the development of ACE's Integrated Fitness Training® Model and many of ACE's live personal-training educational workshops. His previous experiences include collegiate head coaching, strength and conditioning coaching, and opening and managing health clubs for Club One. As a national and international presenter, he is frequently featured on television, radio, internet, and in print publications. He authored chapters in various textbooks and publications, and is presently authoring upcoming academic and consumer books.

ACE-certified Health Coaches assist a variety of individuals with specific goals and needs. Due to the prevalence of inactive lifestyles and increased caloric consumption in modern society, as well as genetic factors that may lead to the excess accumulation of **body fat,** health coaches will most likely serve a high percentage of clientele who are **overweight** or obese. **Obesity** is defined as a **body mass index (BMI)** ≥30 kg/m^2, whereas overweight is classified as a BMI between 25 and 29.9 kg/m^2.

Together, overweight and obesity affect more than two-thirds of the adult population in the United States, which is a trend that has been rising for more than a century, with a substantial increase noted in the past several decades (Ogden et al., 2006; Helmchen & Henderson, 2004).

Obesity is associated with many other adverse health conditions, including **cardiovascular disease (CVD)**, **type 2 diabetes**, and the **metabolic syndrome** [National Heart, Lung, and Blood Institute (NHLBI), 1998]. In addition, chronic obesity may lead to functional impairment (Jensen, 2005) and reduced quality of life (Fontaine & Barofsky, 2001), as well as to greater **mortality** (Fontaine et al., 2003). Fortunately, when treatment is successful at producing even small amounts of weight loss, obese individuals experience many health benefits, including prevention of disease (especially type 2 diabetes) (Knowler et al., 2002) and reduced mortality rate (Bray, 2007). These factors, in combination with the estimated direct and indirect costs of obesity-related conditions, which exceed $117 billion in the United States annually, make treating obesity a national healthcare priority (Stein & Colditz, 2004).

The basis for managing body weight is founded upon energy balance, which is influenced by energy intake (i.e., caloric consumption) and energy expenditure.

Physical activity and structured exercise programs play an important role in weight management because they contribute to long-term weight loss by facilitating energy expenditure. Overweight and obese individuals can achieve weight loss when they expend more daily **calories** on average than they consume.

The energy expenditure provided by increased physical activity and/or structured exercise appears to have minimal impact on weight loss for obese individuals in the initial six months after adopting an intervention program. Only modest reductions in body weight (an average of 2 to 3% decrease) are observed with increased physical activity in overweight and obese adults at the beginning of a weight-reduction program (NHLBI, 1998). This is likely due to the fact that most individuals with excess body fat have low **cardiorespiratory fitness** and cannot tolerate—at least initially—the volume and intensity of exercise required to dramatically impact increases in energy expenditure to drive accelerated weight loss. However, physical activity does appear to be important in the long-term for sustaining significant weight loss and preventing weight regain [American College of Sports Medicine (ACSM), 2009], especially as individuals become more fit and are able to sustain higher volumes of exercise. Furthermore, a review of the literature suggests that diet plus exercise, rather than diet only or exercise only, produces significantly greater weight loss at 12 months, 18 months, and 36 months after the adoption of a weight-loss intervention (Avenell et al., 2004). Thus, the influence of managing caloric intake through healthy eating behaviors is an important factor in long-term weight-loss success that must not be overlooked, and should be coupled with regular physical activity for the greatest impact. It is important to note that an initial weight loss of as little as 10% of body weight can significantly decrease the severity of obesity-associated **risk factors** (e.g., **hypertension** and **insulin resistance**) and is recommended as an appropriate initial goal for obese adults (NHLBI, 2000).

Special Considerations for Overweight/Obese Individuals

Apart from the generally accepted and agreed upon view of obesity as the accumulation of excess body fat, it is an increasingly complex health condition. In their report, *Obesity as a Disease: A White Paper on Evidence and Arguments Commissioned by the Council of the Obesity Society*, Allison and colleagues (2008) unanimously and strongly stated that:

- Obesity is a complex condition with many causal contributors, including many factors that are largely beyond individuals' control.
- Obesity causes much suffering.
- Obesity usually contributes to ill health, functional impairment, reduced quality of life, serious disease, and greater mortality.
- Successful treatment, although difficult to achieve, produces many benefits.
- Obese persons are subject to enormous societal stigma and discrimination.
- Obese persons deserve better.

While it is clear that obesity poses many health challenges, there is controversy as to whether obesity is a disease. Labeling the condition a disease may be beneficial, as it might solicit more resources to the research, prevention, and treatment of obesity, and it could reduce the stigma and discrimination directed at many obese persons. One of the problems with categorizing obesity as a disease is that there are no specific universal symptoms shared among obese individuals and there is only one sign—excess body fat (Allison et al., 2008). Regardless of whether or not obesity is technically called a disease or an adverse health condition, being obese places individuals at an increased risk for **chronic disease** and impaired function.

Common Comorbidities Associated With Overweight/Obesity

The NHLBI (1998) has reported some well-recognized associations between obesity and risk factors for CVD. In individuals with type 2 diabetes, hypertension, or **dyslipidemia**, the percentage of those subjects who were overweight or obese was 82%, 85%, and 84%, respectively (NHLBI, 1998). Of particular importance is the relationship between body fat that is localized in the abdominal area (i.e., **visceral adiposity**) and systemic inflammation. Evidence suggests that CVD, type 2 diabetes, and the metabolic syndrome are all linked to the proinflammatory state associated with abdominal obesity (Lee & Pratley, 2007; Wisse, 2004; Fasshauer & Paschke, 2003). It has been reported that visceral **adipose** tissue secretes several proinflammatory substances (e.g., **interleukin-6**, **tumor necrosis factor-alpha**, and **C-reactive protein**) and that greater levels of visceral adiposity result in higher circulating concentrations of these substances (Panagiotakos et al., 2005; Park, Park, & Yu, 2005). Obese individuals should be carefully screened for **cardiometabolic diseases** (e.g., CVD, type 2 diabetes, and the metabolic syndrome), as these disorders must be taken into consideration when designing exercise programs for this special population.

Fortunately, increased physical activity and/or fitness may attenuate the systemic inflammation associated with visceral adiposity (Mora et al., 2006; Panagiotakos et al., 2004; Church et al., 2002). Evidence also suggests that being physically active can reduce the risk of cardiovascular or all-cause mortality associated with being overweight or obese (Farrell et al., 2002; Lee, Blair, & Jackson, 1999). Additionally, regular exercise (especially moderate to vigorous activity) has been shown to reduce the risk of developing type 2 diabetes (Morrato et al., 2007; Sullivan et al., 2005).

Biomechanical Concerns

In overweight and obese individuals, the musculoskeletal system may experience structural changes that result in low-back pain, decreased **mobility**, modification of the gait pattern, and changes in the relative energy expenditures for a given activity. In addition, **osteoarthritis**, particularly of the knee, is strongly associated with increases in BMI.

Obesity and Low-back Pain

While the association between obesity and low-back pain is unclear, researchers have reported a linear correlation between increasing BMI and low-back pain, especially in large population studies (Leboeuf-Yde, 2000; Toda et al., 2000; Han et al., 1997). There also appears to be a higher incidence of low-back pain in obese women versus obese men (Shiri et al., 2010; Shiri, 2008).

Altered **posture** and a lack of spinal mobility could be underlying causes of low-back pain in obese individuals. Vismara et al. (2010) compared the spines of obese subjects with normal-weight controls and found significant differences at the lumbar, pelvic, and thoracic levels among the groups. Obesity seems to induce an increase in **anterior** pelvic tilt. The increased anterior pelvic tilt induces a greater **flexion** of the sacroiliac joints, which produces undue strain on the L5-S1 joint and surrounding intervertebral discs. This could lead to degenerative deterioration of those discs (i.e., **degenerative disc disease**). There have also been reports of increased lumbar **lordosis** in obese individuals with chronic low-back pain (Vismara et al., 2010; Gilleard & Smith, 2007). At the level of the thoracic spine, Vismara et al. (2010) found that **range of motion (ROM)** during spinal forward flexion was significantly lower in obese subjects and in obese subjects with chronic low-back pain as compared to normal-weight subjects. Stiffness in the thoracic spine translated to forward flexion performed mainly by the lumbar spine, which is most frequently involved in pain **syndromes.**

The postural differences noted above confirm the "kinetic chain" relationship of the musculoskeletal system, such that if a joint experiences stiffness or immobility, nearby joints will sacrifice **stability** and become more mobile to ensure that important bodily movements occur. In the case of obesity, it appears that a rigid thoracic region along with a chronic anterior pelvic tilt forces the lumbar spine (the area located between the thoracic spine and the pelvis) to exceed its normal flexion capabilities, potentially leading to low-back pain. The Vismara et al. (2010) findings, along with others (Lehman, 2004; Nourbakhsh & Arab, 2002), suggest that obese individuals should include strengthening of the lumbar and abdominal muscles as well as mobility exercises for the thoracic spine and pelvis to prevent or reduce chronic low-back pain.

Another biomechanical factor that could contribute to low-back pain in the obese population is increased abdominal circumference and its effect on the function of the muscles that support the spine. In fact, researchers have reported findings that suggest that abdominal obesity is the primary weight-related risk factor for low-back pain (Shiri, 2008; Han et al., 1997). Increased abdominal mass shifts the body's **center of gravity (COG)** forward, farther away from the lumbar spine. The constant efforts of the erector spinae muscles to counteract the pull created by excess abdominal fat may jeopardize the muscles' function of reducing anterior shear forces on the lumbar spine (McGill, Hughson, & Parks, 2000). Other effects of overworked erector spinae muscles include insufficient muscle force output, inappropriate neuromuscular activation, and muscular fatigue (Descarreaux et al., 2008), which are all detrimental to the stability of the spine.

A high concentration of abdominal adiposity could also indirectly increase the likelihood of low-back pain because it leads to the increased production of proinflammatory substances and is associated with dyslipidemia, which results in increased levels of circulating **triglycerides** and **low-density lipoprotein (LDL).** These factors play a major role in the development of **atherosclerosis** (the buildup of plaque in the arteries) in obese individuals (Howard, Ruotolo, & Robbins, 2003). Atherosclerosis could limit the amount of blood distributed to the spine and cause malnutrition of the disc cells (Korkiakoski et al., 2009), which may contribute to disc degeneration. People with severe disc degeneration are more likely to have low-back pain (Cheung et al., 2009). These findings strengthen the argument for weight loss (especially the reduction of abdominal adiposity) in obese individuals as a treatment for low-back pain, because doing so can improve blood lipid profiles, allowing proper nourishment of the discs, and decrease the mechanical strain on the low back. Additionally, strengthening the muscles of the trunk and performing regular **aerobic** endurance exercise are crucial for improving spine health.

Lower-extremity Musculoskeletal Pain

Extra body weight places added stress on the joints, impacts movement, affects gait, and increases foot pressure. In a study investigating forces in the lower extremities, compared to normal-weight individuals (BMI = 24.3 ± 3.0 kg/m^2), obese individuals exhibited higher plantar pressure, especially under the longitudinal arch and on the metatarsal heads, both while standing and walking (Hills et al., 2001). This pressure can contribute to **plantar fasciitis.** In fact, obese individuals are five to six times more likely to have plantar fasciitis than individuals with a normal BMI (18.5 to 25 kg/m^2) (Messier, 2008).

The knee joints in overweight and obese individuals are particularly vulnerable to osteoarthritis and show a greater progression of deterioration from the disease than do the knees of normal-weight individuals. Each excess pound of body weight puts an additional 4-pound stress on the knee (Messier et al., 2005). This additional joint stress represents a viable pathway for the pathogenesis and progression of knee osteoarthritis. Furthermore, the proinflammatory chemicals released by fat cells can also get into the joints and degrade **cartilage** (Messier, 2008).

Due to the pain and disability associated with lower-extremity disorders (e.g., plantar fasciitis and knee osteoarthritis), physical activity can be uncomfortable, which leads to **sedentary** behavior. These factors can cause a vicious cycle, as inactivity can result in even more weight gain. Taking precautions to protect affected, painful joints in overweight and obese clientele will contribute to increased participation in, and **adherence** to, physical activity.

Providing ways for clients with high BMIs to remain active is crucial, not only for cardiometabolic health, but also for quality of life. Weight loss and exercise can improve function and reduce the pain from osteoarthritis. Messier et al. (2005) found that a 5% reduction in body weight, combined with a moderate exercise program (such as walking 30 minutes a day, five days a week), results in a 24% increase in function and a 30% decrease in osteoarthritic knee pain over an 18-month period. For example, an obese client who weighs 250 pounds (114 kg) needs to lose only 12.5 pounds (5.7 kg) to experience these benefits. Conversely, weight gain of approximately 11 pounds (5.0 kg) over a 10-year period has been associated with a 50% increase in the likelihood of developing knee osteoarthritis (Felson et al., 1992).

Impact of Overweight/Obesity on Walking

Changes in lower-extremity musculoskeletal function, such as those described in the previous section, can affect an obese person's gait. Specifically, researchers (DeVita & Hortobágyi, 2003; Messier, 1994; Spyropoulos et al., 1991) report that some overweight and obese individuals have been shown to walk with:

- A shorter step length
- Lower cadence and velocity
- A decreased duration of the single-support phase
- An increased duration of the double-support phase
- Reduced range of motion at the knee and ankle

It is unclear whether these changes are directly related to increases in body weight or if they are an adaptation to reduce pain in the presence of osteoarthritis or to increase dynamic postural stability. Regardless of the causes of abnormal gait observed in obese individuals, these musculoskeletal adaptations should be taken into account when designing exercise programs for this group of clients.

One way to offer joint protection for obese clients who are starting a walking program is to be mindful of the speed at which they begin their training. In their study on the effects of obesity on the **biomechanics** of walking at different speeds, Browning and Kram (2007) found that walking slower reduced **ground reaction forces** and may be an appropriate risk-lowering strategy for obese adults who wish to walk for exercise. When obese subjects walked at 2.2 versus 3.3 miles per hour (mph) [1.0 versus 1.5 meters per second (m/s)], the peak **sagittal plane** forces at the knee were 45% less. Thus, even if an obese client's self-selected walking speed approximates 3.0 mph (1.4 m/s), it might be protective of the lower-extremity joints to recommend that he or she begins walking at a pace closer to 2.0 mph (0.9 m/s), at least initially until a 5% reduction in body weight is achieved.

Impact of Overweight/Obesity on Cycling

While walking may be an appropriate modality to facilitate weight loss, the pain or discomfort associated with it—even at slow cadences—may not be tolerated by some overweight or obese individuals. Consequently, cycling has been used as a non-weight-bearing locomotor activity to promote increased **cardiorespiratory endurance** and caloric expenditure. Research on the biomechanical aspects of cycling in the obese population is surprisingly scarce (Nantel, Mathieu, & Prince, 2010). However, an important physiological consideration is the fact that obese individuals show a higher **oxygen uptake ($\dot{V}O_2$)** for a given cycling intensity when compared to normal-weight individuals (Ofir et al., 2007). In fact, it has been shown that obese individuals expend about 33% more energy than normal-weight subjects during cycling without any external resistance (i.e., zero resistance on the pedal provided by the bike) at 60 revolutions per minute (rpm), which a is a common cycling speed used in clinical settings for physical tests (Anton-Kuchly, Roger, & Varene, 1984). These findings clearly demonstrate that although cycling is a non-weight-bearing activity, the support offered by the bike does not negate all of the difficulty associated with excess body weight. For exercise programming purposes, it is important not to overlook the fact that cycling without external resistance (e.g., at the lowest setting on the bike) can be sufficiently challenging for some obese people.

Another consideration before introducing cycling into an obese person's exercise program is the evidence reported on subject test termination during cycle ergometer assessments in the obese population. Hulens and colleagues (2001) found that reasons to terminate a maximal fitness test on a cycle ergometer differed according to body weight status. Compared to normal-weight subjects, obese participants reported that they terminated the exercise test far more often due to musculoskeletal pain than because of leg fatigue. Thus, musculoskeletal pain is still an important factor to consider for obese clients during cycling, and especially during fitness assessments on a cycle ergometer.

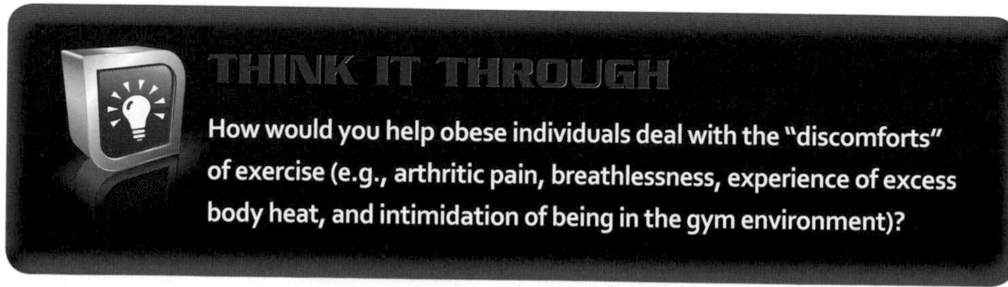

THINK IT THROUGH
How would you help obese individuals deal with the "discomforts" of exercise (e.g., arthritic pain, breathlessness, experience of excess body heat, and intimidation of being in the gym environment)?

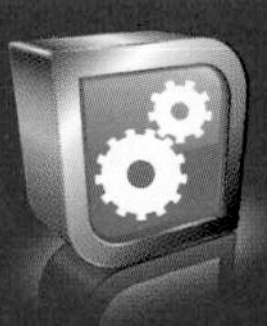

EXPAND YOUR KNOWLEDGE

Obesity Does Not Protect Against Osteoporosis

Until recently, there has been a general consensus that being obese protected women against bone loss. It was thought that carrying extra body weight stimulated the skeleton to produce more bone minerals to support the structural needs of the obese individual. However, a study by Bredella and colleagues (2010) challenged this concept when they found that having too much internal abdominal fat may have a damaging effect on bone health. The researchers investigated abdominal subcutaneous, visceral, and total fat, as well as bone marrow fat and **bone mineral density,** in 50 premenopausal women with a mean BMI of 30 kg/m^2. The results revealed that women with more visceral fat had increased bone marrow fat and decreased bone mineral density. There was no significant correlation between either subcutaneous fat or total fat and bone marrow fat or bone mineral density. Consequently, the authors concluded that having excess visceral fat is more detrimental to bone health than having more superficial fat or fat around the hips.

Evidence from another study that examined complementary investigations in mice and women suggest that extreme obesity in postmenopausal women may be associated with reduced bone mineral density (Núñez et al., 2007). The authors concluded that extreme obesity (BMI > 40 kg/m^2) may increase the risk for osteoporosis. Evidence from animal studies suggest that the dramatically elevated levels of the hormone **leptin,** common in extremely obese individuals, may be associated with impaired bone formation and increased fracture risk (Cock & Auwerx, 2003). These studies suggest that leptin, which is produced primarily by fat cells, may play a role in osteoporosis, and that obese women with high leptin levels may have lower bone mass than overweight and normal-weight women.

Given the worldwide obesity epidemic, and in particular the rising number of obese adult women, the allied healthcare community must be aware of the significant and interrelated public health issues of obesity and osteoporosis. Health and fitness professionals should make it a point to seek out future research in this area as it becomes available.

ACE Integrated Fitness Training® Model Overview

Fitness professionals, including health coaches, are seeing an influx of clientele with an increasingly long list of special needs. What was once a relatively simplistic approach to programming for health-related fitness has become a seemingly complicated process that includes a myriad of training modalities, equipment, and differing schools of thought. The process of learning these new exercise-programming methods and the science behind them seems relatively easy when each is considered individually. It is when determining which training method, or methods, would be most appropriate for each client that the full weight of these rapid advances is felt, often leaving the health coach confused about where to begin and how to progress the client's program (Table 16-1). Both novice and veteran health coaches are well aware of the positive benefits exercise can yield in improving health, fitness, mood, weight management, stress management, and other health-related parameters. The *2008 Physical Activity Guidelines for Americans* reinforce these positive benefits by acknowledging that regular exercise is a critical component of good health and that individuals can reduce their risk of developing chronic disease by staying physically active and participating in structured exercise on a regular basis (U.S. Department of Health & Human Services, 2008). The guidelines specifically state that regular exercise will help prevent many common diseases, such as type 2 diabetes, coronary artery disease, high blood pressure, and the health risks associated with obesity.

Table 16-1

Traditional Physiological Training Parameters versus New Physiological Training Parameters

Traditional Training Parameters	New Training Parameters
• Cardiorespiratory (aerobic) fitness • Muscular endurance • Muscular strength • Flexibility	Traditional Training Parameters plus: • Postural (kinetic chain) stability • Kinetic chain mobility • Movement efficiency • Core conditioning • Balance • Metabolic markers (ventilatory thresholds) • Agility, coordination, and reactivity • Speed and power

The *2008 Physical Activity Guidelines for Americans* suggest that adults should participate in structured cardiorespiratory-related physical activity at a moderate intensity for at least 150 minutes per week or a vigorous intensity for at least 75 minutes per week to experience the health benefits of exercise. In addition, it is recommended that most adults incorporate muscle-strengthening activities at least two days a week. While this document endorses exercise as a means to achieve good health, it does not provide specific instructions for how to exercise.

A summary of general exercise programming guidelines for apparently healthy adults can be found in Table 16-2. These guidelines are based on sound research for providing safe and effective exercise for apparently healthy adults, but they are so broad that health coaches require additional information on how to appropriately implement them for each individual client.

In addition, there are exercise guidelines for many specific groups, including youth, older adults, pre- and postnatal women, and people who have hypertension, dyslipidemia, osteoporosis, and a variety of other special needs. These guidelines are based on medical and scientific research, are published by the governing body of practitioners for each respective special-needs group, and provide specific exercise guidelines to help these individuals improve their health and quality of life. So how does a health coach pull it all together? How

Table 16-2

General Exercise Recommendations for Healthy Adults

Training Component	Frequency (days per week)	Intensity	Time (Duration) or Repetitions	Type (Activity)
Cardiorespiratory	>5 or >3 or 3–5	Moderate (40% to <60% $\dot{V}O_2R$/HRR) Vigorous (≥60% $\dot{V}O_2R$/HRR) Combination of moderate and vigorous	>30 minutes* 20–25 minutes* 20–30 minutes*	Aerobic (cardiovascular endurance) activities and weight-bearing exercise
Resistance	2–3	60–80% of 1 RM or RPE = 5 to 6 (0–10 scale) for older adults	2–4 sets of 8–25 repetitions (e.g., 8–12, 10–15, 15–25; depending upon goal)	8–10 exercises that include all major muscle groups (full-body or split routine); Muscular strength and endurance, calisthenics, balance, and agility exercise
Flexibility	>2–3	Stretch to the limits of discomfort within the ROM, to the point of mild tightness without discomfort	>4 repetitions per muscle group Static: 15–60 seconds; PNF: hold 6 seconds, then a 10–30 second assisted stretch	All major muscle tendon groups Static, PNF, or dynamic (ballistic may be fine for individuals who participate in ballistic activities)

*Continuous exercise or intermittent exercise in bouts of at least 10 minutes in duration to accumulate the minimum recommendation for the given intensity

Note: $\dot{V}O_2R$ = $\dot{V}O_2$ reserve; HRR = Heart-rate reserve; 1 RM = One-repetition maximum; RPE = Ratings of perceived exertion; ROM = Range of motion; PNF = Proprioceptive neuromuscular facilitation

Source: American College of Sports Medicine (2014). *ACMS's Guidelines for Exercise Testing and Prescription* (9th ed.). Philadelphia: Wolters Kluwer/Lippincott Williams & Wilkins.

does a novice or even an experienced health coach know which assessments to perform, when to perform them, which guidelines are most important, when to address foundational imbalances in posture or movement, and how to progress or modify a program based on observed and reported feedback?

To address these questions and more, the American Council on Exercise developed the ACE Integrated Fitness Training (ACE IFT®) Model to provide fitness professionals with a systematic and comprehensive approach to exercise programming that integrates assessments and programming to facilitate behavioral change, while also improving posture, movement, **flexibility**, **balance**, core function, cardiorespiratory fitness, **muscular endurance**, and **muscular strength.**

Function–Health–Fitness–Performance Continuum

The function-health–fitness–performance continuum is based on the premise that exercise programs should follow a **progression** that first reestablishes proper function, then improves health, then develops and advances fitness, and finally enhances performance (Figure 16-1). Each client will have different needs based on his or her personal health, fitness, and goals. Therefore, each client will start his or her exercise program at a unique point along the continuum. The first two components of this continuum involve exercise for improved function and health, which serve as the foundation of every exercise program, even if the

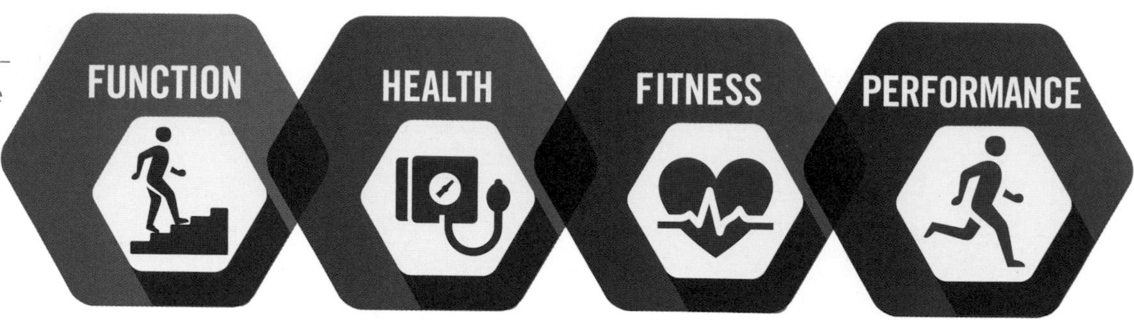

Figure 16-1
The function–health–fitness–performance continuum

client's ultimate goal is to achieve optimal athletic performance for a specific competition. For a client who has been sedentary, improved function and health should be a primary program goal. For clients who have progressed into the fitness or performance domains, their comprehensive training programs should still feature components that maintain or help improve function and health as well as address their specific fitness or athletic goals.

Components of the ACE Integrated Fitness Training Model

The foundation of the ACE IFT Model is built upon **rapport.** Successful health coaches consistently demonstrate excellent communication skills and teaching techniques, while understanding the psychological, emotional, and physiological needs and concerns of their clients. Building rapport is a process that promotes open communication, develops trust, and fosters the client's desire to participate in an exercise program. Rapport should be developed early through open communication and initial positive experiences with exercise, and then enhanced through behavioral strategies that help build long-term adherence.

After establishing an initial rapport, the health coach should collect health-history information to determine if the client has any **contraindications** or requires a physician's evaluation prior to exercise. The collection of health-history information and other pre-exercise paperwork is covered in Chapter 10, while health-related physiological measurements such as **resting heart rate** and blood pressure are covered in Chapter 12. The ACE IFT Model includes functional and physiological assessments that can be performed at specific phases to provide key information for exercise programming in that phase. Some assessments, such as those that focus on functional movement, balance, and range of motion, may be conducted within the first few sessions with a new client, while other assessments might not be conducted until the client has progressed from one phase to another. Ideally, the health coach should utilize a sequential approach to conducting client assessments that begins with reviewing the client's health history; discussing desires, preferences, and general goals; completing a needs assessment; and then determining which assessments are relevant and the timelines in which to conduct them (Figure 16-2). A selection of assessment protocols included in the ACE IFT Model is covered in Chapter 11.

The ACE IFT Model is a comprehensive system for exercise programming that pulls together the multifaceted training parameters required to be a successful fitness professional. It organizes the latest exercise science research into a logical system that helps health coaches determine appropriate assessments, exercises, and progressions for clients based on their unique health, fitness, needs, and goals. The ACE IFT Model has two principal training components:

- Functional movement and resistance training
- Cardiorespiratory training

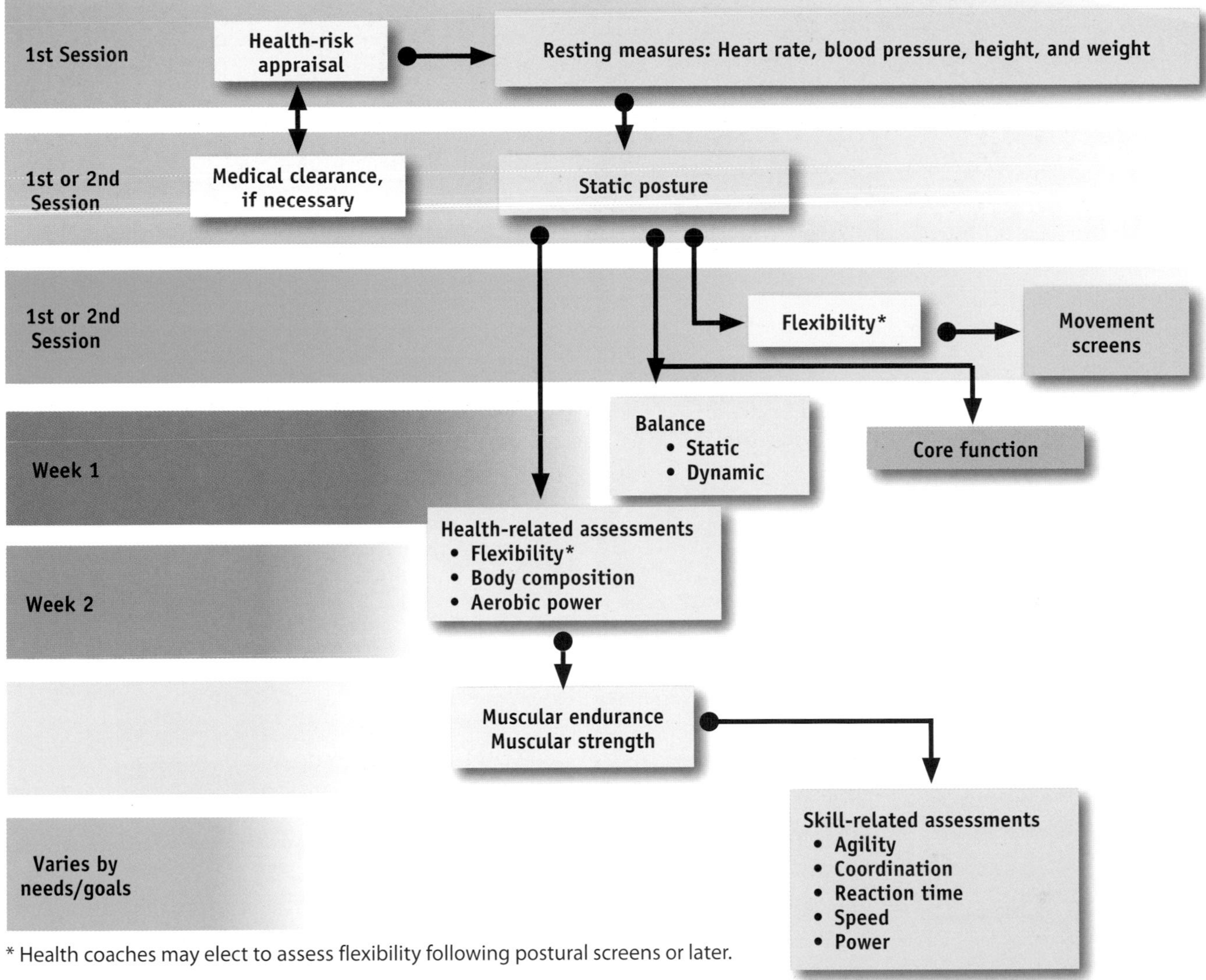

Figure 16-2
Sample assessment sequencing for the general client

Note: Refer to the *ACE Personal Trainer Manual* for information on those assessments not covered in this text.

Each of these components is composed of four phases that provide health coaches with strategies to determine and implement the most appropriate assessments and exercise programs for clients at all levels of fitness. Each phase has a title that is descriptive of the principal training focus during that specific phase (Table 16-3). Rapport is the foundation for success during all phases of training, whether a health coach is working with a highly motivated fitness enthusiast or a sedentary adult looking to adopt more healthful habits.

The four training phases run parallel to the function–health–fitness–performance training continuum that was presented in Figure 16-1 (Figure 16-3). In phase 1, the primary focus is on improving function and health by correcting imbalances through training to improve joint stability and mobility prior to training movement patterns and building an aerobic base to improve parameters of cardiorespiratory health. The primary focus of phase 2 is to progress clients toward improved fitness by introducing aerobic intervals to improve aerobic efficiency and training movement patterns prior to loading the movements. In phase 3, clients progress to higher levels of fitness through load training and the development of **anaerobic** endurance, as cardiorespiratory programming in this phase moves into the performance area of the function–health–fitness–performance continuum. Phase 4 is focused entirely on

Table 16-3				
ACE Integrated Fitness Training Components and Phases				
Training Component	Phase 1	Phase 2	Phase 3	Phase 4
Functional Movement & Resistance Training	Stability and Mobility Training	Movement Training	Load Training	Performance Training
Cardiorespiratory Training	Aerobic-base Training	Aerobic-efficiency Training	Anaerobic-endurance Training	Anaerobic-power Training

Figure 16-3
ACE IFT Model phases and the function–health–fitness–performance continuum

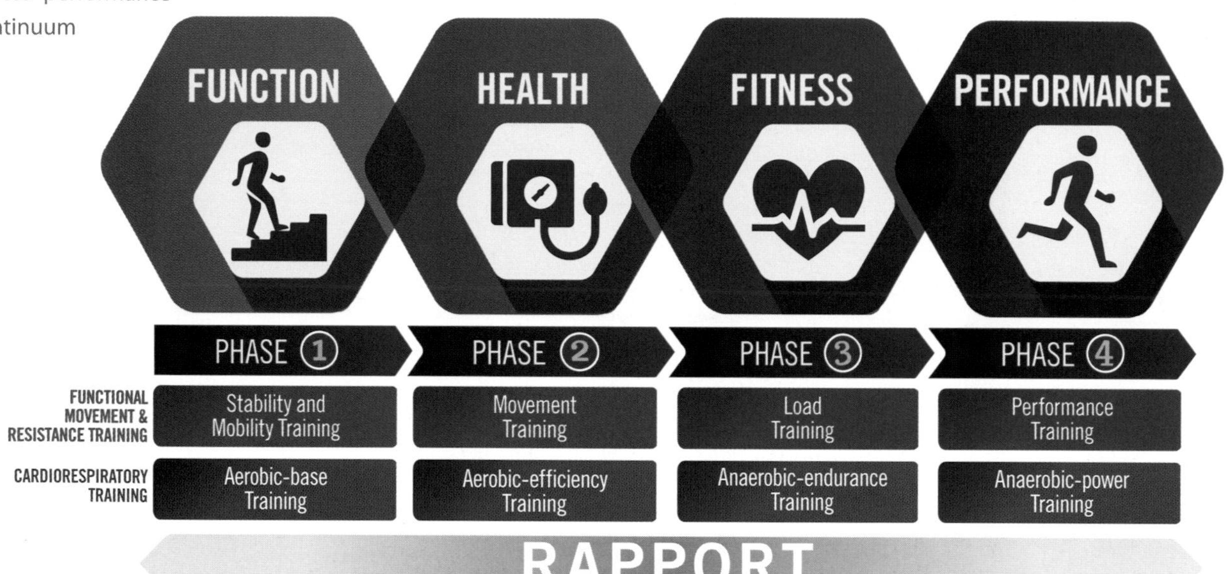

Note: The phases of the ACE IFT Model are not necessarily discrete in terms of their connection to the function–health–fitness–performance continuum. Progression principles should be followed when transitioning from one phase to the next for each training component.

improving performance through training for **muscular power,** speed, agility, reactivity, and anaerobic power. Each client will progress from one phase to the next according to his or her unique needs, goals, and available time to commit to training. Many clients will be at different phases of the two training components based on their current health and fitness, and only clients with performance-oriented goals will reach phase 4.

Applications for Overweight/Obese Individuals

For the purposes of this chapter, the information presented on specific exercise programming will focus primarily on the overweight/obese population. For an in-depth discussion on using the ACE IFT Model for exercise programming and progressions for a wide variety of individuals, refer to the *ACE Personal Trainer Manual.*

There is a general consensus among the U. S. Department of Agriculture, ACSM, and International Association for the Study of Obesity that a weekly energy expenditure of ≥2,000 calories per week, which equates to approximately 60–90 minutes per day of moderate-intensity physical activity, may be required for long-term weight loss (U.S. Department of Agriculture, 2010; ACSM, 2009; Sarris et al., 2003). The basis for these recommendations is also supported by the National Weight Control Registry (NWCR), a cohort of approximately 10,000 "successful losers" who have lost an average of 66 pounds and maintained this loss for approximately 5.5 years. The NWCR found that while dietary control was an important factor in the maintenance of weight loss, one of the most significant findings was that successful losers maintained consistently high daily physical-activity levels. In fact, 90% of the NCWR subjects exercise, on average, about 1 hour per day and 62% report watching fewer than 10 hours of television per week (NCWR, 2012).

The amount of physical activity suggested for weight loss and prevention of weight regain in overweight and obese individuals is clearly greater than that recommended for public health improvement as described in the *2008 Physical Activity Guidelines for Americans*. For improved health, a minimum of 150 minutes of physical activity per week, or 30 minutes of physical activity on most days of the week is advised (U.S. Department of Health & Human Services, 2008; Haskell et al., 2007). For obese individuals, a progression to approximately 250 to 300 minutes of physical activity per week, or 50 to 60 minutes five days each week, may be necessary for long-term weight loss success. In some cases, 60 to 90 minutes of daily exercise may be required (Zoeller, 2007).

The primary mode of initial activity to facilitate weight loss is aerobic, or endurance, exercise. Aerobic conditioning maximizes caloric expenditure in individuals who have obesity or are new to exercise, and reduces the risk of chronic disease associated with obesity (e.g., CVD, type 2 diabetes, and the metabolic syndrome). The ACE IFT Model can be used to adjust exercise selection, intensity, and duration to fit the special needs of overweight and obese clients. Many of these individuals may never progress beyond the aerobic-efficiency phase of cardiorespiratory training (phase 2), and many of them will never progress beyond the loading phase of functional movement and resistance training (phase 3). The most important goal with all clients is to provide them with initial positive experiences that promote adherence through achievable initial successes. Transitioning an obese client into the **action** stage and then on to the **maintenance** stage of change (see Chapter 3) will have a significant impact on that client's health and overall quality of life, and may even have a positive impact on the client's state of physical and mental fitness.

Using Assessment Results to Guide Exercise Programming

After the initial interview and physical assessments have been administered, the health coach can develop a plan of action for the client based on the unique characteristics of the individual and his or her program goals. Keep in mind that fitness assessments may be administered throughout the client's program and may not need to be completed before the client begins his or her first exercise session, especially if performing assessments is contraindicated due to musculoskeletal injury or if the client feels uncomfortable with being measured and compared to standardized norms. A program beginning with simple stabilization exercises, walking, and stretching is an appropriate first-session approach for novice exercisers who are overweight or obese and who feel intimidated by the assessment process. With the exception of a health-history screening, a client does not necessarily have to be assessed immediately upon beginning a program. For early success and to promote feelings of accomplishment, light exercise intensity combined with a tolerable exercise duration works well as an initial plan for introducing physical activity to a deconditioned client. This approach can be incorporated on the first day of engagement with a new client.

When the client and health coach together decide that performing physical-fitness assessments is a good course of action, the information obtained from the process can be valuable to help show progress. The following sections describe how, in general, evaluation data from assessments can be used by the health coach to guide the client's exercise programming.

Cardiorespiratory Fitness

Once the client's cardiorespiratory fitness level has been established and any cardiovascular health risks have been ruled out (see pages 324–337), an appropriate fitness program can be initiated. For novice exercisers, improving on cardiovascular fitness should be addressed in a twofold manner. The first goal is to gradually increase exercise duration. This allows the body to adapt to the new demands of exercise and respond accordingly to the physiological stress of training (e.g., increase in **capillary** density, increase in **mitochondrial** size/number, and enhanced ability to remove **lactic acid**). Initially, training volume can be increased by 10 to 20% per week, until the desired training volume is achieved.

For those who already have a solid cardiorespiratory training base, the second phase of training focuses on increasing exercise intensity, in an effort to increase **$\dot{V}O_2$max.** As long as there are no contraindications to higher-intensity training, it is appropriate to incorporate moderate-intensity steady-state training as well as **interval training.** Health coaches should keep in mind that even among the obese population, physical fitness exists in a continuum, meaning that individuals have different abilities and some are able to tolerate more exertion than others. For clients who are not capable of achieving the minimum recommendation of 150 minutes of weekly moderate-intensity activity (i.e., 30 minutes of endurance exercise, five days per week), reaching this level of activity should be the primary goal during the initial conditioning stage. Overweight and obese adults may find that accumulating 30 minutes of activity in multiple daily bouts of at least 10 minutes in duration is preferable to exerting themselves for longer time periods. This approach is appropriate, at least in the beginning of the training program, as it may be better tolerated and is likely to promote positive feelings associated with successfully accomplishing a healthy task (ACSM, 2014).

Stability and Mobility

A static postural assessment is an excellent test for observing a client's joints and how they relate to each other, and for viewing how those joints maintain their positions against gravity in a relaxed, standing position (see pages 339–341). Individuals who exhibit good posture generally demonstrate an appropriate relationship between stability and mobility throughout the kinetic chain. On the other hand, individuals who exhibit poor posture typically lack the mobility required for normal joint movement, the stability to maintain good posture, or both.

Observing active movement is an effective method to determine the contribution that muscle imbalances and poor posture have on neural control, and also helps identify movement compensations (Whiting & Rugg, 2006; Sahrmann, 2002). Functional movement assessments, such as the body-weight squat test, front plank test, and overhead reach test (see pages 348–352), help health coaches view compensations that occur during a client's movement. If altered movement patterns are present, it is usually indicative of some form of adjusted neural action, commonly referred to as "faulty neural control," which normally manifests itself out of muscle tightness or an imbalance between muscles acting at the joint.

Movement can essentially be broken down and described by five primary movements that people perform during many daily activities (Cook, 2003):

- Bending/raising and lifting/lowering movements (e.g., squatting)
- Single-leg movements (seen in walking and climbing stairs)
- Upper-body pushing movements and resultant movement
- Upper-body pulling movements and resultant movement
- Rotational movements

When mobility is compromised, the following movement compensations typically occur:

- The joint will seek to achieve the desired ROM by incorporating movement into another plane. For example, when a client walks, which requires hip **extension** (sagittal plane movement), and lacks flexibility in the hip flexors, it is possible to see excess **rotation** in the lumbar spine (**transverse plane** movement), thereby producing a compensated movement pattern.
- Adjacent, more stable joints may need to compromise some degree of stability to facilitate the level of mobility needed. For example, if a client exhibits increased **kyphosis** and attempts to extend the thoracic spine, an increase in lumbar lordosis often occurs as a compensation for the lack of thoracic mobility.

A lack of mobility can be attributed to numerous factors, including reduced levels of physical activity, and increased actions that promote muscle imbalance (e.g., repetitive movements, habitually poor posture, side-dominance, poor exercise technique, and imbalanced strength-training programs) (Kendall et al., 2005). This loss of mobility leads to compensations in movement and potential losses of stability at subsequent joints.

It is important to remember that while all joints demonstrate varying levels of stability and mobility, they tend to favor one over the other, depending on their function within the body (Figure 16-4) (Cook & Jones, 2007a; 2007b). For example, while the lumbar spine demonstrates some mobility (approximately 13 degrees of rotation), it is generally stable, protecting the low back from injury. On the other hand, the thoracic spine is designed to be more mobile to facilitate a variety of movements in the upper extremity. The scapulothoracic joint is a more stable union formed by a collection of muscles attaching the scapulae to the ribcage. This arrangement allows the scapulothoracic joint to provide a solid platform for pulling and pushing movements at the shoulder while simultaneously allowing it to tolerate the reactive forces transferred to the body during these movements. The foot is unique, as its level of stability varies during the gait cycle. The foot and ankle joints are more stable when weight-bearing, especially when the foot is flat, and more mobile during the swing phase of the gait cycle, as the ankle moves from **plantar flexion** to **dorsiflexion** and the foot moves from **eversion** to **inversion** as it transitions from pushing off the ground (toe off), moving forward to prepare for heel strike. These stability-mobility relationships of the joints along the kinetic chain should be kept in mind when designing any type of exercise program.

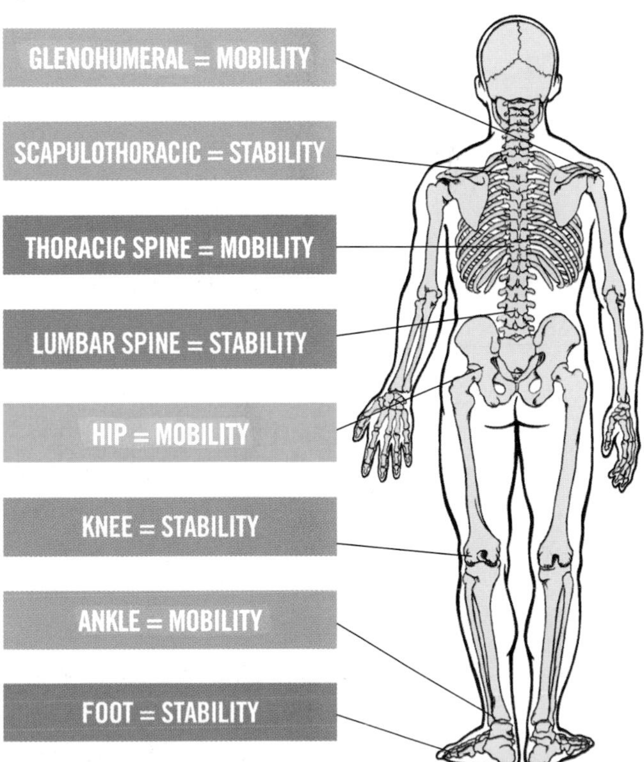

Figure 16-4
Mobility and stability of the kinetic chain

For clients who demonstrate muscle imbalances during a static postural assessment and noticeable compensations during movement screens, their first training objective should be to reestablish appropriate levels of stability and mobility of the joints within the body. This process begins by targeting an important **proximal** region of the body, the lumbar spine, which encompasses the body's **center of mass (COM),** and the core (i.e., the muscles and joints of the trunk, **shoulder girdle,** and hip girdle). As this region is primarily stable, programming should begin by first promoting stability of the lumbar region through the action and function of the core. Once an individual demonstrates the ability to stabilize this region, the program should then progress to the more **distal** segments. Adjacent to the lumbar spine are the hips and thoracic spine, both of which are primarily mobile. As thoracic spine mobility is restored, the program can target stability of the scapulothoracic region. Finally, once stability and mobility of the lumbo-pelvic, thoracic, and shoulder regions have been established, the program can then shift to enhancing mobility and stability of the distal extremities. Attempting to improve mobility within distal joints without developing more proximal stability only serves to compromise any existing stability within these segments. When a joint lacks stability, many of the muscles that normally mobilize that joint may need to alter their true functions to assist in providing stability. For example, if an individual lacks stability in the scapulothoracic joint, the deltoids, which are normally responsible for many **glenohumeral** movements, may need to compromise some of their force-generating capacity and assist in stabilizing glenohumeral movement (Cook & Jones, 2007a). This altered deltoid function decreases force output and may increase the potential for dysfunctional movement and injury.

Figure 16-5 illustrates a programming sequence to promote stability and mobility. It adheres to the basic principle that proximal stability facilitates distal mobility. For each of the five sections of this figure, several exercise examples are provided in Chapter 17 to help health coaches plan and implement programs. Health coaches should feel free to apply

Figure 16-5
Programming components of the stability and mobility training phase

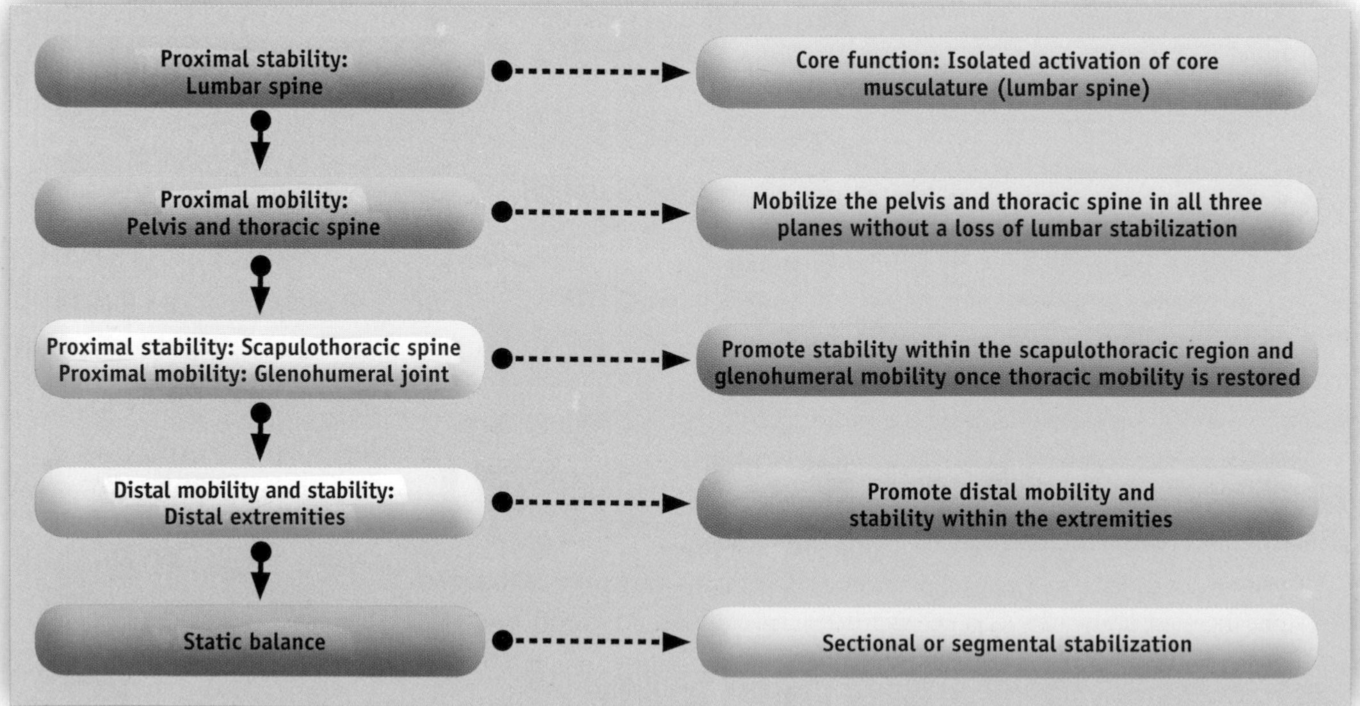

these same principles using different exercises and different programs individualized to a client's specific needs. Based on the postural and movement screen observations, health coaches will identify potential problem areas of the body that need attention (i.e., improvements in stability or mobility). For example, if a client demonstrates a lack of trunk stability during the front plank test (see page 350), a lack of core function should be suspected. Likewise, if a client exhibits an exaggerated anterior pelvic tilt during a static postural assessment due to tight hip flexors, the health coach will need to address a lack of hip flexor mobility.

Flexibility

Static posture assessments and movement screens, such as the body-weight squat test, front plank, and overhead reach (see Chapter 11), can reveal muscles that have become adaptively shortened. If inadequate ROM is found at specific joints or if discrepancies are observed between the right and left sides of the body, a program of focused stretching for the areas in question should be initiated.

The following are some common stretching techniques and general guidelines for their use:

- **Myofascial release:** Clients perform small, continuous, back-and-forth movements (on a foam roller), covering an area of 2 to 6 inches (5 to 15 cm) over the tender region for 30 to 60 seconds (Cook & Jones, 2007b; Barnes, 1999). See page 459 for more information on myofascial release.
  - ✓ Myofascial release should precede static stretching because it realigns the elastic muscle fibers from a bundled position (called a knot or adhesion) into a straighter alignment with the muscle and **fascia,** and resets the proprioceptive mechanisms of the soft tissue (Barnes, 1999). Myofascial release helps reduce hypertonicity (tightness) within the underlying muscles.
- **Static stretching:** Static stretches involve moving a joint to where the targeted muscles reach a point of tension at the end point of the movement. Ideally, clients should perform a minimum of four repetitions on each stretching exercise, holding each repetition for 15 to 60 seconds (Figure 16-6) (ACSM, 2014). However, if following the full recommendation of completing four repetitions is perceived as too time consuming for some clients, even performing just one set of stretching is beneficial.
- **Proprioceptive neuromuscular facilitation (PNF):** PNF stretching involves taking a joint through a movement until the targeted muscles reach a point of tension, holding the stretch for 10 seconds, and then having the client perform an **isometric** contraction of the **agonist** for a minimum of six seconds, followed by a 10- to 30-second assisted or passive static stretch (Figure 16-7) (ACSM, 2014). This type of hold-relax PNF stretch can be performed several times.
- **Active isolated stretching (AIS):** This stretching technique involves moving the joint from the starting position through the motion to the end point, holding for no more than two seconds, and then returning to the starting position to immediately repeat the stretching motion. Clients can perform one or two sets of five to 10 repetitions at a controlled tempo, holding the end range of motion for one to two seconds (Figure 16-8) (Alter, 2004).
- **Dynamic** and **ballistic stretching:** Dynamic stretches prepare the body for the upcoming workout or sport by mimicking movement patterns that will be performed during the actual workout. Dynamic stretches are most effective as part of the warm-up. Ballistic

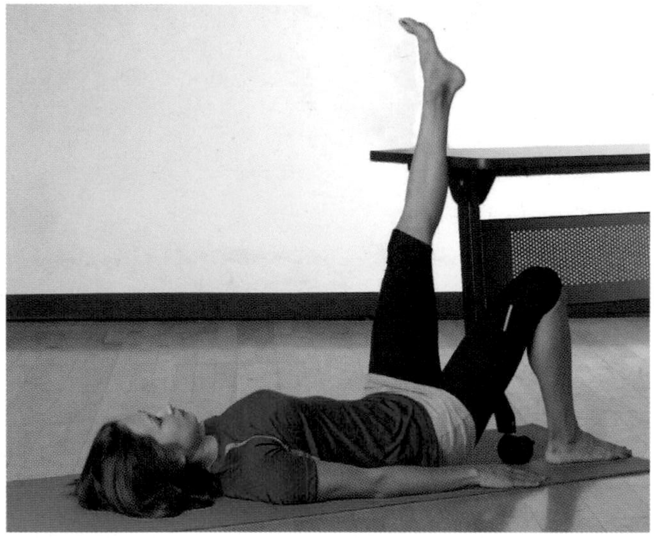

Figure 16-6
Passive static stretch of the hamstrings

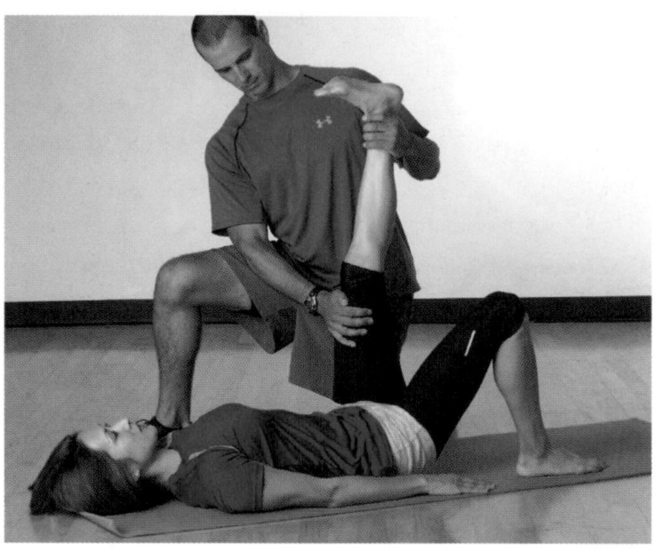

Figure 16-7
Hold-relax hamstrings stretch

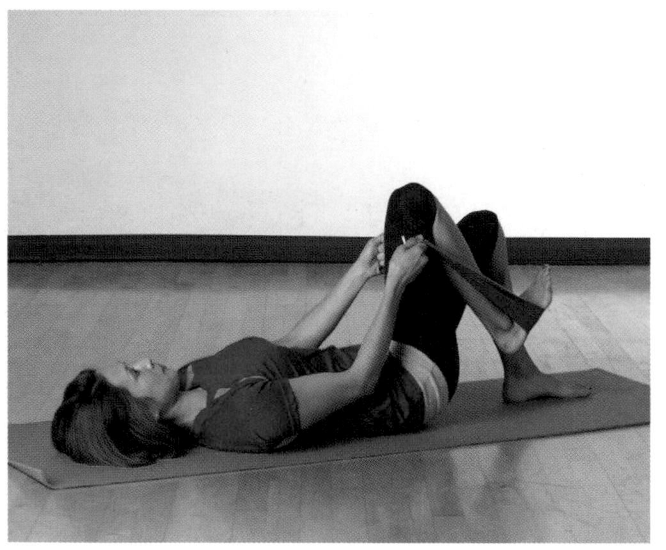

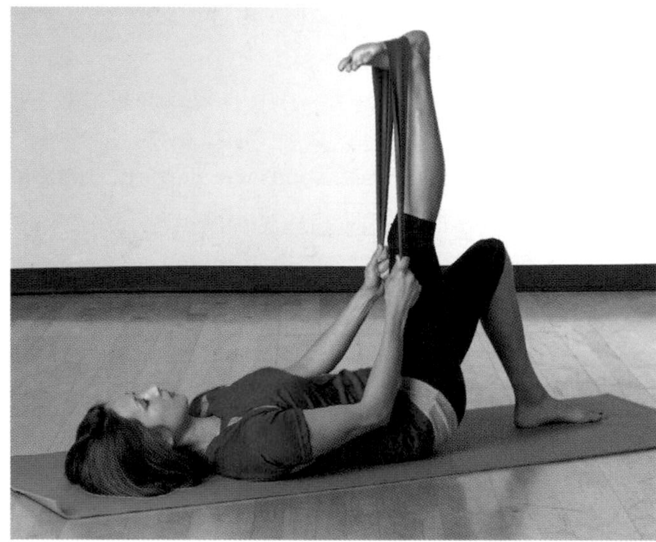

Figure 16-8
Active isolated stretching

stretches incorporate small bouncing movements as part of the dynamic pre-training warm-up. Ballistic stretches usually trigger the stretch reflex, potentially increasing the risk of injury and making them not widely advocated. Clients can perform one or two sets of 10 repetitions of dynamic stretching movements as part of the warm-up, or similar sets of ballistic stretches when appropriate (Cook, 2003).

Balance and Core Function

Given the importance of balance and the condition of the core musculature to fitness and overall quality of life, these baseline assessments should be collected to evaluate the need for comprehensive balance training and core conditioning during the early stages of a conditioning program. Health coaches should feel comfortable evaluating the basic level of **static balance** that a client exhibits by using the sharpened Romberg test or the stork-stand test (see page 342–343).

EXPAND YOUR KNOWLEDGE

Understanding Myofascial Release

Understanding the concept behind myofascial release requires an understanding of the fascial system itself. Fascia is a densely woven, specialized system of **connective tissue** that covers and unites all of the body's compartments. The result is a system where each part is connected to the other parts through this web of tissue. Essentially, the purpose of the fascia is to surround and support the bodily structures, which provides stability as well as a cohesive direction for the line of pull of muscle groups. For example, the fascia surrounding the quadriceps keeps this muscle group contained in the anterior compartment of the thigh (stability) and orients the muscle fibers in a vertical direction so that the line of pull is more effective at extending the knee. In a normal healthy state, fascia has a relaxed and wavy configuration. It has the ability to stretch and move without restriction. However, with physical trauma, scarring, or inflammation, fascia loses its pliability. It becomes tight, restricted, and a potential source of pain. **Acute** injuries, habitual poor posture over time, and repetitive stress injuries can be damaging to the fascia. As a result, the damaged fascia can exert excessive pressure on the underlying structures, producing pain or restriction of motion, which in turn may induce adaptive shortening of the muscle tissue associated with the fascia.

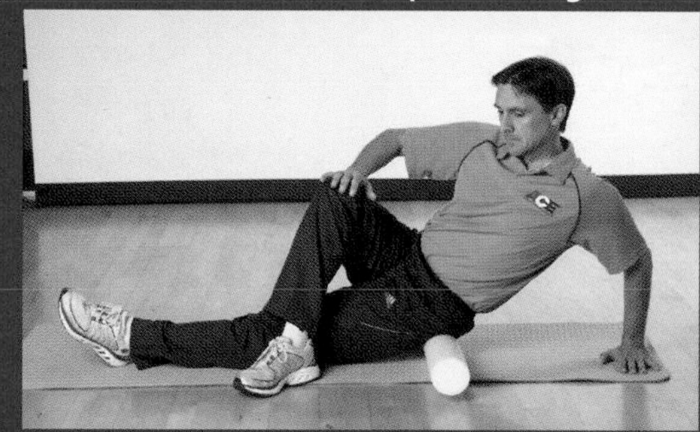

Figure 16-9
Myofascial release for gluteals/external rotators

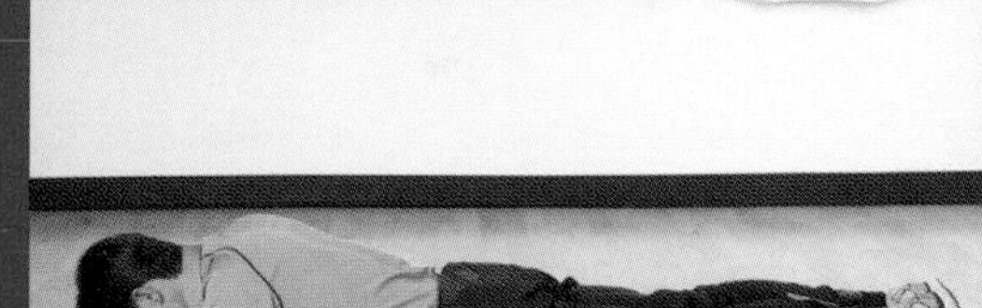

Myofascial release for the quadriceps

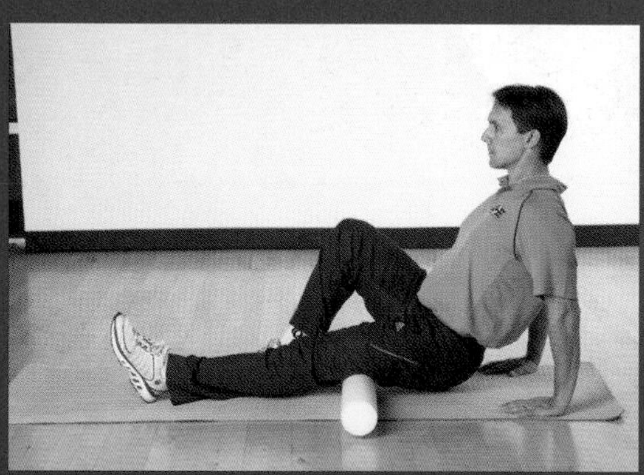

Myofascial release for the hamstrings

Myofascial release is a technique that applies pressure to tight, restricted areas of fascia and underlying muscle in an attempt to relieve tension and improve flexibility. It is thought that applying direct sustained pressure to a tight area can inhibit the tension in a muscle by stimulating the **Golgi tendon organ (GTO)** to bring about **autogenic inhibition.** Tender areas of soft tissue (also called trigger points) can be diminished through the application of pressure (myofascial release) followed by static stretching of the tight area.

The practical application of myofascial release in the fitness setting is commonly done through the use of a foam roller, where the client controls his or her own intensity and duration of pressure. A common technique is to instruct clients to perform small, continuous, back-and-forth movements on a foam roller, covering an area of 2 to 6 inches (5 to 15 cm) over the tender region for 30 to 60 seconds (Figure 16-9). Because exerting pressure on an already tender area requires a certain level of pain tolerance, the intensity of the application of pressure determines the duration for which the client can withstand the discomfort.

For example, a client with a high pain tolerance can position his or her body on the foam roller directly over a tender area and hold the applied pressure for 30 seconds. On the other hand, a client with low pain tolerance can position his or her body near the focal point of the tender area and hold the applied pressure for 60 seconds.

It has been theorized that myofascial release realigns the elastic muscle and connective tissue fibers from a bundled position (called a knot or adhesion) into a straighter arrangement, and resets the proprioceptive mechanisms of the soft tissue, thus reducing hypertonicity within the underlying muscles.

Demonstrated deficiencies in core functional assessments, such as McGill's torso muscular endurance battery (see page 344), should be addressed during exercise programming as part of the foundational exercises for a client. The goal is to create ratios consistent with McGill's recommendations. Muscular endurance, more so than muscular strength or even ROM, has been shown to be an accurate predictor of back health (McGill, 2007). Low-back stabilization exercises have the most benefit when performed daily. When working with clients with low-back dysfunction, it is prudent to include daily stabilization exercises in their exercise plans.

Since most Americans will experience low-back pain at some point in their lives, a comprehensive fitness program should incorporate spinal stabilization exercises. **Core stability** should be a key element in any training program. If the core is not strong, the back may be compromised during a dumbbell shoulder press, creating excessive lumbar lordosis. The same break in position can happen during a squat or a bench press, thus creating excess stress on the lumbar spine. Improper alignment can create a whole host of problems for the lower back, ranging from herniated discs to sciatic pain. While clients' training objectives can vary from post-rehabilitation or prevention of low-back pain to optimizing health and fitness or maximizing athletic performance, all clients will benefit from exercises targeting core stability.

Muscular Fitness

Muscular-endurance testing assesses the ability of a specific muscle group, or groups, to perform repeated or sustained contractions to sufficiently invoke muscular fatigue. While most muscular-endurance tests are designed to measure the ability of a muscle group to maintain a single contraction or produce repeated contractions, the nature of some of the tests are so challenging that deconditioned individuals will fatigue almost immediately. In these cases, the exerciser has to develop a certain level of base strength before muscular-endurance testing can be accomplished properly. Because many overweight and obese individuals are novice exercisers, and as such are likely to be deconditioned, basic muscular-fitness testing for these individuals is enough of a challenge, making muscular-strength testing [such as **one-repetition maximum (1-RM)** testing] unnecessary.

The body-weight squat test (see page 348) and the front plank test (see page 350) are two basic muscular-fitness assessments that are appropriate for most individuals, as long as no injuries of the torso, back, or knees are present. The body-weight squat test assesses muscular fitness of the lower extremity when performing repetitions of a squat-to-stand movement. This test is only suitable for individuals who demonstrate proper form in executing a squat movement. The squat is also a valuable multijoint exercise that can be incorporated into a client's exercise program to develop strength in the lower extremity. If a client performs poorly on the body-weight squat test, it is a sign that he or she is lacking the muscular conditioning required to perform a crucial movement of daily living. In such cases, clients should be taught how to perform a squat correctly and then encouraged to incorporate squats frequently into their exercise programs.

If a client performs poorly on the front plank test, he or she lacks muscular fitness of the core. As such, the client should be given exercises that promote stability of the core and then progressed to performing movement patterns that incorporate distal segments of the body, all while still maintaining appropriate core stability.

Targeting Behaviors for Change in Overweight/Obese Individuals

The two main program components that have been shown to be successful for sustained weight-loss in overweight and obese individuals are modest reductions in energy intake and adequate levels of physical activity (ACSM, 2009; NHLBI, 1998). These two behaviors require a significant lifestyle change, which is perhaps the reason why losing weight and maintaining weight loss proves to be incredibly difficult for most people. Nonetheless, an overweight or obese client who is interested in losing weight must target changing eating and exercise behaviors in order to be successful in the long term.

Setting Goals for Metabolic Success

The following recommendations have been set forth by ACSM (2014) to guide health and fitness professionals in their attempts to assist overweight and obese individuals with weight loss.

- Adults with a BMI ≥25 kg/m^2 should be encouraged to engage in a weight-loss program.
- An initial weight-reduction goal of 5 to 10% of body weight should be targeted over a three- to six-month period.
- Following the initial weight-loss period, clients should be encouraged to enhance communication between their healthcare professionals, nutrition experts, and exercise professionals.
- Dietary changes resulting in a reduction of current caloric intake by 500 to 1,000 calories per day and a decrease in **dietary fat** to <30% of total caloric intake should be targeted.
- Increasing physical activity to a minimum of 150 minutes per week of moderate-intensity exercise should be encouraged.
- A progression to higher amounts of exercise (i.e., 200–300 minutes per week or ≥2,000 calories per week of physical activity) should be recommended to facilitate long-term weight control.
- Resistance training can be implemented as a supplement to the combination of aerobic endurance exercise and modest caloric reduction. While it is not the primary form of exercise recommended for weight loss, a program of regular resistance training can help to preserve muscle mass as a person loses body weight, which has positive implications for improving muscular fitness and **body composition** and helping maintain **resting metabolic rate (RMR).**
- Behavioral modification strategies should be incorporated to promote the adoption and maintenance of the lifestyle changes associated with long-term weight control.

Health coaches can use these recommendations to work together with their clients to set goals that are specific, measurable, attainable, relevant, and time-bound (i.e., **SMART goals**) (see Chapter 13). Furthermore, following up with clients regularly as they achieve short-term goals is a crucial part of maintaining contact with them and guiding them through their weight-loss achievements.

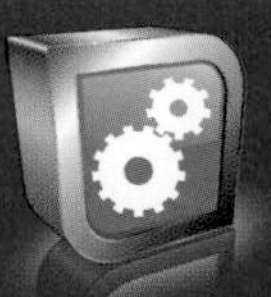

EXPAND YOUR KNOWLEDGE

Not Gaining Is Winning

An important concept that health coaches should consider while implementing weight-loss programs for obese clients is that primary prevention of obesity starts with maintenance of current weight, not weight reduction (ACSM, 2009). In other words, preventing the obese client from gaining any more weight, thus maintaining weight, can be viewed as a successful achievement, especially during the first few weeks of a weight-loss program. The stoppage of additional weight gain means that the behavioral changes the client is attempting to make are working to the extent that the client has stopped the metabolic processes associated with adding on more weight (i.e., caloric intake no longer exceeds caloric expenditure). Providing the client with this insight can be helpful if he or she becomes discouraged due to a lack of weight loss during the initial weeks of a behavior-change program.

Obesity and Weight Regain

Successful weight loss, especially for an obese individual, is a significant achievement and provides numerous health benefits as described earlier in this chapter. Once a weight-loss goal is achieved, clients should have a clearer understanding of the individual strategies that helped them reach their lower body weight. Unfortunately, weight regain remains problematic for those who have lost weight.

A meta-analysis of published research on formerly obese subjects suggests that inherent biological factors could explain the tendency for weight losers to regain weight. For example, it was found that formerly obese persons had a 3–5% lower mean relative RMR than normal-weight control subjects, and the difference could be explained by a low RMR being more frequent among the formerly obese subjects than among the normal-weight control subjects (Arstrup et al., 1999). The authors of the report concluded that the lower RMR among formerly obese subjects could be due to a genetic effect or to an adaptive response to weight loss that may increase the susceptibility of formerly obese persons to regain weight.

Research on obesity-prone rats suggests that lower RMR combined with a progressively increasing appetite appear to be the hallmark of the metabolic tendency to regain weight after weight loss. MacLean and colleagues (2004a) found that a persistent lower RMR explained 60% of the potential energy imbalance, while an elevated appetite explained 40% of weight regain in formerly obese rats. It is likely that these metabolic responses, may explain—at least in part—why sustained weight reduction is so challenging. Accordingly, weight regain after weight loss has been repeatedly shown in both rodents (Levin & Dunn-Meynell, 2004; MacLean et al., 2004b; Levin & Dunn-Meynell, 2002; Levin & Keesey, 1998) and humans (Votruba, Blanc, & Schoeller, 2002; Froidevaux et al., 1993).

Given that regaining lost weight is a likely challenge for clients after they have reached their weight-loss goals, health coaches can help their clients beat the odds by encouraging them to reinforce their commitment to exercise. Although metabolic factors appear to favor weight regain, participation in daily physical activity decreases the rate of weight regain (Chaput et al., 2008). Remember, the NWCR found that while dietary control was an important factor in the maintenance of weight loss, one of the most significant findings was that successful losers maintained consistently high daily physical-activity levels (see page 453).

Similar findings have been reported by Jakicic et al. (2008), who studied obese women randomly assigned to one of four groups based on physical activity energy expenditure (1,000 versus 2,000 kcal/week) and intensity (moderate versus vigorous) with a concomitant decrease in daily dietary energy intake (–1,200 to –1,500 kcal/day). Between the four groups, there was no difference in weight loss at six and 24 months. However, *post hoc* analyses showed that the subjects sustaining a loss of 10% or more of initial body weight at two years reported performing more physical activity (approximately 1,800 kcal/week or 275 min/week) compared to those sustaining a weight loss of less than 10% of initial body weight (who performed approximately 1,000 kcal/week or 170 min/week of physical activity).

While weight regain is a persistent challenge, especially for formerly obese individuals, it does not have to be a certainty. According to the available research, maintaining consistent and permanent high levels of moderate to vigorous daily physical activity seems to be the key for sustained weight loss (Chaput et al., 2008).

Summary

Given current obesity statistics, health coaches will most likely serve a high percentage of clientele who are overweight or obese. Obesity is associated with many other adverse health conditions, including CVD, type 2 diabetes, the metabolic syndrome, functional impairment, reduced quality of life, and greater mortality. Fortunately, when treatment is successful at producing even small amounts of weight loss, obese individuals experience many health benefits, including prevention of disease (especially type 2 diabetes). Health coaches can help their clients overcome obesity and its associated health problems by educating them about the importance of managing body weight by carefully manipulating energy balance, which is influenced by energy intake and energy expenditure. This can be achieved by giving clients the resources to make healthier choices when it comes to dietary intake and physical activity and exercise. Once weight-loss goals are reached, health coaches can play an important role in helping clients maintain their lower body weights by encouraging them to maintain a program of daily, moderate- to vigorous-intensity physical activity.

References

Allison, D.B. et al. (2008). Obesity as a disease: A white paper on evidence and arguments commissioned by the Council of The Obesity Society. *Obesity*, 16, 1161–1177.

Alter, M.J. (2004). *Science of Flexibility* (3rd ed.). Champaign, Ill.: Human Kinetics.

American College of Sports Medicine (2014). *ACSM's Guidelines for Exercise Testing and Prescription* (9th ed.). Philadelphia: Wolters Kluwer/ Lippincott Williams & Wilkins.

American College of Sports Medicine (2009). Position stand: Appropriate physical activity intervention strategies for weight loss and prevention of weight regain for adults. *Medicine & Science in Sports & Exercise*, 41, 459–471.

Anton-Kuchly, B., Roger, P., & Varene, P. (1984). Determinants of increased energy cost of submaximal exercise in obese subjects. *Journal of Applied Physiology*, 56, 18–23.

Astrup, A. et al. (1999). Meta-analysis of resting metabolic rate in formerly obese subjects. *American Journal of Clinical Nutrition*, 69, 1117–1122.

Avenell, A. et al. (2004). Systematic review of the long-term effects and economic consequences of treatments for obesity and implications for health improvement. *Health Technology Assessment*, 21, 1–465.

Barnes, J.F. (1999). Myofascial release. In: Hammer, W.I. (Ed.) *Functional Soft Tissue Examination and Treatment by Manual Methods* (2nd ed). Gaithersburg, Md.: Aspen Publishers.

Bray, G.A. (2007). The missing link–lose weight, live longer. *New England Journal of Medicine*, 357, 818–820.

Bredella, M. et al. (2010). Detrimental effects of visceral obesity on bone health. Presentation at the 96th Scientific Assembly and Annual Meeting of the Radiological Society of North America, Code: SSJ17-05. November 30th.

Browning, R.C. & Kram, R. (2007). Effects of obesity on the biomechanics of walking at different speeds. *Medicine & Science in Sports & Exercise*, 39, 1632–1641.

Chaput, J. et al. (2008). Physical activity plays an important role in body-weight regulation. *Journal of Obesity*, 2011, Article ID 360257, 11 pages doi:10.1155/2011/360257.

Cheung, K.M. et al. (2009). Prevalence and pattern of lumbar magnetic resonance imaging changes in a population study of one thousand forty-three individuals. *Spine*, 34, 934–940.

Church, T.S. et al. (2002). Associations between cardiorespiratory fitness and C-reactive protein in men. *Arteriosclerosis, Thrombosis, & Vascular Biology*, 22, 1869–1876.

Cock, T. A. & Auwerx, J. (2003) Leptin: cutting the fat off the bone. *Lancet*, 362, 1572–1574.

Cook, G. (2003). *Athletic Body in Balance*. Champaign, Ill.: Human Kinetics.

Cook, G. & Jones, B. (2007a). *Secrets of the Shoulder*. www.functionalmovement.com

Cook, G. & Jones, B. (2007b). *Secrets of the Hip and Knee*. www.functionalmovement.com

Descarreaux, M. et al. (2008). Changes in the flexion relaxation response induced by lumbar muscle fatigue. *Biomed Central Musculoskeletal Disorders*, 9, 1.

DeVita, P. & Hortobágyi, T. (2003). Obesity is not associated with increased knee joint torque and power during level walking. *Journal of Biomechanics*, 36, 1355–1362.

Farrell, S.W. et al. (2002). The relation of body mass index, cardiorespiratory fitness, and all-cause mortality in women. *Obesity Research*, 10, 417–423.

Fasshauer, M. & Paschke, R. (2003). Regulation of adipocytokines and insulin resistance. *Diabetologia*, 46, 1594–1603.

Felson, D.T. et al. (1992). Weight loss reduces the risk for symptomatic knee osteoarthritis in women: The Framingham Study. *Annals of Internal Medicine*, 116, 535–9.

Fontaine, K.R. & Barofsky, I. (2001). Obesity and health-related quality of life. *Obesity Reviews*, 2, 173–182.

Fontaine, K.R. et al. (2003). Years of life lost due to obesity. *Journal of the American Medical Association*, 289, 187–193.

Froidevaux, F. et al. (1993). Energy expenditure in obese women before and during weight loss, after refeeding, and in the weight-relapse period. *American Journal of Clinical Nutrition*, 57, 35–42.

Gilleard, W. & Smith, T. (2007). Effect of obesity on posture and hip joint moments during a standing task, and trunk forward flexion motion. *International Journal of Obesity*, 31, 267–277.

Han, T.S. et al. (1997). The prevalence of low back pain and associations with body fatness, fat distribution and height. *International Journal of Obesity & Related Metabolic Disorders*, 21, 600–607.

Haskell, W.L. et al. (2007). Physical activity and public health updated recommendations from the American College of Sports Medicine and the American Heart Association. *Medicine & Science in Sports & Exercise*, 39, 1423–1434.

Helmchen, L.A. & Henderson, R.M. (2004). Changes in the distribution of body mass index of white U.S. men, 1890–2000. *Annals of Human Biology*, 31, 174–181.

Hills, A.P. et al. (2001). Plantar pressure differences between obese and non-obese adults: A biomechanical analysis. *International Journal of Obesity*, 25, 1674–1679.

Howard, B.V., Ruotolo, G., & Robbins, D.C. (2003). Obesity and dyslipidemia. *Endocrinology Metabolism Clinics of North America*, 32, 855–867.

Hulens, H. et al. (2001). Exercise capacity in lean versus obese women. *Scandinavian Journal of Medicine & Science in Sports*, 11, 305–309.

Jakicic, J.M. et al. (2008). Effect of exercise on 24-month weight loss maintenance in overweight women. *Archives of Internal Medicine*, 168, 1550–1559.

Jensen, G.L. (2005). Obesity and functional decline: Epidemiology and geriatric consequences. *Clinics in Geriatric Medicine*, 21, 677–687.

Kendall, F.P. et al. (2005). *Muscles Testing and Function with Posture and Pain* (5th ed.). Baltimore, Md.: Lippincott Williams & Wilkins.

Klem, M.L. et al. (1997). A descriptive study of individuals successful at long-term maintenance of substantial weight loss. *American Journal of Clinical Nutrition*, 66, 239–246.

Knowler, W.C. et al. (2002). Reduction in the incidence of type 2 diabetes with lifestyle intervention or metformin. *New England Journal of Medicine*, 346, 393–403.

Korkiakoski, A. et al. (2009). Association of lumbar arterial stenosis with low back symptoms: A cross-sectional study using two-dimensional time-of-flight magnetic resonance angiography. *Acta Radiologica*, 50, 48–54.

Leboeuf-Yde, C. (2000). Body weight and low back pain: A systematic literature review of 56 journal articles reporting on 65 epidemiologic studies. *Spine*, 25, 226–237.

Lee, C.D., Blair, S.N., & Jackson, A.S. (1999). Cardiorespiratory fitness, body composition, and all-cause and cardiovascular disease mortality in men. *American Journal of Clinical Nutrition*, 69, 373–380.

Lee, Y.H. & Pratley, R.E. (2007). Abdominal obesity and cardiovascular disease risk: The emerging role of the adipocyte. *Journal of Cardiopulmonary Rehabilitation*, 27, 2–10.

Lehman, G.L. (2004). Biomechanical assessments of lumbar spinal function: How low-back pain suffers differ from normals. Implications for outcome measures research. Part I: Kinematic assessments of lumbar function. *Journal of Manipulative & Physiological Therapy*, 27, 57–62.

Levin, B.E. & Dunn-Meynell, A.A. (2004). Chronic exercise lowers the defended body-weight gain and adiposity in diet-induced obese rats. *American Journal of Physiology - Regulatory, Integrative and Comparative Physiology*, 286, 771–778.

Levin, B.E. & Dunn-Meynell, A.A. (2002). Defense of body weight depends on dietary composition and palatability in rats with diet-induced obesity. *American Journal of Physiology - Regulatory, Integrative and Comparative Physiology*, 282, 46–54.

Levin, B.E. & Keesey RE. (1998). Defense of differing body weight set points in diet-induced obese and resistant rats. *American Journal of Physiology - Regulatory, Integrative and Comparative Physiology*, 274, 412–419.

MacLean, P.S. et al. (2004a). Enhanced metabolic efficiency contributes to weight regain after weight loss in obesity-prone rats. *American Journal of Physiology - Regulatory, Integrative and Comparative Physiology*, 287, 1306–1315.

MacLean, P.S. et al. (2004b). Metabolic adjustments with the development, treatment, and recurrence of obesity in obesity-prone rats. *American Journal of Physiology - Regulatory, Integrative and Comparative Physiology*, 287, 288–297.

McGill, S.M. (2007). *Low Back Disorders: Evidence Based Prevention and Rehabilitation* (2nd ed.). Champaign, Ill.: Human Kinetics.

McGill, S.M., Hughson, R.L., & Parks, K. (2000). Changes in lumbar lordosis modify the role of the extensor muscles. *Clinical Biomechanics*, 15, 777–780.

Messier, S.P. (2008). *The Burden of Obesity: A Biomechanical Perspective.* Presented at the ACSM 55th Annual Meeting, Indianapolis, Ind.: May 28, 2008.

Messier, S.P. (1994). Osteoarthritis of the knee and associated factors of age and obesity: Effects on gait. *Medicine & Science in Sports & Exercise*, 26, 1446–1452.

Messier, S.P. et al. (2005). Weight loss reduces knee-joint loads in overweight and obese older adults with knee osteoarthritis. *Arthritis & Rheumatism*, 52, 2026–2032.

Mora, S. et al. (2006). Association of physical activity and body mass index with novel and traditional cardiovascular biomarkers in women. *Journal of the American Medical Association*, 295, 1412–1419.

Morrato, E.H. et al. (2007) Physical activity in U.S. adults with diabetes and at risk for developing diabetes. *Diabetes Care*, 30, 203–209.

Nantel, J., Mathieu, M., & Prince, F. (2010). Physical activity and obesity: Biomechanical and physiological concepts. *Journal of Obesity*, 2011, E-pub Article ID 650230, 10 pages. doi:10.1155/2011/650230.

National Heart, Lung and Blood Institute (2000). *Obesity Education Initiative Expert Panel on the Identification, Evaluation, and Treatment of Overweight and Obesity in Adults: The Practical Guide.* Bethesda, Md.: National Institutes of Health. NIH publication No. 00-4084.

National Heart, Lung and Blood Institute (1998). *Obesity Education Initiative Expert Panel. Clinical Guidelines on the Identification, Evaluation, and Treatment of Overweight and Obesity in Adults: The Evidence Report.* Bethesda, Md.: National Institutes of Health. NIH publication No. 98-4083.

National Weight Control Registry (NCWR) (2012). *NCWR Facts.* National Weight Control Registry www.nwcr.ws/Research/default.htm. Retrieved April 6, 2012.

Nourbakhsh, M.R. & Arab, A.M. (2002). Relation between mechanical factors and incidence of low back pain. *Journal of Orthopaedic Sports & Physical Therapy*, 32, 447–460.

Núñez, N.P. et al. (2007). Extreme obesity reduces bone mineral density: Complementary evidence from mice and women. *Obesity*, 15, 1980–1987.

Ofir, D. et al. (2007). Ventilatory and perceptual responses to cycle exercise in obese women. *Journal of Applied Physiology*, 102, 2217–2226.

Ogden, C.L. et al. (2006). Prevalence of overweight and obesity in the United States, 1999–2004. *Journal of the American Medical Association*, 295, 1549–1555.

Panagiotakos, D.B. et al. (2005). The implication of obesity and central fat on markers of chronic inflammation: The ATTICA study. *Atherosclerosis*, 183, 308–315.

Panagiotakos, D.B. et al. (2004). The associations between leisure-time physical activity and inflammatory and coagulation markers related to cardiovascular disease: The ATTICA study. *Preventive Medicine*, 40, 432–437.

Park, H.S., Park, J.Y., & Yu, R. (2005). Relationship of obesity and visceral adiposity with serum concentrations of CRP, TNF-alpha, and IL6. *Diabetes Research & Clinical Practice*, 69, 29–35.

Sahrmann, S.A. (2002). *Diagnosis and Treatment of Movement Impairment Syndromes*. St. Louis, Mo.: Mosby.

Sarris, W.H. et al. (2003). How much physical activity is enough to prevent unhealthy weight gain? Outcome of the IASO 1st Stock Conference and consensus statement. *Obesity Reviews*, 4, 101–114.

Shiri, R. (2008). Obesity and the prevalence of low-back pain in young adults. *American Journal of Epidemiology*, 167, 1110–1119.

Shiri, R.,et al. (2010). The association between

obesity and low-back pain: A meta-analysis. *American Journal of Epidemiology*, 171, 135–154.

Spyropoulos, P. et al. (1991). Biomechanical gait analysis in obese men. *Archives of Physical Medicine & Rehabilitation*, 72, 1065–1070.

Stein, C.J. & Colditz, G.A. (2004). The epidemic of obesity. *Journal of Clinical Endocrinology & Metabolism*, 89, 2522–2525.

Sullivan, P.W. et al. (2005). Obesity, inactivity, and the prevalence of diabetes and diabetes-related cardiovascular comorbidities in the U.S., 2000–2002. *Diabetes Care*, 28, 1599–1603.

Toda, Y. et al. (2000). Lean body mass and body fat distribution in participants with chronic low back pain. *Archives of Internal Medicine*, 160, 3265–3269.

U.S. Department of Agriculture (2015). *2015-2020 Dietary Guidelines for Americans* (8th ed.). www.health.gov/dietaryguidelines

U.S. Department of Health & Human Services (2008). *2008 Physical Activity Guidelines for Americans: Be Active, Healthy and Happy*. www.health.gov/paguidelines/pdf/paguide.pdf

Vismara, L. et al. (2010) Effect of obesity and low back pain on spinal mobility: A cross sectional study in women. *Journal of NeuroEngineering and Rehabilitation*, 7, 3.

Votruba, S.B., Blanc, S., & Schoeller, D.A. (2002). Pattern and cost of weight gain in previously obese women. *American Journal of Physiology – Endocrinology and Metabolism*, 282, 923–930.

Whiting W.C. & Rugg, S. (2006). *Dynatomy: Dynamic Human Anatomy*. Champaign, Ill.: Human Kinetics.

Wisse, B.E. (2004). The inflammatory syndrome: The role of adipose tissue cytokines in metabolic disorders linked to obesity. *Journal of the American Society of Nephrology*, 15, 2792–2800.

Zoeller, R.F. (2007). Physical activity and obesity: Their interaction and implications for disease risk and the role of physical activity in healthy weight management. *American Journal of Lifestyle Medicine*, 6, 437–446.

Suggested Reading

American College of Sports Medicine (2009). Position stand: Appropriate physical activity intervention strategies for weight loss and prevention of weight regain for adults. *Medicine & Science in Sports & Exercise*, 41, 459–471.

American Council on Exercise (2014). *ACE Personal Trainer Manual* (5th ed.). San Diego, Calif.: American Council on Exercise.

National Heart, Lung and Blood Institute (1998). *Obesity Education Initiative Expert Panel. Clinical Guidelines on the Identification, Evaluation, and Treatment of Overweight and Obesity in Adults: The Evidence Report*. Bethesda, Md.: National Institutes of Health. NIH publication No. 98-4083.

U.S. Department of Agriculture (2015). *2015-2020 Dietary Guidelines for Americans* (8th ed.). www.health.gov/dietaryguidelines

U.S. Department of Health & Human Services (2008). *2008 Physical Activity Guidelines for Americans: Be Active, Healthy and Happy*. www.health.gov/paguidelines/pdf/paguide.pdf

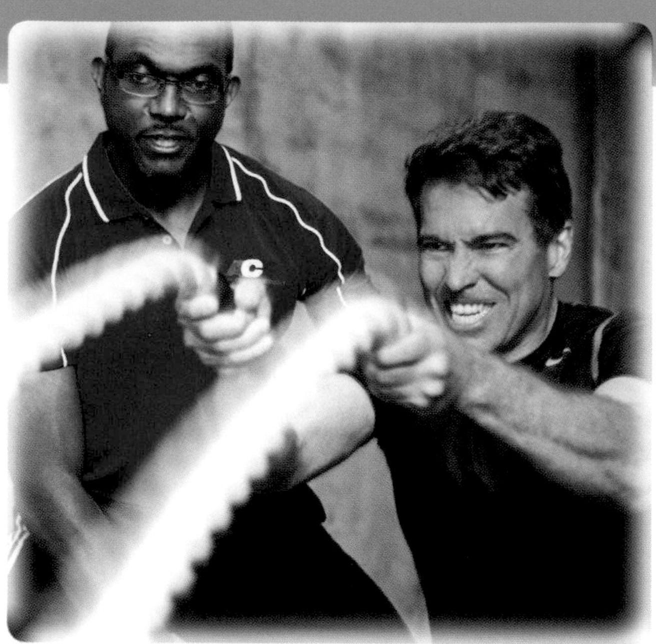

IN THIS CHAPTER:

Fabio Comana, M.A., M.S., is the director of continuing education for the National Academy of Sports Medicine (NASM) and a faculty member in Exercise Science and Nutrition at San Diego State University and UC San Diego. Comana holds numerous fitness certifications from ACE, NASM, the American College of Sports Medicine, and the International Society of Sports Nutrition. Previously, he was an exercise physiologist and certification manager for the American Council on Exercise (ACE) where he played a key role in the development of ACE's Integrated Fitness Training® Model and many of ACE's live personal-training educational workshops. His previous experiences include collegiate head coaching, strength and conditioning coaching, and opening and managing health clubs for Club One. As a national and international presenter, he is frequently featured on television, radio, internet, and in print publications. He authored chapters in various textbooks and publications, and is presently authoring upcoming academic and consumer books.

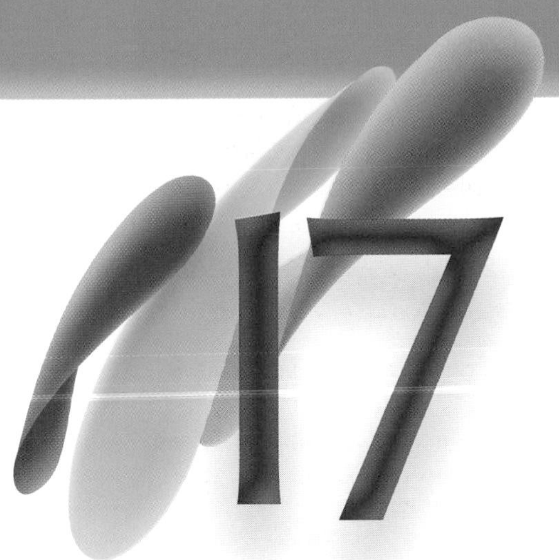

17 Exercise Program Design

FABIO COMANA &
SABRENA JO

Sabrena Jo, M.S., has been actively involved in the fitness industry since 1987, successfully operating her own personal-training business and teaching group exercise classes. Jo is a former full-time faculty member in the Kinesiology and Physical Education Department at California State University, Long Beach. She has a bachelor's degree in exercise science as well as a master's degree in physical education/biomechanics from the University of Kansas. Jo, an ACE-certified Personal Trainer and Group Fitness Instructor, is an author, educator, and fitness consultant who remains very active within the industry.

In Chapter 16, an overview of components and phases of the ACE Integrated Fitness® (ACE IFT®) Training Model was presented. This chapter explores each phase of the ACE IFT Model as it relates to safe and effective exercise programming. Specifically, the programming focus is on the successful facilitation of weight loss in overweight or obese individuals. However, the concepts presented can be applied to any individual as he or she progresses through the function–health–fitness–performance continuum.

Cardiorespiratory Training Based on the ACE IFT Model

Since regular aerobic endurance exercise is the mode of activity that is responsible for the greatest success in long-term weight loss with overweight and obese individuals, the discussion of exercise programming begins with cardiorespiratory training. The basic concept of program design is to create an exercise program with appropriate frequency, intensity, and duration to fit the client's current health and fitness, with adequate progressions to help the client safely achieve his or her goals. The ACE IFT Model has four cardiorespiratory training phases:

- Phase 1: Aerobic-base training
- Phase 2: Aerobic-efficiency training
- Phase 3: Anaerobic-endurance training
- Phase 4: Anaerobic-power training

Clients are categorized into a given phase based on their current health, fitness levels, and goals. By utilizing the assessment and programming tools in each phase, ACE-certified Health Coaches can develop individualized cardiorespiratory programs for clients ranging from sedentary to endurance athletes. Programming in each phase will be based on the **heart rate (HR)** training three-zone model shown in Figure 17-1, using HR at the **first ventilatory threshold (VT1)** and the **second**

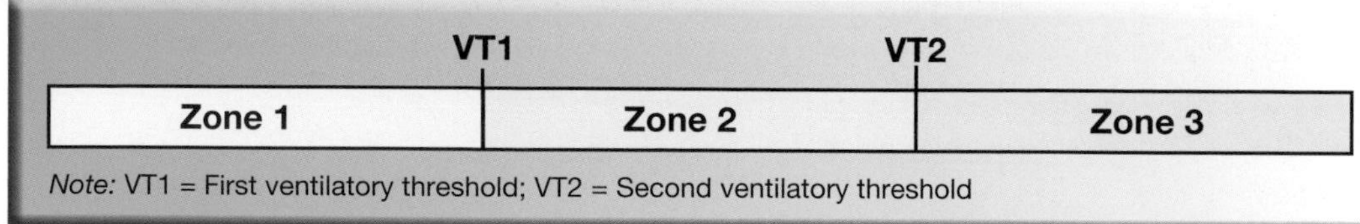

Figure 17-1
Three-zone training model

> Stated simply, if a client can talk comfortably, he or she is training in zone 1. If the client is not sure if he or she can talk comfortably, he or she is working in zone 2. If the client definitely cannot talk comfortably while training, he or she is working in zone 3.

ventilatory threshold (VT2) to develop individualized programs based on each client's unique metabolic responses to exercise (see pages 329–332). These two metabolic markers provide a convenient way to divide intensity into training zones that are determined without any use of, or reference to, **maximal heart rate (MHR):**

- Zone 1 (relatively easy exercise) reflects heart rates below VT1.
- Zone 2 reflects heart rates from VT1 to just below VT2.
- Zone 3 reflects heart rates at and above VT2.

It is important to note that training principles in the ACE IFT Model's cardiorespiratory training phases can be implemented using various exercise intensity markers, including ones based on predicted values such as a percentage of **heart-rate reserve** (%**HRR**) or a percentage of maximal heart rate (%MHR), but the exercise intensities will not be as accurate for individual clients as when they utilize measured HR at VT1 and VT2 (Table 17-1).

Table 17-1

Three-zone Training Model Using Various Intensity Markers

Intensity Markers	Zone 1	Zone 2	Zone 3	Advantages/Limitations
Metabolic markers: VT1 and VT2* (HR relative to VT1 and VT2)*	Below VT1 (HR <VT1)	VT1 to just below VT2 (HR ≥VT1 to <VT2)	VT2 and above (HR ≥VT2)	• Based on measured VT1 and VT2 • Ideally, VT1 and VT2 are measured in a lab with a metabolic cart and blood lactate • Field tests are relatively easy to administer, require minimal equipment, and provide accurate corresponding HRs at VT1 and VT2 • Programming with metabolic markers allows for individualized programming
Talk test*	Can talk comfortably	Not sure if talking is comfortable	Definitely cannot talk comfortably	• Based on actual changes in ventilation due to physiological adaptations to increasing exercise intensities • Very easy for practical measurement • No equipment required • Can easily be taught to clients • Allows for individualized programming
RPE (terminology)*	"Moderate" to "somewhat hard"	"Hard"	"Very hard" to "extremely hard"	• Good subjective intensity marker • Correlates well with talk test, metabolic markers, and measured %$\dot{V}O_2$max • Easy to teach to clients

Table 17-1 *continued*

Three-zone Training Model Using Various Intensity Markers

Intensity Markers	Zone 1	Zone 2	Zone 3	Advantages/Limitations
RPE (0 to 10 scale)*	3 to 4	5 to 6	7 to 10	• Good subjective intensity marker • Correlates well with talk test, metabolic markers, and measured % $\dot{V}O_2$max • 0 to 10 scale is easy to teach to clients
RPE (6 to 20 scale)	12 to 13	14 to 16	17 to 20	• Good subjective intensity marker • Correlates well with talk test, metabolic markers, and measured % $\dot{V}O_2$max • 6 to 20 scale is not as easy to teach to clients as the 0 to 10 scale • *Note:* An RPE of 20 represents maximal effort and cannot be sustained as a training intensity.
%$\dot{V}O_2$R	40 to 59%	60 to 84%	≥85%	• Requires *measured* $\dot{V}O_2$max for most accurate programming • Impractical due to expensive equipment and testing • Increased error with use of *predicted* $\dot{V}O_2$max or *predicted* MHR • Relative percentages for programming are population-based and not individually specific
%HRR	40 to 59%	60 to 84%	≥85%	• Requires *measured* MHR and RHR for most accurate programming • Measured MHR is impractical for the vast majority of health coaches and clients • Use of RHR increases individuality of programming vs. strict %MHR • Use of *predicted* MHR introduces potentially large error; the magnitude of the error is dependent on the specific equation used • Relative percentages for programming are population-based and not individually specific
%MHR	64 to 76%	77 to 93%	≥94%	• Requires *measured* MHR for accuracy in programming • Measured MHR is impractical for the vast majority of health coaches and clients • Use of *predicted* MHR introduces potentially large error; the magnitude of the error is dependent on the specific equation used • Does not include RHR, as is used in %HRR • Relative percentages for programming are population-based and not individually specific
METs	3 to 6	6 to 9	>9	• Requires *measured* $\dot{V}O_2$max for most accurate programming • Can use in programming more easily than other intensity markers based off $\dot{V}O_2$max • Limited in programming by knowledge of METs for given activities and/or equipment that gives MET estimates • Relative MET ranges for programming are population-based and not individually specific (e.g., a 5-MET activity might initially be perceived as vigorous by a previously sedentary client)
Category terminology for exercise programming	Low to moderate	Moderate to vigorous	Vigorous to very vigorous	

Note: VT1 = First ventilatory threshold; VT2 = Second ventilatory threshold; HR = Heart rate; RPE = Ratings of perceived exertion; $\dot{V}O_2$max= $\dot{V}O_2$maximum; $\dot{V}O_2$R = VO_2 reserve; HRR = Heart-rate reserve; MHR = Maximal heart rate; RHR = Resting heart rate; METs = Metabolic equivalents

*These are the preferred intensity markers to use with the three-zone model when designing, implementing, and progressing cardiorespiratory training programs using the ACE Integrated Fitness Training Model.

Table 17-2 provides an overview of the cardiorespiratory training phases of the ACE IFT Model. This is followed by detailed descriptions that explain the training focus of each stage and strategies for implementing and progressing exercise programs to help clients reach

Table 17-2

Cardiorespiratory Training Phase Overview

Phase 1—Aerobic-base Training

- The focus is on creating positive exercise experiences that help sedentary clients become regular exercisers.
- No fitness assessments are required prior to exercise in this phase.
- Focus on steady-state exercise in zone 1 (below HR at VT1).
- Gauge by the client's ability to talk (below talk test threshold) and/or RPE of 3 to 4 (moderate to somewhat hard).
- Progress to phase 2 once the client can sustain steady-state cardiorespiratory exercise for 20 to 30 minutes in zone 1 (RPE of 3 to 4) and is comfortable with assessments.

Phase 2—Aerobic-efficiency Training

- The focus is on increasing the duration of exercise and introducing intervals to improve aerobic efficiency, fitness, and health.
- Administer the submaximal talk test to determine HR at VT1. There is no need to measure VT2 in phase 2.
- Increase workload at VT1 (increase HR at VT1), then introduce low zone 2 intervals just above VT1 (RPE of 5) to improve aerobic efficiency and add variety in programming.
- Progress low zone 2 intervals by increasing the time of the work interval and later decreasing the recovery interval time.
- As client progresses, introduce intervals in the upper end of zone 2 (RPE of 6).
- Many clients will stay in this phase for many years.
- If a client has event-specific goals or is a fitness enthusiast looking for increased challenges and fitness gains, progress to phase 3.

Phase 3—Anaerobic-endurance Training

- The focus is on designing programs to help clients who have endurance performance goals and/or are performing seven or more hours of cardiorespiratory exercise per week.
- Administer the VT2 threshold test to determine HR at VT2.
- Programs will have the majority of cardiorespiratory training time in zone 1.
- Interval and higher-intensity sessions will be very focused in zones 2 and 3, but will make up only a small amount of the total training time to allow for adaptation to the total training load.
- Many clients will never train in phase 3, as all of their non-competitive fitness goals can be achieved through phase 2 training.
- Only clients who have very specific goals for increasing speed for short bursts at near-maximal efforts during endurance or athletic competitions will move on to phase 4.

Phase 4—Anaerobic-power Training

- The focus is on improving anaerobic power to improve phosphagen energy pathways and buffer large accumulations of blood lactate in order to improve speed for short bursts at near-maximal efforts during endurance or athletic competitions.
- Programs will have a similar distribution to phase 3 training times in zones 1, 2, and 3.
- Zone 3 training will include very intense anaerobic-power intervals.
- Clients will generally only work in phase 4 during specific training cycles prior to competition.

Note: HR = Heart rate; VT1 = First ventilatory threshold; RPE = Ratings of perceived exertion; VT2 = Second ventilatory threshold their goals within the phase, and then advance to the next phase if desired. It is important to note that not every client will start in phase 1, as some clients will already be regularly participating in cardiorespiratory exercise, and only clients with very specific performance or speed goals will move into phase 3 and reach phase 4. In addition, the submaximal **talk test** for VT1 (see page 329) is recommended for introduction in phase 2, while the field test for VT2 (see page 332) should ideally be introduced during phase 3. Also, clients may be in different phases for cardiorespiratory training and functional movement and resistance training based on their current health, fitness, exercise-participation levels, and goals.

Phase 1: Aerobic-base Training

Phase 1 has a principal focus of getting clients who are either sedentary or have little cardiorespiratory fitness to begin engaging in regular cardiorespiratory exercise of low-to-moderate intensity with a primary goal of improving health and a secondary goal of building fitness. These clients may have long-term goals for fitness and possibly even sports performance, but they need to progress through phase 1 first. The primary goal for the health coach during this phase should be to help the client have positive experiences with cardiorespiratory exercise and to help him or her adopt exercise as a regular habit. The intent of this phase is to develop a stable aerobic base upon which the client can build improvements in health, endurance, energy, mood, and caloric expenditure.

Once regularity of exercise habits is established, the duration of exercise is extended until the individual can perform 20 to 30 continuous minutes of cardiorespiratory exercise on most days with little residual fatigue, at which point they can progress to phase 2. This approach to training ensures the safety of exercise, while at the same time allowing some of the potential physiologic adaptations and most of the health benefits to occur. Within this general design is recognition that the benefit-to-risk ratio of low-intensity zone 1 training is very high for the beginning exerciser, with the possibility for very large gains in health and basic fitness and almost no risk of either cardiovascular or musculoskeletal injury. As the exerciser develops more ambitious goals, more demanding training (either longer or more intense) can be performed.

Program Design for Phase 1: Aerobic-base Training

The primary goal of this phase is to help clients have positive experiences with exercise to facilitate program adherence and success. Cardiorespiratory fitness assessments are not necessary at the beginning of this phase, as they will only confirm low levels of fitness and potentially serve as negative reminders about why the sedentary client with low levels of fitness may not have good **self-efficacy** regarding exercise. All cardiorespiratory exercise during this phase falls within zone 1 (sub-VT1), so the health coach can use the client's ability to talk comfortably as the upper exercise-intensity limit. The health coach can also teach the client to use the 0 to 10 category ratio scale, with the client exercising at a **rating of perceived exertion (RPE)** of 3 to 4 (moderate to somewhat hard) (Table 17-3). It is not necessary to conduct the submaximal talk test assessment to determine HR at VT1 until phase 2.

As a general principle, exercise programs designed to improve the aerobic base begin with zone 1–intensity exercise with HR below VT1 performed for as little as 10 to 15 minutes two to three times each week. However, this should be progressed as rapidly as

Table 17-3

Ratings of Perceived Exertion (RPE)

RPE	Category Ratio Scale
6	0 Nothing at all
7 Very, very light	0.5 Very, very weak
8	1 Very weak
9 Very light	2 Weak
10	3 Moderate
11 Fairly light	4 Somewhat strong
12	5 Strong
13 Somewhat hard	6
14	7 Very strong
15 Hard	8
16	9
17 Very hard	10 Very, very strong
18	• Maximal
19 Very, very hard	
20	

Data from: Borg, G. (1998). *Borg's Perceived Exertion and Pain Scales.* Champaign, Ill.: Human Kinetics.

tolerated to 30 minutes at moderate intensity (zone 1; below "talk test" with HR below VT1), performed at least five times each week. Changes in duration from one week to the next should not exceed a 10% increase versus the week prior. Once this level of exercise can be sustained on a regular basis, the primary adaptation of the aerobic base will be complete.

For the most part, early training efforts should feature continuous exercise at zone 1 intensity. Depending on how sedentary a person was prior to beginning the program, this level of easy exercise may be continued for as little as one to two weeks or for as long as six weeks. The beginning duration of exercise should match what the client is able to perform. For some, this might be 15 continuous minutes, while for others it might be only five to 10 continuous minutes. From that point, duration should be increased at a rate of no more than 10% from one week to the next until the client can perform 30 minutes of continuous exercise. Once the client is comfortable with assessments and can sustain steady-state cardiorespiratory exercise for 20 minutes in zone 1 (RPE of 3 to 4), he or she can move onto phase 2.

A sample aerobic-base (phase 1) training progression for a client exercising four days per week is illustrated in Table 17-4. This sample shows appropriate progressions for weekly duration with different options for session duration during most weeks to add variety and accommodate other program goals.

Table 17-4

Sample Phase 1 Cardiorespiratory-training Progression

Training Parameter	Week 1	Week 2	Week 3	Week 4	Week 5
Frequency	4 times/week	4 times/week	4 times/week	4 times/week	4 times/week
Duration—Total for Week: (10% weekly increase)	60 min/week	66 min/week	72 min/week	80 min/week	88 min/week
Duration of Sessions (continuous)	4 x 15 min	4 x 16.5 min or 2 x 15 min 2 x 18.5 min	4 x 18 min or 2 x 17 min 2 x 19 min	4 x 20 min or 2 x 18 min 2 x 22 min	4 x 22 min or 2 x 20 min 2 x 24 min
Intensity	<VT1 HR RPE = 3	<VT1 HR RPE = 3	<VT1 HR RPE = 3	<VT1 HR RPE = 3 to 4	<VT1 HR RPE = 3 to 4
Zone	1	1	1	1	1
Training Format	Steady state	Steady state	Steady state	Steady state	Steady state
Work-to-Recovery Intervals (active recovery)	None	None	None	None	None

Note: VT1 = First ventilatory threshold; RPE = Ratings of perceived exertion

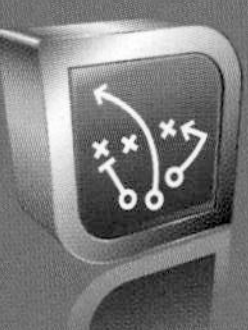

APPLY WHAT YOU KNOW

Using Technology to Your Advantage—ACE IFT Model Phase 1: Special Considerations for Overweight/Obese Individuals

Two important considerations related to aerobic exercise training for overweight and obese clients are the appropriateness of the exercise equipment and the individual's ability to tolerate the duration of activity. In both cases, the use of technological advances in exercise equipment or devices can be useful.

Both upright and recumbent cycling are popular modes of aerobic activity for obese individuals. However, the seats on many of the cycles are too narrow and not supportive enough for exercisers with higher BMIs. Before having an obese client embark on a cycling program, the health coach should ensure that the seat is wide enough for proper support and has enough cushioning for added comfort. Typically, recumbent models have adequate seat size and cushioning, as well as the added benefit of back support. A relatively unique type of exercise equipment called recumbent cross trainers are also excellent options for obese exercisers. These machines are a cross between a stair climbing machine with moveable handles and a recumbent bike. They allow the exerciser to work the upper and lower body at the same time without stressing the joints, and they can accommodate a variety of body types and sizes (Figure 17-2).

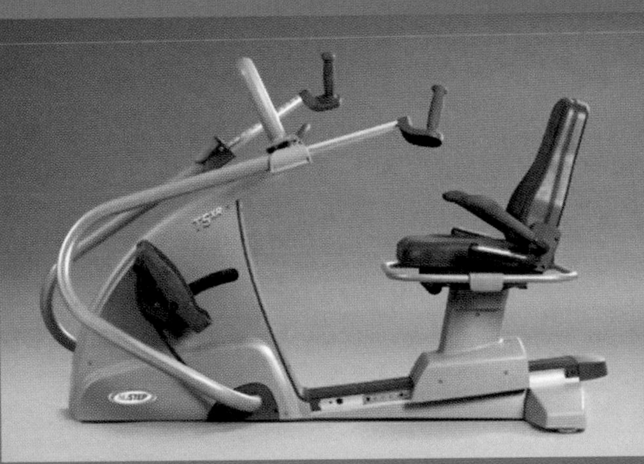

Figure 17-2
Recumbent cross trainer
Photo courtesy of www.nustep.com.

The musculoskeletal discomfort associated with obesity can make a prolonged exercise session (e.g., 30 minutes or more) intolerable. During the initial period of training, recommending that obese clients accumulate the desired number of minutes of exercise throughout the day, rather than all at once, might help ease any muscle or joint pain associated with physical activity. Even if the client has no other option but to walk for exercise, splitting up the session can reduce the musculoskeletal demands of the activity.

Pedometers track the number of steps an individual takes throughout a given time period. They can be an exceptionally motivating tool to help obese clients accumulate meaningful physical activity, especially if they sit at a desk for most of their workday.

One option for utilizing pedometers is to have the client set an alarm to go off every hour as a prompt to get up and move. Once the alarm sounds, the client takes a walk around the building. For even more accountability, the client can log in an exercise journal the total number of steps taken each day with a goal of getting in at least 50 to 100 steps every hour. More advanced pedometers also allow the user to download the data and keep track of the number of steps taken on a computer so that additional journal materials are unnecessary. Eventually, the client can add in extra challenges like taking the stairs during the walk and pacing for increased speed, as long as these challenges do not induce undue musculoskeletal pain.

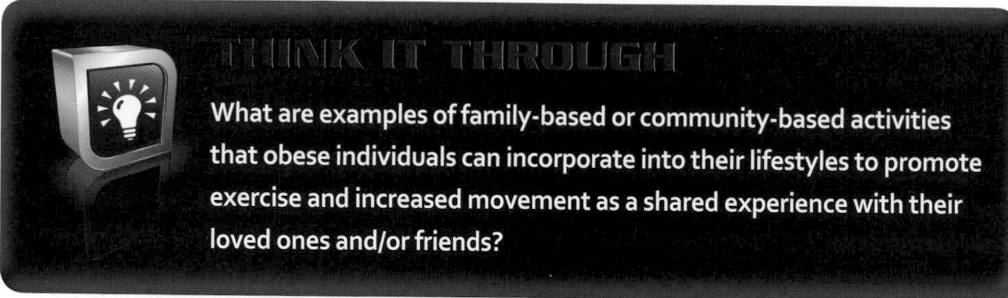

THINK IT THROUGH
What are examples of family-based or community-based activities that obese individuals can incorporate into their lifestyles to promote exercise and increased movement as a shared experience with their loved ones and/or friends?

Phase 2: Aerobic-efficiency Training

Phase 2 has a principal training focus of increasing the time of cardiorespiratory exercise while introducing intervals to improve the ability to exercise at greater workloads to improve fitness and increase caloric expenditure. However, it is important to understand that after an aerobic base has been achieved, additional gains in fitness will require increases in training intensity, frequency, or duration. At this time, the health coach should review the goals of the client. What are the client's exercise goals—health and basic fitness benefits, improved appearance, and/or weight-loss benefits?

Phase 2 is the primary cardiorespiratory training phase for regular exercisers in a fitness facility who have goals for improving or maintaining fitness and/or weight loss. Cardiorespiratory training in this phase includes increasing the workload by modifying frequency, duration, and intensity, with intervals introduced that go into zone 2 and eventually approach HR at VT2. The zone 2 intervals in this phase provide a stimulus that will eventually increase the HR at VT1, resulting in the client being able to exercise at a lower HR when at the same level of intensity, and also allowing the client to exercise at higher intensities, expending more calories per minute, while at the VT1 HR.

Clients training in phase 2 who have a goal to complete an event, such as a 10K run, can reach their goal of completing the event within the training guidelines of this phase. Once a client begins working toward multiple endurance performance goals, trains to improve his or her competitive speed, begins training seven or more hours per week, or simply wants to take on the challenge of training like an athlete, the client should move on to phase 3 of cardiorespiratory training.

For the many clients who never develop competitive goals or the desire to train like an endurance athlete, training in phase 2 will provide very adequate challenges to help them improve and maintain cardiorespiratory fitness for many years. The workouts in most non-athletically focused group exercise classes fall into this phase. Phase 2 covers the principles for building aerobic efficiency that are implemented with most health coach clients and fitness enthusiasts.

Program Design for Phase 2: Aerobic-efficiency Training

At the beginning of phase 2, the health coach should have the client perform the submaximal talk test to determine HR at VT1 (see page 329). This HR will be utilized for programming throughout the phase, and will need to be reassessed periodically as fitness improves to see if the HR at VT1 has increased and training intensities need to be adjusted.

This phase of cardiorespiratory training is dedicated to enhancing the client's aerobic efficiency by progressing the program through increased duration of sessions, increased frequency of sessions when possible, and the introduction of zone 2 intervals. In phase 2, the warm-up, cool-down, recovery intervals, and steady-state cardiorespiratory exercise segments are performed at or just below VT1 at an RPE of 3 to 4 (0 to 10 scale) to continue advancing the client's aerobic base. Aerobic intervals are introduced at a level that is just above VT1, or an RPE of 5 (0 to 10 scale). The goal of these intervals is to improve aerobic efficiency by raising the intensity of exercise performed at VT1, improve the client's ability to utilize fat as a fuel source at and just above VT1, improve exercise efficiency at VT1, and add variety to the exercise program.

As a general principle, intervals should start out relatively brief (initially about 60 seconds), with an approximate hard-to-easy ratio of 1:3 (e.g., a 60-second work interval followed by a 180-second recovery interval), eventually progressing to a ratio of 1:2 and then 1:1. The duration of these intervals can be increased in regular increments, depending on the goals of the exerciser, but should be increased cautiously over several weeks depending on the client's fitness level. As a general principle, the exercise load (calculated from the session RPE or the integrated time in the zone) should be increased by no more than 10% per week. Early in phase 2, exercise bouts with a session RPE greater than 5 (e.g., hard exercise) should be performed infrequently. As the client's fitness increases, steady-state exercise sessions with efforts just above VT1 (RPE of 5) can be introduced.

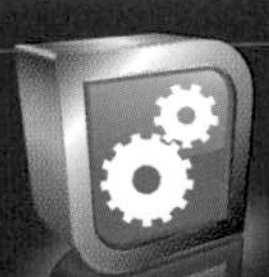

EXPAND YOUR KNOWLEDGE

Session RPE

Selecting an appropriate intensity is always a major challenge for health coaches who seek proper levels of overload, yet want to create an optimal experience, especially when working with newer, deconditioned clients, clients who are apprehensive about undergoing cardiorespiratory fitness testing, and individuals for whom heart-rate measures are invalid (e.g., those taking beta blockers).

The "session RPE" was developed as a method of monitoring the combined intensity and duration of an exercise session (Herman et al., 2006; Foster et al., 1995). If an individual is asked to rate the overall intensity of an exercise bout about 30 minutes after the conclusion of that bout using the category ratio (0 to 10) scale, and then multiplies this rating by the duration of the bout, a score representing the combined intensity and duration of the bout is generated (i.e., the training load) (Foster et al., 2001; Foster, Daniels, & Seiler, 1999; Foster et al., 1996). In practice, this daily score can be summated on a weekly basis, generating a weekly training load for self-monitoring purposes. This is an effective programming and monitoring tool that promotes appropriate initial exercise intensities, creates some ownership of programming on the part of the client, and allows a limited degree of training flexibility to facilitate adherence.

This model can be used exclusively and indefinitely to monitor exercise intensity, or health coaches may opt to use it during only the initial stage of a clients' program, perhaps before conducting any cardiorespiratory tests for aerobic fitness. Health coaches should adhere to the following guidelines when using the session RPE model:

- Spend time helping the client become familiar with the 0 to 10 RPE scale.
- Determine appropriate RPE intensities for each exercise session based on the client's current activity levels, while providing a small overload challenge (e.g., a 5-out-of-10 effort for someone who has been exercising at a 4-to-4½ effort).

- Identify the frequency and duration that is appropriate for the client's current conditioning level and feasible within his or her schedule (e.g., three times a week for 15 minutes).
- Implement a RPE-training volume model (i.e., RPE x frequency x duration).
  - ✓ For example, Joe's key goal is to improve his cardiorespiratory fitness, and he and his health coach mutually decide that a feasible start is for him to participate in cardiovascular training sessions three times each week for approximately 20 minutes each, at a 5-out-of-10 effort.
  - ✓ His total weekly training volume is 3 x 20 minutes = 60 minutes, and his target goal for week one = 60 minutes x RPE of 5 = 300 points.
  - ✓ Joe's progression over three weeks at a 10% progression rate per week:
    - Week 1 = 300 points
    - Week 2 = 330 points
    - Week 3 = 365 points
  - ✓ The health coach can provide Joe options on how he can achieve his target number by manipulating any of the three variables (i.e., intensity, frequency, and duration) (Table 17-5). While allowing Joe some flexibility and ownership of his program, the health coach should subscribe to the K.I.S.S. principle (keep it simple and short) to avoid confusion and potential drop-out.

Table 17-5

Training Progression and Options Using Frequency x Duration x Intensity (RPE)

	Frequency	Duration	Intensity (RPE)	Total Points
Week 1 goal				300
Options	3 sessions	x 20	x 5	= 300
	2 sessions 1 session	x 20 x 18	x 5 x 5.5	= 200 = 99 299
	2 sessions 2 sessions	x 16 x 13	x 5 x 5.5	= 160 = 143 303
Week 2 goal				330
Options	3 sessions	x 22	x 5	= 330
	2 sessions 1 session	x 22 x 18	x 5 x 6	= 220 = 108 328
	2 sessions 2 sessions	x 19 x 16.5	x 4 x 5.5	= 152 = 181 333

Note: RPE = Ratings of perceived exertion

Low zone 2 intervals should first be progressed by increasing the time of each interval and then moving to a 1:1 work-to-recovery (hard-to-easy) interval ratio. As the client progresses, intervals can progress into the upper end of zone 2 (RPE of 6) at a 1:3 work-to-recovery ratio, progressing first to longer intervals and then eventually moving to intervals with a 1:1 work-to-recovery ratio. Well-trained and motivated non-athletes can progress to where they are performing as much as 50% of their cardiorespiratory training in zone 2. Once the well-trained non-athlete reaches seven or more hours of training per week or develops performance goals, he or she should progress to phase 3. Clients with advanced fitness who are training for a one-time event or are preparing to advance to phase 3, can perform brief intervals (up to 30 seconds) that go just above VT2 (RPE of 7) to further develop aerobic power and provide additional variety.

It is not necessary to measure VT2 during this phase, as an RPE of 5 to 6 (0 to 10 scale) can be used to represent intensities in zone 2, and an RPE of 7 (very hard) can be used to identify efforts just above VT2. Programming variables and variety during phase 2 are diverse enough for clients who do not have competitive goals to train in this phase for many years. A sample cardiorespiratory-training progression for a client in phase 2 is presented in Table 17-6. This sample shows appropriate progressions for weekly duration with different options for session duration during most weeks to add variety and accommodate other program goals.

Table 17-6

Sample Phase 2 Cardiorespiratory-training Progression

Training Parameter	Week 1	Week 2	Week 3	Week 4	Week 5
Frequency	3 times/week	3–4 times/week	3–4 times/week	4 times/week	4–5 times/week
Duration (10% weekly increase)	"X" minutes	10% increase	10% increase	10% increase	10% increase
Intensity	Below VT1 HR	Below and above VT1 HR	Below and above VT1 HR	Below and above VT1 HR	Above VT1 HR
Zone	1	1 and 2	1 and 2	1 and 2	1 and 2
Training Format	Steady state	Aerobic intervals	Aerobic intervals	Aerobic intervals	Aerobic intervals
Work-to-Recovery Intervals (active recovery)	None	1:2 2–3 minute intervals	1:2 3–4 minute intervals	1:1½ 3–4 minute intervals	1:1 4–5 minute intervals

Note: VT1 = First ventilatory threshold; HR = Heart rate

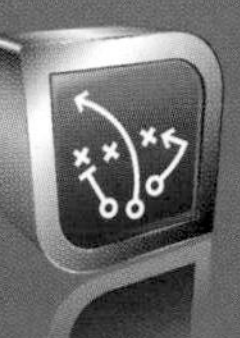

APPLY WHAT YOU KNOW

Using Technology to Your Advantage—ACE IFT Model Phase 2: Special Considerations for Overweight/Obese Individuals

An effective way to introduce aerobic-interval training to overweight and obese clients is to make the activity enjoyable and relevant. The use of a personal digital music player can be a simple tool that makes performing the more intense work required during an aerobic interval more fun and meaningful to the client. This strategy can be used with any type of land-based aerobic endurance exercise modality (e.g., cycling, walking on the treadmill, walking outdoors, and elliptical training).

- The first step is to ask the client to make a continuous playlist using five to 10 songs that he or she finds particularly uplifting and motivating. Given that most songs are approximately three minutes in duration, the playlist will most likely be 15 to 30 minutes long.
- The second step is to instruct the client to identify the chorus of each song and commit to working harder during the chorus. Thus, each time the chorus starts to play, the client has an opportunity to exert a little more energy with the knowledge that when the chorus is finished, he or she can revert back to the less-intense work that should be performed for the majority of the song. Typically, the chorus segments of most radio-edit music last about 20 to 45 seconds.

This method allows clients to explore their limits of intensity while listening to their favorite music. For added interest and motivation, clients can be encouraged to create more playlists so that they have a variety of music from which to choose. Additionally, as clients progress in their endurance capabilities, more songs can be added to the playlist to increase the duration of the exercise session.

Phase 3: Anaerobic-endurance Training

Phase 3 is designed for clients who have endurance-performance goals and are performing seven or more hours of cardiorespiratory training per week. The training principles in phase 3 are for clients who have one or more endurance-performance goals that require specialized training to ensure that adequate training volume and appropriate training intensity and recovery are included to create performance changes that help the client reach his or her goals. Clients do not need to be highly competitive athletes to train in zone 3. They need only to be motivated clients with endurance-performance goals and the requisite fitness from phase 2 to build upon.

A variety of studies with different types of athletes, including Nordic skiers, cyclists, and runners, have suggested that 70 to 80% of training is performed at intensities lower than VT1 (zone 1) (Seiler & Kjerland, 2006; Esteve-Lanao et al., 2005). These same studies suggest that athletes typically perform 5 to 10% of their training above VT2 (zone 3). Thus, even though zone 3 training can be very effective in terms of provoking improvements, only a small amount is tolerable, even in competitive athletes. Surprisingly, very little training is actually performed in the intensity zone between the two thresholds (zone 2). This intensity has been called "the black hole" (where there is a psychological push to do more, but a physiologic pull to do less), since it is the zone where exercise is hard enough to make a person fatigued, but not hard enough to really provoke optimal adaptations (Seiler & Kjerland, 2006).

In individuals who are already routinely exercising and who desire to move toward their optimal biological potential, most training (approximately 80%) should be performed at intensities where speech is comfortable (zone 1), and about 10% of training should be performed at intensities above VT2 (zone 3), where the physiological provocation to make large gains is present.

With the increase in training load during phase 3, consideration must also be given to the amount of recovery training. Where the regular recreational exerciser in the aerobic base phase of training (phase1) can safely and comfortably perform essentially the same training bout every day, the competitive-level exerciser will need to use a decidedly hard/easy approach to training, or he or she will be at risk for problems from accumulating fatigue and loss of training benefit from the inability to repeatedly do really hard training sessions. In any case, even in the most seriously trained athlete, it is probably not productive to perform more than three or four high-intensity or very long training sessions per week.

Program Design for Phase 3: Anaerobic-endurance Training

Program design during this phase should be focused on helping the client enhance his or her aerobic efficiency to ensure completion of goal events, while building anaerobic endurance to achieve endurance-performance goals. Improved anaerobic endurance will help the client perform physical work at or near VT2 for an extended period, which will result in improved endurance, speed, and power to meet primary performance goals.

To program effective intervals for improving anaerobic endurance, the health coach should have the client perform the field test for VT2 to determine the client's HR at VT2 (see page 332). Once the health coach has current values for the client's HR at VT1 and VT2, he or she can establish a three-zone model that is specific to the client. For example, if a client's HR at VT1 is 143 bpm and HR at VT2 is 162 bpm, the client's HR zones would be as follows:

- Zone 1 = less than 143 bpm
- Zone 2 = 143 to 161 bpm
- Zone 3 = 162 bpm and above

These HR zones can then be used as intensity markers to help the client stay within the correct zone for the desired training outcome of a given workout.

Training intensity should be varied, with 70 to 80% of training in zone 1, approximately 10% to 20% of training in zone 3, and only brief periods (less that 10%) in zone 2. This large volume of zone 1 training time is critical to program success for clients with endurance-performance goals, as exercise frequency, intensity, and time all add to the total load. Individuals who increase each of these variables too quickly are at risk for burnout and overuse injuries. Table 17-7 illustrates the work in zones 1, 2, and 3 that might be performed by a client training for a marathon during a four-week training period.

Table 17-7

Sample Phase 3 Cardiorespiratory-training Program: Four-week Period for Marathon Training

Training Parameter	Week 1— Increase Intensity	Week 2— Increase Intensity	Week 3— Increase Intensity	Week 4— Recovery Week
Training Volume	Total training time = 9 hours	Total training time = 9.5 hours	Total training time = 10 hours	Total training time = 6.5 to 7.5 hours
Zone 1 (~80% of volume)	1 time/week Long run = 2 hours 30 min	1 time/week Long run = 2 hours 45 min	1 time/week Long run = 3 hours	1 time/week Long run = 2 hours
3 workouts per week plus warm-up, cool-down, and rest intervals during zone 2 and 3 workouts	1 time/week 90-min run (RPE = 4)	1 time/week 90-min run (RPE = 4)	1 time/week 90-min run (RPE = 4)	1 time/week 60-min run (RPE = 4)
	1 time/week 60-min run (RPE = 3–4)	1 time/week 60-min run (RPE = 3–4)	1 time/week 60-min run (RPE = 3–4)	1 time/week 45-min run (RPE = 3)
Zone 2 (~10% of volume)	3 x 5-min intervals 1:1½ work:rest ratio	4 x 5-min intervals 1:1½ work:rest ratio	5 x 5-min intervals 1:1½ work:rest ratio	2 x 8-min intervals 1:2 work:rest ratio
1 workout per week	60-min workout with long warm-up and cool-down	70-min workout with long warm-up and cool-down	75-min workout with long warm-up and cool-down	60-min workout with long warm-up and cool-down
Zone 3 (~10% of volume)	2 sets: 3 x 60-second intervals	3 sets: 3 x 45-second intervals	3 sets: 3 x 60-second intervals	2 sets: 3 x 30-second intervals
1 workout per week	1:3 work:rest ratio	1:3 work:rest ratio	1:3 work:rest ratio	1:3 work:rest ratio
	10 min between sets	10 min between sets	10 min between sets	10 min between sets
	60-min workout with long warm-up and cool-down	70-min workout with long warm-up and cool-down	75-min workout with long warm-up and cool-down	45-min workout with long warm-up and cool-down
Strength Training	Circuit training 2 days/week 1 hour/session	Circuit training 2 days/week 1 hour/session	Circuit training 2 days/week 1 hour/session	Circuit training 1–2 days/week 1 hour/session

If the client begins showing signs of overtraining (e.g., increased RHR, disturbed sleep, or decreased hunger on multiple days), the health coach should decrease the frequency and/or intensity of the client's intervals and provide more time for recovery. Also, if the client cannot reach the desired intensity during an interval, or is unable to reach the desired recovery intensity or heart rate during the recovery interval, the interval session should be stopped and the client should recover with cardiorespiratory exercise at an RPE of 3, and no more than 4, to prevent overtraining.

Phase 4: Anaerobic-power Training

The fourth phase of the ACE IFT Model for cardiorespiratory training focuses on anaerobic power. Only highly fit and competitive clients with very specific goals related to high-speed performance during endurance events will require exercise programming in phase 4. Some examples of athletes that might perform phase 4 training include track and road cyclists who compete in events that require repeated sprinting and recovery throughout the race and during the final sprint finish, competitive kayakers who need to paddle vigorously for short periods to navigate through difficult sections of rapids, and cross-country runners who need to be able to repeatedly surge up and recover following multiple hills during the course of a race.

This anaerobic-power training phase can essentially be thought of as strength training, although it is specific to the mode of activity (e.g., running or cycling). The intent is to perform very high-intensity training of nearly maximal muscular capacity, but with enough recovery to prevent the rapid accumulation of fatigue, so that the muscular system can be taxed maximally.

This is very specialized training intended to be performed by individuals preparing for competition. It is intended to increase the tolerance for the metabolic by-products of high-intensity exercise, including exercise performed at intensities greater than $\dot{V}O_2$max. Since this kind of training is very uncomfortable and, in older individuals, potentially dangerous, it should be performed only after a long period of training accommodation.

Program Design for Phase 4: Anaerobic-power Training

Most clients will never reach phase 4 training, as only clients with very specific goals for achieving high sprinting speed and/or short bursts of very high levels of power for challenges such as short hills, will require anaerobic-power training. Some health coaches who work with more highly competitive clients may work with several clients per year who train in phase 4, while others may not work with anyone in phase 4 for several years. Even elite athletes will only spend part of a given year performing phase 4 training cycles to prepare for specific competitions.

Obviously, this kind of training is only designed for individuals interested in competition, and can be tolerated only on a limited basis. Examples might include 6 x 100-meter acceleration runs, where the middle 40 meters are performed at absolute maximal intensity. There might be five minutes of recovery between runs, allowing for full recovery. This type of training should not generally be viewed as cardiorespiratory training. It is entirely supplemental and designed for muscular accommodation.

The total weekly exercise program for a client training in phase 4 will look similar to a client training in phase 3, with 70 to 80% of the training time in zone 1, approximately 10% to 20% of training in zone 3, and only brief periods (less that 10%) in zone 2. The difference will be in the types of intervals performed during some of the zone 3 workout time. Intervals for the phase

4 client will be very short sprints or hill sprints designed to tax the **phosphagen** stores in the muscles and create a rapid rise in blood **lactate** levels. These short, highly intense intervals (RPE of 9 to 10) will be followed by long recovery intervals that may be 10 to 20 times longer than the work intervals. For example, a client could perform 5 x 10-second accelerations while cycling on a relatively flat road with little traffic, with each acceleration followed by a 2- to 3-minute recovery interval (10-second work interval with 120- to 180-second recovery interval). These anaerobic-power intervals are supplementary to the full training program performed by a client who has endurance-performance goals. As such, these intervals should be performed only once per week as a complement to the full endurance-training program.

Functional Movement and Resistance Training Based on the ACE IFT Model

There are two essential prerequisite stages to training clients that are frequently overlooked. Traditional training focuses on strengthening muscles or improving their endurance capacity in isolation and generally disregards the relationship of the entire kinetic chain (stability-mobility relationship) with reference to postural alignment of the joints. Health coaches should always emphasize these two stages (ACE IFT Model phases 1 and 2) during the initial portion of a client's training program to "straighten the body before strengthening it," and restore good joint alignment and muscle balance across joints. Good joint alignment facilitates effective muscle action and joint movement, serving as the platform from which good exercise technique is built. Given the complexity of current exercise equipment and the advanced nature of many exercises, health coaches must stress the importance of learning how to perform the five primary movement patterns correctly, as they represent the foundation to all movement (see Figure 17-23, page 503). Proper execution of these movements enhances the potential to promote movement efficiency, as well as long-term maintenance and integrity of the joint structures, muscles, connective tissues, and nerves of the musculoskeletal system.

Once the functional aspects of movement have been adequately addressed, clients can progress on to resistance training with increasing weightloads. Strength training improves the client's fitness level by placing emphasis on muscle force production and manipulating the variables of training to address a variety of specific exercise goals. For many clients, phase 3 (load training) will be the final phase they will reach in their exercise programming, as phase 4 (performance training) of the ACE IFT Model involves training techniques and methods designed to enhance athletic performance. While a number of clients will welcome the challenge of incorporating athletic-training techniques into their programs for variety and possibly improved performance in team or individual competitions, many clients will not want to take this extra step.

Phase 1: Stability and Mobility Training

Strengthening muscles to improve posture should initially focus on placing the client in positions of good posture and begin with a series of low-grade isometric contractions [<50% of maximal effort or **maximal voluntary contraction (MVC)**], with the client completing two to four repetitions of five to 10 seconds each. The goal is to condition the postural (tonic) muscles that typically contain greater concentrations of **type I muscle fibers** with volume as opposed to intensity (Kendall et al., 2005). Higher intensities that require greater amounts of force will generally evoke faulty recruitment patterns. The exercise volume can be gradually increased (overload) to improve strength and endurance, and to reestablish muscle balance at the joints.

Because many deconditioned individuals lack the ability to stabilize the entire kinetic chain, the initial emphasis should be placed on muscle isolation using supportive surfaces and devices (e.g., floor, wall, or chair backrest) prior to introducing integrated (whole-body, unsupported) strengthening exercises. For example, to help a client strengthen the **posterior** deltoids and rhomboids, which are associated with forward-rounded shoulders, a health coach could start by having the client perform reverse flys in a **supine** position, isometrically pressing the backs of the arms into the floor, rather than sets of dynamic high-back rows using external resistance. The use of support offers the additional benefit of kinesthetic and visual feedback, which is critical to helping clients understand the alignment of specific joints (e.g., when lying on the floor, the individual can feel and see the contact points with the floor when joints are placed in ideal postural positions). The strengthening exercises should ultimately progress to dynamic movement, initially controlling the ROM to avoid excessive muscle lengthening before introducing full-ROM movement patterns. An important concept to keep in mind is that while a muscle may be strong in a lengthened position, it needs strength at a normal and healthy resting length (Lieber, 2009; MacIntosh, Gardiner, & McComas, 2006; Williams & Goldspink, 1978). For example, to strengthen the rhomboids using more dynamic movements, the client should hold the scapulae in a good postural position and avoid scapular **protraction** and **retraction** during the movement. Dynamic strengthening exercises for good posture do not involve heavy loads, but rather volume training to condition the type I fibers. Consequently, health coaches should plan on one to three sets of 12 to 15 repetitions when introducing dynamic strengthening exercises. To summarize, the strengthening of weakened muscles follows a progression model beginning with two to four repetitions of isometric muscle contractions, each held for five to 10 seconds at less than 50% of MVC in a supported, more isolated environment. The next progression is to dynamic, controlled ROM exercises incorporating one to three sets of 12 to 15 repetitions.

Addressing Mobility Needs in the Obese Population

Many of the stability and mobility exercises presented in the following sections require the client to lie down or sit on the floor. This can be challenging for obese clients who find it difficult to transition from standing to lying or sitting on the floor, and vice versa. Painful joints or other musculoskeletal problems combined with increased body mass might make performing floor-based exercises a poor choice for obese clients. Alternatively, floor exercises can be performed on an elevated platform or on a sturdy athletic training table. These options allow obese clients to perform the necessary movements while lying down or being seated without the uncomfortable, and perhaps intimidating, task of transitioning to the floor. Health coaches who consistently work with obese clients should make an effort to obtain some type of elevated exercise surface for this special population.

Proximal Stability: Activating the Core

The goal of functional movement and resistance training is to promote stability of the lumbar spine by improving the reflexive function of the core musculature that essentially serves to stabilize this region during loading and movement. The core functions to effectively control the position and motion of the trunk over the pelvis, which allows optimal production, transfer, and control of force and motion to more distal segments during whole-body movements (Willardson, 2007; Kibler, Press, & Sciascia, 2006). The term "core" generally refers to the muscles of the lumbo-pelvic region, hips, abdomen, and lower back. Table 17-8 provides guidelines for exercise progression for core activation when a client is lying supine (Figure 17-3). Table 17-9 provides an exercise progression for core stabilization when a client is on the hands-and-knees (Figure 17-4).

Table 17-8

Exercise Progression for Core Activation

Pelvic floor contractions ("Kegels," or the contraction to interrupt the flow of urine)	Perform 1-2 sets x 10 repetitions with a 2-second tempo, 10-15 second rest intervals between sets
TVA contractions (drawing the belly button toward the spine)	Perform 1-2 sets x 10 repetitions with a 2-second tempo, 10-15 second rest intervals between sets
Combination of both contractions	Perform 1-2 sets x 10 repetitions with a 2-second tempo, 10-15 second rest intervals between sets
Contractions with normal breathing	Perform 1-2 sets x 5-6 repetitions with slow, 10-second counts while breathing independently, 10-15 second rest intervals between sets Progress to 3-4 sets x 10-12 repetitions, each with a 10-second count, 10-15 second rest intervals between sets

Note: TVA = Transverse abdominis

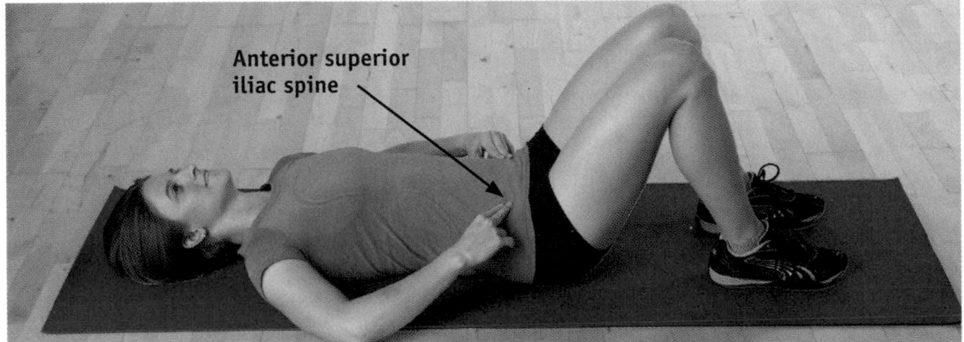

Figure 17-3
Supine drawing-in body position

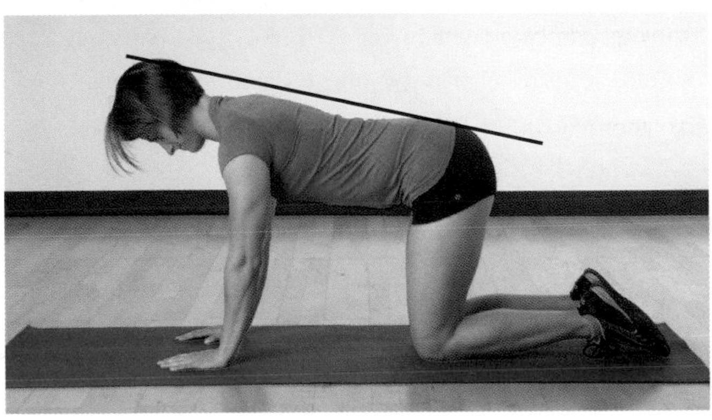

a.

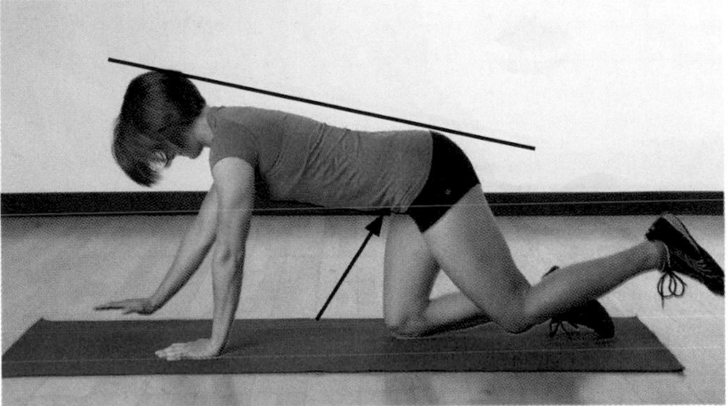

b.

Figure 17-4
Quadruped drawing-in with extremity movement

Table 17-9	
Exercise Progression for Core Stabilization	
1. Raise one arm 0.5 to 1 inch (1.25 to 2.5 cm) off the floor and perform the sequence of controlled shoulder movements: • 6–12 inch (15–30 cm) sagittal plane shoulder movements (flexion/extension) • 6–12 inch (15–30 cm) frontal plane shoulder movements (abduction/adduction) • 6–12 inch (15–30 cm) transverse plane shoulder movements (circles or circumduction)	Perform 1-2 sets x 10 repetitions with a 2-second tempo, use 10–15 second rest intervals between sets
2. Raise one knee 0.5 to 1 inch (1.25 to 2.5 cm) off the floor and perform the sequence of controlled hip movements: • 6–12 inch (15–30 cm) sagittal plane hip movements (flexion/extension) • 6–12 inch (15–30 cm) frontal plane hip movements (abduction/adduction) • 6–12 inch (15–30 cm) transverse plane hip movements (circles)	Perform 1-2 sets x 10 repetitions with a 2-second tempo, use 10–15 second rest intervals between sets
3. Raise contralateral limbs (i.e., one arm and the opposite knee) 0.5 to 1 inch (1.25 to 2.5 cm) off the floor and perform the sequence of movements: • Repeat the above movements in matching planes (i.e., simultaneous movement in the same plane with both limbs) or alternating planes (i.e., mixing the planes between the two limbs). • This contralateral movement pattern mimics the muscle-activation patterns used during the push-off phase portion of walking and is an effective exercise to train this pattern.	Perform 1-2 sets x 10 repetitions with a 2-second tempo, use 10–15 second rest intervals between sets

Proximal Mobility: Hips and Thoracic Spine

Improving mobility of the two joints immediately adjacent to the lumbar spine is the focus of proximal mobility. Based on observations made during the postural assessment and movement screens, limitations in mobility within these two areas in any of the three planes should become the focus. Health coaches should follow some fundamental principles when programming to improve mobility in these body regions:

- Although these two regions should exhibit good mobility in all three planes, they are typically prone to poor mobility. Consequently, some static stretching to improve muscle flexibility (or extensibility) should precede dynamic mobilization exercises.
- When attempting to improve muscle flexibility or joint mobility, clients must avoid undesirable or compensated movements at successive joints (e.g., avoid any increases in lumbar lordosis associated with a tight latissimus dorsi muscle during an overhead stretch).
- Because the body may lack the ability to effectively stabilize the entire kinetic chain, supportive surfaces should be utilized while promoting mobility (e.g., floor, benches, and backrests).
- Because muscles contribute to movement in all three planes, health coaches should incorporate flexibility exercises that lengthen the muscles of the hips and thoracic spine in all three planes.

Figures 17-5 through 17-9 present exercises that promote mobility of the hips, while Figures 17-10 and 17-11 present exercises that promote mobility of the thoracic spine.

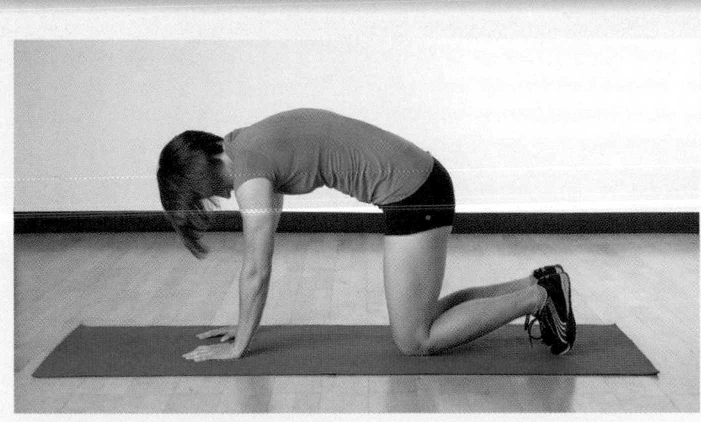

a.

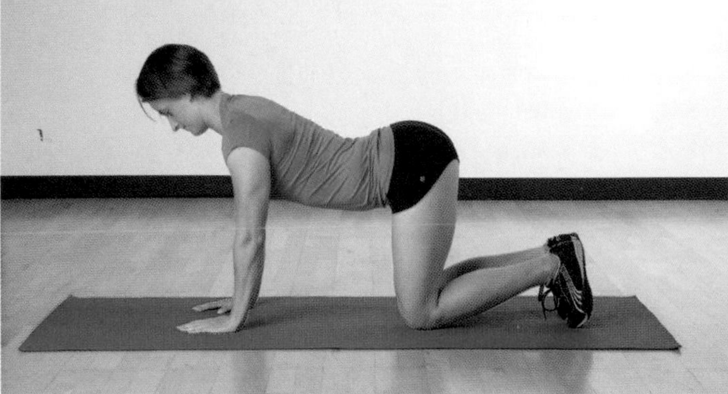

b.

Figure 17-5
Cat-camel

Objective: To improve extensibility within the lumbar extensor muscles

Preparation and position:

- Assume the quadruped position with the hands positioned directly under the shoulders (shoulder-width apart) and the knees positioned directly under the hips (hip-width apart).
- Engage the core muscles to create a neutral spine in this starting position.
- The elbows should remain extended throughout the exercise.

Exercise:

- From this starting position, exhale slowly while contracting the abdominals [draw the belly button toward the spine (i.e., "hollowing")], gently pushing and rounding the entire back upward. Drop the head, bringing the chin toward the chest (a).
- Hold this position for 15 seconds.
- Slowly inhale, relax, and return to the starting position, but allow the stomach and spine to sag toward the floor. Allow the shoulders to collapse (adduct) toward the spine, and tilt the head upward (b).
- Hold this position for 15 seconds.
- Perform two to four repetitions.

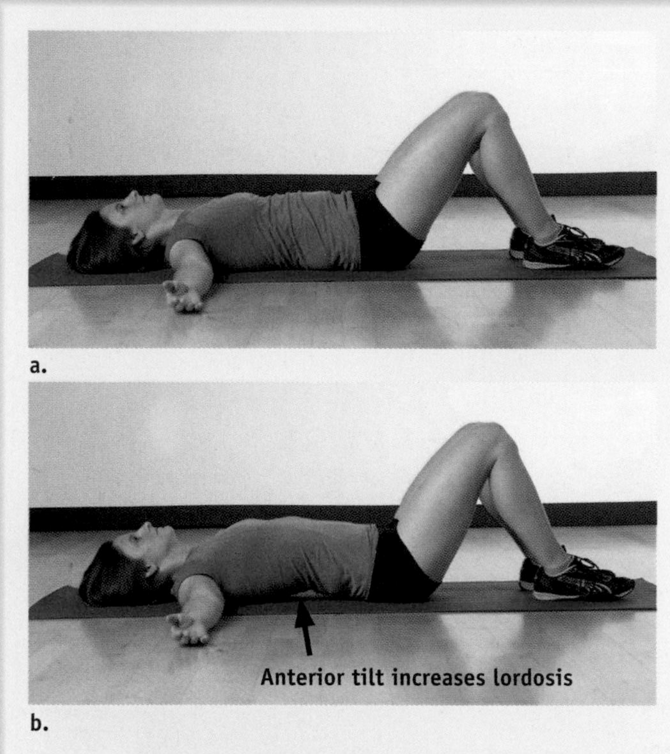

a.
b.

Figure 17-6
Pelvic tilts

Objective: To improve hip mobility in the sagittal plane

Preparation and position:

- Lie supine with the knees bent and the feet placed flat on the floor, aligning the anterior superior iliac spine (ASIS) with the knee and second toe.
- Abduct the arms to shoulder height, resting them on the floor with the arms externally rotated (palms facing upward) (a).

Exercise:

- Slowly contract the abdominals to tilt the pelvis posteriorly, hold briefly, relax and then contract the erector spinae muscles and hip flexors to tilt the pelvis anteriorly (b).
- Perform one or two sets of five to 10 controlled repetitions, holding the end position for one or two seconds with 30-second rest intervals between sets.

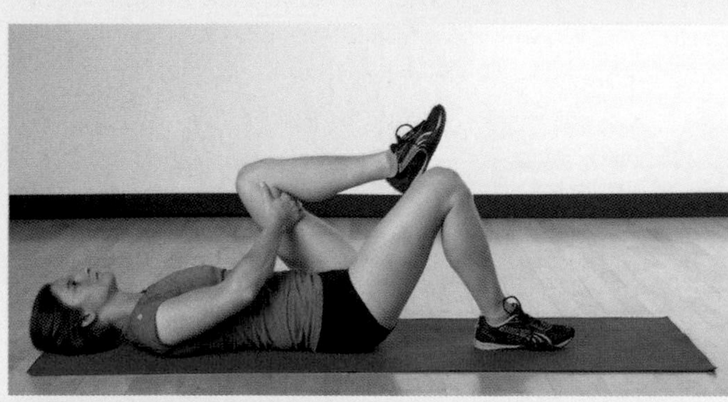
a.

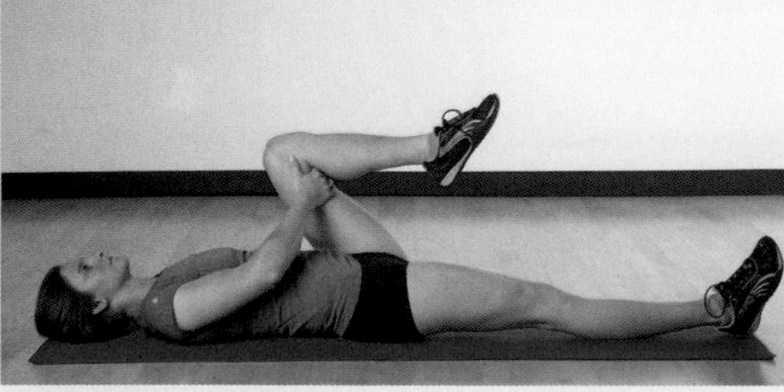
b.

Figure 17-7
Hip flexor mobility: Lying hip flexor stretch

Objective: To improve mobility of the hip flexors in the sagittal plane without compromising lumbar stability

Preparation and position:

- Lie supine with the knees bent and the feet placed flat on the floor, aligning the anterior superior iliac spine (ASIS) with the knee and second toe.
- Engage the core muscles to stabilize the lumbar spine in the neutral position and maintain this position throughout the exercise.

Exercise:

- Reach both hands behind one knee and gently pull the knee toward the chest (a).
- Slowly extend the opposite leg until it is either fully extended or lumbar stability is compromised (b).
- Perform two to four repetitions per side, each for a minimum of 15 seconds.

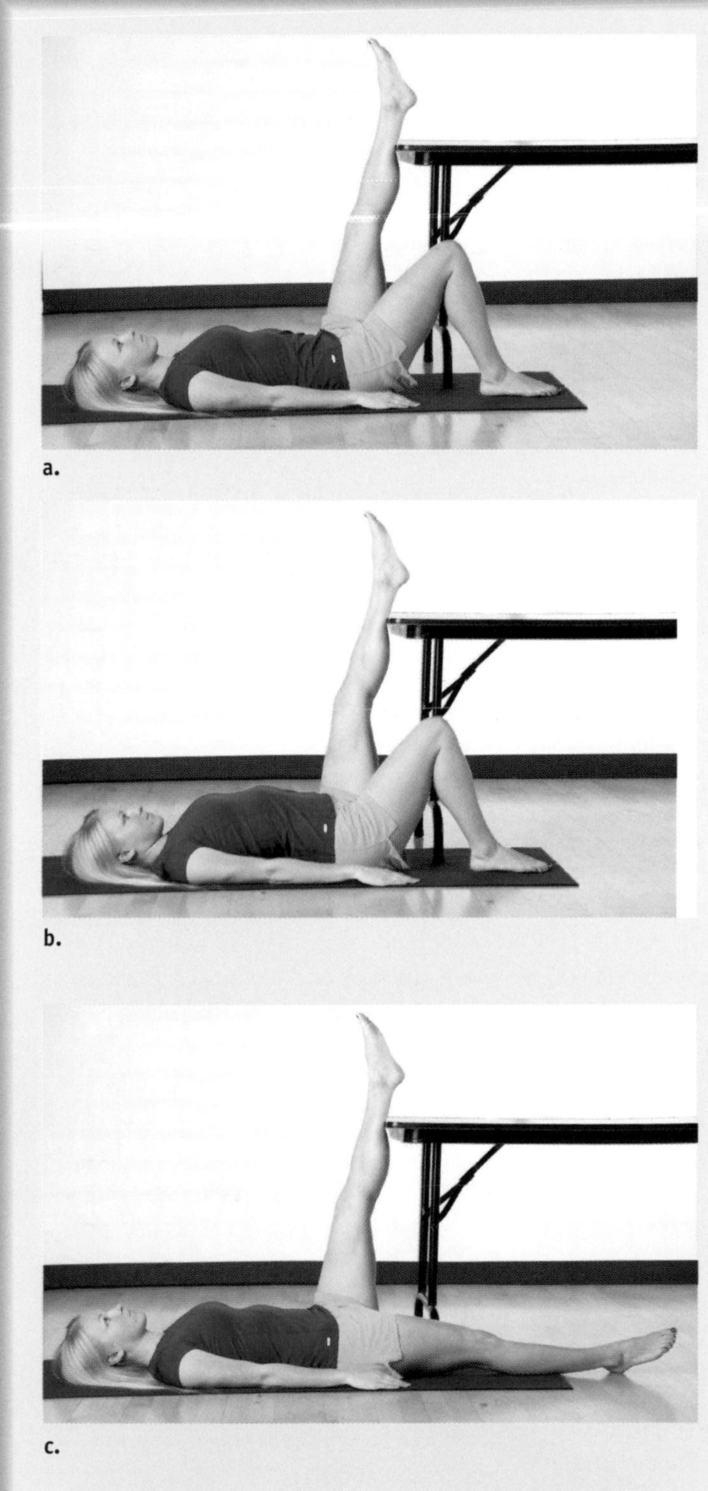

a.

b.

c.

Figure 17-8
Hamstrings mobility: Lying hamstrings stretch

Objective: To improve mobility of the hamstrings in the sagittal plane without compromising lumbar stability

Preparation and position:

- Lie supine inside a door jamb or beside a sturdy table with one knee bent and the foot placed flat on the floor, aligning the anterior superior iliac spine (ASIS) with the knee and second toe.
- Engage the core muscles to stabilize the lumbar spine in the neutral position, and maintain this position throughout the exercise.
- Raise the opposite leg to rest it on the table or door jamb with slight flexion in the knee and plantar flexion at the ankle (to remove any limitation from the gastrocnemius during the stretch) (a).

Exercise:

- Exhale and slowly extend the raised leg, stretching the hamstrings.
- The objective is to promote hamstrings flexibility with the extended leg positioned at an 80- to 90-degree angle with the floor.
- Perform two to four repetitions per side, each for a minimum of 15 seconds.

Progression: Perform a series of pelvic tilts, holding the anterior pelvic tilt to increase the magnitude of he stretch (b).

Progression: Extend the lower leg for the duration of the stretch without compromising lumbar stability (c).

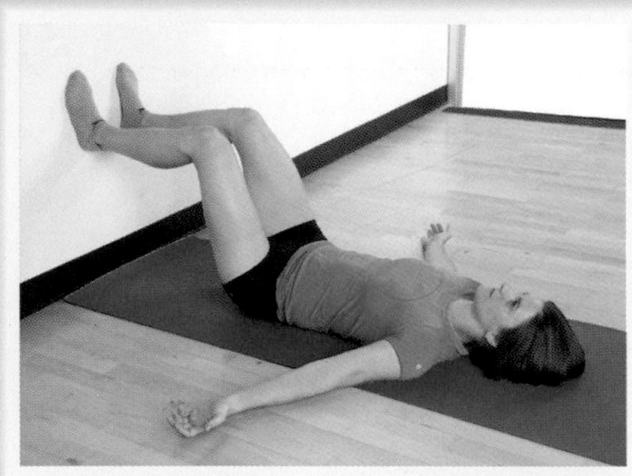

a.

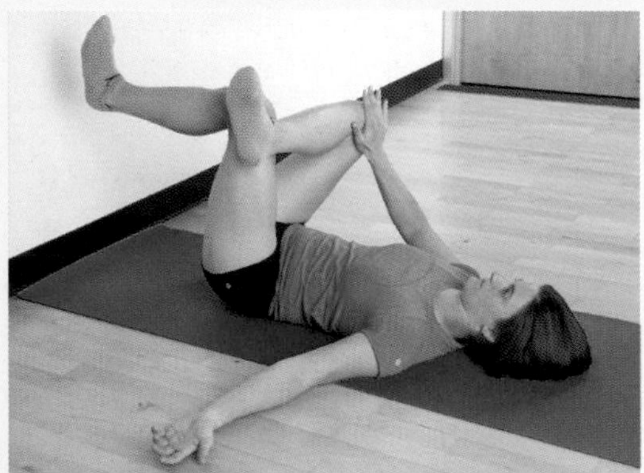

b.

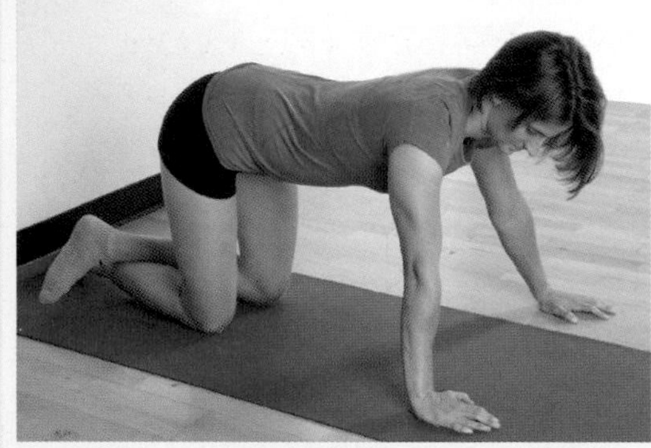

c.

Figure 17-9
Hip mobilization: Supine 90-90 hip rotator stretch

Objective: To improve hip mobility in the transverse plane

Preparation and position:

- Lie supine with both feet placed against a wall, with an approximately 90-degree bend at the knees and 60 to 80 degrees of flexion at the hips (a).
- Cross one leg over the opposite knee, resting that ankle on the knee.
- Engage the core muscles to stabilize the lumbar spine in the neutral position and maintain this position throughout the exercise.
- Place one hand on the crossed knee.

Exercise:

- Exhale and gently push the crossed knee away from the body while simultaneously lifting the opposite foot off the wall, increasing the degree of hip flexion (b).
- Perform two to four repetitions per side.
- Hold each stretch for a minimum of 15 seconds.

Progression: Assume the quadruped position, crossing the lower part of the left leg over the right leg (externally rotating the left leg). Position the left arm 1 to 2 feet (30 to 61 cm) out to the side of the body (c). Slowly lean the body out to that side, supporting the weight on the outspread hand (d). Perform two to four repetitions per side and hold each stretch for a minimum of 15 seconds (Tumminello, 2007).

Progression: Assume the quadruped position, engaging the core muscles to stabilize the lumbar spine. Lift the left leg slightly, extend it backward while sliding it across the right leg and behind the body, and drop the hips toward the floor during the movement while avoiding hip rotation (e) (Tumminello, 2007). Perform one or two sets of five to 10 controlled repetitions per side, holding the end range of motion for one or two seconds, with 30-second rest intervals between sets.

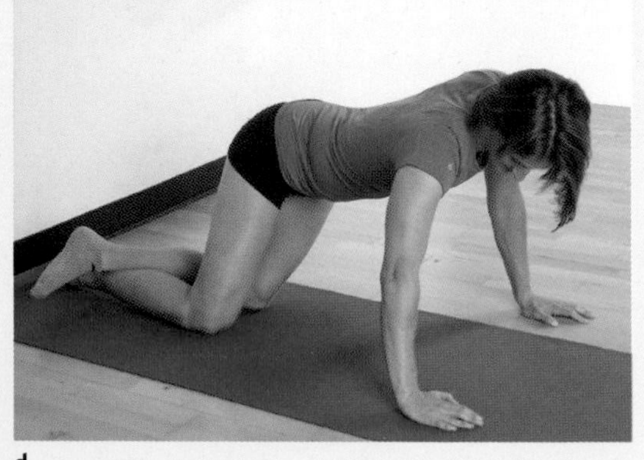

d.

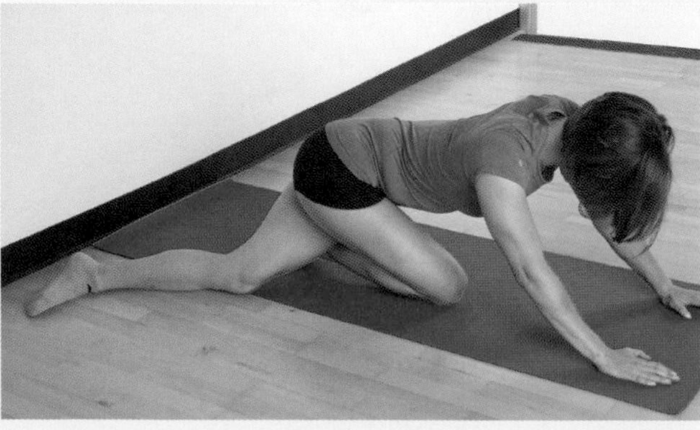

e.

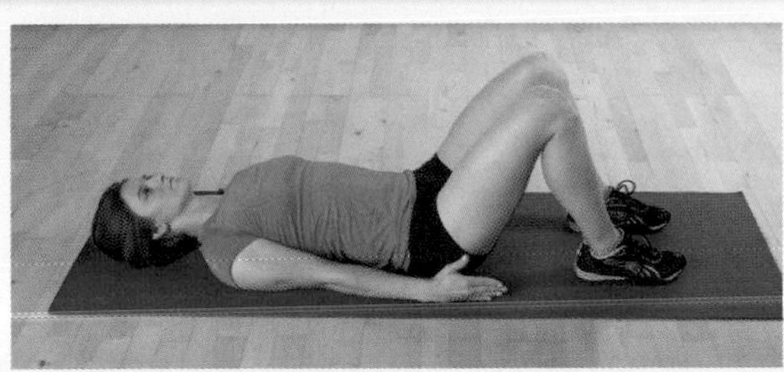

a.

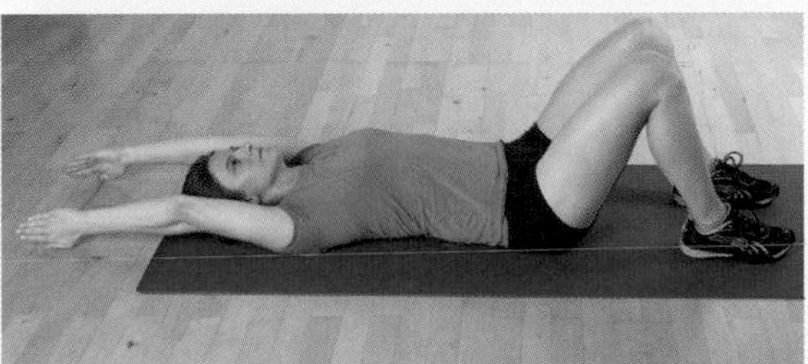

b.

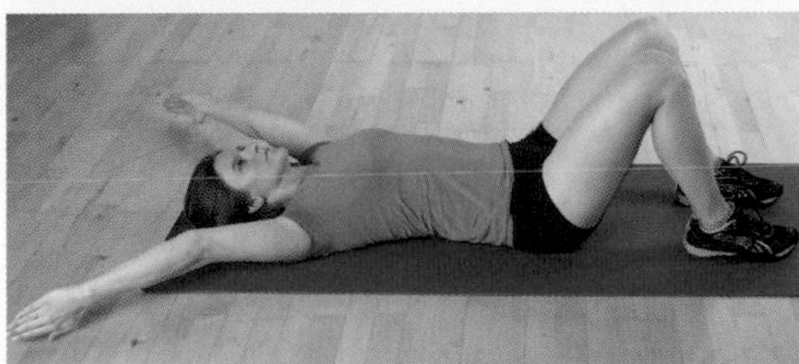

c.

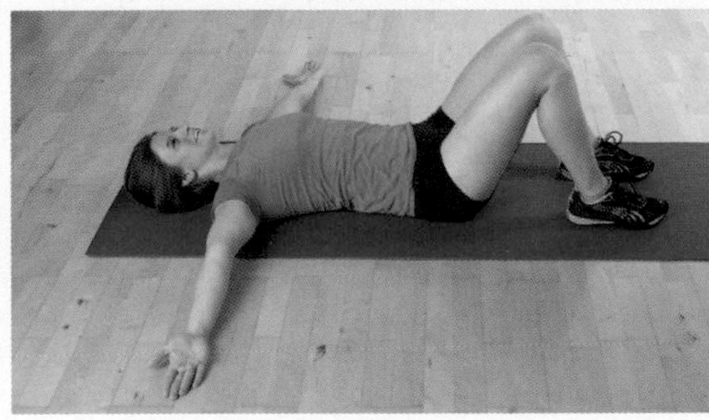

d.

Figure 17-10

Thoracic spine (T-spine) mobilization exercises: Spinal extensions and spinal twists

Spinal Extensions

Objective: To promote thoracic extension

Preparation and position:

- Lie supine with the knees bent and feet placed flat on the floor, aligning the anterior superior iliac spine (ASIS) with the knee and second toe.
- Position the arms at the sides with elbows extended.
- Engage the core muscles to stabilize the lumbar spine (avoiding increased lordosis during the exercise) and maintain this contraction throughout the exercise.
- Depress and retract the scapulae while stabilizing the low back (a).

Exercise:

- Exhale and slowly flex the shoulders, raise both arms overhead, and attempt to bring both hands to touch the floor overhead ("I" position) (b). Since the arms tend to internally rotate during shoulder flexion, and shrugging of the shoulders often occurs, attempt to depress the scapulae and keep the arms in a neutral or externally rotated position.
- Slowly return to the starting position.
- Perform one or two sets of five to 10 controlled repetitions, holding the end range of motion for one to two seconds, with 30-second rest intervals between sets.
- Repeat the entire movement from the starting position, but move into a "Y" formation, abducting the arms to 135 degrees (c).
- Repeat the entire movement from the starting position, but move in a "T" formation, sliding the arms along the floor and abducting them to 90 degrees (d).
- Repeat the entire movement from the starting position, but, with the elbows bent, move in a "wiper formation," sliding the arms along the floor from the sides to an overhead position.

Continued on next page

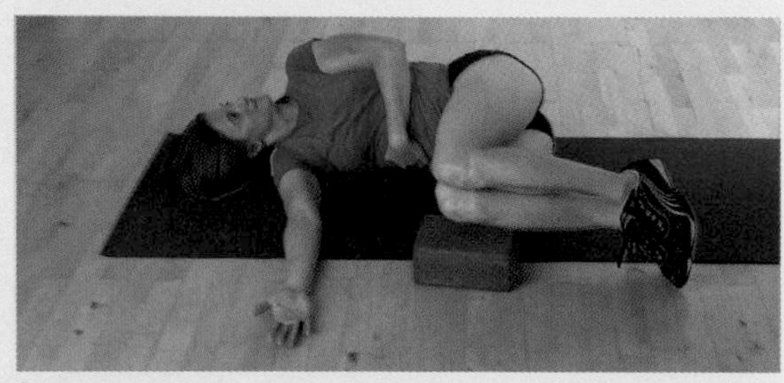
e.

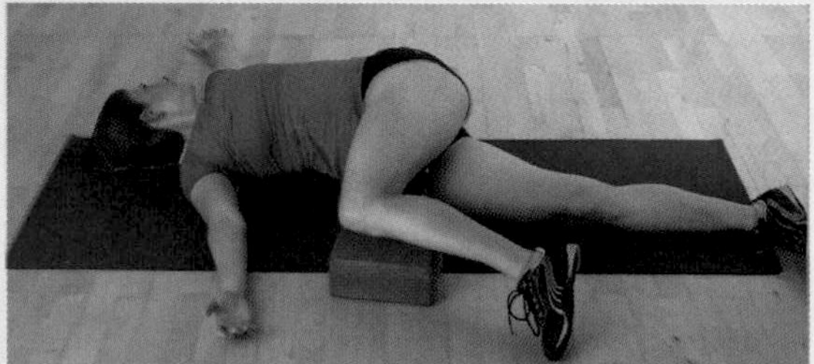
f.

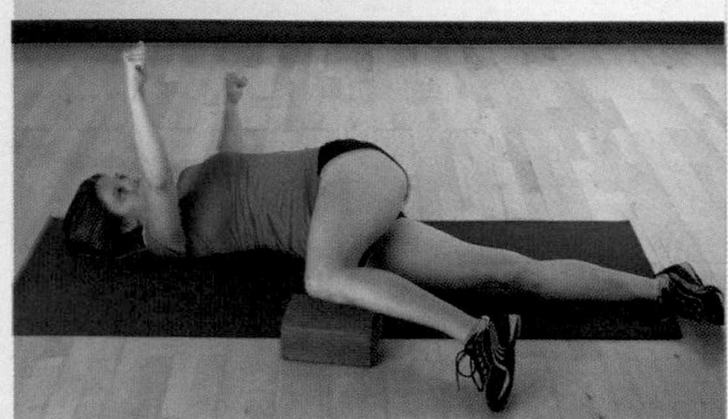
g.

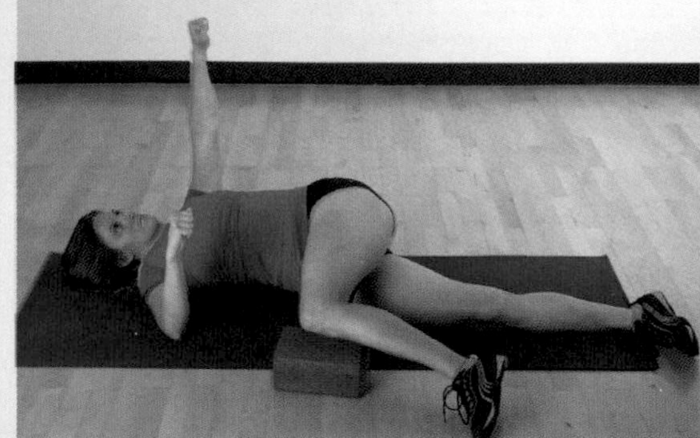
h.

Spinal Twists

Objective: To promote trunk rotation, primarily through the thoracic spine with some lateral hip mobility

Preparation and position:

- Lie on one side, bending both knees to 90 degrees, flexing the hips to 90 to 100 degrees, and aligning both knees together, resting them on a ball or riser. Keep the lower knee on the ball or riser throughout this first exercise progression and keep both knees aligned. Engage the core muscles to stabilize the lumbar spine (avoiding increased lordosis) and maintain this contraction throughout the exercise.
- Reach the upper arm across and in front of the body, grasping the ribcage on the opposite side of the trunk (e).

Exercise:

- Exhale and slowly rotate the torso by pulling on the ribcage. Attempt to avoid any rotational movement of the hips and knees.
- Perform two to four repetitions to each side.
- Hold each pull for 15 to 30 seconds.

Progression: Repeat the same stretch, but place a squeezable object (e.g., a soft ball or yoga block) between the knees, positioning the lower knee on the floor.

Progression: Repeat the same stretch, but extend the lower leg and rest the inside of the upper knee on a squeezable object.

Progression: Repeat the same stretch, but change the upper arm from the rib-grab position to abducting the arm to 90 degrees with an extended elbow, and attempt to bring the upper arm down to touch the floor (f).

Progression—push-pull: Assume any of the starting positions for the lower extremity on one side. Depress and retract both scapulae, then move the upper arm to the start position of a press movement (e.g., bench press), while the lower arm moves into the start position of a pull movement (without protracting the scapula) (g & h). Simultaneously perform an upward press with the upper arm and a high-back row with the lower arm. Perform one or two sets of five to 10 controlled repetitions per side, holding the end range of motion for one or two seconds, with 30-second rest intervals between sets.

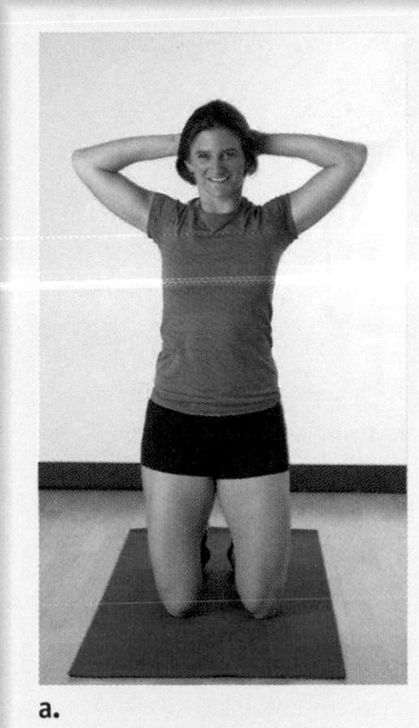

a.

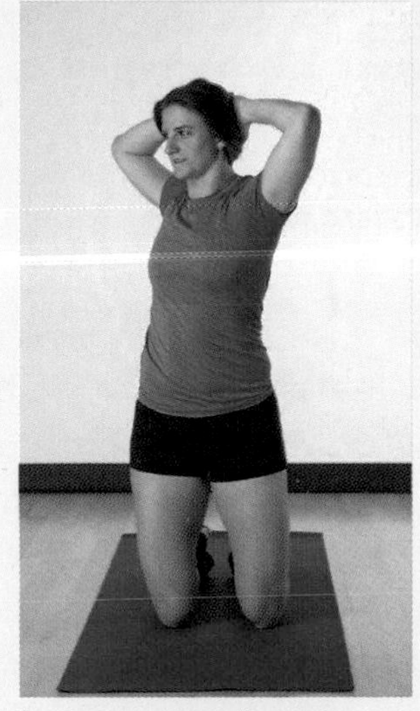

b.

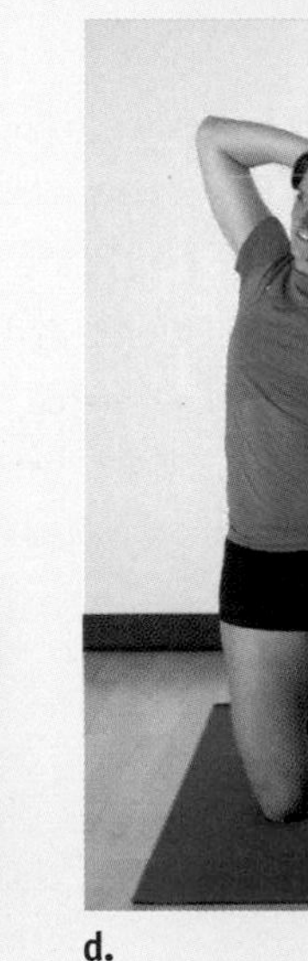

c.

d.

Figure 17-11

Thoracic spine (T-spine) mobilization: Prisoner rotations

Objective: To promote thoracic spine mobility in the transverse plane

Preparation and position:

- Assume a kneeling position and interlock the hands lightly behind the head without pulling the head forward into neck flexion (a).
- Engage the core muscles to stabilize the lumbar spine, and maintain this contraction throughout the exercise.
- The exercise objective is to promote trunk rotation, primarily within the thoracic spine without rotating the hips.

Exercise:

- Exhale and slowly rotate the arms to the right until a point of resistance is reached (no bouncing movement) (b). Avoid rotating the hips.
- Hold this position for 15 seconds and then laterally flex the trunk, pointing the right elbow toward the floor (c). Hold this position for five seconds.
- Return to an upright position and then laterally flex in the opposite direction (d). Hold this position for five seconds.
- Return to the upright position and allow the trunk to rotate further into the movement.
- Perform two to four repetitions to each side.

Source: Tumminello, N. (2007). *Warm-up Progressions—Volumes 1 and 2*. Baltimore, Md.: Performance University.

Proximal Stability of the Scapulothoracic Region and Distal Mobility of the Glenohumeral Joint

Improving stability within the scapulothoracic region during upper-extremity movements (e.g., push- and pull-type motions), while promoting movement at the glenohumeral joint, is an important focus of exercises for the shoulder and shoulder girdle. The glenohumeral joint is a highly mobile joint and its ability to achieve this degree of movement is contingent upon the stability of the scapulothoracic region (i.e., the ability of the scapulae to maintain appropriate proximity against the ribcage during movement) (Houglum, 2010; Sahrmann, 2002). It is the synergistic actions of muscle groups working through **force-couples** in this region that help achieve this stability, considering that the scapulae only attach to the **axial skeleton** via the clavicle. Promoting stability within this joint, therefore, requires muscle balance within the force-couples of the joint. Additionally, as many of these muscles also cross the glenohumeral joint, they require substantial levels of mobility. This implies that a program promoting scapulothoracic stability may need to include stretches to promote extensibility of both the muscle and joint structures. Therefore, static stretches to improve tissue extensibility should precede dynamic movement patterns and strengthening exercises.

To enhance tissue extensibility, clients can employ several different stretching modalities. Myofascial release using a stick or foam roller—moving across the tender spots—will help realign the elastic fibers and reduce hypertonicity (see page 459 for more information on myofascial release) (Barnes, 1999). This should precede static stretching of the shoulder capsule and of specific muscles of the scapulae. When stretching the shoulder capsule with a client, health coaches must address the **inferior**, posterior, anterior, and **superior** components.

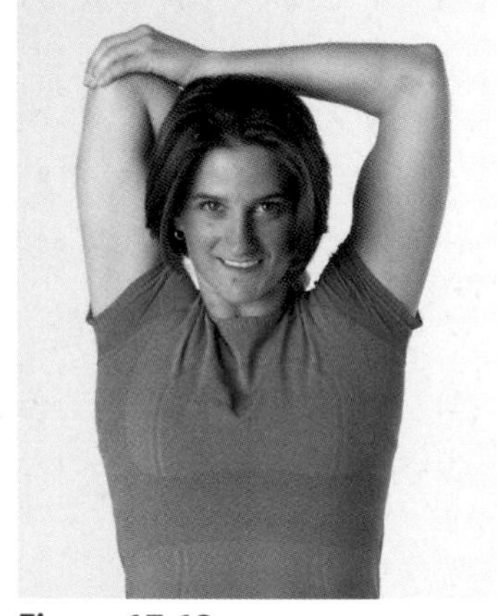

Figure 17-12
Overhead triceps stretch

- Stretch the inferior capsule using an overhead triceps stretch (Figure 17-12).
- Stretch the posterior capsule by bringing the arm across and in front of the body (Figure 17-13a). An alternative position for this stretch is to stand adjacent to a wall, flexing the arm in front of the body to 90 degrees and resting the full length of the arm against the wall (Figure 17-13b), then slowly rotate the trunk inward toward the wall (Figure 17-13c). Since this movement also produces scapular abduction, and since it is common for clients to have abducted scapulae as a postural deviation, it should be a minimal focus during shoulder stretching.
- Stretch the anterior capsule using a pectoralis stretch (Figure 17-14).
- Stretch the superior capsule by placing a rolled-up towel 2 inches above the elbow against the trunk (bent-elbow position at the side of the body), grasping the base of the elbow and pulling it downward and inward (Figure 17-15).

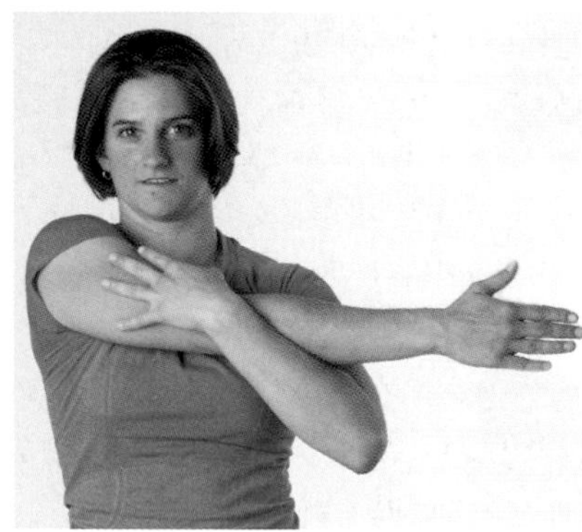

a.

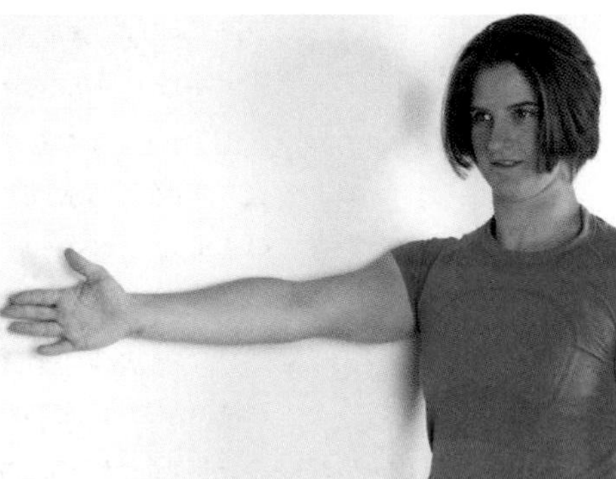

b.

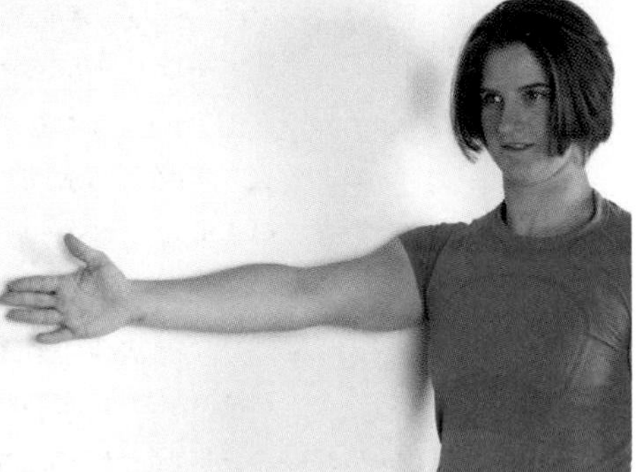

c.

Figure 17-13
Posterior capsule stretches

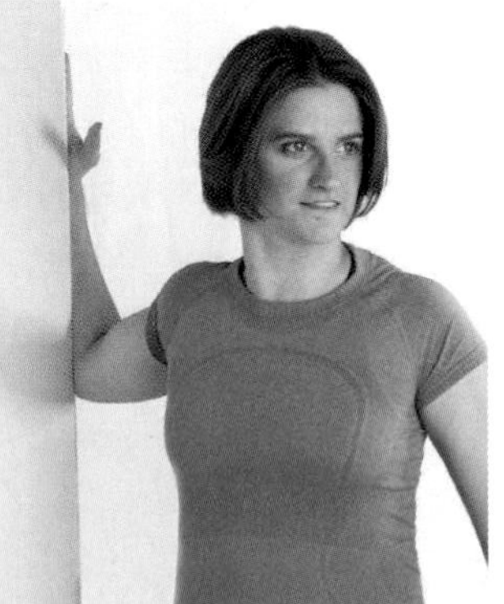

Figure 17-14
Anterior capsule (pectoralis) stretch

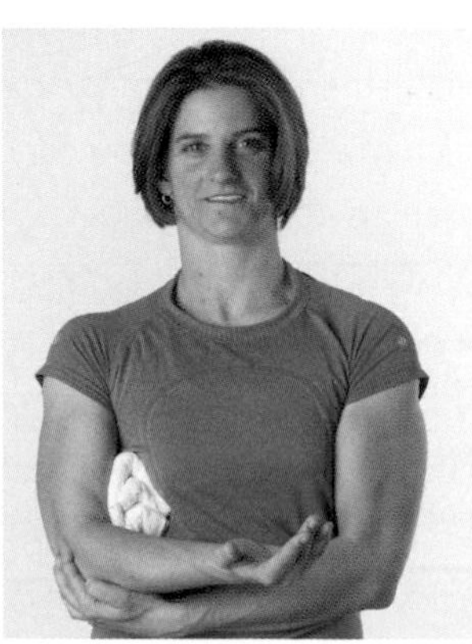

Figure 17-15
Superior capsule stretch

One important consideration for promoting scapulothoracic stability revolves around the type of exercises selected (i.e., closed-chain or open-chain exercises). During **closed kinetic chain (CKC)** movements where the distal segment is more fixed (e.g., pull-ups and push-ups), a key role of the serratus anterior is to move the thorax toward a more fixed, stable scapulae (Houglum, 2010; Cook & Jones, 2007a). During **open kinetic chain (OKC)** movements (e.g., front raises and side lateral raises), however, a key role of the serratus anterior is to control movement of the scapulae about the ribcage (Houglum, 2010; Cook & Jones, 2007a). CKC movements are generally considered more functional, as they mimic daily activities closely. CKC exercises load and compress joints, increasing kinesthetic awareness and **proprioception,** which translates into improved parascapular and shoulder stability (Cook & Jones, 2007a). Isolated OKC exercises, on the other hand, are not as effective in restoring coordinated parascapular control. One challenge with CKC exercises is that many are too challenging for deconditioned individuals. Thus, it is important to initially use the floor to provide kinesthetic feedback as the client lies supine and OKC movements to improve control and movement efficiency and increase kinesthetic awareness of shoulder position. Health coaches can start by first helping the individual recognize the normal resting position of the scapulae kinesthetically (i.e., feel the correct scapulae position against the floor). The exercise presented in Figure 17-16 helps achieve this awareness by instructing the client on how to "pack" the scapulae.

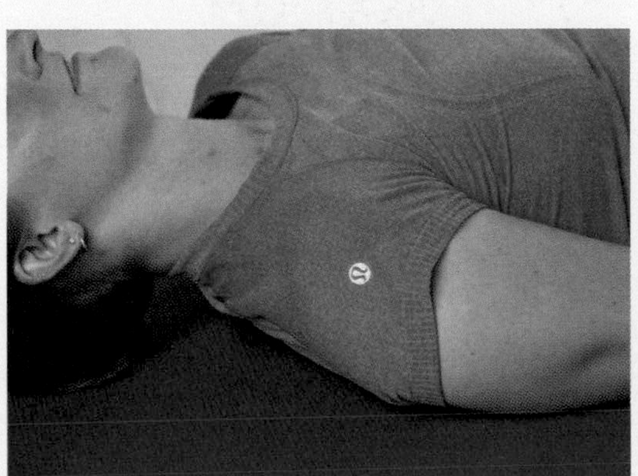

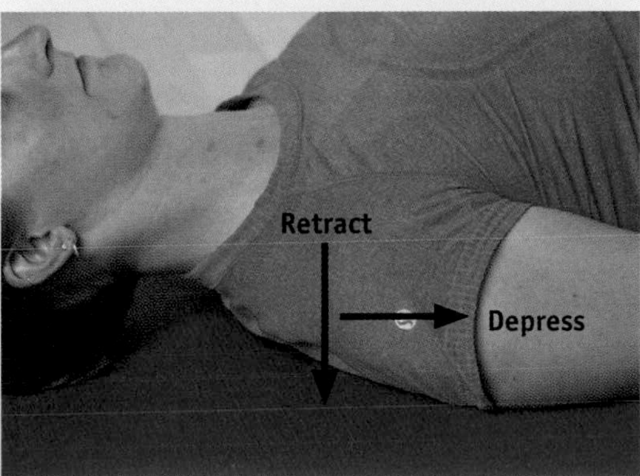

b.

Figure 17-16
Shoulder packing

Objective: To kinesthetically improve awareness of good scapular position, improving flexibility and strength of key parascapular muscles

Preparation and position:

- Lie supine on a mat with knees bent to 90 degrees and the feet placed flat on the floor, aligning the anterior superior iliac spine (ASIS) with the knee and second toe.
- Position the arms at the sides of the trunk with the palms facing upward.
- Engage the core muscles to stabilize the lumbar spine in the neutral position. Maintain this position throughout the exercise (a).

Exercise:

- Exhale and perform two to four repetitions of each of the following, holding each contraction for five to 10 seconds (b):
  - ✓ Scapular depression
  - ✓ Scapular retraction
- Using passive assistance from the opposite arm, gently push down on the shoulder (posterior tilt on scapula) without losing lumbar stability. Hold this position for 15 to 60 seconds.
- Relax and repeat two to four times on each shoulder.

A variety of exercises can be used to condition the rotator cuff muscles, but whichever exercises are selected, the client must perform them from the packed shoulder position. Figures 17-17 through 17-20 provide examples of OKC and CKC rotator cuff exercises that promote scapulothoracic stability.

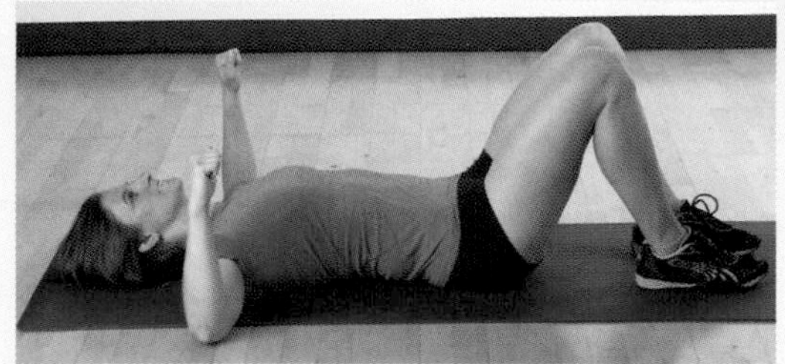
a.

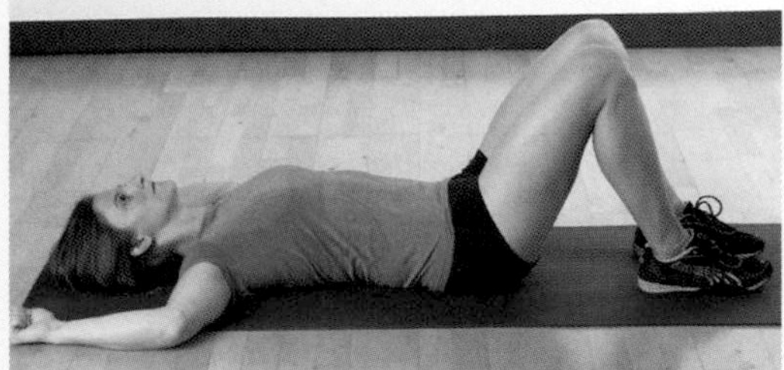
b.

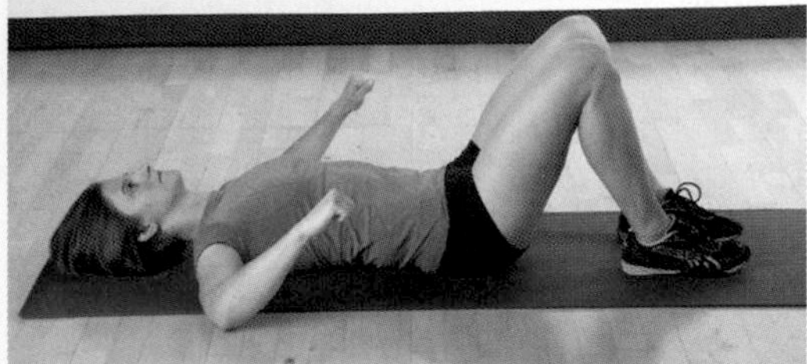
c.

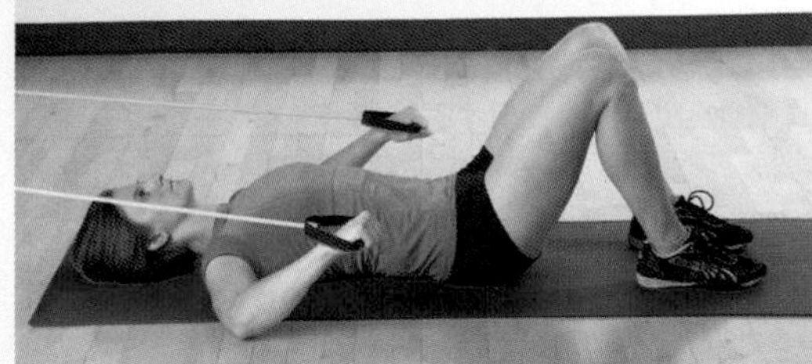
d.

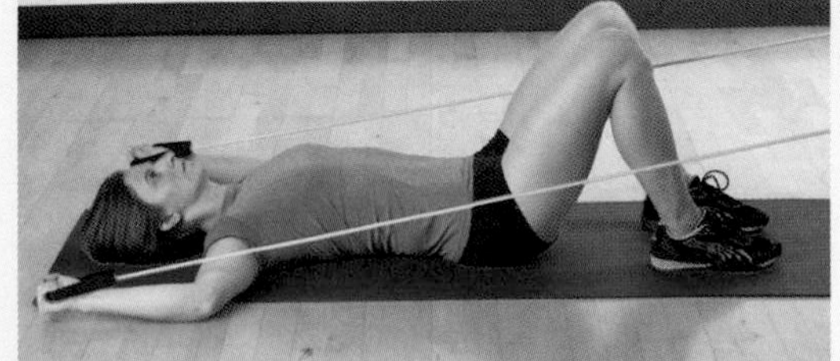
e.

Figure 17-17
Internal and external humeral rotation

Objective: To improve rotator cuff function while maintaining good scapular position

Preparation and position:

- Lie supine on a mat with knees bent and feet placed flat on the floor, aligning the anterior superior iliac spine (ASIS) with the knee and second toe.
- Engage the core muscles to stabilize the lumbar spine in the neutral position and maintain this position throughout the exercise.
- Pack both scapulae and maintain this position throughout the exercise.
- Abduct the arms to 90 degrees (shoulder height), resting the backs of the upper arms on the mat, and bend the elbows 90 degrees so that the forearms are perpendicular to the floor (a).

Exercise:

- *External rotation:* Slowly externally rotate the arms backward, bringing the forearms toward the floor. The ultimate goal is to achieve movement so that the back of the forearms rest on the floor (90 degrees of movement) (b).
- Hold this position for 15 to 60 seconds and repeat two to four times.
- *Internal rotation:* From the starting position, internally rotate the arms forward, bringing the forearms toward the floor. The ultimate goal is to achieve movement so that the forearms reach an angle of 20 to 30 degrees above the floor (60 to 70 degrees of movement) (c).
- Hold this position for 15 to 60 seconds, and repeat two to four times.

Progression: Once the end ranges can be reached, add resistance to condition these muscles (d & e). Remember, these are small muscles with higher concentrations of type 1 fibers, so they respond best to volume training. Add no more than 5 pounds (2.3 kg) of external resistance (cable or dumbbell) and build volume toward three sets of 12 to 15 repetitions with 30-second rest intervals between sets.

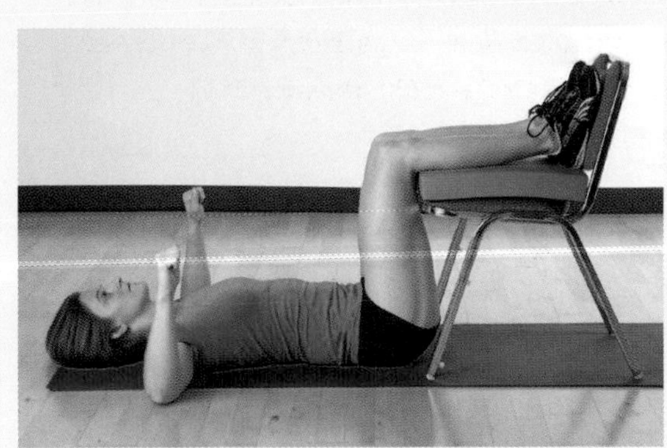
a.

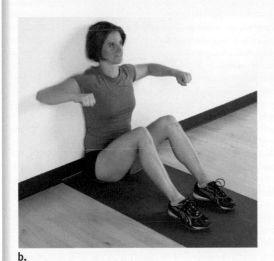
b.

Figure 17-18
Reverse flys with supine 90-90

Objective: To strengthen the posterior muscles of the shoulder complex

Preparation and position:

- Lie supine on the floor with both legs draped over a chair or riser. The height of the chair or riser should allow the knees and hips to flex to 90 degrees without elevating the hips off the floor.
- Align the anterior superior iliac spine (ASIS) with the knee and second toe and use supports to hold the feet in this position (e.g., pillows), preventing any external or internal rotation of the feet and lower legs, which would alter pelvic and low-back position.
- Abduct the arms to 90 degrees (shoulder height), resting the backs of the upper arms on the mat and bending the elbows 90 degrees so that the forearms are perpendicular to the floor.
- Engage the core muscles to stabilize the lumbar spine in the neutral position and maintain this position throughout the exercise (a).
- Pack both scapulae and maintain this position throughout the exercise.

Exercise:

- Exhale and press the back of the arms into the floor with less than 50% of maximal voluntary contraction, without altering the position of the lumbar spine.
- Perform two to four repetitions, holding each isometric contraction for five to 10 seconds.

Progression: Lying supine, build exercise volume toward three sets of 12 to 15 repetitions, with 30-second rest intervals between sets.

Progression: Seated with the back flat against a wall and knees bent, perform three sets of 12 to 15 repetitions, with 30-second rest intervals between sets. Maintain contact between the sacrum, low back, scapulae, and back of the head and the wall (b).

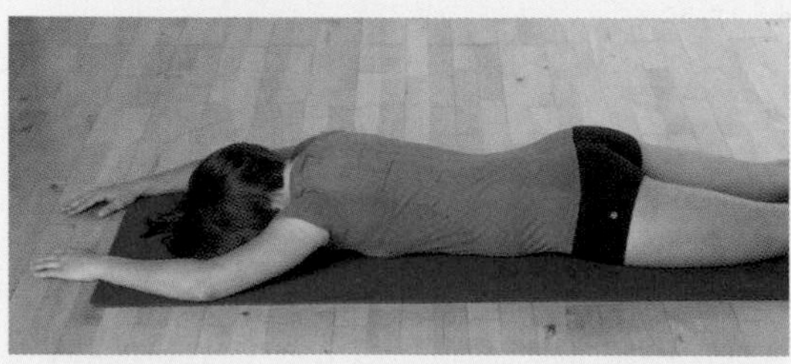
a.

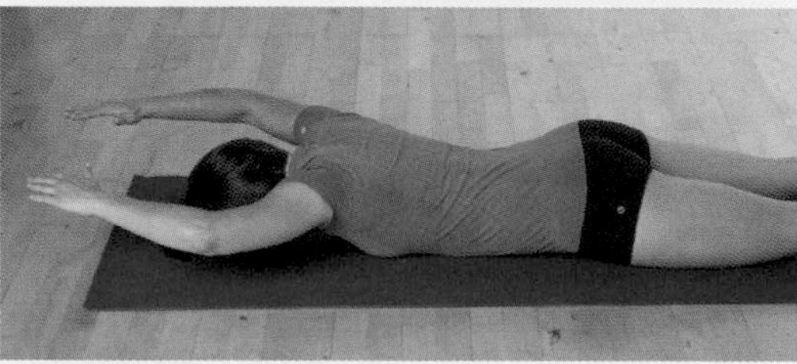
b.

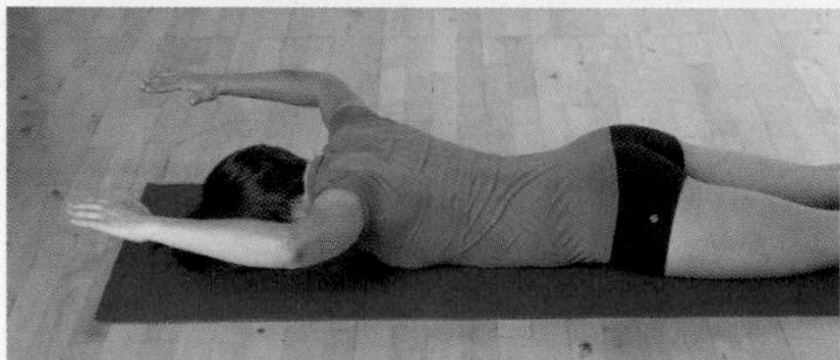
c.

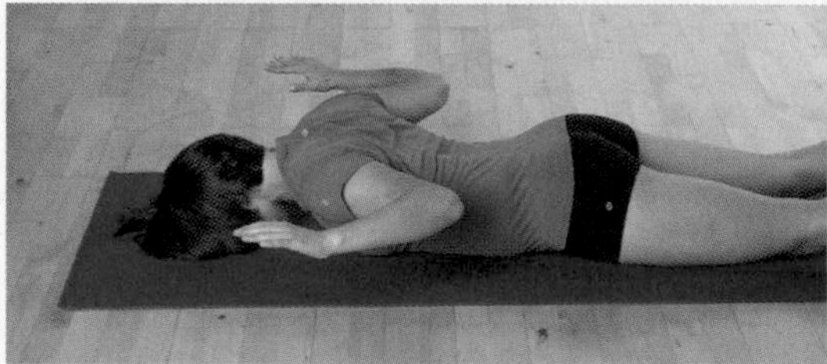
d.

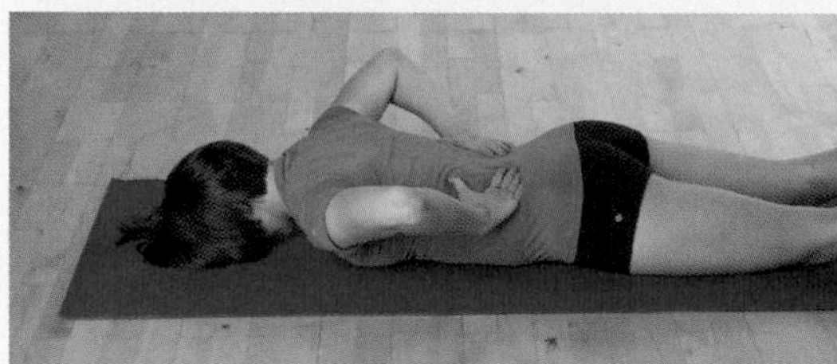
e.

Figure 17-19
Prone arm lifts

Objective: To strengthen the parascapular muscles

Preparation and position:

- Lie prone on a mat with both legs extended and arms positioned overhead with bent elbows, resting the back of the upper arms on a mat.
- Engage the core muscles to stabilize the lumbar spine in the neutral position and maintain this position throughout the exercise.
- Pack both scapulae and maintain this position throughout the exercise (a).

Exercise:

- *"I" formation:* Exhale and lift both arms 2 to 4 inches (5 to 10 cm) off the floor (keeping the elbows bent), while maintaining a depressed scapular position (avoiding scapular elevation) (b).
- Perform two to four repetitions, holding each repetition for five to 10 seconds.
- *"Y" formation:* Slide both arms out to a 135-degree position, keeping the elbows bent, but resting the arms on the mat (forming the letter "Y"). Exhale and lift both arms 2 to 4 inches (5 to 10 cm) off the floor while maintaining a depressed scapular position (avoiding scapular elevation) (c).
- Perform two to four repetitions, holding each repetition for five to 10 seconds.
- *"W" formation*: Slide both arms out to 90 degrees (shoulder height), resting the arms on the mat (forming the letter "W"). Exhale and lift both arms 2 to 4 inches (5 to 10 cm) off the floor while maintaining a depressed scapular position (avoiding scapular elevation) (d).
- Perform two to four repetitions, holding each repetition for five to 10 seconds.
- *"0" formation:* Reach behind the back and interlock the fingers, if possible, forming a giant letter "0" on the back, resting both forearms on the back. Exhale and lift both arms 2 to 4 inches (5 to 10 cm) off the back, while maintaining a depressed scapular position (avoiding scapular elevation) (e).
- Perform two to four repetitions, holding each repetition for five to 10 seconds.

Progression: Repeat the "I", "Y," and "W" formations with fully extended arms (note that the "W" formation becomes a "T" formation with the arms fully extended). Build the exercise volume toward three sets of 12 to 15 repetitions with 30-second rest intervals between sets. These exercises can ultimately be progressed to an incline position on a stability ball, standing, or in a hip-hinge or forward-bending position (hips flexed 90 degrees).

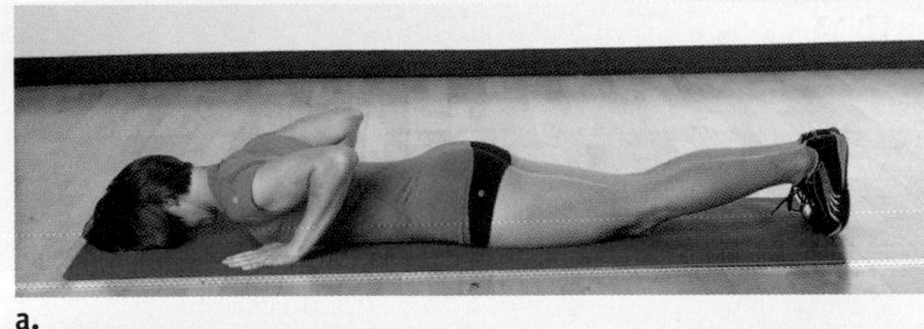
a.

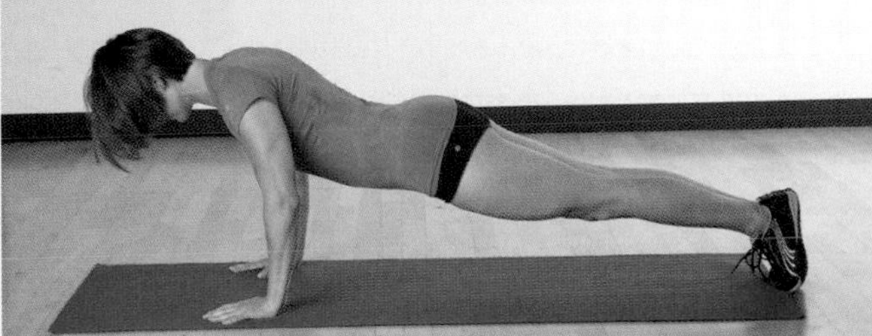
b.

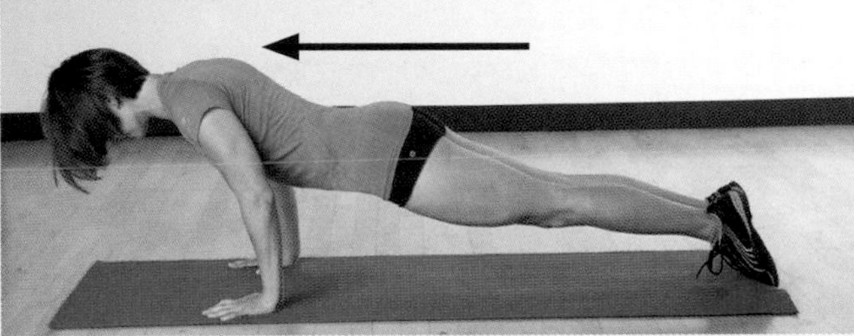
c.

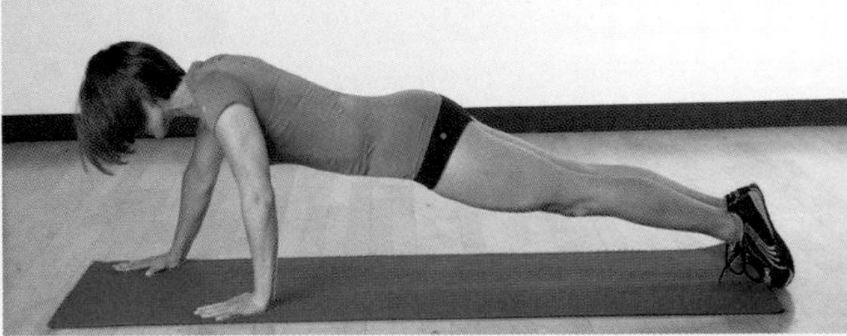
d.

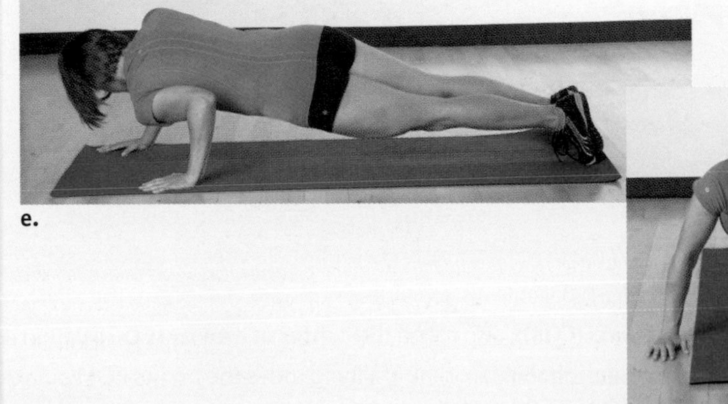
e.

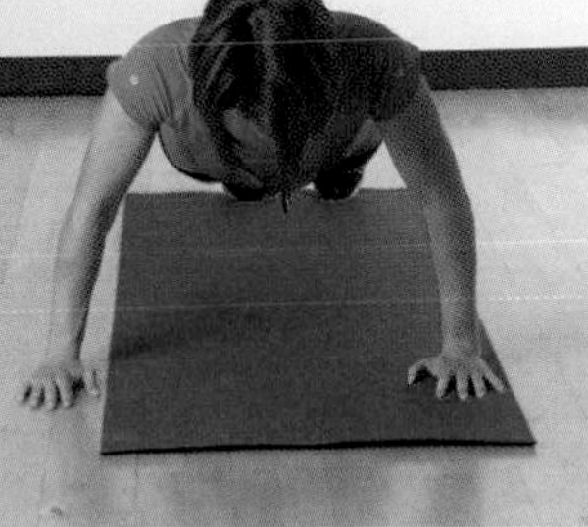
f.

g.

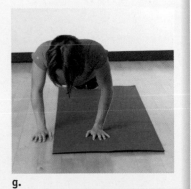

Figure 17-20
Closed kinetic chain weight shifts

Objective: To stabilize the scapulothoracic joint and lumbar spine in a closed kinetic chain (CKC) position

Preparation and position:

- Lie prone on a mat, placing the hands directly under the shoulders and extending both legs.
- Engage the core muscles to stabilize the lumbar spine in the neutral position. Maintain this position throughout the exercise.
- Pack the shoulders (see Figure 17-16) and maintain this position throughout the exercise (a).
- Press the body upward to assume a full or bent-knee press-up position (b).

Exercise:

- Slowly shift the body weight 3 to 6 inches (8 to 15 cm) forward without moving the hands (c).
- Perform two to four repetitions, holding each for five to 10 seconds.

Progression: Offset one hand into a staggered position by moving it 6 to 12 inches (15 to 30 cm) forward of the shoulder and repeat the movement (d). Perform two to four repetitions, holding each for five to 10 seconds. Repeat to the opposite side.

Progression: Drop the shoulder of the hand positioned under the shoulder toward the floor (e). Perform one or two sets of five to 10 repetitions to each side.

Progression: Perform side shuffles, moving the hands 6 to 12 inches (15 to 30 cm) side-to-side (f & g). Perform one or two sets of five to 10 repetitions to each side.

Distal Mobility

Within the distal segments of the body, the gastrocnemius and soleus muscles (triceps surae) are often problematic, exhibiting tightness and limited mobility. During a squatting movement, many individuals demonstrate a lack of adequate ankle dorsiflexion and are unable to keep their heels down during the lowering phase. An individual who is unable to keep the heels down during a squat movement will need to improve ankle mobility and calf flexibility, which will promote stability within the foot (if he or she stands in a pronated position).

After reestablishing flexibility within the calf muscles through myofascial release and static stretching techniques, individuals can progress to performing the dynamic ankle mobilization exercise presented in Figure 17-21, which mimics the ankle's role during walking and running activities (Gray & Tiberio, 2007).

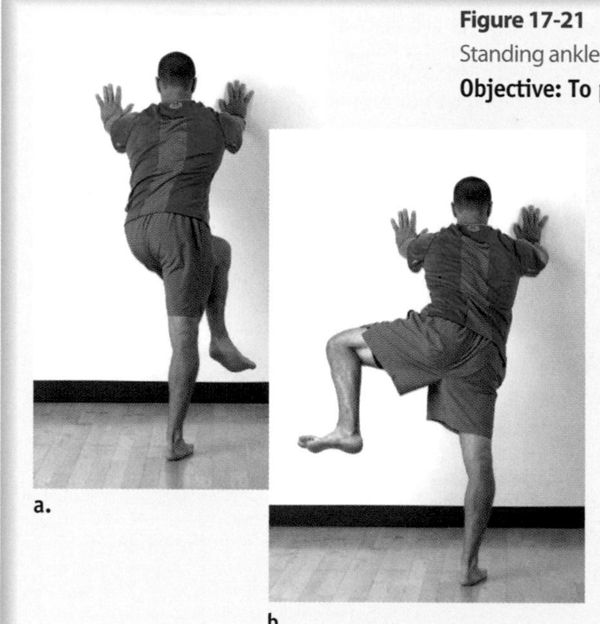

Figure 17-21
Standing ankle mobilization
Objective: To promote ankle mobility during a dynamic movement pattern

Preparation and position:
- Remove shoes and stand in front of a wall with the feet placed a few inches apart. Lean forward and support the upper extremity with the arms by placing the hands on the wall while stretching the calf muscles.
- Engage the core muscles to stabilize the lumbar spine in the neutral position. Maintain this position throughout the exercise.

Exercise:
- Slowly lift one foot off the ground, flexing the hip and bending the knee close to 90 degrees.
- While stabilizing the body over the stance leg and continuing to lean forward, swing the raised leg across the front of the body in the transverse plane (a), and then swing that same leg back out in the opposite direction (b).
- Perform one or two sets of five to 10 repetitions with each leg, holding each end position for one or two seconds.

Static Balance: Segmental

Movement is essential to complete all **activities of daily living (ADL)**, and the ability to move efficiently requires control of the body's postural alignment or balance. Balance is a foundational element of all programming and should be emphasized early in the training program once core function is established and an individual shows improvements in stability and mobility throughout the kinetic chain. Balance not only enhances physical performance, but also contributes to improving the psychological and emotional states by building self-efficacy and confidence (Rose, 2010). Balance is subdivided into static balance, or the ability to maintain the body's **center of mass (COM),** also called the **center of gravity (COG),** within its **base of support (BOS)**, and **dynamic balance**, or the ability to move the body's COM outside of its BOS while maintaining postural control and establishing a new BOS (Whiting & Rugg, 2006; Shumway-Cook & Woollacott, 2001).

COM represents that point around which all weight is evenly distributed (Kendall et al., 2005). It is generally located about 2 inches (5 cm) anterior to the spine in the location of the first and second sacral joints (S1 and S2), but varies in individuals by body shape, size, and gender, being slightly higher in males due to greater quantities of musculature in the upper body (Rose, 2010; Kendall et al., 2005). A person's COM constantly shifts as he or she changes position, moves, or adds external resistance. BOS is defined as the two-dimensional distance between and beneath the body's points of contact with a surface (Houglum, 2010).

After the client performs exercises to reestablish core function, static balance training, beginning with segmental or sectional stabilization training, can be introduced. This entails the use of specific static-balance exercises performed over a fixed BOS that impose small balance challenges on the body's core. The client adopts a seated position and engages the core musculature. By following the training guidelines and manipulating the variables listed in Table 17-10, health coaches can gradually progress exercises by increasing the balance challenge until the client experiences difficulty in maintaining postural control, yet does not fall (Rose, 2010). The objective with these progressions is to increase the exercise challenge until a threshold of balance or postural control becomes evident, and then continue gradually from that point by manipulating any of the variables.

Table 17-10

Training Guidelines for Static Balance

Training Variables	Training Conditions
2–3 times per week Perform exercises toward the beginning of workouts before the onset of fatigue (which decreases concentration) Perform 1 set of 2–4 repetitions, each for 5–10 seconds	Narrow BOS (e.g., wide to narrow) Raise COM (e.g., raising arms overhead) Shift LOG (e.g., raising arms unilaterally, leaning or rotating trunk) Sensory alteration [e.g., shifting focal point to a finger 12 inches (30 cm) in front of one's face, performing slow hand-eye tracking, or performing slow head movements such as looking up and down] Sensory removal (e.g., closing eyes)

Note: BOS = Base of support; COM = Center of mass; LOG = Line of gravity

After incorporating the variables covered in Table 17-10, health coaches can introduce two more challenging variables, but only if they are considered appropriate and consistent with the client's goals:

- Reduce the points of contact (e.g., move from balancing on two feet to one foot).
- Add additional unstable surfaces (e.g., air discs, Airex™ pad, BOSU®, or Step 360®).

Each of these challenges should be introduced separately, gradually increasing the exercise difficulty by manipulating the variables provided in Table 17-10 under this new challenge. Next, health coaches can introduce the second challenge in a similar manner (e.g., move to one foot and reintroduce the variables listed in Table 17-10 before implementing additional unstable surfaces, which should be introduced with two feet).

Static Balance: Integrated (Standing)

The natural progression from seated exercises is to standing exercises, thereby integrating the entire kinetic chain, which represents more function and mimics many ADL. During integrated movements, the effects of external loads, gravity, and reactive forces all increase, thereby necessitating a greater need to stabilize the spine. McGill (2006) introduced the concept of bracing, explaining how it improves spinal stability by providing a wider BOS. To teach a client how to brace, a health coach can have the client stand in a relaxed position and engage the core muscles. The client can then imagine a person standing in front of him or her who is about to deliver a quick jab to the stomach. In anticipation of the jab, the individual should stiffen up the trunk region by co-contracting both layers of muscles. This represents bracing, which, unlike centering (or drawing in the navel) that acts reflexively, is a conscious contraction used for short time periods during external loading on the spine (e.g., when performing a weighted squat or picking up a box).

The health coach can introduce standing static-balance training on stable surfaces before progressing to static unstable (e.g., air discs, Airex pad, BOSU, or Step 360) or dynamic unstable surfaces (e.g., Coretex®), both of which gradually increase the balance challenge. Both forms of training are important to developing efficiency within the **proprioceptive, vestibular**, and **ocular systems,** but the decision regarding which training surfaces to use depends primarily on the client's needs, capabilities, and goals. Regardless, all balance exercises should ultimately incorporate some form of dynamic balance training on stable surfaces (e.g., movement on the ground) to mimic ADL. When designing static balance-training programs, health coaches should follow the stance-position progressions illustrated in Figure 17-22. The health coach should identify which stance position challenges the client's balance threshold and then repeat the exercises with progressions outlined in Table 17-10.

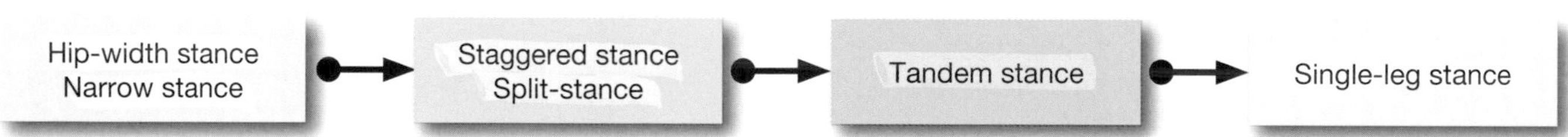
Hip-width stance
Narrow stance
Staggered stance
Split-stance
Tandem stance
Single-leg stance

Figure 17-22
Stance-position progressions

Phase 2: Movement Training

While phase 1 (stability and mobility training) includes some static-balance training (segmental and static whole-body stabilization), it is during the next level of training (phase 2: movement training) that the entire kinetic chain is integrated into more dynamic movement. During this phase, the dynamic nature of the movement patterns, especially when adding external resistance, will demand a greater need for bracing.

As noted earlier in the chapter, human movement can essentially be broken down into five primary movements that encompass all ADL (Figure 17-23). Movements can be as simple as one primary movement or as complex as the integration of several of them into a single motion. The five primary movements are as follows:

- Bend-and-lift movements (e.g., squatting)
- Single-leg movements (e.g., single-leg stance and lunging)
- Pushing movements (primarily in the vertical/horizontal planes)
- Pulling movements (primarily in the vertical/horizontal planes)
- Rotational (spiral) movements

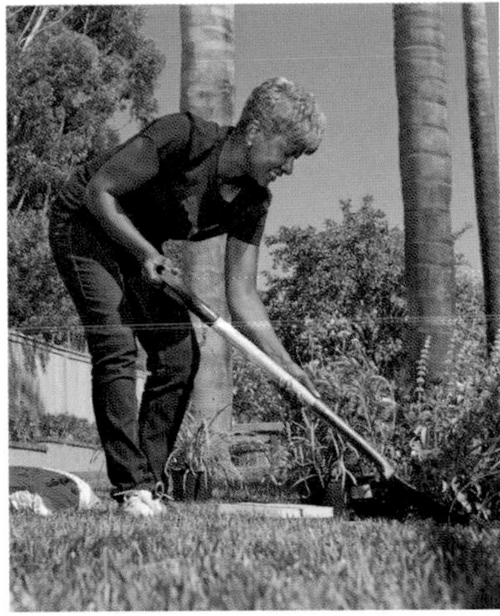
a. Bend-and-lift movement

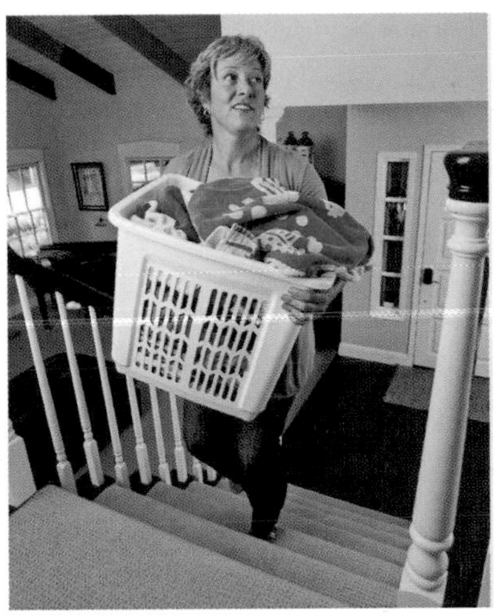
b. Single-leg movement

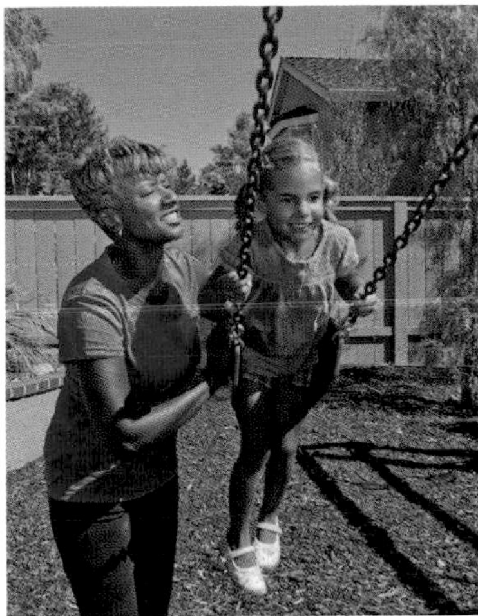
c. Pushing movement

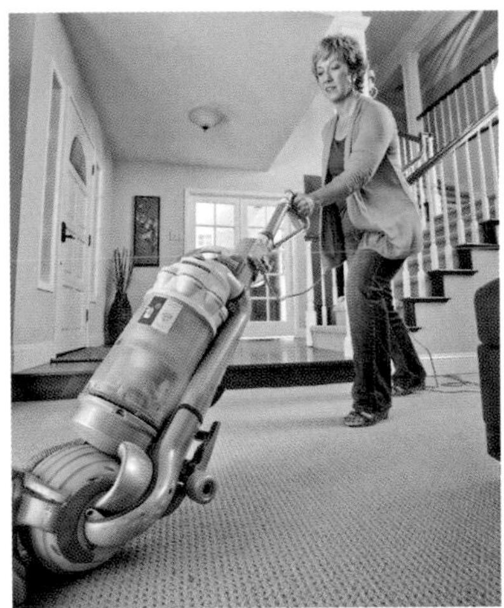
d. Pulling movement

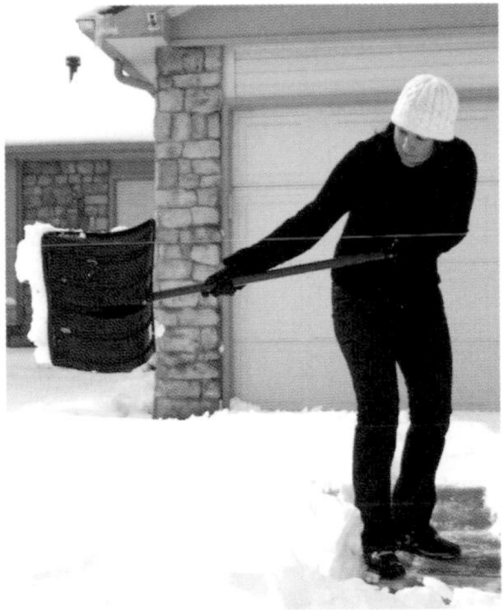
e. Rotational movement

Figure 17-23
Five primary movement patterns

What is universal to all clients is the need to train these movement patterns as a prerequisite to all resistance-training exercises that involve an external load. In essence, if a client can perform these five primary movements effectively and possesses the appropriate levels of stability and mobility throughout the kinetic chain, it improves his or her potential for efficient movement and decreases the likelihood for compensation, pain, or injury (Gray & Tiberio, 2007). This phase of training follows stability and mobility training and involves teaching patterns for these five movements, using body weight as resistance and the **levers** within the body (e.g., the arms) as drivers to increase exercise intensity (Gray & Tiberio, 2007).

Bend-and-lift Movements

The bend-and-lift movement associated with the squat is perhaps one of the most prevalent activities used in strength training and throughout most individuals' ADL (e.g., sitting and standing), yet this movement is subject to much controversy given its potential for harm to the knees and low back, especially when an external load is added. Faulty movement patterns associated with poor technique will disrupt muscle function and joint loading, compromising performance and ultimately leading to overload and potential injury (Kendall et al., 2005; Sahrmann, 2002). Proper technique is therefore the key differentiator. One limiting factor to good technique is a lack of ankle mobility, which, according to Kendall et al. (2005), is normally between 15 and 20 degrees of ankle dorsiflexion. To evaluate this limitation, the health coach can have the client place one foot on a low riser [<12 inches (30 cm)], positioning the tibia perpendicular to the floor. The client leans slowly forward, dorsiflexing the ankle until the heel lifts off the floor or the ankle falls into pronation. The health coach can then determine the degree of motion achieved. Mobility of less than 15 degrees merits a need to improve ankle mobility prior to teaching the full bend-and-lift movement.

The bend-and-lift maneuver begins with a solid platform of good posture and bracing of the abdominal region (when using external loads). As the exercises in this training phase (phase 2: movement training) utilize body weight as the primary form of resistance, bracing might not be necessary, but clients should be reminded to brace the core when lifting external loads. Figures 17-24 through 17-26 provide examples of exercises that train the bend-and-lift movement pattern.

Throughout their daily activities, people often find themselves bending down to lift objects off the floor, and rarely do they use proper deadlift technique. Split- or staggered-stance positions, internal or external foot rotation, and even variations in arm position are common. Considering that these variations represent most individuals' daily movements, clients should be trained functionally to mimic these patterns. Therefore, once a client demonstrates proficiency with the bend-and-lift movement, progress the movement patterns to incorporating variations in foot position coupled with various arm movements (Figure 17-27). From a standpoint of functionality, people normally bend down to lift objects with their hands

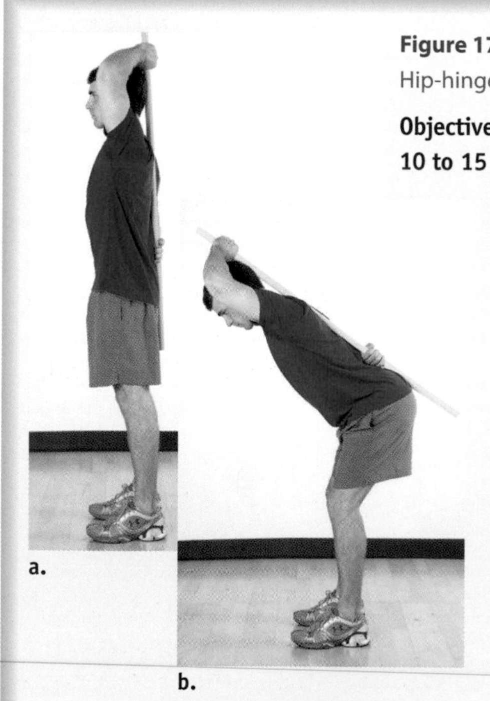

Figure 17-24
Hip-hinge

Objective: To emphasize "glute dominance" over "quad dominance" during the initial 10 to 15 degrees of movement

Preparation and position:

- Stand in a neutral stance position with the feet hip-width apart and place a light bar or dowel along the back that makes contact with the head, thoracic spine, and sacrum (three-point contact).
- Hold the bar above the head in one hand and around the low-back region with the other hand.
- Engage the core muscles to stabilize the lumbar spine in the neutral position and maintain this position throughout the exercise (a).

Exercise:

- While pressing the dowel into the three points, slowly perform a forward bend, pushing the hips backward with slight knee flexion, while maintaining contact with the dowel on all three points at all times (b).
- The goal is to emphasize moving backward while minimizing the downward movement of the hips toward the floor.
- Perform one to three sets of 15 repetitions.

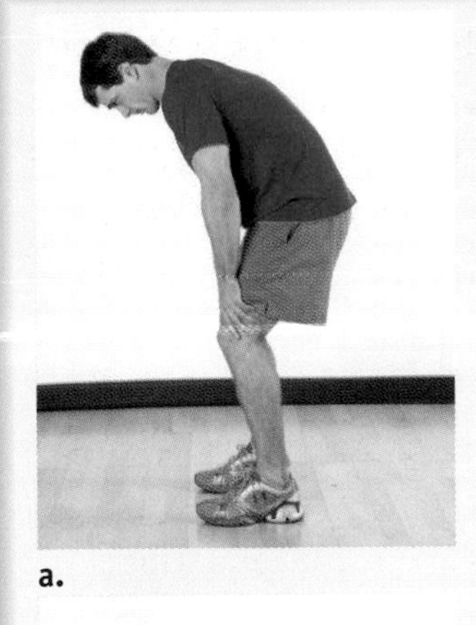
a.

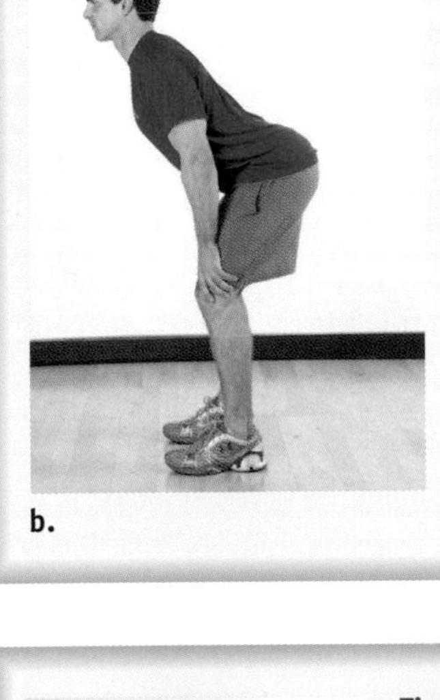
b.

Figure 17-25
Pelvic tilts and back alignment

Objective: To promote pelvic control and lumbar stability throughout the lowering phase

Preparation and position:

- Stand in a neutral position with the feet hip-width apart, and, with the hands on the upper thighs, hip-hinge 10 to 15 degrees.
- Engage the core muscles to stabilize the lumbar spine in the neutral position.

Exercise:

- While holding this position, perform a series of pelvic tilts, changing the low-back position between flexion (rounding) and extension (arching).
- Perform one or two sets of five to 10 repetitions, holding each end position for one to two seconds.
- Move the hands down to rest on the knees, dropping deeper into the bend, and perform the same number of repetitions (a & b).
- Lower the body further, resting the elbows on the lower thighs and perform the same number of repetitions.
- Lower the hands toward the floor or to a low riser [<12 inches (30 cm)] and perform the same number of repetitions.
- Lower the hands to the floor to touch the underside of the front of the feet or shoes. (*Note:* Some heavier clients may not be physically able to achieve this position.) Once this position is achieved, perform full repetitions pushing through the heels to a full standing position, then return to this lowered position. Perform the same number of repetitions.

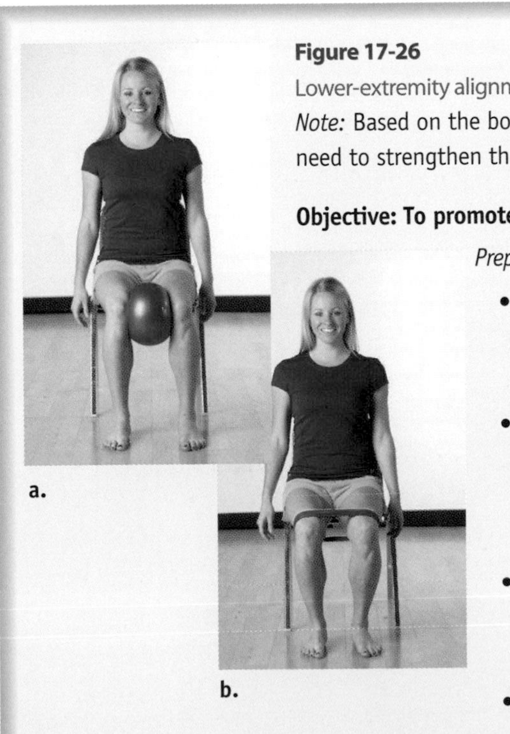
a.
b.

Figure 17-26
Lower-extremity alignment
Note: Based on the body-weight squat assessment (see page 348), health coaches can determine the need to strengthen the hip abductors or adductors.

Objective: To promote alignment among the hips, knees, and feet during a bend-and-lift movement

Preparation and position:

- Start seated in a chair, aligning the anterior superior iliac spine (ASIS) with the knee and second toe.
- Clients who need to strengthen the hip adductors can place a soft squeezable ball between the knees (a).
- Clients who need to strengthen the hip abductors can wrap an elastic band around the knees (b).
- Engage the core muscles to stabilize the lumbar spine in the neutral position and maintain this position throughout the exercise.

Exercise:

- Perform one or two sets of five to 10 contractions, holding each contraction in the specific direction for one or two seconds.

Progression: Hold the isometric contraction while standing up out of the chair to full-standing position and returning into the chair. Perform one or two sets of 10 repetitions, holding the contraction in the specific direction throughout the movement.

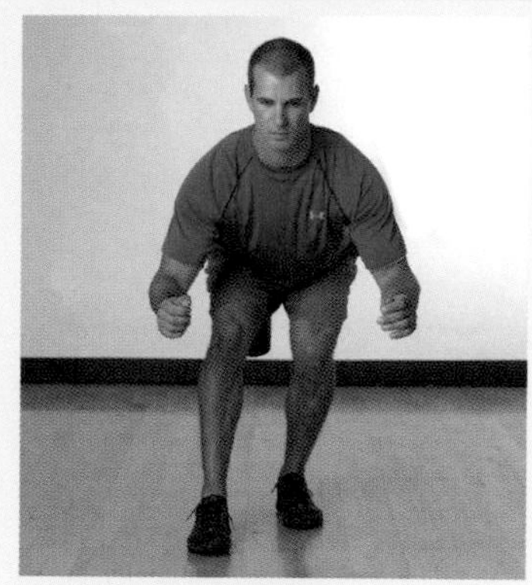
a.

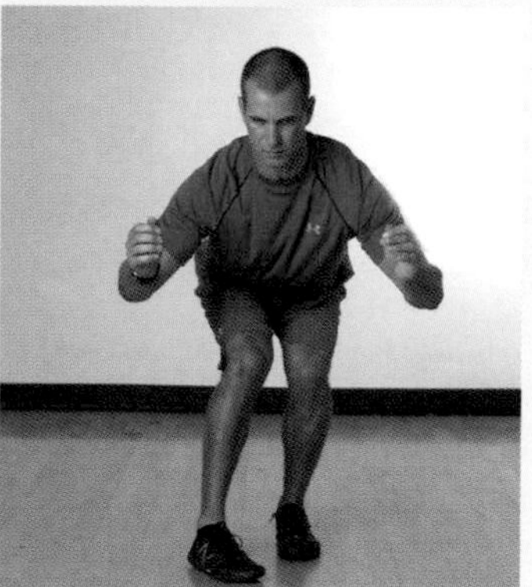
b.

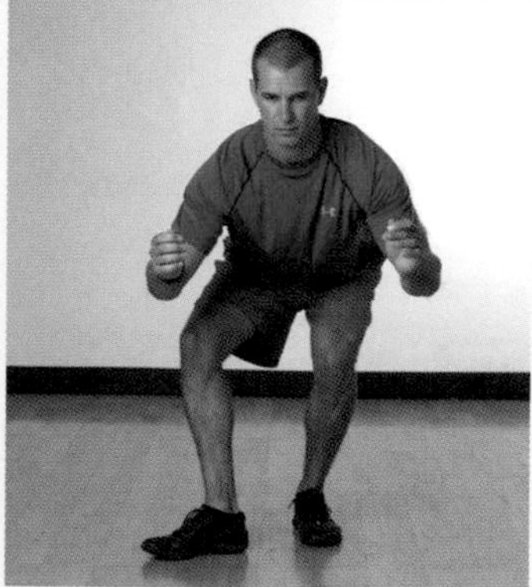
c.

Figure 17-27

Squat variations

Note: Health coaches should progress to these exercises only when a client demonstrates good technique with a standard squat.

Objective: To promote stability and mobility throughout the kinetic chain with variations of the standard squat movement

Preparation and position:

- Start in the standing (neutral) position with the feet hip-width apart, but vary the position of the feet as follows:
  - ✓ *Staggered stance:* Right or left foot forward (a)
  - ✓ *Internal rotation:* Right or left foot rotated inward from neutral (always maintain knee alignment over the second toe) (b)
  - ✓ *External rotation:* Right or left foot rotated outward from neutral (always maintain knee alignment over the second toe) (c)
- Engage the core muscles to stabilize the lumbar spine in the neutral position. Maintain this position throughout the exercise.

Exercise:

- Hip-hinge and drop into a squat, ideally lowering the body to an end-range where the thighs are parallel with the floor or where the fingertips touch the floor.
- Perform one to three sets of 10 to 15 repetitions at a controlled tempo, varying foot positions.

Progressions: Adding the arms as drivers (bilaterally or unilaterally) increases the exercise intensity and the need for additional stability and mobility along the kinetic chain. For example, begin by driving the arms toward the floor during the lowering phase prior to driving the arms in all three planes with a high-arm position.

- Add the following drivers:
  - ✓ *Sagittal plane:* Drive both arms toward the floor or toward the ceiling during the lowering phase (d).
  - ✓ *Frontal plane:* Drive both arms to either side (lateral lean) during the lowering phase (e).
  - ✓ *Transverse plane:* Drive both arms in rotation to either side during the lowering phase (f).

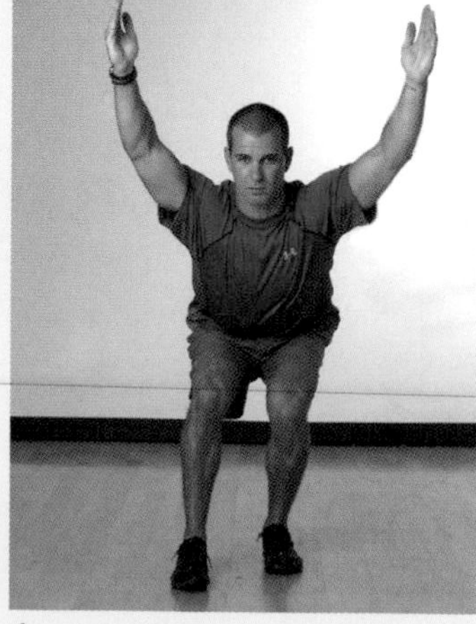
d.

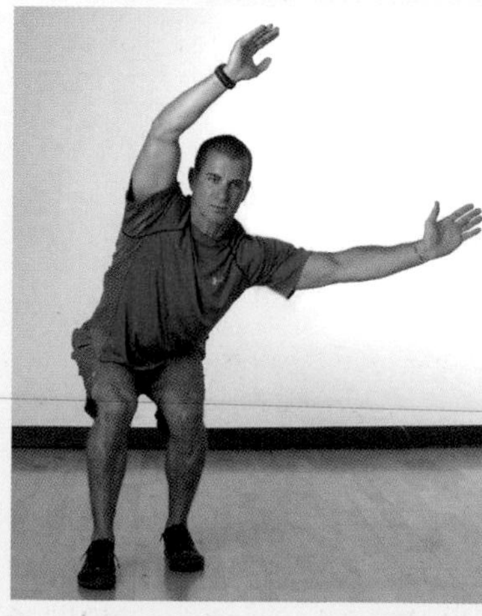
e.

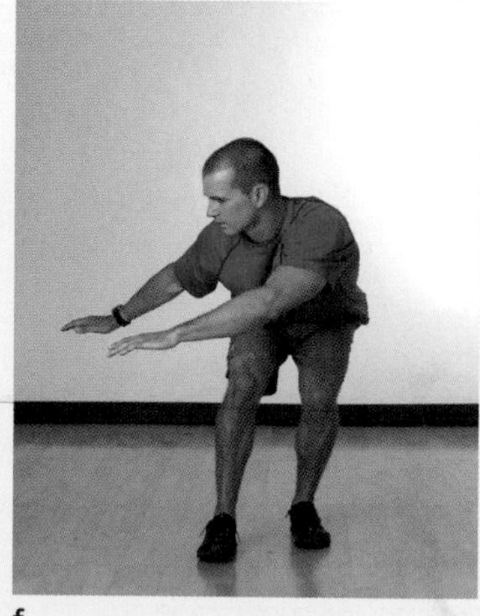
f.

by their sides, so health coaches should teach these variations beginning with the most simplistic position (i.e., arms at the sides) prior to moving into high-arm positions (e.g., front squat, back squat, or overhead positions). Keep in mind that these high-arm positions require a greater degree of thoracic mobility, which many clients may lack. Thus, clients should be taught the bend and lift in the deadlift position first (i.e., arms at sides), before being introduced to the front-squat position and then the back and overhead positions.

Single-leg Movement Patterns

Walking, the default movement pattern of human locomotion, puts the body into a single-leg stance position during each step as the raised leg swings forward (swing phase) just prior to the heel striking the ground. Standing efficiently on a single leg mandates stability in the stance leg, hip, and torso, while simultaneously exhibiting mobility in the raised leg if stepping is involved. Weakness in the hip abductors reflects an inability to control **lateral** hip shift, placing additional stress on the knee. Some clients will demonstrate this compensation during the balance assessments (i.e., sharpened Romberg test or stork-stand test—see pages 342–343) as their stance-leg hip hikes upward and the opposite hip drops downward. Sometimes clients with a lateral hip-shift weakness will only demonstrate their compensations during movement on a single leg. To check this, the health coach can have clients stand on one leg and slowly swing the free leg forward and backward in the sagittal plane. Lateral hip-shift weakness is present if, during the leg swing movement, the stance-leg hip shifts laterally more than a few millimeters. Clients who have this movement compensation should first strengthen the hip abductors in isolation (e.g., side-lying leg raise) before integrating full-body, weight-bearing movements. Before learning any single-leg exercises (e.g., lunges), clients should learn how to effectively control hip adduction to prevent excessive lateral shift of the hip. Ultimately, individuals should demonstrate control of this lateral shift during gait, where the feet are positioned approximately 3.0 to 3.5 inches (7.6 to 8.9 cm) apart. However, clients should first be taught to do so from a feet-together position before progressing to the normal gait-width distance (Figure 17-28).

Static Balance on a Single Leg

Once an individual demonstrates the ability to effectively stand on one leg, the health coach can introduce dynamic movements of the upper and lower extremity over a static base of support. Next, various forms of resistance (e.g., medicine balls, cables, or bands) that increase the stabilization demands and the potential need for bracing during movement can be introduced. This is where the health coach's creativity in programming becomes important—to heighten the fun factor. Programming can be creative, but should always be progressed with common sense to keep the drills and exercises skill- and conditioning-level appropriate. The basic, but very functional, series of movement patterns presented in Table 17-11 and Figure 17-29 is based off the Balance Matrix created by Gary Gray, and incorporates both isolated and integrated upper- and lower-extremity movement in all three planes, all over a static base of support (Gray, 2008).

Progression for the single-leg stance involves adding external resistance and increasing the balance challenge. Holding a medicine ball or dumbbell, or introducing partial single-leg squats, adds resistance to the kinetic chain and increases the balance challenge. As resistance

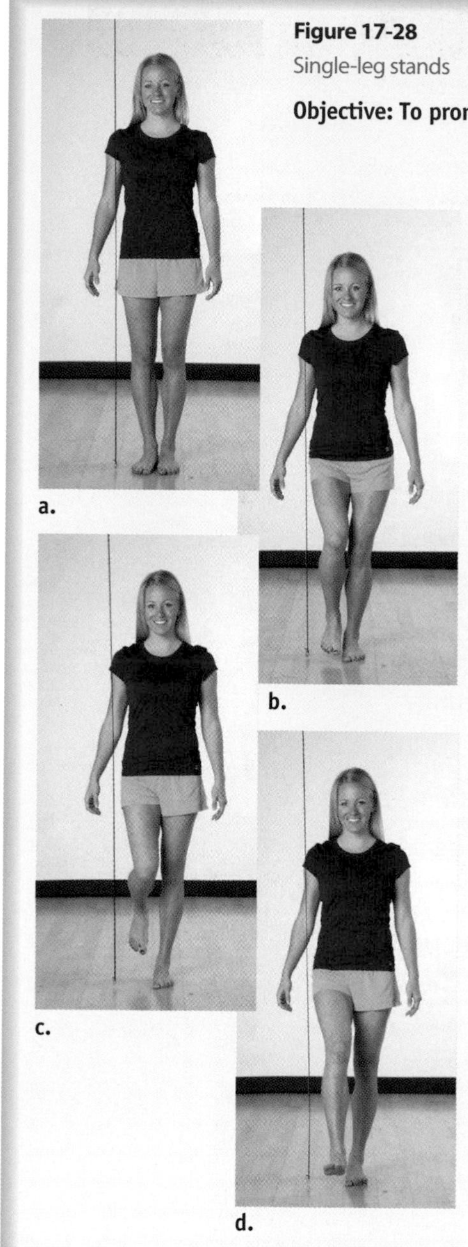

Figure 17-28
Single-leg stands

Objective: To promote stability within the stance-leg and hip during a single-leg stand

Preparation and position:

- The health coach hangs a plumb line from the ceiling or high fixed point, attaching a small weighted object (e.g., washer or nut) to the other end and suspending it 1 to 2 inches (2.5 to 5.1 cm) from the floor.
- Stand facing a mirror with feet together, positioning the right hip immediately adjacent to the plumb line (the plumb line should lightly touch the right hip).
- Engage the core muscles to stabilize the lumbar spine in the neutral position and maintain this position throughout the exercise (a).

Exercise:

- Hip-hinge 10 to 15 degrees, transferring the body weight into the heels.
- Contract the adductor and abductor muscle groups in the left thigh, then slowly raise the right heel 1 inch (2.5 cm) off the floor (do not raise the entire foot yet) (b).
- Briefly hold this position, then slowly unload the entire foot, lifting it 1 to 3 inches (2.5 to 7.6 cm) off the floor while watching the hip position in the mirror. Attempt to control the lateral hip shift away from the plumb line (to the exerciser's left). The goal is to prevent the space that appears between the line and hips from exceeding 2 inches (5.1 cm) [smaller individuals should aim for approximately 1 inch (2.5 cm) of space, while taller individuals should aim for 2 inches (5.1 cm)].
- Briefly hold this position, then slowly extend the hips and stand vertically, again controlling the spacing. The torso should not move and the stance-leg should remain stable.
- Perform one or two sets of five to 10 repetitions per leg, resting for 30 seconds between sets. Repeat with the opposite leg.

Progression: Perform a leg swing to mimic gait (i.e., from the hip-hinge position, swing the leg with each standing vertical stand) (c & d).

Progression: Repeat the same exercise with the feet positioned at the normal gait-width distance.

Note: This exercise can be performed without a plumb line if one is not available.

Table 17-11

Dynamic Movement Patterns Over a Static Base of Support

Introduce upper-extremity movements • Movements: ✓ Arms can move unilaterally (one arm at a time) ✓ Arms can move bilaterally (both arms move together) ✓ Arms can move reciprocally (alternating arm directions) ✓ Position the feet in any stance indicated in Figure 17-22 (except single-leg stance) • Directions: ✓ Move arm(s) in the sagittal plane (flexion/extension) ✓ Move arm(s) in the frontal plane (lateral flexion from an overhead position) ✓ Move arm(s) in the transverse plane (rotation from the shoulder-height position with a bent elbow)	Perform the following: • 1-2 sets of 10–20 repetitions per side • Slow, controlled tempos [avoid bouncing at the end-ROM—the transition zone between movement in one direction and movement in another direction (also known as the transformational zone)] • Less than 30-second rest intervals between sets
Introduce lower-extremity movements • Movements: ✓ Assume a single-leg stand ✓ Start by swinging the leg forward and backward, touching the toes to the floor at each end-ROM (transformational zone), then progress to unsupported leg swings. • Directions: ✓ Move the leg in the sagittal plane (flexion/extension) ✓ Move the leg in the frontal plane (abduction/adduction) ✓ Move the leg in the transverse plane (rotation in front or behind the stance leg)	Perform the following: • 1-2 sets of 10–20 repetitions per side • Slow, controlled tempos (avoid bouncing at the end-ROM—the transformational zone) • Less than 30-second rest intervals between sets
Integrate upper- and lower-extremity movements • Move limbs ipsilaterally (same side) or contralaterally (opposite side) • Move limbs "in synch"—moving in the same direction (e.g., the leg and arm move forward together) • Move limbs "out of synch"—moving in opposite directions	Perform the following: • 1-2 sets of 10–20 repetitions per side • Slow, controlled tempos (avoid bouncing at the end-ROM—the transformational zone) • Less than 30-second rest intervals between sets

Note: ROM = Range of motion

Figure 17-29
Dynamic movement patterns

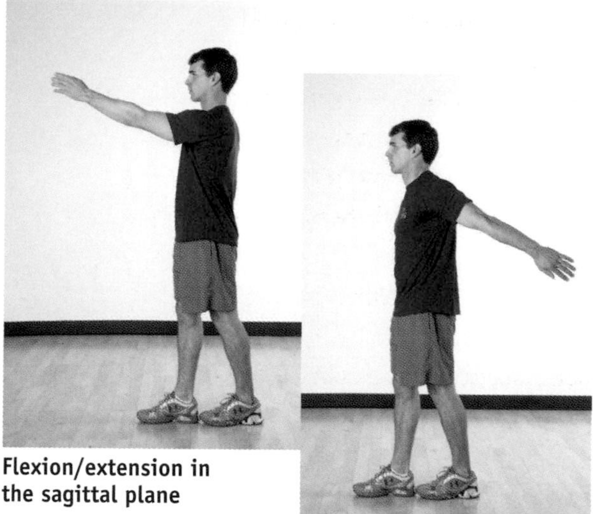

Flexion/extension in the sagittal plane

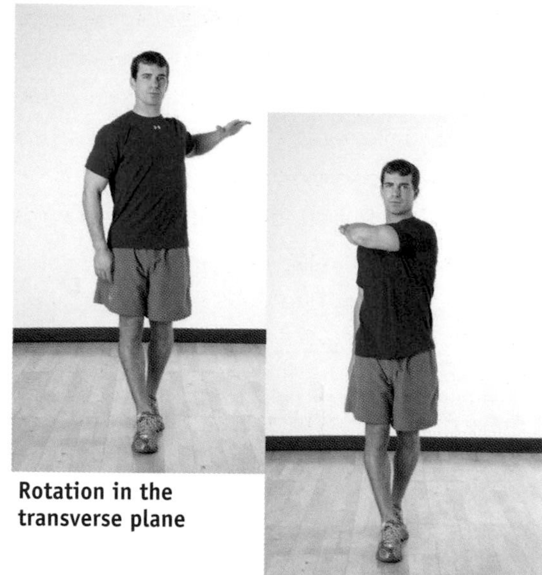

Rotation in the transverse plane

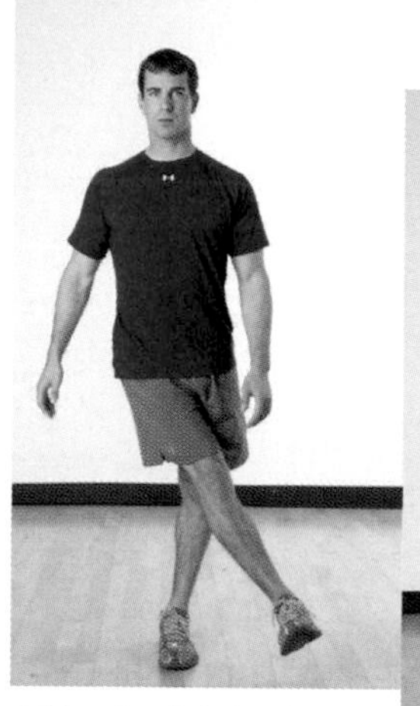

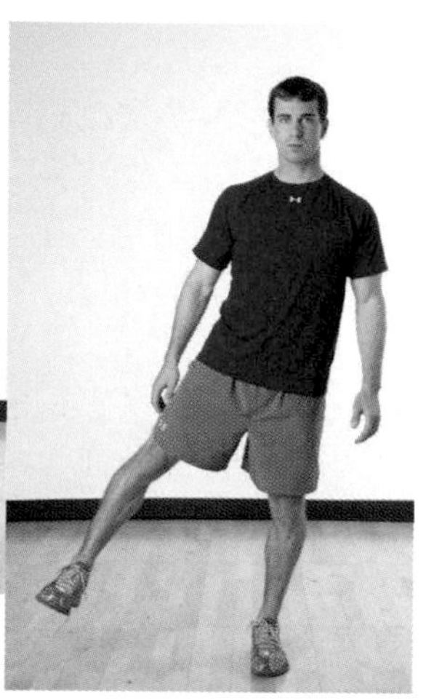

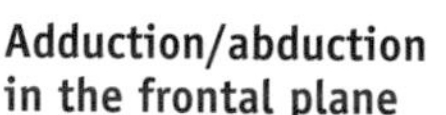

Adduction/abduction in the frontal plane

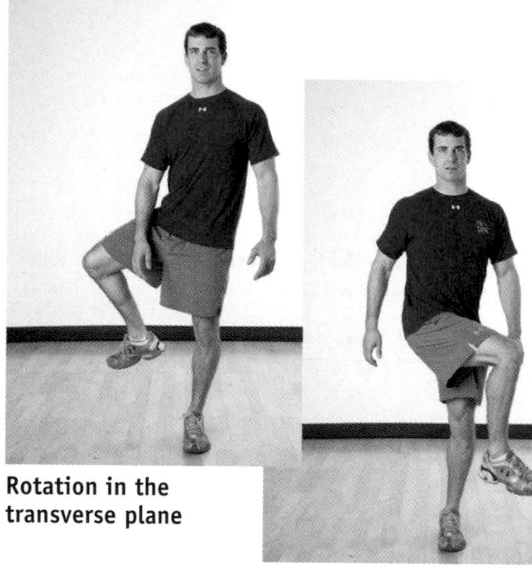

Rotation in the transverse plane

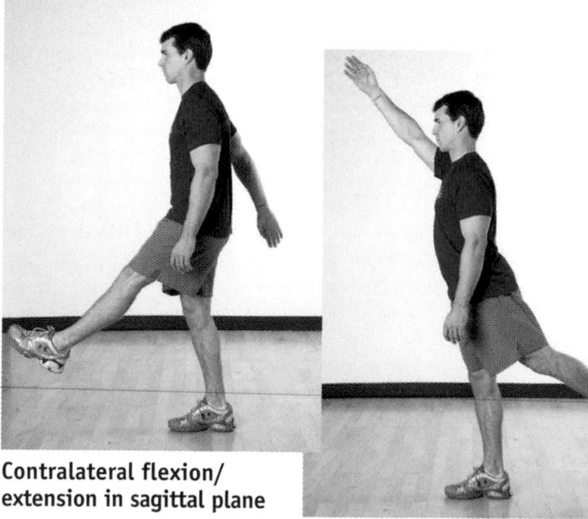

Contralateral flexion/ extension in sagittal plane

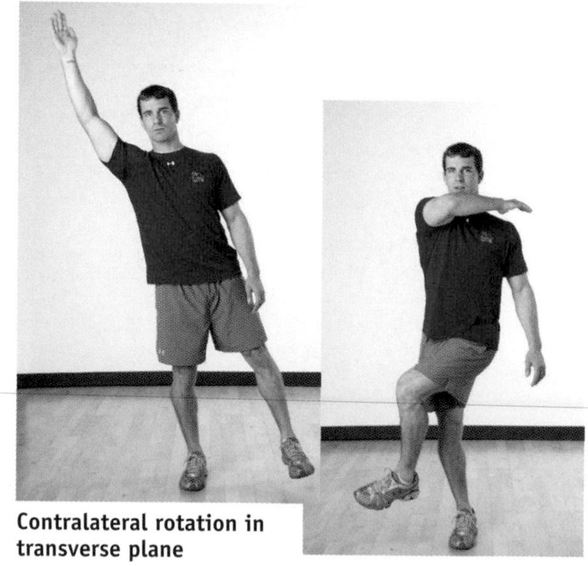

Contralateral rotation in transverse plane

(load) increases, the number of repetitions per set, and possibly total number of sets, should be reduced with longer rest intervals between sets (e.g., 30 to 60 seconds).

A primary single-leg pattern involves teaching clients how to lunge effectively, a movement pattern that is often performed poorly in any plane. While lunge mechanics are very similar to the squat or bend-and-lift mechanics, many individuals deviate from basic movement principles (Cook & Jones, 2007b). The exercises presented in Figure 17-30 teach the mechanics of the lunge and variations to the basic lunge.

As with squats, people often find themselves performing variations to the traditional lunge during their daily activities, workouts (e.g., side lunges), or even during sports (e.g., cutting and sidestepping). These variations involve directional lunges, foot-position variations, and movements with the upper extremities in all three planes of movement. Considering these

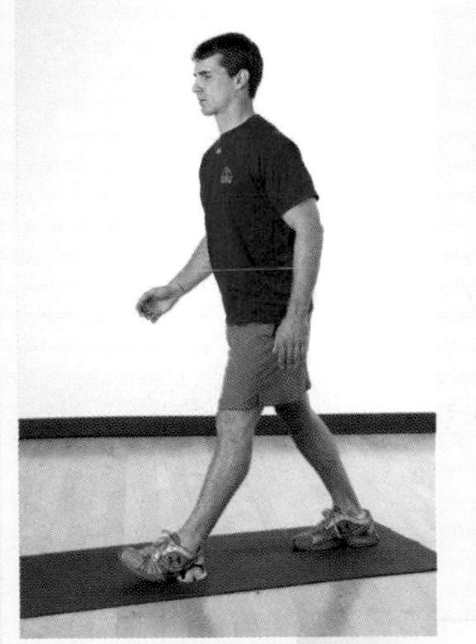

a.

b.

c.

Figure 17-30
Lunges

Objective: To teach the proper mechanics of the full lunge

Preparation and position:

- Start in the standing position, with the feet hip-width apart, shoulders packed (see Figure 17-16), head neutral, and weight distributed toward the heels.
- Engage the core muscles to stabilize the lumbar spine in the neutral position and maintain this position throughout the exercise.

Exercise:

- Slowly lift one leg, controlling the lateral hip shift and reaching forward to take a small step [<24 inches (61 cm)], lightly touching the heel on the floor. Briefly hold this position (a).
- Allow the entire foot to make contact. Once it is firmly positioned on the ground, initiate a hip-hinge movement to begin the downward phase of the lunge (b). This allows for a more natural hinge motion at the knee and reduces the shearing forces.
    - Lower the hips and shoulders together, allowing a slight forward torso lean, but maintain strong core engagement to avoid lumbar lordosis (c).
    - Avoid any misalignment of the knee over the foot, as well as hip adduction and torso rotation.
    - In the lowered position, the health coach can check for the following:
        - ✓ Alignment in the frontal plane of the anterior superior iliac spine (ASIS), knee, and second toe
        - ✓ The figure-4 position with the leading leg and torso in parallel, with the leading leg near perpendicular to the floor (exhibiting a slight forward lean—tibial translation)
        - ✓ No lateral weight shifting or torso rotation
- Perform one to three sets of 12 to 15 repetitions with a controlled tempo, allowing 30-second rest intervals between sets.
- Use the glute "push" and hamstrings "pull" to rise out of the lunge.

variations represent daily movements, clients should be trained functionally to mimic these patterns. Once a client demonstrates proficiency with the standard lunge pattern, the health coach can progress the exercise to include directional changes, different foot positions, and upper-extremity movement (Figure 17-31). Bear in mind that high-arm positions require a greater degree of thoracic and hip mobility, which a client may lack. Therefore, clients should begin by driving the arms in the low position prior to incorporating the high-arm-position movements.

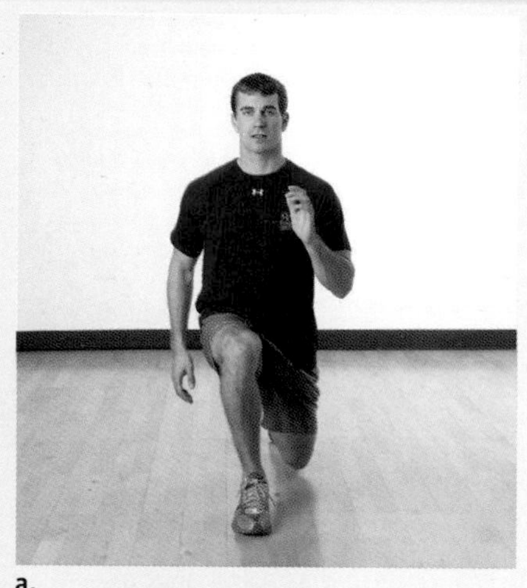

a.

Figure 17-31
Lunge matrix

Note: Health coaches should progress to this exercise only after a client demonstrates good technique with a standard forward lunge.

Objective: To promote stability and mobility throughout the kinetic chain using variations of the standard lunge movement

Preparation and position:

- Using the grid presented in the illustration (next page), the health coach can teach the client to move in all eight directions, starting and ending each repetition from the center position.
- Engage the core muscles to stabilize the lumbar spine in the neutral position and maintain this position throughout the exercise.

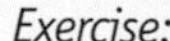

Exercise:

- The health coach teaches the directional movements with stepping prior to introducing lunges.
- When lunging forward, backward, and sideways, align the feet and hips forward (a, c, e, & g).
- When lunging to the oblique angles, align the feet and hips in that direction (b, d, f, & h).
- Follow the same technique instructions outlined in Figure 17-30.
- Perform one to three sets to each direction with each leg.

Source: Gray, G. & Tiberio, D. (2007). *Chain Reaction Function.* Adrian, Mich.: Gray Institute.

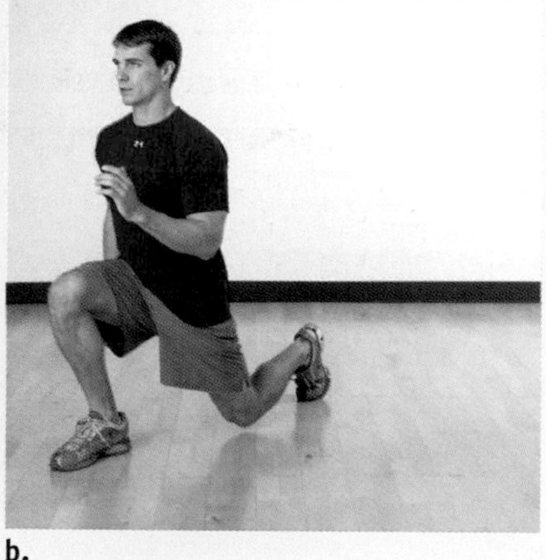

b.

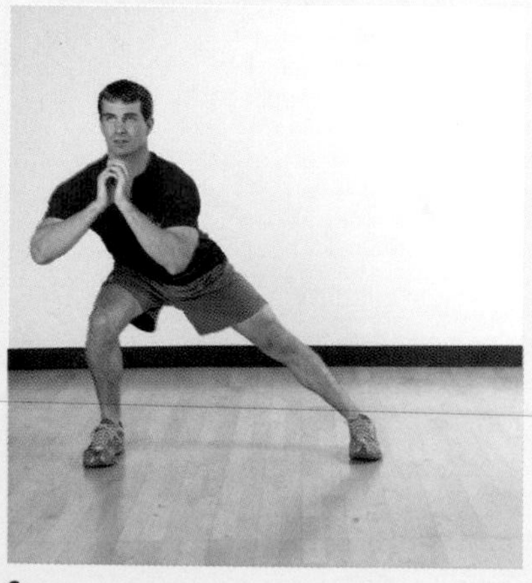

c.

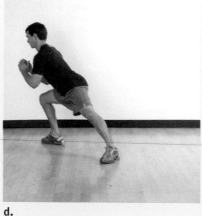

d.

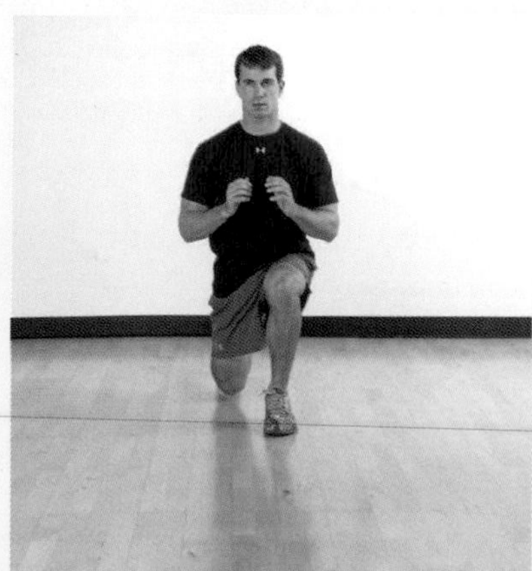

e.

Continued on next page

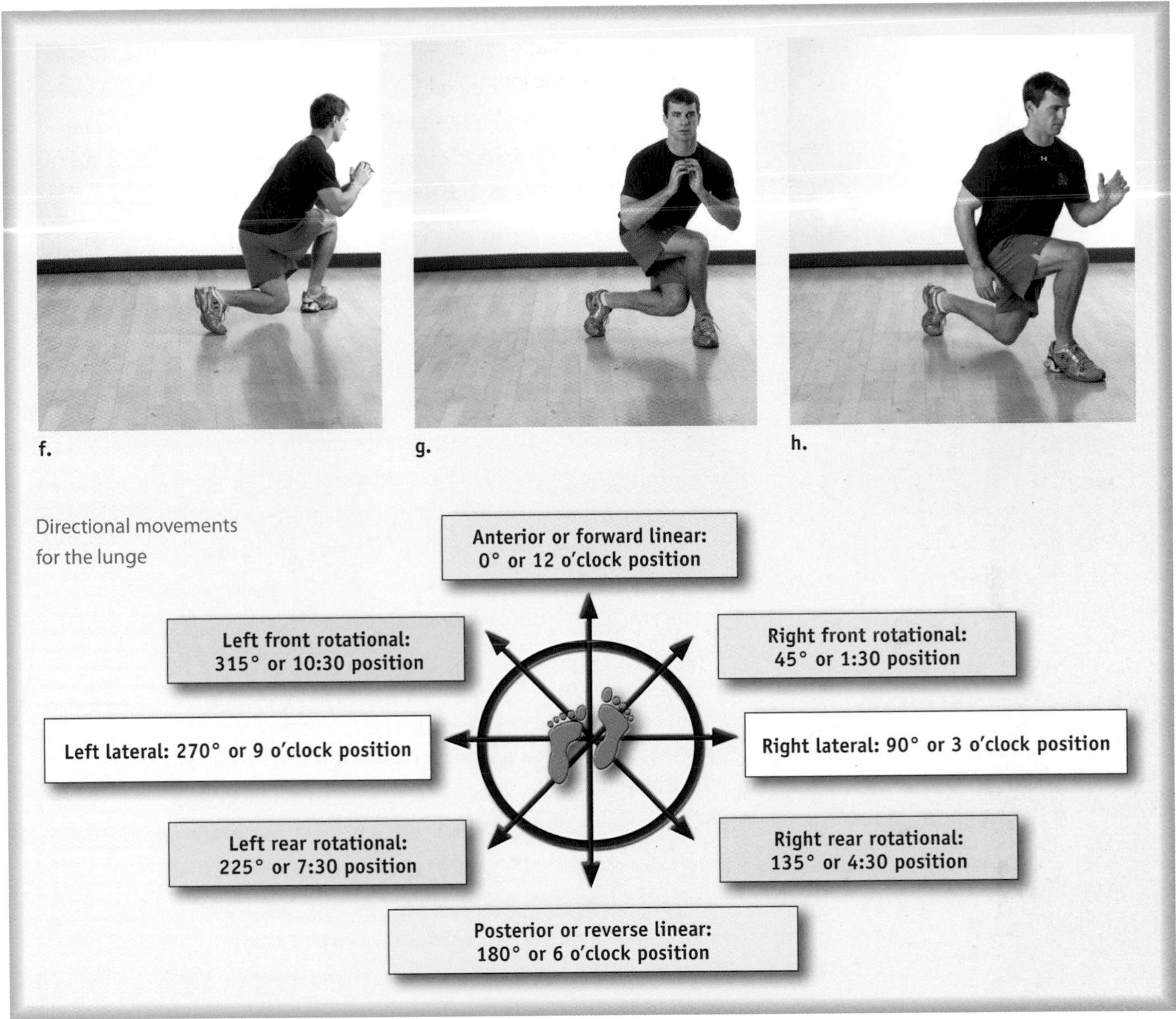

Directional movements for the lunge

When working with more athletic individuals, these same movement patterns can progress to jumps, hops, or bounds. However, individuals should never begin jumping, bounding, or hopping activities until they can effectively demonstrate correct landing technique and the ability to decelerate the impact forces of landing.

Pushing Movements

In everyday activities, pushing movements are pervasive, as they move the arms in front of the body or over the head. If the shoulder joint and shoulder girdle muscles work together properly, pushing actions can be performed effectively with minimal stress to the upper-extremity joints. When altered joint mechanics are present, such as the case when muscles have become adaptively shortened or lengthened due to repetitive use or poor posture, the risk for injury increases.

During shoulder flexion (e.g., front raise exercise or pushing open a door) and overhead presses (e.g., dumbbell press exercise or putting luggage into an overhead compartment

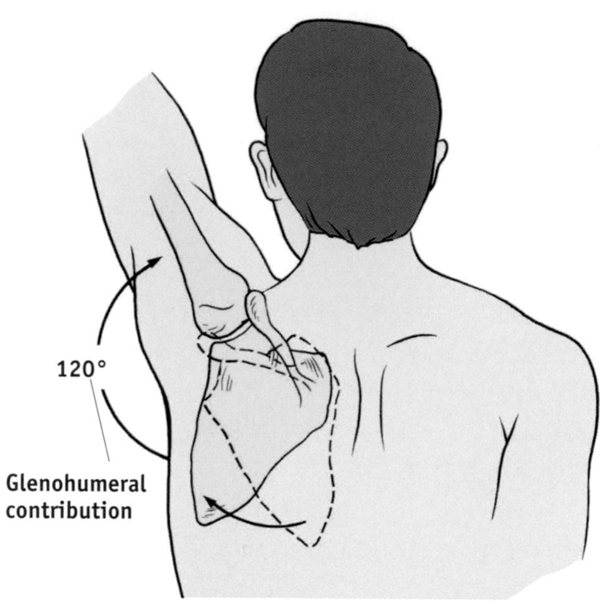

Figure 17-32
The movement of the arm is accompanied by movement of the scapula—a ratio of approximately 2° of arm movement for every 1° of scapular movement occurs during shoulder abduction and flexion; this relationship is known as scapulohumeral rhythm.

on an airplane), movement to 180 degrees is achieved by the collaborative effort of the scapulae rotating against the ribcage and the humerus rotating within the glenoid fossa. The movement generally requires approximately 60 degrees of scapular rotation and 120 degrees of glenohumeral rotation (Figure 17-32) (Sahrmann, 2002). While the scapulae require some degree of mobility to perform the various movements of the arm, they fundamentally need to remain stable to promote normal mobility within the glenohumeral joint. During these movements, insufficient, premature, or excessive activation of specific scapular muscles (e.g., dominant rhomboids resisting upward scapular rotation or overactive upper trapezius forcing excessive scapular elevation) will compromise scapular stability, which in turn affects the ability of the muscles around the glenohumeral joint to execute their function effectively. For example, if the scapulae cannot sink slightly while the arms extend overhead, this may interfere with scapular rotation and scapular stability. This forces the glenohumeral joint to assume greater loads, reducing its force-generating capacity and increasing the potential for injury (Cook & Jones, 2007a). This illustrates the importance of setting or packing the scapulae prior to shoulder flexion or abduction movements.

Exercises during this phase of training progress beyond stability and shift toward integrating whole-body movement patterns. Exercises can begin with more traditional pushing and pulling movements that primarily target the shoulder girdle in a bilateral or unilateral fashion, using supported backrests, then progress to becoming unsupported (e.g., standing in a normal or split-stance position), which better mimics most ADL (Figure 17-33).

Another common mistake made when performing overhead presses is the tendency to simply yield to gravity during the **eccentric** or downward phase of a shoulder press. This creates instability within the shoulder joint, given the changing roles of the deltoids between the starting and overhead position (Cook & Jones, 2007a). This overhead shoulder press position may increase the potential for anterior displacement of the humerus, given the lack of support from the anterior deltoid in the overhead position. However, the latissimus dorsi wraps around the anterior capsule from behind and, when elongated or loaded, can offer stability to the anterior shoulder (Cook & Jones, 2007a). Therefore, if the latissimus dorsi is engaged to begin the lowering phase, anterior containment is provided to help stabilize the shoulder and precipitate greater force production during the lifting phase. Thus, clients should be coached to engage the latissimus dorsi during the lowering phase and not simply yield to gravity (Figure 17-34).

Pulling Movements

The common actions of pulling open a door or lifting objects to hold them close to the body are examples of how people use pulling movements in their everyday activities. Similar to the body mechanics of pushing, when the shoulder and shoulder girdle are functioning within their ideal ranges of motion, pulling movements are effective actions that transfer minimal stress to the joints. However, muscles that do not provide the

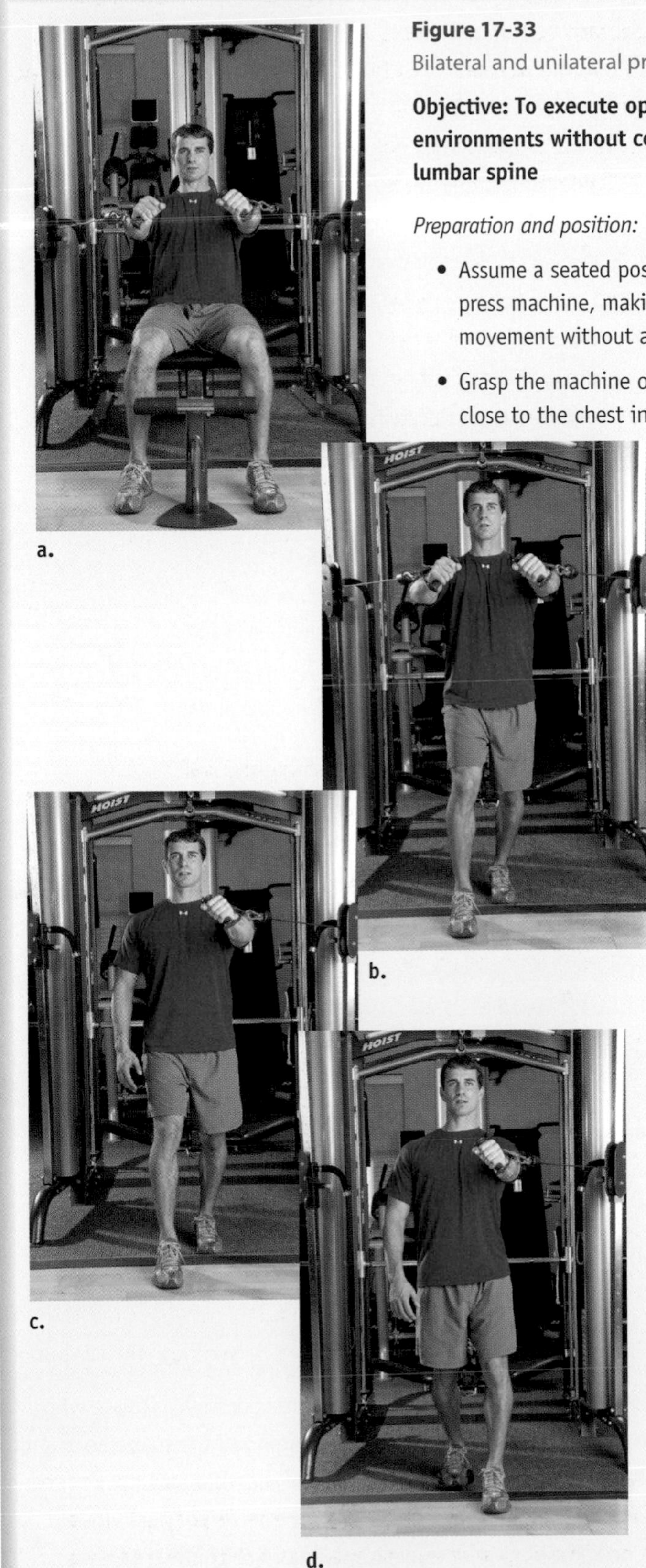

Figure 17-33

Bilateral and unilateral presses

Objective: To execute open-chain pushing movements in unsupported environments without compromising stability in the scapulothoracic joint and lumbar spine

Preparation and position:

- Assume a seated position on a seat or bench of any weightstack or cable-press machine, making contact with the backrest. Progress by repeating the movement without any contact against the backrest.
- Grasp the machine or cable handles firmly in both hands, positioning the hands close to the chest in a starting press position.
- Pack both shoulders (see Figure 17-16) and brace the core, holding these positions throughout the exercise.

Exercise:

- Exhale and gently press the load away bilaterally from the chest, preventing any change to the position of the lumbar spine or scapulae (do not perform a push-plus by protracting the scapulae when the elbows fully extend or elevate the scapulae). The goal is to reach full elbow extension, yet maintain a stable trunk and shoulder girdle (a).
- Slowly return to the starting position by adducting the scapulae (maintain the same starting position).
- Perform one or two sets of 12 to 15 repetitions with a controlled tempo, allowing 30-second rest intervals between sets.

Progression—Standing press: Repeat the same bilateral movement, but from a standing, split-stance position, alternating the forward leg with each set (b). A cable press or TRX® are suitable pieces of equipment to introduce for these progressions.

Progression—Single-arm press with a contralateral stance: Repeat the same movement, but pushing unilaterally with one arm, while the opposite leg is positioned forward in the split-stance position (c).

Progression—Single-arm press with an ipsilateral stance: Repeat the same movement, but pushing unilaterally with one arm, while the same-side leg is positioned forward in the split-stance position (d). The challenge is to resist the body's tendency to rotate during the push movement.

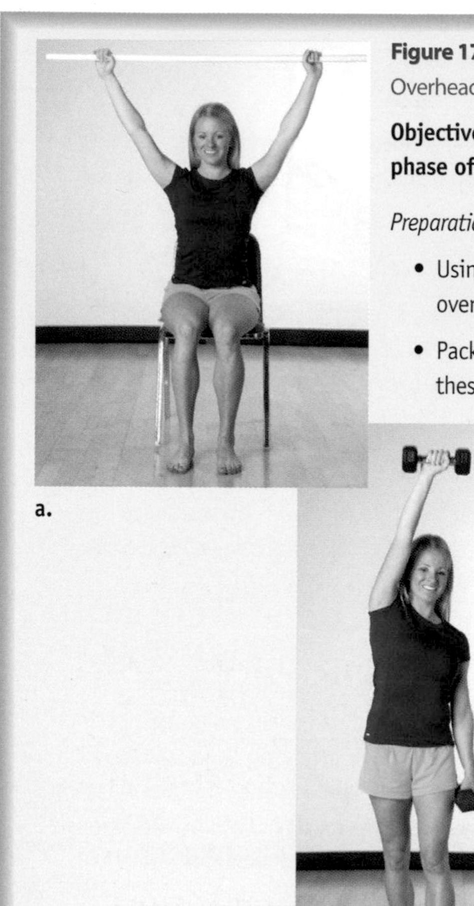

a.

b.

Figure 17-34
Overhead press

Objective: To provide additional stability to the shoulder capsule during the lowering phase of overhead pressing movements

Preparation and position:

- Using a dowel or lightly weighted bar, assume a seated position to perform a seated overhead press.
- Pack both shoulders (see Figure 17-16) and brace the core, holding these positions throughout the exercise.
- Press the bar overhead to the fully extended arm position, ensuring that the scapulae are not elevated (a).

Exercise:

- Actively engage the latissimus dorsi to initiate the pull-down sequence, lowering the bar to the starting position.
- Perform one or two sets of 12 to 15 repetitions with a controlled tempo, allowing 30-second rest intervals between sets.

Progression: Holding dumbbells, perform a variety of shoulder-press movements while introducing changes in the plane of movement:

- Add a trunk rotation, pressing upward across and even behind the body (b).
- Add lateral trunk movements (e.g., side lunge) and press overhead or across the front of the body.
- Assume a squat position, holding the dumbbells closer to waist level, and perform a series of uppercuts, driving the dumbbells across and behind the body to an end-point just above shoulder level.

appropriate strength or stability in the upper extremity—especially those that have attachments on the scapulae, ribcage, and humerus—can end up adding excess wear on the joints as they cannot effectively transfer mechanical forces.

Pulling movements follow many of the same principles as pressing movements with regard to stabilizing the scapulothoracic region, which helps promote effective glenohumeral function (Figure 17-35). Health coaches should identify whether they want to train a client to pull from a position of scapular stability, implying that the movement is purely from the shoulder (i.e., glenohumeral or shoulder extension/horizontal extension), or whether they are intentionally incorporating scapular retraction and adduction into the pulling motion. Clients whose scapular stability is compromised, such as those who exhibit forward-rounded shoulders, abducted scapulae, or winging of the scapulae, should perform pulling exercises—at least initially—from a position of scapular stability with very little resistance (external load). This means that the scapulae are in the set position and they do not move as the glenohumeral joint acts in extension or horizontal extension. Once the client has demonstrated that he or she is able to maintain the scapular set position for various pulling movements, scapular retraction and adduction can be added to the pulling exercises to ensure that the scapulothoracic and glenohumeral joints have the opportunity to move as they should during normal daily activities.

Exercises to promote effective pulling can begin with more traditional movements that primarily target the shoulder girdle in a bilateral or unilateral fashion, using supported backrests, then progress to becoming unsupported (e.g., standing in a normal, split-stance, or lunge position) that mimic most ADL.

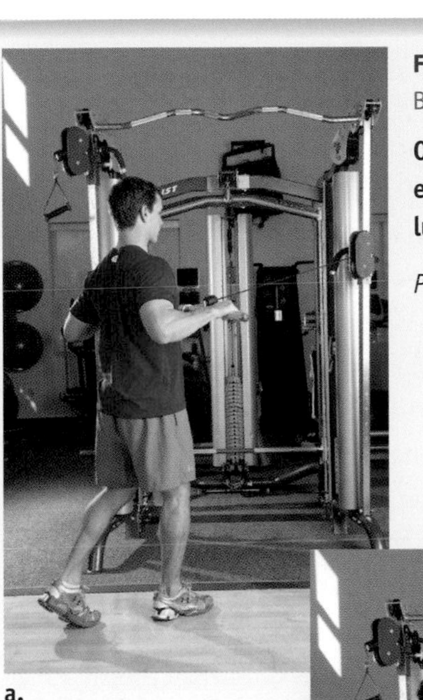

a.

b.

c.

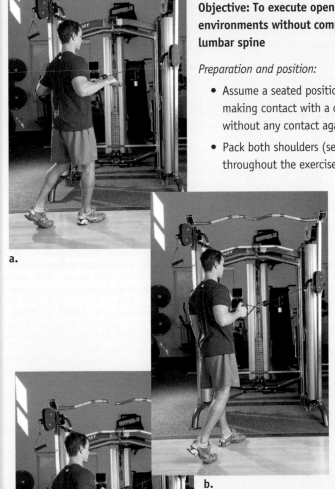

Figure 17-35
Bilateral and unilateral rows

Objective: To execute open-kinetic-chain pulling movements in unsupported environments without compromising stability of the scapulothoracic joint and lumbar spine

Preparation and position:

- Assume a seated position on a seat or bench of any weightstack or cable machine, making contact with a chest plate or rest. Progress by repeating the movement without any contact against a rest.
- Pack both shoulders (see Figure 17-16) and brace the core, holding these positions throughout the exercise.
- Grasp the machine or cable handles firmly in both hands, in a shoulder-flexed, elbow-extended position without protracting the scapulae.

Exercise:

- Exhale and gently pull the load bilaterally toward the body, preventing any change to the position of the lumbar spine or scapulae (avoid retracting or squeezing the shoulder blades together). The goal is to continue pulling until the elbows are bent 90 degrees, yet maintain a stable trunk and shoulder girdle.
- Slowly return to the starting position by extending the arms.
- Perform one or two sets of 12 to 15 repetitions with a controlled tempo, allowing 30-second rest intervals between sets.

Progression—Standing pull: Repeat the same bilateral movement, but from a standing, split-stance position, alternating the forward leg with each set (a). A cable pull or TRX are suitable pieces of equipment to introduce for these progressions.

Progression—Single-arm pull with a contralateral stand: Repeat the same movement, but pulling unilaterally with one arm while the opposite leg is positioned forward in the split-stance position (b).

Progression—Single-arm pull with an ipsilateral stand: Repeat the same movement, but pulling unilaterally with one arm, while the same-side leg is positioned forward in the split-stance position (c). The challenge is to resist the body's temptation to rotate during the pulling movement.

Rotational Movements

Rotational movements represent the last of the primary movements and are perhaps some of the most complex movements, given how many follow spiral or diagonal patterns throughout the body. These movements generally incorporate movement into multiple planes simultaneously (e.g., a golf backswing requires transverse plane rotation, thoracic and lumbar extension, and some lateral flexion). Many of these movements increase the forces placed along the vertebrae, so health coaches must exercise care when teaching these movements and only do so after the client has conditioned the core effectively.

Consideration of good technique and appropriate levels of mobility and stability in the thoracic and lumbar spine is critical in facilitating synchronous movement and dissipating the generated ground reactive forces over larger surface areas (e.g., upward toward the cervical vertebra and downward toward the hips, knees, and ankles) (Gray & Tiberio, 2007). The ability to dissipate ground reactive forces reduces the impact on local areas and decreases the potential for injury.

Two key movements involving diagonal or spiral patterns of movement within the arms, shoulders, trunks, hips, and legs are the wood chop and the hay bailer:

- *Wood chops*: This exercise involves a pulling action to initiate the movement down across the front of the body, followed by a pushing action in the upper extremity as the arms move away from the body (Figure 17-36). In addition, it requires stabilization of the trunk in all three planes (i.e., during flexion, rotation, and side-bending), and weight transference through the hips and between the legs to gain leverage and maintain balance (Cook & Jones, 2007b). **Concentric** action during the downward chop is achieved by using a high anchor point (e.g., high cable pulley or band).
- *Hay bailers*: This exercise involves a pulling action to initiate the movement up across the front of the body, followed by a pushing action in the upper extremity as the arms move away from the body (Figure 17-37). In addition, it requires stabilization of the trunk in all three planes (extension in the sagittal plane, rotation in the transverse plane, and side-bending in the frontal plane), and weight transference through the hips and between the legs to gain leverage and maintain balance (Cook & Jones, 2007b).

The need for thoracic mobility is greater during these movements than with the pushes and pulls, given the three-dimensional nature of the movement patterns. Performing these exercises without thoracic mobility or lumbar stability may compromise the shoulders and hips, and increase the likelihood for injury. The thoracic spine offers greater mobility than the lumbar spine. Therefore, lumbar stability and control of lumbar rotation should be emphasized while promoting movement within the thoracic spine.

Program Design for Beginners

The basic programming guidelines in the movement-training phase are to give clients exercises to help them develop proper control and adequate ROM while performing the five basic movements. The timeframe for movement training is two weeks to two months, depending on each client's initial level of movement ability and his or her rate of progression. The FIRST acronym can be used to guide exercise program design: frequency, intensity, repetitions, sets, and type.

- *Frequency*: Two to three days per week is adequate for the beginning stages of a movement-training program. Considering that many clients who are deconditioned

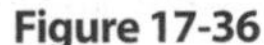

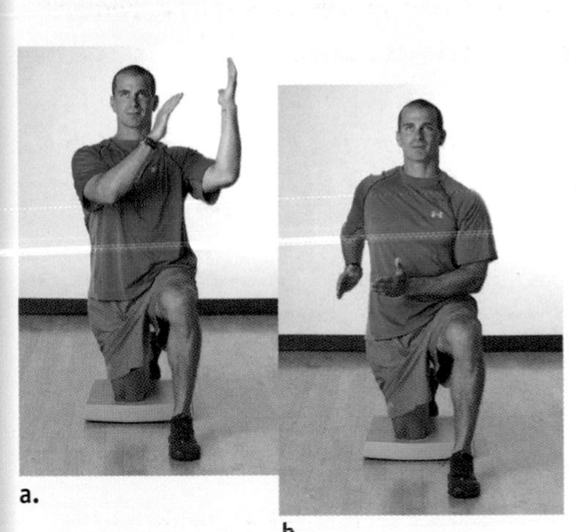

a. b.

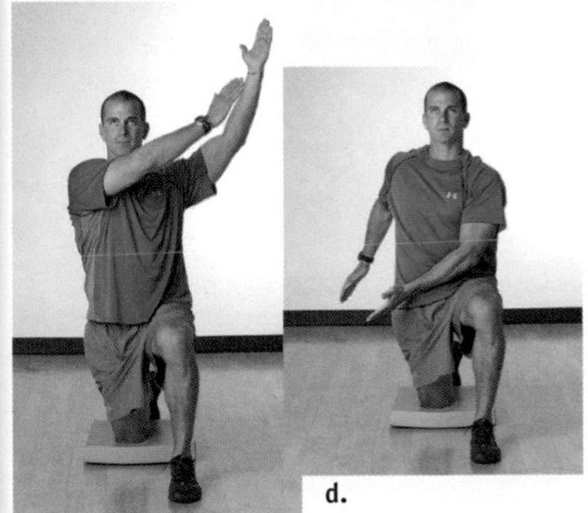

c. d.

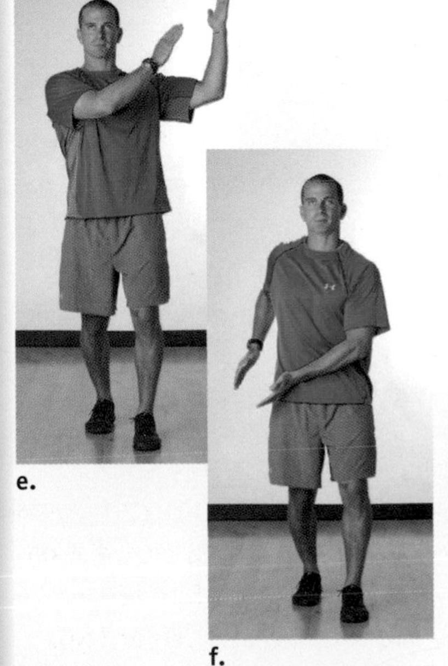

e. f.

g. h.

Figure 17-36

Wood-chop spiral patterns

Note: Given the complexity of the wood-chop movement, the individual should first learn basic spiral patterns without placing excessive loads upon the spine.

Objective: To introduce basic spiral patterns with small, controlled forces placed along the spine

Preparation and position:

- Assume a half-kneeling position, placing the rear knee directly under the hips. This position engages both the hip flexors and extensors to help stabilize the spine.
- An unstable surface may be placed under the rear knee to increase the stability demands on the core. *Note:* Clients should only progress to the unstable surface after demonstrating good core strength and stability.
- Pack both shoulders (see Figure 17-16) and brace the core, holding these positions throughout the exercise.
- Imagine holding a short handle that positions the hands 6 to 12 inches (15 to 30 cm) apart and raise the handle toward the shoulder on the same side as the leading leg, keeping both hands close to the body (a).
- The hips and torso (chest) should remain aligned forward.

Exercise:

- Exhale and slowly perform a downward movement across the front of the body, moving the handle toward the opposite hip and keeping both arms close to the body to shorten the length of the lever (called the moment arm) (b).
- The hips and torso (chest) should remain aligned forward.
- Return to the starting position and repeat.
- Perform one or two sets of 12 to 15 repetitions in each direction, alternating the knee position with each directional change.

Progression—Long moment arm: Repeat the same movement, but extend the arms (acting as a driver) to increase the range of motion and leverage, but keep both arms close the body during the movement (c & d). The hips and torso (chest) should remain aligned forward.

Progression—Standing short moment arm: Assume a split-stance position, placing the leg on the same side as the chop start position forward. Bend both elbows, placing the hands 6 to 12 inches (15 to 30 cm) apart and raise the handle toward the shoulder on the same side as the leading leg, keeping both hands close to the body (e & f). Repeat the same chopping movement with bent elbows. The hips and torso (chest) should remain aligned forward.

Progression—Standing long moment arm: Assume the same split-stance position and repeat the same chopping movement, but extend the arms (g & h). The hips and torso (chest) should remain aligned forward.

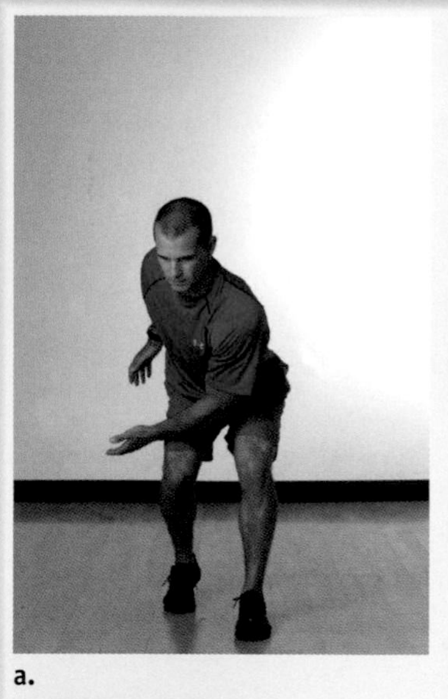
a.

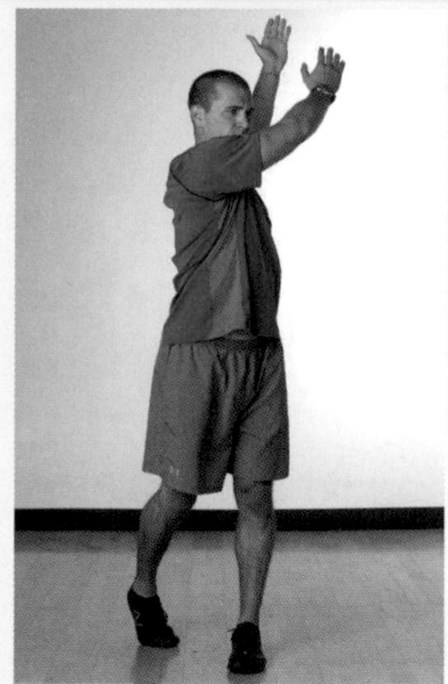
b.

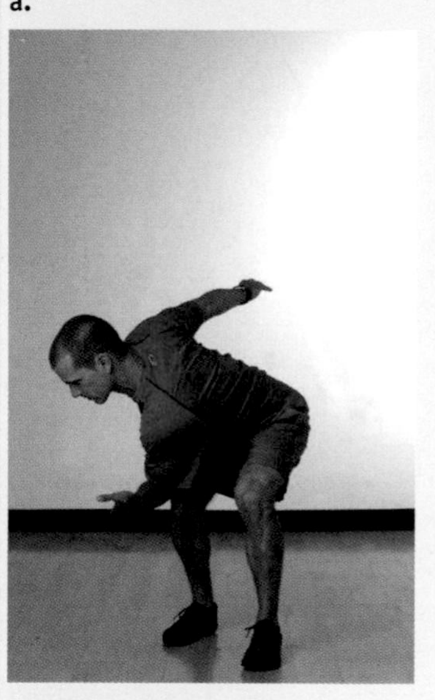
c.

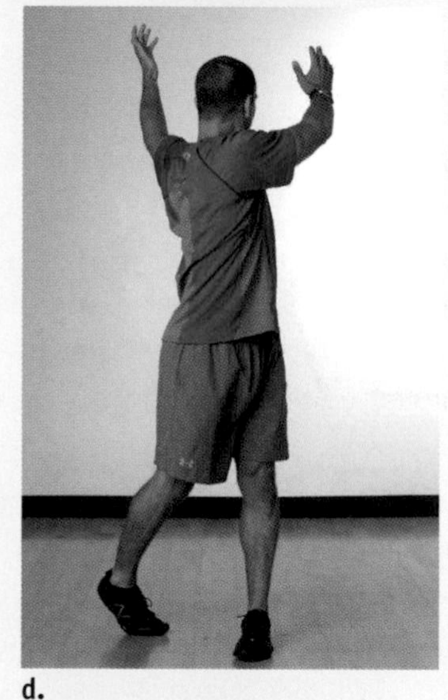
d.

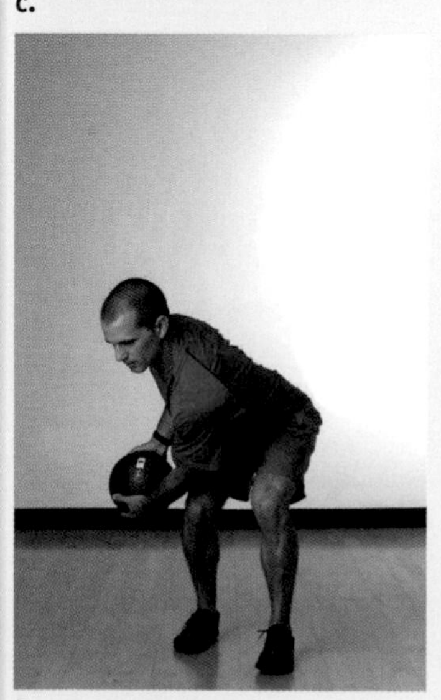
e.

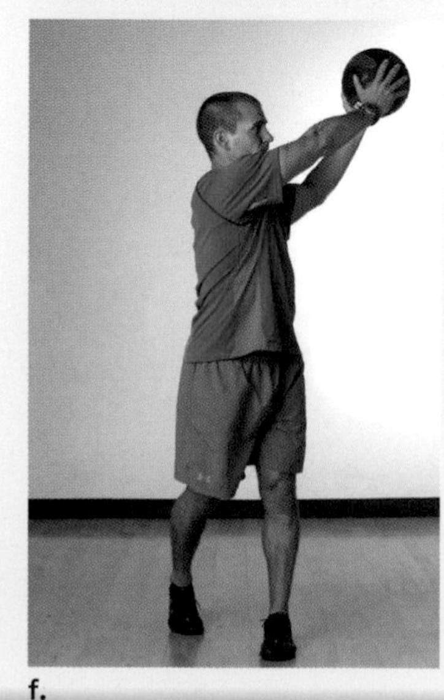
f.

Figure 17-37
Full wood-chop and hay-bailer patterns

Objective: To introduce the full multiplanar wood-chop and hay-bailer movement patterns while controlling forces placed along the spine

Preparation and position (a & b):

- Assume a staggered position, placing the inside leg 6 to 12 inches (15 to 30 cm) forward.
- Pack both shoulders (see Figure 17-16) and brace the core, holding these positions throughout the exercise.
- Imagine holding a short handle that positions the hands 6 to 12 inches (15 to 30 cm) apart and raise the handle toward the inside shoulder on the same side as the leading leg, keeping both hands close to the body.
- Load 60 to 70% of the body weight onto the inside leg.

Exercise:

- Exhale, hip-hinge (hip flex), and squat while rotating the hips outward, transferring 60 to 70% of the body weight onto the outside leg.
- While the hips rotate, the chest and shoulders should remain aligned over the pubis (center of the pelvis).
- Return to the starting position and repeat.
- Perform one or two sets of 12 to 15 repetitions in each direction, alternating the stance position with each directional change.

Progression—Long moment arm: Repeat the same movement, but extend the elbows and move the hands 2 to 3 feet (0.6 to 0.9 m) apart (the use of a dowel might prove useful). A wide, extended grip concentrates force-generation from the hips and not from the shoulder or arms. Repeat the movement and, while the hips rotate, the chest and shoulders should remain aligned over the pubis (center of the pelvis).

Progression—Full chop (c & d): Repeat the same movement, but allow the torso to rotate further into the start position and rotate past the hips at the end position. Allow the unloaded leg to pivot during the movement to help transfer and dissipate forces.

Progression (e & f): Add external resistance in the form of a medicine ball, kettle bell, cable, or elastic tubing.

and have a weight-loss goal will also be engaging in regular cardiorespiratory training, a frequency of two days per week may be a more appropriate recommendation.

- *Intensity*: Since the goal is to focus on coordination and muscular conditioning for the basic movement patterns, clients should not use any external load while performing the exercises.
- *Repetitions*: An appropriate repetition range for movement training is 12 to 20 repetitions.
- *Sets*: A range of two to three sets is appropriate for each movement-training exercise.
- *Type*: Exercise selection should focus on the five basic movement patterns: squats, lunges, pushes (both in the horizontal plane and overhead), pulls, and rotational movements.

Adding Resistance to Movement Training

When the five primary movements can be performed with proper form, external resistance may be applied for progressive strength development. It is essential that the external loads are increased gradually so that correct movement patterns are not altered during the exercise performance. See the following section on program design for load training (phase 3) for specific guidelines for safely and effectively increasing weight loads.

- *Squat:* External loading may be applied with various types of resistance equipment. A client may begin by holding a medicine ball while doing squats. Another resistance option is placing an elastic band under the feet and holding each end of the band while performing squats. A third resistance tool is free weights, beginning with dumbbells and progressing to barbell squats when the legs can handle more resistance than the hands can hold. An alternative exercise to the barbell squat is the leg press, which trains the same pattern of movement without the direct pull of gravity, while strengthening the quadriceps, hamstrings, and gluteus maximus muscles.
- *Lunge:* Lunge movements (in any direction) may be performed with external loads by holding a medicine ball or dumbbells. Initially, resistance bands and barbells are not recommended tools for lunge movements, as lunging is a high balance-challenge activity and the unpredictable forces of elastic resistance and the awkward length of barbells might make it too difficult for clients who have minimal experience with lower-extremity exercise.
- *Pushing movements:* Pushing movements may be performed with added resistance by using resistance bands or cables in a standing position, by performing machine chest presses from a seated position, or by lifting free weights (dumbbells or barbells) from a lying (supine) position. Medicine balls may also be used for pushing movements from a supine position, and from a standing position by performing a chest pass (releasing the medicine ball).
- *Pulling movements:* Pulling movements may be performed with external loads by using resistance bands or cables in a standing position, by performing machine rows and pull-downs from a seated position, and by lifting dumbbells from a bent-over standing position with the torso parallel to the floor and supported by one arm (bent-over row exercise). Medicine balls and barbells are not recommended for beginners for rowing exercises, because one arm is not free for torso support.
- *Rotational movements:* External resistance may be applied to rotational movements by using resistance bands or cables in a standing position, by using machines from a seated position, or by lifting medicine balls from a variety of positions (standing, seated, and lying). It can be difficult to use barbells in rotational movements, but dumbbells can be used in movements that directly oppose gravity's line of pull.

Program Design for Beginners

The acronym FIRST may be used to designate the five key components of resistance-training program design: frequency, intensity, repetitions, sets, and type of exercise. During the initial weeks of resistance training, motor learning plays a major role in the desired physical development and movement patterns. Consequently, during this training period, exercise repetition should be emphasized over exercise intensity.

- *Frequency:* Beginning exercisers experience excellent results by strength training two to three days a week, and this is the recommended training frequency during the movement-training phase.
- *Intensity:* Due to the emphasis on proper movement patterns, the training intensity is lower during this phase. Start with a light resistance that allows clients to learn proper movement techniques and then progress resistance to a maximum of 60 to 70% of maximal resistance.
- *Repetitions:* The number of repetitions performed varies inversely with the intensity of the exercise set. That is, fewer repetitions can be performed with a higher resistance and more repetitions can be completed with a lower resistance. During the movement-training phase, the lower training intensity permits more repetitions in each exercise set. Most people can perform about 12 repetitions with 70% of maximal resistance and about 16 repetitions with 60% of maximal resistance. It is therefore recommended that movement-training phase exercises first be performed with light resistance that allows for proper movement patterns to be learned, and then progressed to weightloads that allow the movement to be completed for between 12 and 16 repetitions. Generally, if the resistance does not permit at least 12 repetitions, it should be reduced. When 16 repetitions can be properly performed, the resistance should be increased by approximately 5%.
- *Sets:* Studies have demonstrated that one set of resistance exercise is as effective as multiple training sets (Carpinelli & Otto, 1998; Starkey et al., 1996), especially for beginning exercisers. For movement-training phase workouts, one set of each exercise is certainly a good starting point. As training progresses, more sets of each exercise may be performed as determined by the client's desire to do so. During the first 10 to 12 weeks of resistance exercise, both single- and multiple-set training have been shown to increase lean (muscle) weight by approximately 3 pounds (1.4 kg) (Westcott, 2009; Campbell et al., 1994). Single-set programs are an effective way to help previously sedentary clients become comfortable with the challenges of resistance training. When the client demonstrates consistent adherence and initial adaptations to a single-set program, the volume of sets can increase.
- *Type:* The type of exercise should be selected to help the client learn and improve movement patterns with respect to his or her muscular fitness and strength-training experience. Clients with less muscle strength and training experience should begin with basic exercises performed with external resistance and relatively stable conditions. Exercise selection can begin with machines, which utilize the basic movement patterns of exercise but provide stability and control the path of motion. Once a client demonstrates progress with motor control and muscular strength, he or she can begin performing ground-based standing exercises that emphasize muscle integration.

Such exercises include dumbbell squats, overhead dumbbell presses, standing cable rows, and standing cable presses. As strength increases, emphasis may be placed on multiplanar movements that require higher levels of muscle integration. Movements may be performed from unsupported postures, with closed-kinetic-chain exercises for the lower-body muscles and open-kinetic-chain exercises for the upper-body muscles. Free-moving lever-action exercises are appropriate during movement training.

Appropriate Rates of Progression for Beginners

The standard recommendation for progression is a 5% resistance increase whenever the end range number of repetitions can be completed. However, during the early stages of resistance training, the motor-learning effect enhances strength gains by facilitating muscle-fiber recruitment and contraction efficiency. Therefore, during the movement-training phase, resistance increases may be more than 5% if the exerciser experiences a relatively fast rate of progression. For example, when a client completes 16 repetitions with 100 pounds (45 kg), the weightload may be increased up to 110 pounds (50 kg) (10% increase), as long as at least 12 repetitions can be performed with the heavier resistance.

Once the exercises can be executed with correct movement patterns while maintaining neutral posture, a stable center of gravity, and controlled movement speed, clients may progress to the load-training phase (phase 3).

Phase 3: Load Training

In the load-training phase, the training emphasis progresses from stability and mobility and movement training to muscle force production, which can be addressed in different ways to attain specific developmental objectives. The training objectives may include increased muscular endurance, increased muscular strength, increased muscle **hypertrophy,** as well as improved body composition, movement, function, and health. Regardless of the specific objective of the load-training program, it is recommended that stability and mobility training and movement training exercises be included in the warm-up and cool-down activities.

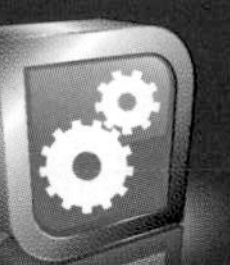

EXPAND YOUR KNOWLEDGE

Resistance Training Is Not a Factor in Weight Loss

The reason that resistance training is not included as a major factor in the exercise recommendations for weight loss for overweight and obese individuals is because there is a lack of evidence to support weight training for weight loss and maintenance. While it is true that resistance training may increase muscle mass, which can create positive changes in body composition and may in turn increase daily energy expenditure, it does not seem to be effective for weight reduction in the initial months of training, nor does it add to weight loss when combined with diet restriction [American College of Sports Medicine (ACSM), 2009].

However, it is important that health coaches do not discount the role of resistance training in health improvement. In addition to the functional movement and performance benefits provided by regular resistance training, lifting weights has been associated with improvements in CVD risk factors, even in the absence of significant weight loss. Regular resistance training has been shown to increase **high-density lipoprotein (HDL) cholesterol** (Hurley et al., 1988), decrease **low-density lipoprotein (LDL)** (Hurley et al., 1988; Goldberg et al., 1984), and decrease triglycerides (Goldberg et al., 1984). Reductions in both **systolic** and **diastolic blood pressure** have also been reported as a result of participation in a resistance-training program (Kelley, 1997; Norris, Carroll, & Cochrane, 1990).

Perhaps the most revealing evidence to support to the health benefits of weight training is related to its association with improvements in type 2 diabetes. Improved **insulin** sensitivity has been reported in individuals who engage in resistance-training programs (Di Pietro et al., 2006; Ibanez et al., 2005). In addition, Church and colleagues (2010) found that performing a combination of aerobic exercise and resistance training was associated with improved glycemic levels among patients with type 2 diabetes, compared to patients who did not exercise. The level of improvement was not seen among patients who performed either aerobic exercise or resistance training alone. Taken together, these findings suggest that both aerobic endurance exercise and resistance training must be included in a well-rounded exercise program.

Program Design for Improving Muscular Strength

Muscular strength is a measure of the maximal force that can be produced by one or more muscle groups, and is typically assessed by the **one-repetition maximum (1-RM)** weightload in an exercise (e.g., leg press and bench press). If a client increases his or her 1-RM bench press from 200 pounds (91 kg) to 250 pounds (114 kg), he or she has experienced a 25% improvement in bench press strength. Although some of the weightload increase may be attributed to motor learning, much of the improvement would be due to strength development in the pushing muscles—pectoralis major, anterior deltoids, and triceps—as a result of a progressively challenging training program. Although increases in muscular strength are accompanied by increases in muscular endurance, preferred protocols for strength development place more emphasis on training intensity.

The FIRST recommendations for improving muscular strength are as follows:

- *Frequency:* High-intensity resistance training causes significant tissue microtrauma that typically requires 72 hours for muscle remodeling to higher strength levels (McLester et al., 2003). Consequently, clients who complete total-body workouts should schedule two training sessions per week. Clients who prefer to perform split routines (working different muscle groups or movement patterns on different days) should take at least 72 hours between workouts for the same muscles. For example, clients who do pushing movements for the chest, shoulders, and triceps on Mondays and Thursdays, pulling movements for the upper back and biceps on Tuesdays and Fridays, and squat, lunge, and rotational movements for the legs and trunk on Wednesdays and Saturdays have six weekly workouts, but provide at least 72 hours of recovery time between exercises for the same muscle groups.
- *Intensity:* The initial stages of muscular-strength training may be successfully conducted with a range of weightloads (e.g., 70 to 90% of maximal resistance). However, for optimal strength development, most authorities recommend weightloads between 80 and 90% of the 1 RM. Exercises with near-maximal weightloads that allow one to three repetitions with more than 90% of maximal resistance are highly effective for developing muscular strength. However, these exercises are not appropriate for the average client unless he or she has a training goal directly related to increased strength. Because these are relatively heavy weightloads, a periodized approach that progressively increases the training intensity over several weeks is recommended.

- *Repetitions:* Repetition ranges are essentially determined by the exercise resistance. Because exercises with relatively high exercise weightloads cannot be performed for many repetitions, training for muscular strength involves fewer repetitions than training for muscular endurance. Most individuals can complete about four repetitions with 90% of maximal resistance and about eight repetitions with 80% of maximal resistance. Therefore, the recommended repetition range for muscular strength development is four to eight repetitions. When nine repetitions can be completed with correct training technique, the weightload should be increased by approximately 5%.
- *Sets:* Muscular strength can be significantly increased through either single-set or multiple-set training (Carpinelli & Otto, 1998; Starkey et al., 1996). It may be prudent to start clients with one hard set of each exercise (after performing progressively challenging warm-up sets), and increase the number of stimulus sets in accordance with clients' interest and ability to performing additional sets. Generally, muscular-strength programs do not exceed three to four sets of each training exercise. To perform repeated exercise sets with relatively heavy weightloads, clients must take longer recovery periods between successive sets. Unlike muscular-endurance training, which features one- to two-minute rests between sets, muscular-strength training generally features three- to four-minute recovery periods between sets of the same exercise. The longer rests lead to longer workouts for muscular-strength training programs. For example, a standard 10-exercise workout could require about two hours (125 minutes) for completion (3 sets x 10 exercises x 40-second performance plus 30 x 210 seconds recovery time). Fortunately, single-set training programs can effectively increase muscular strength in much shorter exercise sessions. For example, a single set of 10 exercises would require about 20 to 25 minutes for completion, and the inclusion of a warm-up set for each exercise would make the workout about 45 to 50 minutes in duration on the high end. Single-set programs using an appropriate warm-up and a challenging training intensity are effective means of helping clients maintain adherence to their programs when they have other demands for their time, such as a hectic schedule at work or managing the needs of a busy household.
- *Type:* Muscular-strength training may be performed with many types of resistance equipment. However, like muscular-endurance training, the consistency and incremental weightloads provided by standard machine and free-weight exercises make these the preferred training modes for developing higher strength levels. Generally, linear exercises that involve multiple muscle groups utilized in the basic movements are the preferred method for increasing total-body strength. These exercises include squats, deadlifts, or leg presses for the squat pattern; step-ups and lunges for the lunge pattern; bench presses, incline presses, shoulder presses, and bar dips for the push pattern; and seated rows, lat pull-downs, and pull-ups for the pulling pattern. Rotary exercises that isolate specific muscle groups (e.g., leg extensions, leg curls, hip adductions, hip abductions, lateral raises, chest crosses, pull-overs, arm extensions, arm curls, trunk extensions, and trunk curls) should not be excluded from muscular-strength workouts, but these typically play a lesser role than the movement-based exercises that challenge multiple muscles at the same time.

Appropriate Rates of Progression in Strength Training

The recommended procedure for improving muscular strength is the double-progressive training protocol. There are numerous factors that affect the rate of strength development, and progress varies considerably among individuals. Consequently, it is not practical to suggest weekly weightload increases, as some clients will progress more quickly and others will progress more slowly than the recommended resistance increments. To facilitate individual stimulus–response relationships and to reduce the risk of doing too much too soon, health coaches should factor both repetitions and resistance into the training progression. First, the client's repetition range, such as four to eight repetitions per set, must be established. Second, the client can continue training with the same exercise resistance until the terminal number of repetitions (eight repetitions) can be completed with proper technique. When this is accomplished, the health coach should raise the resistance by approximately 5%, which will reduce the number of repetitions the client can perform.

EXPAND YOUR KNOWLEDGE

Obesity Does Not Result in Increased Muscle Strength

While it might be common to think that a person who weighs more due to excess body fat is consequently stronger than a normal-weight individual, the opposite is true. Obesity lessens a person's strength because excessive body fat infiltrates and weakens muscle tissue. When strength relative to body weight is considered, obese individuals tend to be much weaker (Messier, 2008). This lack of physical strength relative to total body weight can negatively impact the performance of ADL. Thus, while resistance training may not be the primary recommended mode of activity for weight loss for the obese population, it certainly is an important adjunct to the overall exercise program and should not be overlooked.

Prerequisite Muscular Strength Prior to Performance Training

Some athletically oriented clients will want to progress to performance-training to prepare for a specific athletic event or competition. The performance training phase (phase 4) focuses specifically on enhancing athletic skills for sports through the application of power exercises that emphasize the speed of force production, and the performance of specific drills that improve speed, agility, quickness, and reactivity. Clients who progress to performance training should have successfully completed both the movement- and load-training phases (phases 2 and 3). They should demonstrate good postural stability, proper movement patterns, and relatively high levels of muscular strength before initiating the performance-training phase. To facilitate maintenance and progress of posture techniques and movement training, these exercises can be incorporated in dynamic warm-up activities prior to performing performance-training workouts.

> It is important for health coaches to understand that power training for performance involves advanced exercise techniques that can place greater stress on the musculoskeletal system than standard strength training. Consequently, health coaches should be certain that their clients have both the movement abilities and muscular strength to properly and safely execute the performance-training progressions.

Phase 4: Performance Training

This phase of training emphasizes specific training related to performance enhancement. Power training during the performance-training phase is an important component of sports-conditioning programs that helps prepare athletes for the rigors of their specific sport. Typically, this type of program is not appropriate for the average exerciser who is interested in improving general health and fitness. However, there are individuals who could benefit from adding power training to their fitness programs, such as middle-aged clients who have been strength training for months and are looking to improve their performance enough to participate in recreational sport activities. Older-adult clients can also benefit from certain forms of power training that emphasize power and quickness to help avoid falls. Furthermore, if designed and progressed appropriately, power training can add interest and fun to an existing exercise program.

Strength training performed during the load-training phase (phase 3) increases muscular force production, but does not specifically address the period of time during which the force is produced. Power training enhances the velocity of force production by improving the ability of muscles to generate a large amount of force in a short period of time. Power is needed in all sports and activities that require repeated acceleration and deceleration. Power can be defined as both the velocity of force production and the rate of performing work:

Power Equations

Power = Force x Velocity

Power = Work/Time

Where:

- Force = Mass x Acceleration
- Velocity = Distance/Time
- Work = Force x Distance

If a client meets all of the prerequisites for performance training and expresses an interest in amplifying his or her training regimen through high-intensity sports conditioning, the next step is to determine the purpose of the program. That is, the health coach must learn which fitness parameters or sports skills the client hopes to improve and then set out to design a safe and effective program to meet the client's goals. Answering the following questions may be helpful in determining an appropriate power-based performance-training program for a client:

- Which movement patterns and activities (aerobic vs. anaerobic) are required for the client to be successful in reaching his or her performance goals?
- What are the athletic skills and abilities the client currently lacks?
- What are the common injuries associated with the activity? For example, lateral ankle sprains are common in soccer, especially if the athlete has high arches, so incorporating drills designed to enhance a client's ankle reactivity, and thus stability, would be appropriate.

Plyometric Training Overview

To improve the production of muscular force and power, a conditioning format called **plyometric exercise** can be implemented. Plyometric exercise incorporates quick, powerful movements and involves the stretch-shortening cycle [an active stretch (eccentric contraction) of a muscle followed by an immediate shortening (concentric contraction) of that same muscle]. Lower-body plyometrics are appropriate for clients who play virtually any sport, as well as for those who want to enhance their reaction and balance abilities, as long as the client has developed the prerequisite strength to begin plyometric training and has learned first how to land correctly. Lower-body plyometric exercises include jumps and bounds (involving one leg or both legs) (Table 17-12).

Table 17-12

Lower-body Plyometric Exercises

Type of Jump	Description
Jumps in place	Jumps require taking off and landing with both feet simultaneously. Jumps in place emphasize the vertical component of jumping and are performed repeatedly with no rest between jumps.
Single linear jumps or hops	These exercises emphasize the vertical and horizontal components of jumping and are performed at maximal effort with no rest between actions.
Multiple linear jumps or hops	These exercises move the client in a single linear direction, emphasize the vertical and horizontal components of jumping or hopping, and are performed repeatedly with no rest between actions.
Multidirectional jumps or hops	These exercises move the client in a variety of directions, emphasize the vertical and horizontal components of jumping, and are performed repeatedly with no rest between actions.
Hops and bounds	Hops involve taking off and landing with the same foot, while bounds involve the process of alternating feet during the take-off and landing (e.g., taking off with the right foot and landing with the left foot). Hops and bounds emphasize horizontal speed and are performed repeatedly with no rest between actions.
Depth jumps or hops	These exercises involve jumping or hopping off of a box, landing on the floor, and immediately jumping or hopping vertically, horizontally, or onto another box.

Jumping and Hopping Tips

- Clients should land softly on the midfoot, and then roll forward to push off the ball of the foot. Landing on the heel or ball of the foot must be avoided, as these errors increase impacting forces. Landing on the midfoot also shortens the time between the eccentric and concentric actions (i.e., the amortization phase), thus increasing the potential for power development if another jump follows.
- Ensure alignment of the hips, knees, ankles, and toes due to the potential for injury, especially in women.
- Encourage clients to drop the hips to absorb the impact forces and develop gluteal dominance. Clients must avoid locking out the knees upon landing, which leads to the development of quadriceps dominance. Poor landing technique may lead to knee injuries, particularly in women. Proper hip mechanics during flexion and extension, along with the requisite muscular strength, is extremely important for developing lower-body power, which is why it is recommended that a client go through both the movement- and load-training phases (phases 2 and 3) before progressing to power-based exercises in the performance training phase.
- Instruct clients to engage the core musculature, which stiffens the torso, protects the spine during landing, and allows for increased force transfer during the subsequent concentric contraction (or jump).
- Clients should land with the trunk inclined slightly forward, the head up, and the torso rigid. Health coaches can cue clients to keep their "chests over their knees" and their "nose over their toes" during the landing phase of jumps.

For a more in-depth discussion about performance training, including assessments and program design suggestions for plyometrics, speed, agility, and reactivity training, refer to the *ACE Personal Trainer Manual*.

Summary

The primary mode of activity to facilitate weight loss is aerobic, or endurance, exercise. Aerobic conditioning maximizes caloric expenditure and reduces the risk of chronic disease. Health coaches can use the ACE IFT Model to program exercise selection, intensity, and duration to fit the special needs of overweight and obese clients. Many of these individuals may never progress beyond the aerobic-efficiency phase of cardiorespiratory training (phase 2), and many of them will never progress beyond the load-training phase of functional movement and resistance training (phase 3). Helping an obese client transition into the **action** stage and then on to the **maintenance** stage of change will have a significant impact on that client's health and overall quality of life, and may even have a positive impact on the client's state of physical and mental fitness.

References

American College of Sports Medicine (2014). *ACSM's Guidelines for Exercise Testing and Prescription* (9th ed.). Philadelphia: Wolters Kluwer/Lippincott Williams & Wilkins.

American College of Sports Medicine (2009). Position stand: Appropriate physical activity intervention strategies for weight loss and prevention of weight regain for adults. *Medicine & Science in Sports & Exercise*, 41, 459–471.

Barnes, J.F. (1999). Myofascial release. In: Hammer, W.I. (Ed.) *Functional Soft Tissue Examination and Treatment by Manual Methods* (2nd ed). Gaithersburg, Md.: Aspen Publishers.

Borg, G. (1998). *Borg's Perceived Exertion and Pain Scales.* Champaign, Ill.: Human Kinetics.

Campbell, W. et al. (1994). Increased energy requirements and changes in body composition with resistance training in older adults. *American Journal of Clinical Nutrition,* 60, 167–175.

Carpinelli, R.N. & Otto, R.M. (1998). Strength training: Single versus multiple set. *Sports Medicine*, 26, 2, 73–84.

Church, T.S. et al. (2010). Effects of aerobic and resistance training on hemoglobin A1c levels in patients with type 2 diabetes. *Journal of the American Medical Association*, 304, 2253–2262.

Cook, G. & Jones, B. (2007a). *Secrets of the Shoulder*. www.functionalmovement.com

Cook, G. & Jones, B. (2007b). *Secrets of the Hip and Knee*. www.functionalmovement.com

Di Pietro, L. et al. (2006). Exercise and improved insulin sensitivity in older women: Evidence of the enduring benefits of higher intensity training. *Journal of Applied Physiology*, 100, 142–149.

Esteve-Lanao, J. et al. (2005). How do endurance runners actually train? Relationship with competition performance. *Medicine & Science in Sports & Exercise,* 37, 496–504.

Foster, C., Daniels, J., & Seiler, S. (1999). Perspectives on correct approaches to training. In: Lehmann, M. et al. (Eds.) *Overload, Performance Incompetence and Regeneration in Sport*. New York: Kluwer Academic/Plenum Publishers.

Foster, C. et al. (2001). Monitoring exercise training during non-steady state exercise. *Journal of Strength Conditioning Research,* 15, 109–115.

Foster, C. et al. (1996). Athletic performance in relation to training load. *Wisconsin Medical Journal,* 95, 370–374.

Foster, C. et al. (1995). Effects of specific vs. cross training on running performance. *European Journal of Applied Physiology,* 70, 367–372.

Goldberg, L. et al. (1984). Changes in lipid and lipoprotein levels after weight training. *Journal of the American Medical Association*, 252, 504–506.

Gray, G. (2008). *The Thoracic Spine.* Adrian, Mich.: Gray Institute.

Gray, G. & Tiberio, D. (2007). *Chain Reaction Function*. Adrian, Mich.: Gray Institute.

Herman, L. et al. (2006). Validity and reliability of the session RPE method for monitoring exercise training intensity. *South African Journal of Sports Medicine,* 18, 14–17.

Houglum, P.A. (2010) *Therapeutic Exercise for Musculoskeletal Injuries* (3rd ed.). Champaign, Ill.: Human Kinetics.

Hurley, B.F. et al. (1988). Resistive training can reduce coronary risk factors without altering $\dot{V}O_2$max or percent bodyfat. *Medicine & Science in Sports & Exercise*, 20, 150–154.

Ibanez, J. et al. (2005). Twice-weekly progressive resistance training decreases abdominal fat and improves insulin sensitivity in older men with type 2 diabetes. *Diabetes Care*, 28, 662–667.

Kelley, G. (1997). Dynamic resistance exercise and resting blood pressure in adults: A meta-analysis. *Journal of Applied Physiology*, 82, 1559–1565.

Kendall, F.P. et al. (2005). *Muscles Testing and Function with Posture and Pain* (5th ed.). Baltimore, Md.: Lippincott Williams & Wilkins.

Kibler, W.B., Press, J., & Sciascia, A. (2006). The role of core stability in athletic function. *Sports Medicine,* 36, 189–198.

Lieber, R.L. (2009). *Skeletal Muscle Structure, Function, and Plasticity: The Physiological Basis of*

Rehabilitation (3rd ed.). Baltimore, Md.: Wolters Kluwer/ Lippincott Williams & Wilkins.

MacIntosh, B.R., Gardiner, P.F., & McComas, A.J. (2006). *Skeletal Muscle Form and Function* (2nd ed.). Champaign, Ill.: Human Kinetics.

McGill, S.M. (2006). *Ultimate Back Fitness and Performance* (3rd ed.). Waterloo, Canada: Backfitpro.

McLester, J. et al. (2003). A series of studies: A practical protocol for testing muscle endurance recovery. *Journal of Strength and Conditioning Research,* 17, 2, 259–273.

Messier, S.P. (2008). The Burden of Obesity: A Biomechanical Perspective. Presented at the ACSM 55th Annual Meeting, Indianapolis, IN. May 28, 2008.

Norris, R., Carroll, D., & Cochrane, R. (1990). The effect of aerobic and anaerobic training on fitness, blood pressure, and psychological stress and well-being. *Journal of Psychosomatic Research,* 34, 367–375.

Rose, D.J. (2010). *FallProof!* (2nd ed.). Champaign, Ill.: Human Kinetics.

Sahrmann, S.A. (2002). *Diagnosis and Treatment of Movement Impairment Syndromes*. St. Louis, Mo.: Mosby.

Seiler, K.S. & Kjerland, G.O. (2006). Quantifying training intensity distribution in elite athletes: Is there evidence for an 'optimal' distribution. *Scandinavian Journal of Medicine & Science in Sports,* 16, 49–56.

Shumway-Cook, A. & Woollacott, M.H. (2001). *Motor Control: Theory and Practical Applications* (2nd ed.). Philadelphia: Lippincott Williams & Wilkins.

Starkey, D. et al. (1996). Effect of resistance training volume on strength and muscle thickness. *Medicine & Science in Sports & Exercise,* 28, 10, 1311–1320.

Tumminello, N. (2007). *Warm-up Progressions—Volumes 1 and 2.* Baltimore, Md.: Performance University.

Westcott, W.L. (2009). ACSM strength training guidelines: Role in body composition and health enhancement. *ACSM's Health & Fitness Journal,* 13, 4, 1–9.

Whiting W.C. & Rugg, S. (2006). *Dynatomy: Dynamic Human Anatomy*. Champaign, Ill.: Human Kinetics.

Willardson, J.M. (2007). Core stability training: Applications to sports conditioning programs. *Journal of Strength and Conditioning Research,* 21, 3, 979–985.

Williams, P. & Goldspink, G. (1978). Changes in sarcomere length and physiologic properties in immobilized muscle. *Journal of Anatomy,* 127, 459.

Suggested Reading

American College of Sports Medicine (2009). Position stand: Appropriate physical activity intervention strategies for weight loss and prevention of weight regain for adults. *Medicine & Science in Sports & Exercise,* 41, 459–471.

American Council on Exercise (2014). *ACE Personal Trainer Manual* (5th ed.). San Diego, Calif.: American Council on Exercise.

Carey, A. (2005). *The Pain-Free Program*. Hoboken, N.J.: John Wiley & Sons.

Kreighbaum, E. & Barthels, K.M. (1996). *Biomechanics: A Qualitative Approach for Studying Human Movement* (4th ed.). Needham, Mass.: Pearson Education.

Myers, T. (2009). *Anatomy Trains: Myofascial Meridians for Manual and Movement Therapists* (2nd ed.). Edinburgh: Churchill Livingstone.

Sahrmann, S.A. (2002). *Diagnosis and Treatment of Movement Impairment Syndromes*. St. Louis, Mo.: Mosby.

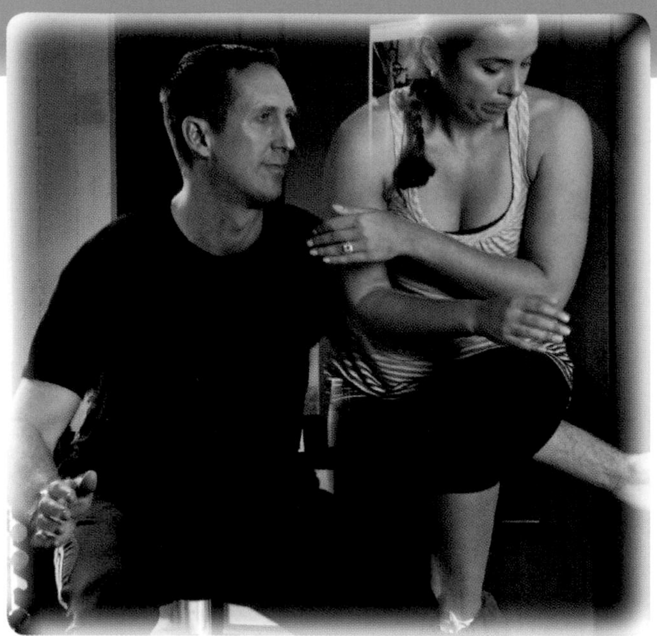

IN THIS CHAPTER:

Helping Clients Establish Self-reliance

MICHELLE MURPHY ZIVE

Michelle Murphy Zive, M.S., R.D., is the executive director of the UC San Diego initiatives for Communities Putting Prevention to Work, locally known as Healthy Works, and the Network for a Healthy California. Both projects are focused on improving the health of the community through nutrition education and by changing the environment, systems, and policies so the community has access to affordable locally grown food. Zive has been with the Division of Child Development and Community Health at UCSD for almost 25 years. She studies nutrition-related issues, including obesity prevention, food security, and access to healthy foods and physical activity, and has published more than 50 peer-reviewed articles. Zive co-wrote, with Dr. Philip Nader, You Can Prevent Childhood Obesity: Practical Ideas from Pregnancy to Adolescence, A Legacy of Health for Our Children, *which translates the authors' research into useful information for the general public.*

Self-reliance is the dependence on one's own powers, capabilities, and resources. Without exception, this should be the goal of ACE-certified Health Coaches for all of their clients. In other words, health coaches should be designing lifestyle-modification programs that instill and support self-reliant skills and capabilities, such as self-monitoring and goal-setting, throughout the program. When a client has been successful at maintaining a healthy lifestyle for more than six months, he or she should be self-reliant (Glanz et al., 2008).

This may seem counterintuitive, and some health coaches may be hesitant to coach this way, saying, "What happens if every one of my clients becomes self-reliant? They will not need me and then what will happen to my business?"

These are similar to questions every parent ponders: What happens if my child leaves for college and does not need me anymore? It is the job of parents to teach children to grow confident in their own abilities to navigate the world successfully. If a child is allowed his or her independence, he or she will be back to get more "coaching" when issues or challenges arise.

The Importance of Self-reliance in Making Behavioral Changes and Maintaining Lifestyle Modifications

It is important to note that self-reliance is a goal, not an outcome. Self-reliance is fluid. For instance, even when lifestyle-modification goals have been achieved and maintenance has occurred, there can be a **relapse** to an unhealthy behavior. For example, Bob has a client, Mary, who he has been training for more than a year. When Mary first came to Bob, she wanted to lose 50 pounds (22.7 kg) by increasing her cardiovascular activity and eliminating sodas and French fries from her diet. Mary has achieved these goals and kept up these changes for the past seven months.

Mary says, "The reason I've been able to lose the weight is because Bob and I have set realistic goals and I feel confident that I can maintain the weight loss with the changes I've made."

A month passes and Mary has been skipping her biweekly trainings with Bob. The next time Bob sees Mary, she complains that she is started to drink soda again and has not been doing her daily walks.

Bob's coaching is still important to help Mary discover why she is having these relapses and what she can do to get herself back to living a healthy life.

In Chapter 14, behavioral theory models are explained to help health coaches better understand how lifestyle behavioral modifications are complex, how unhealthy behaviors are changed to healthy ones, and how these changes are maintained. It is worth revisiting two of these theories in the context of self-reliance. The **socio-ecological model (SEM)** (Glanz et al., 2008) explains the contribution of multiple levels and contexts that influence health, including eating and physical-activity behaviors. The other behavioral model is the **transtheoretical model of behavioral change (TTM),** which focuses on the client's readiness to make and maintain the change (Prochaska & DiClemente, 1984).

Sallis et al. (2006) conducted research using the SEM to explain factors and contexts that affect physical activity and how certain environments and communities support active living (Figure 18-1).

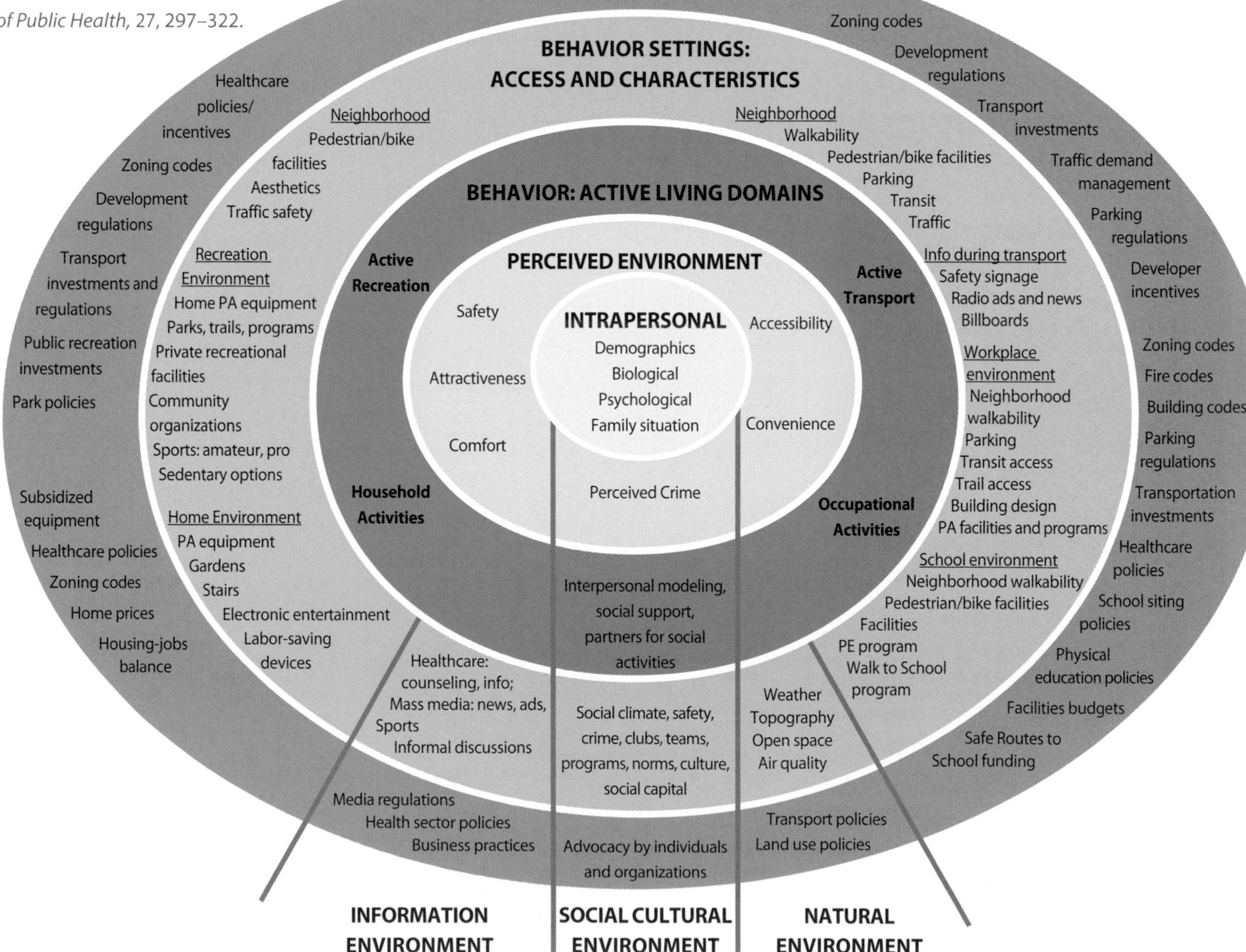

Figure 18-1
Ecological model of four domains of active living

Sallis, J.F. et al. (2006). An ecological approach to creating active living communities. *Annual Review of Public Health,* 27, 297–322.

The authors propose a model identifying potential environmental and policy factors within four spheres of influence, including recreation, transport, occupation, and household.

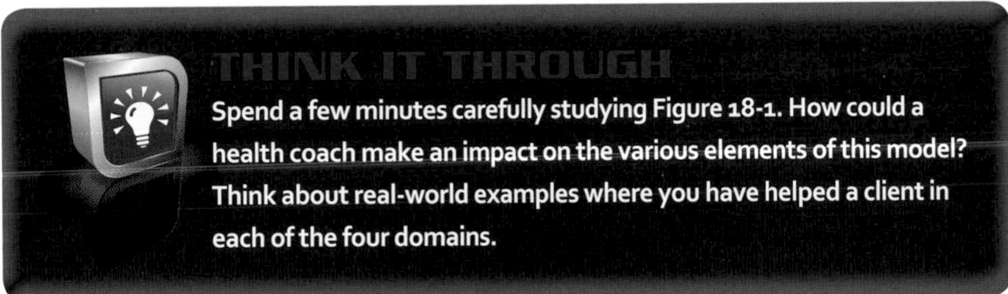

THINK IT THROUGH
Spend a few minutes carefully studying Figure 18-1. How could a health coach make an impact on the various elements of this model? Think about real-world examples where you have helped a client in each of the four domains.

Research supports that there are multiple levels of influence on physical activity (Booth et al., 2001; King et al., 1995). What does the SEM mean to health coaches and the self-reliance of their clients? There are many influences involved in changing an individual's behavior, including the individual's knowledge, attitude, and skills, the interpersonal domain (social networks, including family and health coaches), schools/institutions (environment and ethos), community (cultural values and norms), and public policy (Figure 18-2). It is up to the health coach to help the client be aware of and understand this concept.

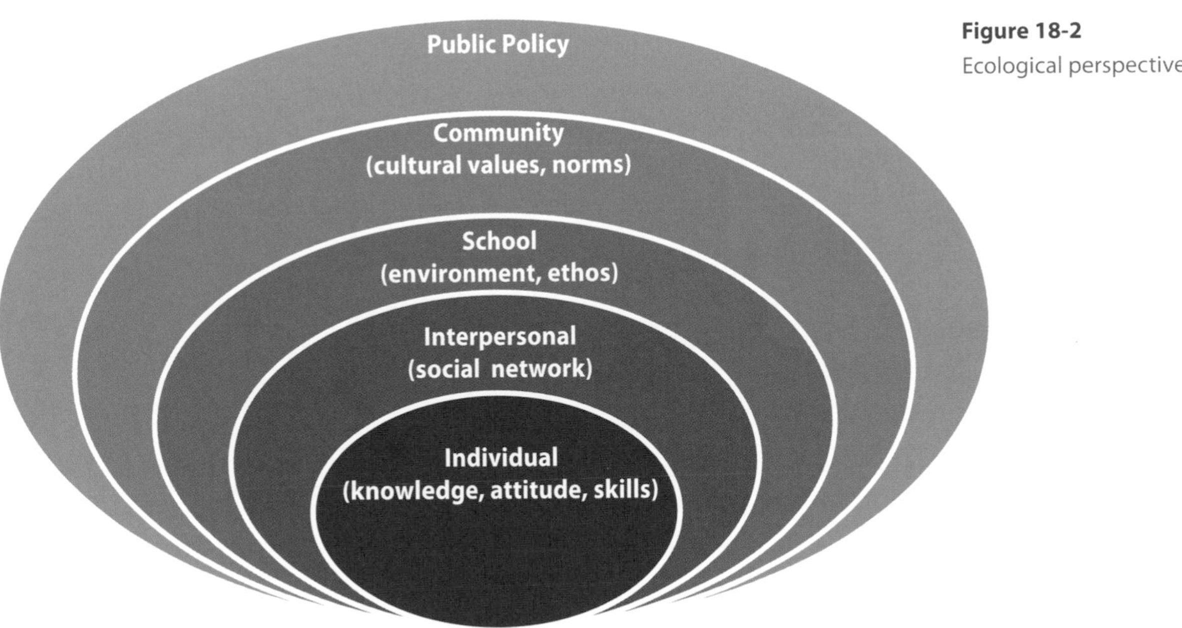

Figure 18-2
Ecological perspective

The sphere in which the health coach has the greatest influence is the interpersonal area—those interactions in the gym, on the phone, through email, the Internet, and so on. However, the health coach can help the client be more successful throughout the various levels of influence. For example, a health coach can increase a client's knowledge, help with developing skills, and troubleshoot how to be successful in eating healthy or being physically active when the health coach is not around by changing the client's environment, such as having healthy snacks in the desk drawer at work or asking one of the client's coworkers to walk during lunch (see Chapter 14). By helping the client come up with solutions to hurdles, relapses, or barriers to healthy living, the health coach will increase the success of the client in maintaining a healthy lifestyle and improving **self-efficacy** to be able to continue these healthy behaviors into the future (Kong et al., 2010). Refer to Chapter 3 for more information on self-efficacy.

The TTM consists of five stages of behavioral change—**precontemplation, contemplation, preparation, action,** and **maintenance.** Precontemplation is the stage where people are **sedentary** and are not considering an activity program or healthier lifestyle. The contemplation stage is where people are still sedentary, but are considering the importance of activity and a healthier lifestyle and the negative implications of remaining sedentary. Yet, they are still unable to commit to making a change. In the preparation stage, people are doing some kind of physical activity, such as the occasional walk or visit to the gym, and are ready to adopt an active and healthier lifestyle. During the action stage, people are engaged in a physical-activity program and actions that involve a healthier lifestyle, like eating more fruits and vegetables, but have been doing so for less than six months. Maintenance is the stage where people have established a healthy behavior for more than six months.

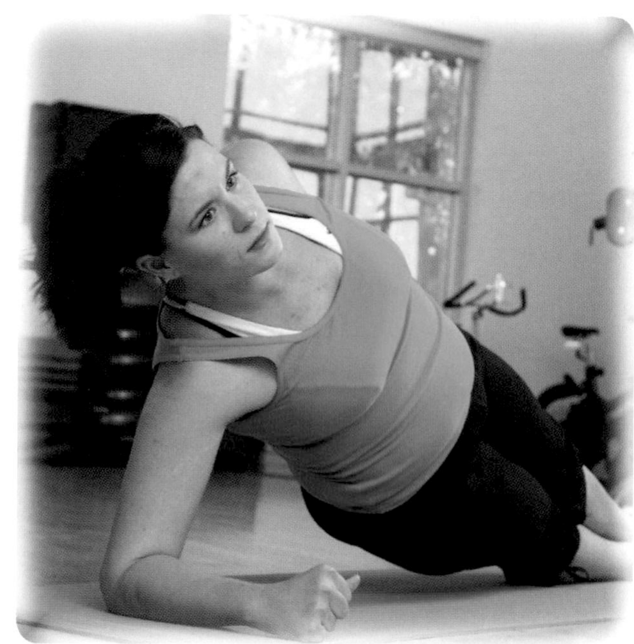

The second component of the TTM is the process of how to make changes and how to move from one stage to another (see Table 3-1, page 60). The health coach should help clients identify in which stage they belong based on their readiness to change and level of motivation, and then implement stage-specific interventions. The goal of any intervention is to advance the client to the next stage of change.

The third component of the TTM is self-efficacy. Bandura (1986) defines self-efficacy in this context as the belief in one's own capabilities to maintain a healthy lifestyle through adopting and maintaining a physical-activity program and healthy nutrition. Self-efficacy is the most important component of a client being self-reliant or feeling confident in his or her ability to adopt and maintain a healthy lifestyle. The final component of the TTM is **decisional balance**, which is the number of perceived pros and cons related to adopting and/or maintaining a healthy behavior. In summary, precontemplators and contemplators perceive more cons than pros in adopting a healthy lifestyle. As people move through the stages, the balance changes to more pros than cons. The active and healthy nutrition behaviors of people in the later stages of the TTM—the action and maintenance stages—is a testament to this fact. See Chapter 3 for more information on the TTM and how to successfully implement it with clients.

It is important for health coaches to understand the difference between a lapse and a relapse. Consider a client who, over the course of several weeks, has broken a bad habit of eating junk food at night. One evening, he eats a few cookies, but successfully fights the urge to eat more and does not continue the behavior on subsequent evenings. This client had a brief lapse and quickly got himself back on track. If that client had continued to eat the whole bag of cookies and then decided that he is simply unable to regulate his evening snacking, a relapse would be imminent, where he gives up on the healthy behaviors and goes back to eating junk food every night. In other words, a lapse is a temporary "fall off the wagon," but a relapse involves a return to unhealthy behaviors.

Life happens, jobs are stressful, family situations change, and people run out of time and motivation to exercise and eat healthy. The health coach's role is to help the client identify these challenges and the causes of a relapse and to remind the client of his or her successes and self-efficacy in order to get back on the right path. For example, a health coach has a client, Lisa, who has identified that her nine-year-old son is causing a lot of stress because of his attention deficit disorder (ADD), and this is why Lisa has stopped walking every morning. The health coach might say, "Lisa, I know that dealing with your son's ADD has added stress to your life. Remember, you've said in the past that your walking program has helped reduce your stress levels. Do you think walking could do that for you again in this situation?" This type of discussion will help reinforce the client's self-reliance.

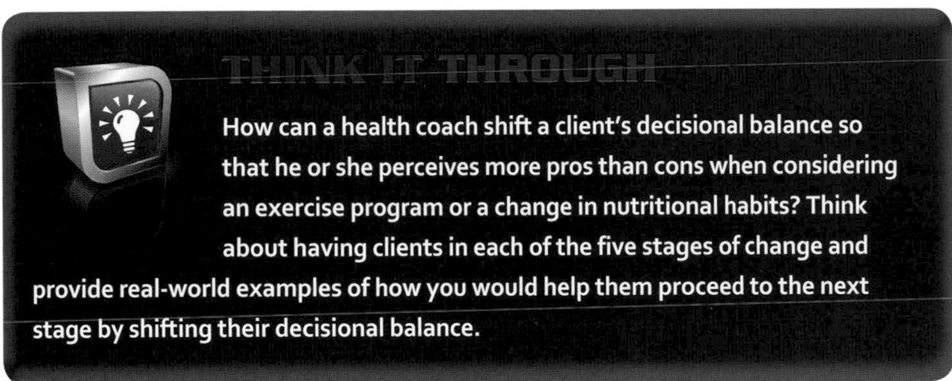

THINK IT THROUGH
How can a health coach shift a client's decisional balance so that he or she perceives more pros than cons when considering an exercise program or a change in nutritional habits? Think about having clients in each of the five stages of change and provide real-world examples of how you would help them proceed to the next stage by shifting their decisional balance.

Self-efficacy

Self-efficacy cannot be underestimated in predicting the success of a client to initiate and maintain a healthy lifestyle. While the TTM and SEM include self-efficacy as important in initiating and maintaining health behaviors, there are also cognitive-behavioral theories focused on self-efficacy. The **self-efficacy model** hypothesizes that all sustained changes in behaviors are mediated by self-efficacy (Bandura, 1997). Research suggests that self-efficacy predicts adherence to healthy behaviors, such as being physically active and eating healthfully, and is improved through perceived incremental successes (Williams & French, 2011; Lee, 2008) (Figure 18-3).

The self-efficacy construct has been expanded on by its developer, Albert Bandura, into the **social-cognitive theory** (Bandura, 1986). The main principle of the theory is called **triadic reciprocal situation.** The components of the triad, which greatly influence each other, are as follows:

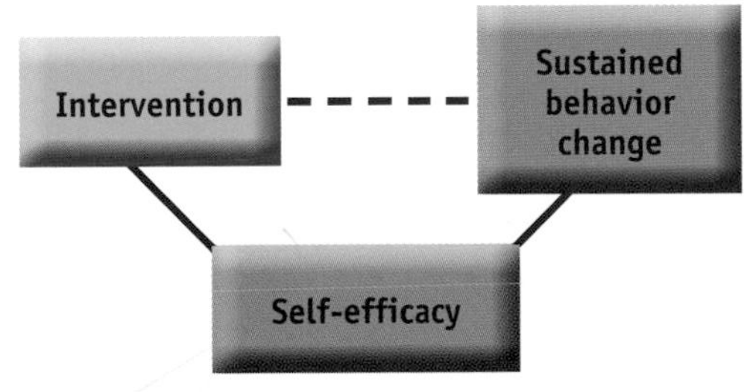

Figure 18-3
Proposed mediation effects of self-efficacy

- *Cognitions:* Thoughts that allow one to consider present situations based on previous experiences and expected outcomes
- *Behaviors:* Previous actions
- *Environment:* Social and physical situations in which people act

The social-cognitive theory posits that all health behaviors are goal-driven through anticipation of outcomes. Self-efficacy interacts with these goals through the simultaneous influence of cognitions, behaviors, and environment on each other. What does the social-cognitive theory have to do with the health coach? Individuals are capable of self-regulating their actions and choosing situations and environments that will positively influence and promote healthful behaviors. The theory reinforces that individuals are active participants in maintaining their own behaviors. This is the definition of self-reliance: the belief that an individual is capable of maintaining his or her own healthy lifestyle.

Strategies for Establishing Self-reliance

Establish Self-efficacy Through Goal-setting

There are many strategies that health coaches can use to help clients establish self-efficacy and self-reliance, beginning with helping them set realistic goals (see Chapter 13). From the outset of the client–health coach relationship, realistic goals should be established so the client can accomplish them and feel confident in his or her ability to set, implement, and achieve the goals. Research shows that realistic goal-setting involves the following components (Shilts et al., 2004).

- Goals should be specific and action-oriented. A vague goal of "try your hardest to eat healthy" is not very helpful. "Eat one more serving of vegetables per day" is a better goal.
- Long-term goals, such as lose 45 pounds (20.4 kg), should be broken down into incremental, short-term goals, such as, "Run on the treadmill for 30 minutes, five days this week."
- Goals should be time-sensitive. For example, consider a client who does not usually eat breakfast but knows she will be better able to stop overeating throughout the day if she starts off the day with breakfast. A time-specific goal for this client would be "I will eat breakfast four days this week." Without a timeframe, it will be difficult for the client to get motivated.
- Goals should be made with, and be acceptable to, the client. The health coach's role is to help set and then adjust individualized goals so they can be attained.
- Tracking goals is imperative to success. As with tracking eating and exercise habits, tracking of goals gives a client a road map to success. This tool should be used by the client to review successes, lapses, and barriers and then discussed with the health coach to plan other goals.
- A formal plan of action, such as an exercise program or eating plan, is necessary to accomplish the goals.
- Goals should be prioritized. Again, keep in mind that the health coach's job is to guide the client in prioritizing his or her own goals while knowing which ones the client will be able to attain.

It is important that realistic goals involve the following principles (Figure 18-4):

- Long-term goals (i.e., six months or longer) are broken into attainable short-term (e.g., one- to two-months) goals.
- A plan of action is established that is challenging, but realistic, for the client.
- There is a process for **feedback** between the health coach and the client to assess progress.

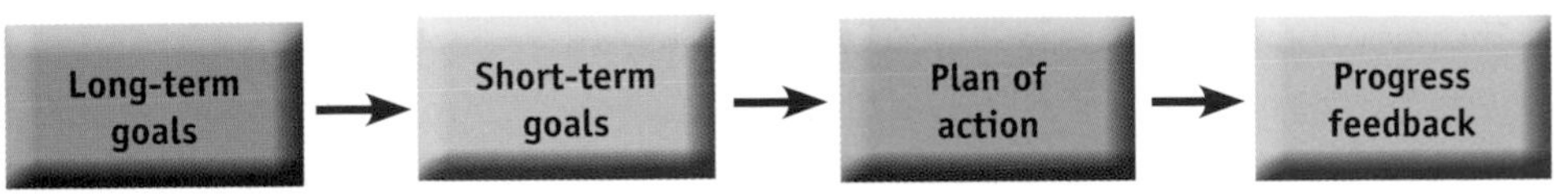

Figure 18-4
Essential components of the goal-setting process

This goal-setting process, including feedback, should be an integral part of a health coach's coaching, from helping a new client adopt an exercise program to seeing that client reach the maintenance stage. Setting and attaining goals will build self-reliance. Remember, attaining a goal, even a long-term goal, and reaching the maintenance stage does not mean that a client should be set off on his or her own. It is important to remind clients that the ultimate goal is making a true lifestyle change. Therefore, a health coach should be coaching clients on goal-setting, providing feedback, and helping find solutions to relapses for many years to come.

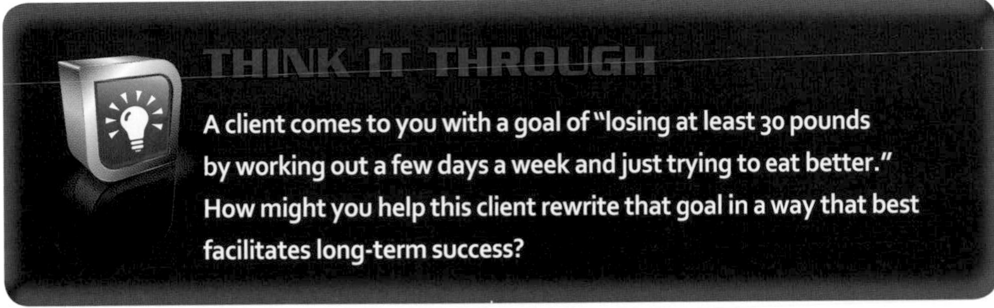

A client comes to you with a goal of "losing at least 30 pounds by working out a few days a week and just trying to eat better." How might you help this client rewrite that goal in a way that best facilitates long-term success?

EXPAND YOUR KNOWLEDGE

Health at Every Size

Over the past 30 years, an obesity epidemic has taken place. Today, two-thirds of American adults are overweight or obese (Ogden & Carroll, 2010). This epidemic has caused the public health establishment to develop policies aimed at helping individuals reduce their **body mass index (BMI)** (Marketdata Enterprises, 2009). Yet, these policies, coupled with the fact that Americans spend $58.6 billion annually for solutions from the private weight-loss industry, have done little to help the majority of individuals maintain weight loss over a long period of time or to realize the recognized benefits of improved health and mortality that come from maintaining a healthy weight (Mann et al., 2007). Further, this focus on weight has caused unprecedented levels of body dissatisfaction (Monteath & McCabe, 1997) and repeated attempts to lose weight.

A growing transdisciplinary movement called Health at Every Size (HAES) challenges the significance of promoting weight loss and dieting behavior and argues for a shift in focus to weight-neutral outcomes. Randomized controlled clinical trials indicate a HAES approach is associated with statistically and clinically relevant improvements in physiological measures (e.g., blood pressure and blood lipids), health behaviors (e.g., eating and activity habits and dietary quality), and psychosocial outcomes (e.g., self-esteem and body image), and HAES achieves these health outcomes more successfully than weight-loss treatment and without the contraindications associated with a weight focus (Provencher et al., 2009; Bacon et al., 2005). Bacon and Aphramor (2011) evaluated the evidence and rationale that justify shifting the healthcare paradigm from a conventional weight focus to HAES. What would it look like if a health coach focused on supporting improved health behaviors, such as eating more lean protein and fruits and vegetables and/or being active most days of the week, instead of on weight loss?

Since this is a shift from focusing on weight to health promotion, there may be some resistance from both the client and health coach. Remember, two of the main reasons clients come to a health coach are to "get toned" and lose weight. Concrete numbers such as body-composition measurements, weight, and BMI are easier to focus on because clients see the change in the numbers. However, based on Bacon and Aphramor (2011) and other research (Provencher et al., 2009; Bacon et al., 2005), a health coach and the client may be more successful in promoting health rather than focusing on weight loss. Health coaches should consider the following guidelines when focusing on HAES:

- Continue to help set healthy behavioral goals that are specific, measurable, attainable, relevant, and time-bound, such as adding an additional high-intensity workout to the week.
- Long-term goals should focus on health, not weight.
- Interventions should have a holistic focus and consider the physical, emotional, social, occupational, intellectual, spiritual, and ecological aspects of health.
- Programs should focus on promoting self-esteem, self-efficacy, body satisfaction, and body-size diversity.
- Interventions should focus on modifiable behaviors to improve health and not weight. Weight is not a behavior.

Encourage Clients to Practice Behaviors on Their Own

Once a health coach has helped a client set realistic goals, including short-term behavioral goals of physical activity and healthy eating and long-term goals focused on process (e.g., the client will increase the number of steps walked in a week), an agreement can be considered. A **behavioral contract** is a formal agreement between the health coach and the client that outlines a set of behaviors by the client to complete within a certain timeline (Figure 18-5). The components of the contract that promote health-behavior maintenance are:

- Clarity
- Commitment from both the client and the health coach
- A formal commitment that promotes accountability
- Rewards outlined once goals are achieved

Examples of the types of behaviors that could be in a contract include:

- Commit to eat between 1,500 and 1,800 kcal/day
- Complete four 45-minute sessions per week on the elliptical machine
- Ask one's spouse to walk twice a week
- Commit to be at the gym with the health coach two times per week

Visit www.ACEfitness.org/HealthCoachResources to download a free PDF of a behavioral contract, as well as other forms and assessment tools that you can use throughout your career as a health coach.

Using Behavioral Contracting to Promote Lifestyle Change

Behavioral contracting is an effective behavior-modification strategy. In behavioral contracting for exercise adherence, the health coach and the client set up a system of rewards for sticking to the lifestyle-modification program. Behavioral contracting is most effective when the rewards are outlined by, and meaningful to, the client. If the rewards are not meaningful, the client may not find them to be worth working toward. Behavioral contracting works differently for each individual and health coaches have to be careful not to push certain rewards on clients. Additionally, behavioral contracting is most effective when it is used consistently. Once certain goals are met, contracts need to be reconstructed throughout the duration of program participation.

Below are the elements of a typical behavioral contract.

I Will: (Do what) ____________________

(When) ____________________

(How often)____________________

(How much)____________________

How confident am I that I will do this? _______ *(on a scale of 0 to 10, with 0 being not at all confident and 10 being completely confident)*

If I successfully make this positive lifestyle change by _______, I will reward myself with ____________

____

____________________.

If I fail to successfully make this positive lifestyle change, I will forfeit this reward.

I, ____________________, have reviewed this contract and I agree to discuss
(Client)

the experience involved in accomplishing or not accomplishing this health behavior improvement with

____________________ on ____________________.
(Health Coach) (Date)

Signed (Client): ____________________

Signed (Health Coach):____________________

Figure 18-5
Behavioral contract

Self-rewards, those the client identifies and gives to him- or herself, are important for adopting and maintaining healthy behaviors. The key is that these rewards are intrinsic, or coming from within the client, and not extrinsic, or given by someone else. Examples of "good" self-rewards upon completion of the goal are a massage, a new outfit, or time doing a favorite hobby. When people are first adopting healthy behaviors and achieving goals, especially long-term ones, rewards are usually bigger and more frequent. Once the client is in the maintenance phase (i.e., implementing a healthy behavior for more than six months), rewards may become less integral to maintaining the behavior. However, it is important to note that positive self-talk is an effective reward no matter where the client is in terms of making or maintaining healthy behavioral changes. Transitioning a client's negative self-talk, such as, "I will never stop eating ice cream" or "I will not be able to keep up with an exercise program," to positive self-talk, such as "I will have fruit instead of ice cream," "I've done this before and I can do it again," or "I can keep being physically active since I like the feeling of accomplishment I get after the workout" is an important strategy for health coaches to use to help reinforce self-efficacy and self-reliance in their clients.

Finding ways for the client to self-monitor is not only imperative to successful behavioral change and maintenance but also for promoting self-reliance (Burke et al., 2011). Whether it is a food/exercise diary or an "app" on a Smartphone, the following variables need to be tracked: the goal(s), targeted behaviors, successes and barriers to the goals, and self-rewards.

Throughout the client–health coach relationship, the health coach should give the client the tools, confidence, and support to go home and implement the behaviors in order to develop self-reliance. Remember that providing feedback keeps the client motivated to continue with the lifestyle modifications, in addition to fostering a desire to look to the health coach for continued help with the process. When providing feedback and reviewing the client's self-monitoring tool, the health coach needs to ask:

- What were your successes this week?
- What helped you be successful?
- Did you reward yourself for your success? How?
- Were there any barriers or hurdles to your goals? If so, what were they?
- What would you like to do about the barriers?

APPLY WHAT YOU KNOW

Be a Coach, Not a Sage

Cheryl has been coming to Molly for personal training and weight-loss coaching for the past year. Cheryl has been successful in implementing and maintaining several healthy lifestyle behaviors, including giving up her late-night snacks, eating breakfast every day, and doing 45 minutes of moderate to vigorous physical activity five days a week.

Last week, Cheryl and Molly had the following conversation:

- Cheryl: "I'm starting to eat at night again. My kids and job are stressing me out."
- Molly: "What would you like to have happen?"

- Cheryl: "I'd like to stop eating at night."
- Molly: "What do you need to stop eating at night?"
- Cheryl: "I need to get rid of the junk food in my cupboards. I need to track all my food, including my late night snacking, and I need to start doing yoga to relieve my stress."
- Molly: "Can you get rid of the junk food, track your food, and start yoga?"
- Cheryl: "Yes, I can."
- Molly: "Will you do those three things over the next week to stop the snacking at night?"
- Cheryl: "Yes, I will."

Does this conversation seem too easy? Perhaps, but there are a couple of key principles highlighted in the scenario to improve Cheryl's self-reliance. Molly encourages Cheryl to come up with her own solutions to snacking at night. Molly is not judging or giving advice on what works for her in her own life, but allows Cheryl to do this on her own. Imagine if the scenario had played out like this:

- Cheryl: "I'm starting to eat at night again. My kids and job are stressing me out."
- Molly: "What? After all the hard work we've done together? You know what you need to do is just stop. Just don't snack. Go exercise like I do."

What do you think would happen if this was the way Molly handled Cheryl's admission to late night snacking? Would Cheryl feel good about herself? Would she trust herself to make the necessary changes or would she succumb to the slippery slope and continue her snacking? Do you imagine Cheryl would come back to Molly if this was the way she was coached?

This may be an exaggeration, but it highlights how essential it is for the health coach to coach and not preach. Reinforce those tools that have helped in the success, such as self-monitoring, rewards, or social support. Encourage clients to come up with their own strategies. This allows a client to develop self-reliance.

Help Clients Find and Implement a Support System

Positive social support by the people around the client cannot be underestimated. In the SEM, this is the sphere just outside the individual level (see Figure 18-2). The interpersonal sphere involves the relationships between family members, spouses/partners, friends, coworkers, workout buddies, and health coaches. Research shows that social support is positively related to maintaining physical-activity and weight-management programs (Dahn et al., 2011). For example, people who participated in group physical-activity sessions reported more enjoyment, support, camaraderie, and a personal sense of commitment to continue with their physical-activity programs (Dahn et al., 2011). There is little doubt that those people who surround a client can positively influence his or her lifestyle and support the client's efforts to make and maintain healthy behaviors. Nonetheless, why is it so difficult for people to ask those around them for what they need to be successful? It is as if some people feel like it is a sign of weakness to ask for help.

It is up to the health coach to encourage clients to ask for support by using some of the following techniques:

- Role play. The client asks the health coach for help, with the health coach acting as the client's friend or spouse. Sometimes just saying it out loud helps the client feel confident about asking for the help. It is important to role play a negative response. Ask the client, "What's the worse that happens if the person says 'no'? Who else can you ask?" The majority of the people will say "yes." In fact, many times the response will be, "Why didn't you just ask?"
- Help identify people who are interested in the same kind of help. Are there other clients looking to start a walking club on the weekends?
- Start a group session at the health coach's facility. The health coach facilitates these sessions, whether they are group exercise classes, discussions about healthy eating, goal-setting sessions, or cooking classes. In a national weight-loss program, the facilitator only speaks about 25% of the time. The rest of the time features the participants exchanging ideas, tips, and solutions to stay on course. The health coach simply guides the discussion.

Since every client is different, the health coach has to understand which of these strategies for getting social support will work for each client.

Help Clients Create or Maintain an Environment That Fosters Success

The sphere outside of the individual and interpersonal levels in the SEM diagram is the environment (see Figure 18-2). Both the TTM and SEM focus on the importance of creating successes (self-efficacy) to continue to motivate a client and to develop and support self-reliance. Having access to physical activities and healthy food can only build up these successes for the client. Unfortunately, in most communities it is easier to get cheap, energy-dense food than healthy food. There are numerous and easy ways to be entertained while sitting, such as the TV, computer, and video games. This highlights the importance of clients changing their immediate environment. The client's home, office, and car are the places where the client has the most control over the environment.

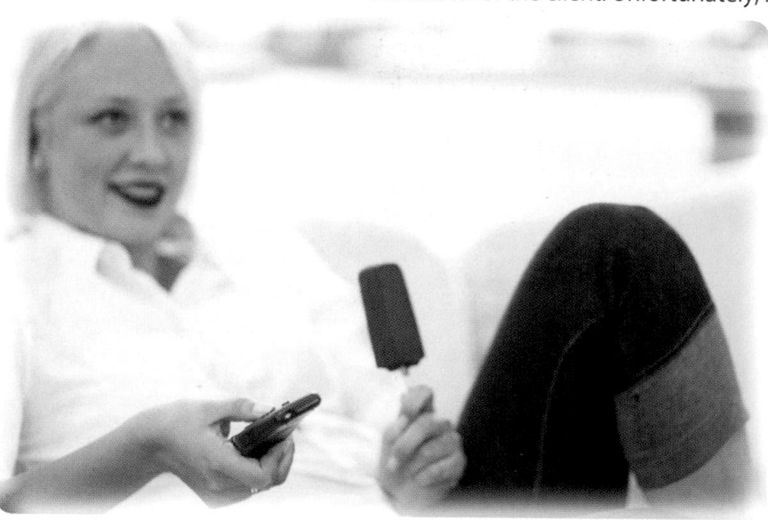

Health coaches should introduce the following strategy for changing a negative, unhealthy environment to a healthy one. First, have the client identify those places or cues that encourage unhealthy behaviors. Have the client take an inventory of his or her home, especially the kitchen, as well as his or her car and office or workspace. Are there cookies, cake, and chips on the kitchen counter for the kids? Are there unhealthy snacks in the glove compartment or a soda in the cup holder? At work, does the client keep a candy stash in a desk drawer? In terms of physical activity, is the treadmill covered by clothes? Are the workout shoes buried underneath slippers? It is the health coach's job to help the client identify these negative environmental cues by asking the right questions and having an open conversation that takes into account the client's past struggles and successes.

Second, encourage the client to clean up those places where there are negative, unhealthy temptations. The instinct of both the health coach and the client is to throw out all the "junk" food, but remember, this is a lifestyle. Is it realistic to not have any sweets or salty snacks in the house for the rest of the client's life? Instead of getting rid of food, designate a place for "junk" food that is not as accessible as having it displayed on the kitchen counter. Prepackaged snacks are a good idea. This will encourage the client to only grab one portion and then have to think about going back for another one. Does the client have a hard time getting up in the morning? Does he or she hit the snooze button on the alarm clock and go back to sleep? Encourage the client to put the alarm clock somewhere in the room where he or she has to walk to turn it off. Also suggest that the client pack a gym bag the night before.

Finally, the health coach should support the client's effort to change the negative into positive. Remember, the bottom line is to make the healthy choice the easiest one. Some suggestions include putting washed fruit in a bowl in the middle of the kitchen table, placing cut-up vegetables in prepackaged baggies in the refrigerator, or posting encouraging notes at home and at the office such as, "Get up and walk." The client should consider posting a workout/eating calendar. The client can use the calendar to track diet and physical activity and check off those days where he or she worked out and ate well. Seeing a month full of check marks will continue to encourage the client's healthy lifestyle.

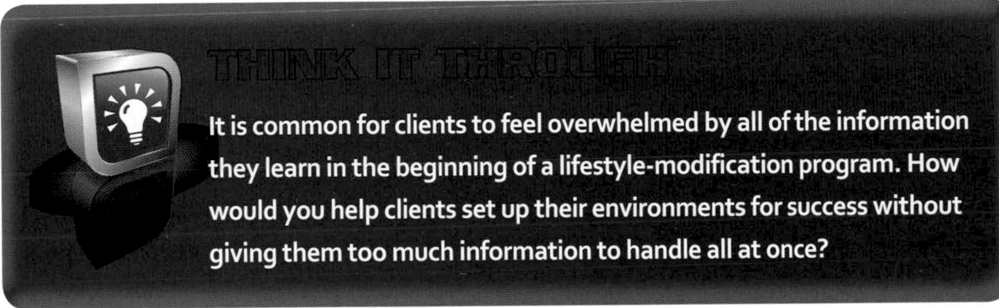

THINK IT THROUGH
It is common for clients to feel overwhelmed by all of the information they learn in the beginning of a lifestyle-modification program. How would you help clients set up their environments for success without giving them too much information to handle all at once?

Find Ways to Cope With Setbacks

Setbacks—both lapses and relapses—will happen. Sometimes the easiest part of a healthy exercise and eating lifestyle is the beginning. This is the time when the client is very motivated and sees some of the most dramatic results. Often, the hardest part is to keep the client motivated when those dramatic results are not happening and life takes over. After all, living a healthy lifestyle is not a sprint; it is a marathon. When setbacks occur, it is the role of the health coach to be a sincere coach and educator by reminding the client of past successes, including those successful strategies for maintaining healthy behaviors.

Self-monitoring

The self-monitoring tool that helped clients make those dramatic changes in the first place can help put them back on track again. Tracking diet and exercise can be tedious and is an easy behavior to let slide. The health coach should encourage the client to break out the food/exercise diary when there are setbacks. Have the client write down three days of diet and exercise. Review the completed diary with the client and ask questions so the client can recognize those areas to be focused on to get back on track. For instance, if after reviewing the diary it is obvious the client is eating on the go and not planning meals or snacks, the health coach should ask, "What's happening in your life that you're eating on the run?" "What is this doing to your planning?" "What would you like to have happen?" Self-monitoring holds the client accountable, not only to the health coach, but also, and more importantly, to him- or herself. Furthermore, it is easier to see those opportunities the client can take advantage of to get back on track.

Reinforce Successes

The primary role of the health coach is to be a supporter to the client. This means reminding clients of their successes throughout the process of improving their lifestyles. The health coach should review his or her notes on the client regarding those accomplishments. Celebrate successes with the client. Encourage clients to visualize being successful when they are experiencing setbacks. Promote positive self-talk. Instead of the client saying to him- or herself, "I've gained 5 pounds," the client can say, "I've taken off those 5 pounds before and I'll do it again." By focusing on successes, the client develops more self-efficacy to tackle barriers and setbacks.

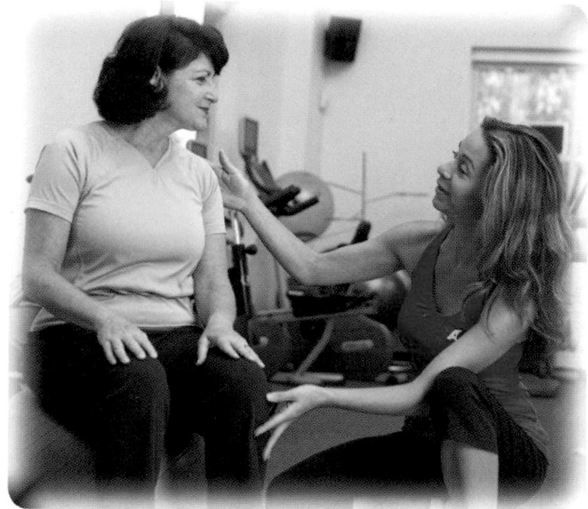

Motivational Interviewing

Motivational interviewing (MI) is a client-focused, semi-directive counseling approach focused on exploring and resolving ambivalence around behavioral change and/or maintenance (see Chapter 5). The goal of MI is to enhance clients' motivation for change and adherence to a healthy lifestyle. MI has been effective in the addictions field, and more recently for weight loss and weight-loss maintenance (Rieger, 2009). Armstrong et al. (2011) reviewed 11 randomized control trials using MI as a strategy to impact weight loss in overweight or obese patients. They found that MI was significantly related to a greater reduction in weight.

There are four MI principles:

- *Express empathy:* The health coach needs to see the world through the client's eyes.
- *Support self-efficacy:* MI is about the client having the power and motivation to make and sustain behavioral changes.
- *Roll with resistance:* This is the part of MI where the health coach listens to the client's struggles and excuses for not making or maintaining the behavioral change. The struggles usually involve the client's ambivalence about the change. The health coach helps identify what the ambivalence is about and coaches the client to identify barriers and solutions. Therefore, the conversation is never a confrontation between the health coach and the client, but rather the health coach supporting the client in discovering solutions.
- *Develop discrepancy:* Motivation for change occurs when the client sees the difference between where he or she is now and where he or she wants to be in the future. The health coach helps the client recognize how current behaviors conflict with those self-identified goals, such as losing 50 pounds (22.7 kg). Once the client sees this discrepancy, his or her motivation to change will be heightened.

MI is based on the TTM stages—precontemplation, contemplation, preparation, action, and maintenance—as well as the avoidance of relapse. This means the health coach has to meet the client where he or she is in changing the behavior and not try to force the client to change if he or she has not expressed a desire to do so.

Additional Strategies to Encourage Self-reliance

Using Technology to Keep Connected While Still Encouraging Self-reliance

Coons and others (2011) found that handheld devices offered a potent and portable platform to support self-regulation. Health coaches should identify what kind of technological tools their clients want to use. Older clients may not want a phone app or text messages, but would like encouraging phone calls. The following are some examples of tools available to keep clients on track when the health coach is not around.

Phone Apps

Platforms on Smartphones include diet trackers, energy calculators, tools for making healthy shopping lists and finding restaurants that offer healthy, low-fat food, workout videos, activity trackers, and relaxation and inspirational videos (see www.ACEfitness.org/healthapps). These applications are meant to provide support for the client when the health coach is not around—in essence serving as a personal health coach that is available at all times.

Text Messaging/Emails

Text messages and emails are easy ways to remind clients to keep on track and give encouraging words throughout the day. They can also be used with a large group around a general topic, such as "Have you done your 30 minutes of cardio yet?" or "Have you tracked your food intake yet?" Text messages and emails can also be a way to touch base and write a quick personal reminder to an individual client about whatever particular struggle he or she is dealing with.

Websites, Blogs, and Vlogs

Website, blogs, and vlogs (i.e., video logs) are excellent ways to keep clients motivated: "Thinking of you. Here is a link to the kettlebell exercise we were talking about." The ACE website (www.ACEfitness.org) is a great resource filled with how-to videos, articles summarizing the latest research, and references about a variety of fitness topics. If the health coach is computer savvy, then creating a website, blog, or vlog could help keep clients connected. However, it is important to remember that content should be updated frequently. If the health coach cannot update the site every week or so, finding other sites to use is the better option.

Phone Calls and Personal Notes

For all the wonderful things technology has brought, the world has lost something: personal contact. Again, the health coach should ask each client how he or she would like to be contacted. A personal phone call of encouragement or a handwritten note can go long way to supporting a client's healthy lifestyle (Wu, 2010; Digenio, et al., 2009).

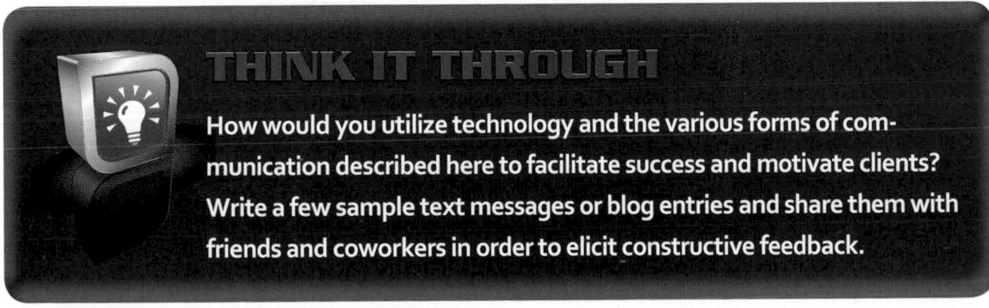
THINK IT THROUGH
How would you utilize technology and the various forms of communication described here to facilitate success and motivate clients? Write a few sample text messages or blog entries and share them with friends and coworkers in order to elicit constructive feedback.

Products for Clients

Tip Sheets

Tip sheets can come from sources like the ACE website, the Academy of Nutrition and Dietetics, and www.ChooseMyPlate.gov. Important topics such as how to track diet and exercise, estimate portion sizes, utlilize positive self-talk, or do a new exercise are just some examples of the tip sheets health coaches have access to that will help support clients in continuing on their path to maintaining a healthy lifestyle. If the health coach cannot find a tip sheet for a specific topic, he or she can create one. These can be posted on the health coach's website, blog, or vlog.

Food/Exercise Journals

Some clients will want to use the old-fashioned paper and pencil method to track their food and exercise. There are many stores (online and otherwise) that have these types of journals. Again, if the health coach cannot find the "perfect" journal, he or she can develop one with inspirational quotes, tips, and reminders. The health coach is the expert. Use this expertise to find or create the right journal for a client (see Chapter 14).

Books

The health coach should have a reading list of books to support and encourage the client. Refer to the Suggested Reading lists throughout this manual for additional ideas and resources.

Support Groups

Health coaches should provide opportunities to have support groups. The health coach should facilitate these groups and have discussion topics such as how to create a healthy refrigerator/pantry, handle stress without eating, or keep active in bad weather. However, 75% of the class should be devoted to time in which people can discuss hurdles, successes, and ideas. Again, the idea is to have the health coach stay connected to these clients, but not be the lecturer or expert, thereby allowing the group members to be the experts for each other.

It is best when starting out to have the group meet on a weekly basis. Any more than that and the clients could get burned out or find it difficult to attend; any less than once a week and motivation and group cohesion will suffer.

Special Classes/Workshops

Workshops can be conducted either in person or via web conferencing. Topics could include staying motivated, what to do about relapses, or demonstrating and practicing a new exercise or exercise program. This is an opportunity for the health coach to teach a group of people who are in the maintenance stage about important topics that impact this group.

Partnerships With Allied Healthcare Professionals

Health coaches should consider partnering with other health professionals. A **registered dietitian (R.D.)** can create a diet plan for clients, something that the health coach cannot do. Consider having a psychologist give presentations about the importance of "mind over matter" when it comes to creating and living a healthy lifestyle. Partnering with a medical doctor (M.D.) means the health coach's clients can have a number of physiological and physical measurements done that impact health. These measurements can be taken throughout the year to keep the client on track and ensure that BMI, skinfolds, and other measurements are in the normal ranges (see Chapter 11). Other partnerships to be considered by the health coach are with a chef to show clients how to prepare healthy, tasty foods, or with a yoga instructor or other specialized fitness professional. By partnering with others, the health coach is providing a more comprehensive lifestyle program that will keep clients excited and motivated to come back for more, even though they have proven they can do the work on their own.

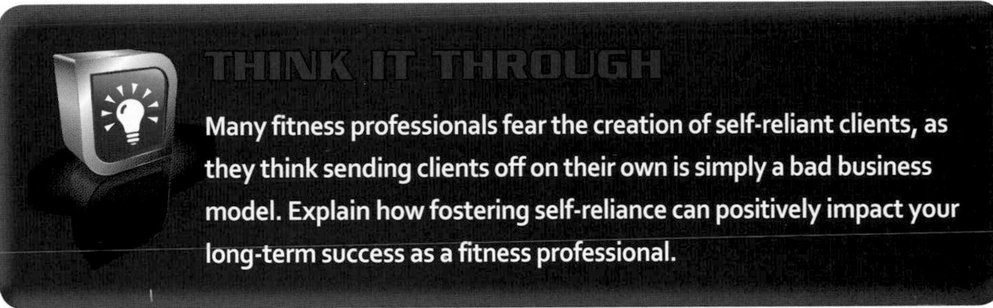

THINK IT THROUGH
Many fitness professionals fear the creation of self-reliant clients, as they think sending clients off on their own is simply a bad business model. Explain how fostering self-reliance can positively impact your long-term success as a fitness professional.

Summary

A client's self-reliance is necessary to the success of maintaining a healthy lifestyle. Health coaches should help develop and support those skills and capabilities that give the client the confidence to undertake and succeed at physical-activity and weight-management programs. While this is a key role for the health coach, it does not stop when the client is in the maintenance phase. Self-reliance is a goal; it is not the outcome or the end. There will be lapses and relapses. Most people have a problem with maintaining physical activity, nutrition, and lifestyle behavioral changes. In fact, most people fall back into bad habits and behaviors and gain back lost weight. The health coach should continue to support each client's self-reliance and increase his or her motivation to maintain a healthy lifestyle.

References

Armstrong, M.J. et al. (2011). Motivational interviewing to improve weight loss in overweight and/or obese patients: A systematic review and meta-analysis of randomized controlled trials. *Obesity Review,* 12, 709–712.

Bacon, L. & Aphramor, L. (2011). Weight science: Evaluating the evidence for a paradigm shift. *Nutrition Journal,* 9, 10–23.

Bacon, L. et al. (2005). Size acceptance and intuitive eating improve health for obese, female chronic dieters. *Journal of the American Dietetic Association,* 105, 929–936.

Bandura, A. (1997). The anatomy of stages of change. *American Journal of Health Promotion,* 12, 1, 8–10.

Bandura, A. (1986). *Social Foundations of Thought and Action: A Social Cognitive Theory*. Englewood Cliffs, N.J: Prentice Hall.

Booth, S.L. et al. (2001). Environmental and societal factors affect food choice and physical activity: Rationale, influences, and leverage points. *Nutrition Reviews,* 3, 21–39.

Burke, L.A. et al. (2011). Self-monitoring in weight loss: A systematic review of the literature. *Journal of the American Dietetic Association*, 111, 92–102.

Coons, M.J. et al. (2011). The potential of virtual reality technologies to improve adherence to weight loss behaviors. *Journal of Diabetes Science and Technology*, 5, 2, 340–344.

Dahn, J.R. et al. (2011). Weight management for veterans: Examining change in weight before and after MOVE! *Obesity,* 19, 5, 977–981.

Digenio, A.G. et al. (2009). Comparison of methods for delivering a lifestyle modification program for obese patients: A randomized trial. *Annals of Internal Medicine,* 150, 4, 255–262.

Glanz, K. et al. (2008). *Health Behavior & Health Education: Theory, Research and Practice.* San Francisco: John Wiley & Sons.

King, A.C. et al. (1995). Environmental and policy approaches to cardiovascular disease prevention through physical activity: Issues and opportunities. *Health Education Quarterly,* 22, 499–511.

Kong, W. et al. (2010). Predictors of success to weight-loss intervention program in individuals at high risk for type 2 diabetes. *Diabetes Research and Clinical Practice,* 90, 147–153.

Lee, L.L. et al. (2008). Using self-efficacy theory to develop interventions that help older people overcome psychological barriers to physical activity: A discussion paper. *International Journal of Nursing Studies*, 45, 11, 1690–1699.

Lorig, K. & Fries, J.F. (1990). *The Arthritis Helpbook: A Tested Self-Management Program for Coping with Your Arthritis.* Reading, Mass.: Addison-Wesley.

Mann, T. et al. (2007). Medicare's search for effective obesity treatments: Diets are not the answer. *The American Psychologist,* 62, 3, 220–233.

Marketdata Enterprises (2009). *The U.S. Weight Loss & Diet Control Market*. Tampa, Fla.: Marketdata Enterprises.

Monteath, S.A. & McCabe, M.P. (1997). The influence of societal factors on female body image. *Journal of Social Psychology,* 137, 708–727.

Ogden, C.L. & Carroll, M.D. (2010). *Prevalence of Overweight, Obesity, and Extreme Obesity Among Adults: United States Trends 1960–1962 through 2007–2008.* Washington D.C.: Centers for Disease Control and Prevention, National Center for Health Statistics.

Prochaska, J.O. & DiClemente, C.C. (1984). *The Transtheoretical Approach: Crossing Traditional Boundaries of Therapy.* Homewood, Ill.: Dow Jones/Irwin.

Provencher, V. et al. (2009). Health-at-every-size and eating behaviors: 1-year follow-up results of a size acceptance intervention. *Journal of the American Dietetic Association,* 109, 1854–1861.

Rieger, E. (2009). The use of motivational enhancement strategies for the maintenance of weight loss among obese individuals: A preliminary investigation. *Diabetes, Obesity and Metabolism,* 11, 637–640.

Sallis, J.F. et al. (2006). An ecological approach to creating active living communities. *Annual Review of Public Health,* 27, 297–322.

Shilts, M.K. et al. (2004). Goal setting as a strategy

for dietary and physical activity behavior change: A review of the literature. *American Journal of Health Promotion*, 19, 81–93.

Williams, S.L. & French, D.P. (2011).What are the most effective intervention techniques for changing physical activity self-efficacy and physical activity behavior—and are they the same? *Health Education Research*, 26, 2, 308–322.

Wu, L. (2010). Patients' experience of a telephone booster intervention to support weight management in type 2 diabetes and its acceptability. *Journal of Telemedicine and Telecare,* 16, 4, 221–223.

Suggested Reading

Cornier, M.A. (2011). Is your brain to blame for weight regain? *Physiology & Behavior,* 104, 608–612.

Glanz, K. et al. (2008). *Health Behavior & Health Education: Theory, Research and Practice.* San Francisco: John Wiley & Sons.

Machowicz, R. (2011). *Unleash the Warrior Within: Develop the Focus, Discipline, Confidence and Courage You Need to Achieve Unlimited Goals.* New York: Da Capo Lifelong Books.

Sciamanna, C.N. et al. (2011). Practices associated with weight loss versus weight-loss maintenance. *American Journal of Preventative Medicine,* 41, 2, 159–166.

Tribole, E. & Resch, E. (2003). *Intuitive Eating: A Revolutionary Program That Works.* New York: St. Martin's Press.

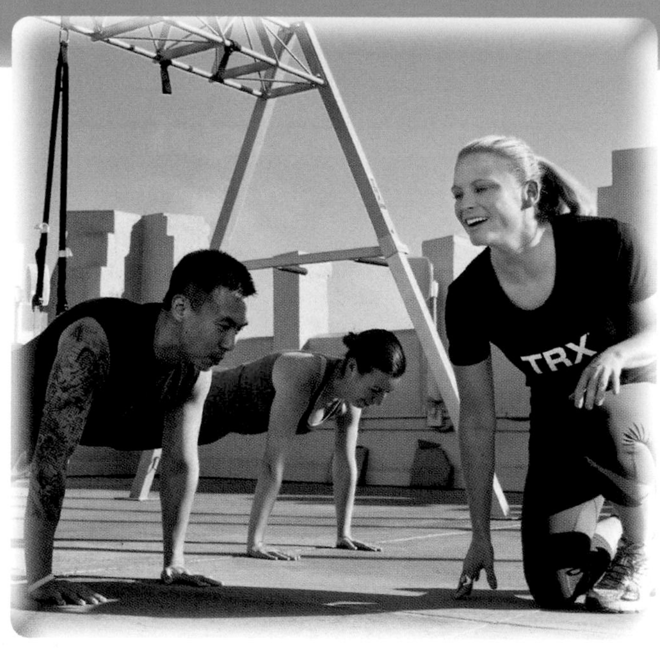

IN THIS CHAPTER:

Michael R. Mantell, Ph.D., earned his Ph.D. at the University of Pennsylvania and his M.S. at Hahnemann Medical College, where he wrote his thesis on the psychological aspects of obesity. His career includes serving as the Chief Psychologist for Children's Hospital in San Diego and as the founding Chief Psychologist for the San Diego Police Department. Dr. Mantell is a member of the Scientific Advisory Board of the International Council on Active Aging, the Chief Behavior Science Consultant to the Premier Fitness Camp at Omni La Costa, a best-selling author of two books, including the 1988 original Don't Sweat the Small Stuff, P.S. It's All Small Stuff, *an international behavior science fitness keynote speaker, an advisor to numerous fitness-health organizations, and is featured in many media broadcasts and worldwide fitness publications. He has been featured on Oprah, Good Morning America, the Today Show, and has been a contributor to many major news organizations including Fox and ABC News. Dr. Mantell is a nationally sought after behavioral science coach for business leaders, elite amateur and professional athletes, individuals, and families. He is included in the greatist.com's 2013 list of "The 100 Most Influential People in Health and Fitness."*

19

Case Studies: From Theory to Practice

MICHAEL R. MANTELL &

SABRENA JO

Sabrena Jo, M.S., has been actively involved in the fitness industry since 1987, successfully operating her own personal-training business and teaching group exercise classes. Jo is a former full-time faculty member in the Kinesiology and Physical Education Department at California State University, Long Beach. She has a bachelor's degree in exercise science as well as a master's degree in physical education/biomechanics from the University of Kansas. Jo, an ACE-certified Personal Trainer and Group Fitness Instructor, is an author, educator, and fitness consultant who remains very active within the industry.

In this chapter, three case studies are presented to illustrate how ACE-certified Health Coaches can use their skills, knowledge, and tools to help clients with differing needs and lifestyle issues. The examples provide opportunities for the health coach to see how different models of intervention may be of use and reflect the most contemporary approaches from which to draw. Of course, health coaches are strongly encouraged to stay current with new findings in professional practice by attending ACE and other continuing education programs; reading relevant professional literature; networking with healthcare, coaching, fitness, and nutrition specialists; and being aware of popular literature.

The health coach will learn how to do an initial **rapport**-building interview (including how to determine the client's stage of behavioral change), what assessments are appropriate, how to apply the ACE Integrated Fitness Training® (ACE IFT®) Model, (particularly the first two stages), how to deal with **relapse** potential to help clients stay on track, and how to provide social and environmental support to clients. The case studies are simplified versions of the complex realities of real-life clients that should be viewed as teaching tools, not strict guidelines to follow. When the health coach meets his or her first real-life client, these basics will serve as a lens through which the myriad of human issues can be best understood. Every client provides the health coach with an opportunity to creatively apply the foundation of knowledge developed in this manual, within the appropriate scope of ethical and professional practice, and to develop and grow as a certified health coach.

Rick: Obese and Sedentary

Rick is a 60-year-old retired assembly-line worker who contacted a health coach to help him reach his health-related goals. Rick was diagnosed with **type 2 diabetes** one year ago and has been prescribed an oral medication to control it. He also had his gallbladder removed five years ago due to repeated bouts of gallstone accumulation, most likely exacerbated by his consumption of high-fat foods. Rick is 50 pounds (22.7 kg) overweight and was classified as obese two weeks ago at his last doctor's visit. Rick also mentions that he has chronic low-back pain. He has been cleared for exercise by his physician, who informed Rick that losing weight will help alleviate his back pain and improve his blood **glucose** levels. Currently, Rick is **sedentary,** but admits that he has plenty of time to exercise now that he is retired.

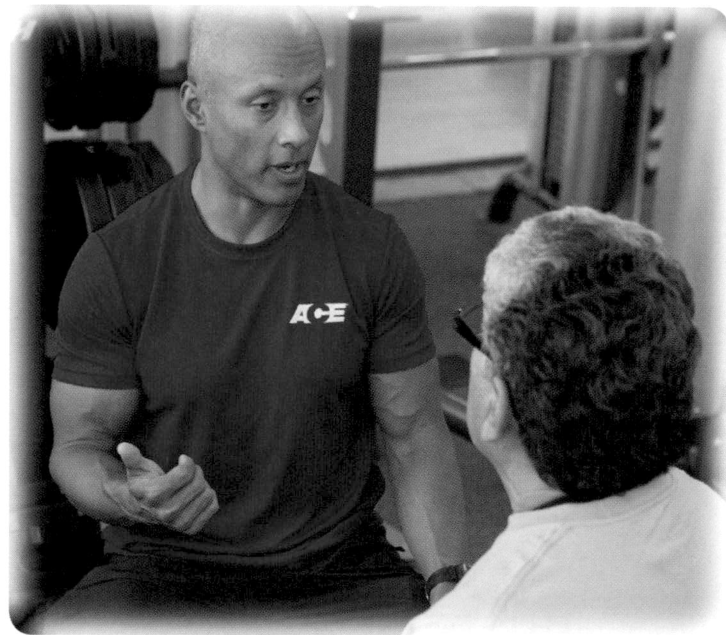

What do we know about Rick?

- He is a 60-year-old retiree.
- He initiated contact with the health coach.
- Health history includes:
  - ✓ Type 2 diabetes
  - ✓ Oral medication for diabetes
  - ✓ Gallbladder surgery five years ago
  - ✓ 50 pounds (22.7 kg) overweight
  - ✓ Chronic low-back pain
  - ✓ Physician cleared him for exercise
  - ✓ Sedentary lifestyle
- His goals are to lose weight, improve blood-sugar control, and decrease lower-back discomfort.

The first step in dealing with this type of health history is for the health coach to realize that feeling a bit inundated with information is reasonable and provides the justification for carefully using a structured approach to understand what is known about the client. The health coach would also be wise to acknowledge that his or her coaching skills, along with well-anchored self-confidence, can be invaluable to the client as he or she begins the journey of behavioral change.

Initial Contact

The health coach should schedule the first available and convenient appointment with Rick. It would be helpful for the health coach to spend a few minutes either in person or on the phone asking basic questions, getting to know Rick, and establishing the business side of the relationship:

- "May I ask how you were referred to me?"
- "Please tell me a bit about what led you to decide to call for assistance at this time?" The health coach may also ask, "Can you tell me briefly what general goals you had in mind that prompted you to contact me?"
- Make several reflective comments back to the client based on what he said to ensure that the client begins to think and feel that he is heard and understood, and that a connection has begun to be built.

- "I'd like to discuss my fees with you. My fee per 60-minute session is $________. Ordinarily I am paid at the end of each session and I accept checks, cash, and credit cards. I'm happy to discuss other arrangements, such as packages and payment plans, if you are interested."
- "Do you have any questions I might be able to answer for you now, before we get together?"
- Summarize what you heard and then close with, "I appreciate Dr. Jones (or whoever referred the client to the health coach) suggesting my name to you and I'm delighted you called. That's a great first step on the road to reaching your goals of __________. I've had the privilege of working with other clients facing similar issues and I look forward to helping you. You may want to arrive a bit early to complete some initial paperwork, or if you prefer I can email it to you. Which is more convenient for you? I look forward to seeing you on (date) at (time). Feel free to give me a call before then with any additional questions."

If the appointment is set for more than a week away, a reminder call may be appropriate to confirm the meeting.

Interview and Screening

After a warm, professional greeting, the health coach can use the first few minutes of the session explaining to Rick what to expect. Some health coaches find it of value to ask, "May I ask what you anticipated our visits would be like?" This type of question provides the health coach and the client an opportunity to immediately deal with erroneous expectations that may need to be cleared up. It may help Rick clarify his thinking about the reality of what the health coach will be doing to help him reach his goals.

The initial history-gathering discussion is designed to help build rapport (i.e., develop **empathy,** warmth, and genuineness between the client and health coach). During this process, the health coach can demonstrate professionalism in environment, appearance, speech, body language, and attentiveness. The health coach should ask appropriate, thought-provoking questions to demonstrate concern, care, and an organized approach to the investigation part of the initial meeting. The following list provides examples of open-ended (and a few relevant closed-ended) questions that would help the health coach build rapport with Rick.

- "You say you are retired. Tell me a bit about the nature of the work you did previously."
- "You mentioned on the phone that you've been diagnosed with type 2 diabetes and take medication for that. Tell me when you were diagnosed, and what medications you've taken and are currently taking for it. How is the medication working for you? Do you experience any side effects? Will you authorize me to speak with your doctor if necessary?"
- "You mentioned that five years ago you had gallbladder surgery. Can you tell me about that experience?"
- "You described low-back pain. Please tell me more about that pain. Where do you feel it? When do you feel it? Can you describe how it feels? Are there any things you do that make it feel better or worse?"
- "You said your doctor diagnosed you with obesity and said you were 50 pounds overweight. Tell me about your weight history as a child, teen, and adult. What have you done about it in the past that was helpful and not helpful?"

Visit www.ACEfitness.org/HealthCoachResources to download a free PDF of the readiness to change questionnaire, as well as other forms and assessment tools that you can use throughout your career as a health coach.

The health coach should focus on identifying the client's readiness to change and stage of behavioral change. The health coach may use a **motivational interviewing** technique to assess readiness to change. For example, the health coach can ask Rick, "On a scale of 1–10, where 1 is 'not at all important to change,' and 10 is 'I am ready to do whatever it takes to change my lifestyle and get healthier,' how would you rate how important it is for you to change now?" When Rick offers the number, the health coach asks him why he gave that number. Next, the health coach asks Rick, "Why didn't you choose a lower number and why not a higher number?" Lastly, the health coach asks Rick, "What would it take for you to move one or two numbers up on this measure?" The health coach can summarize what he or she heard Rick say. Finally, in this approach, the health coach should pose the same scale and questions again, this time regarding Rick's *confidence* in changing behavior.

Given that Rick has been to his physician and called the health coach for assistance, it is likely he is in the **preparation** stage of readiness, with thoughts such as, "I want to be healthier, lose weight, and eat healthier, but I've had a poor history of doing so. I'm ready to change that." If the health coach is not certain about Rick's stage, a Readiness to Change Questionnaire may be used (Figure 19-1).

Figure 19-1
Readiness to change questionnaire

	YES	NO
Are you looking to change a specific behavior?	❑	❑
Are you willing to make this behavioral change a top priority?	❑	❑
Have you tried to change this behavior before?	❑	❑
Do you believe there are inherent risks/dangers associated with not making this behavioral change?	❑	❑
Are you committed to making this change, even though it may prove challenging?	❑	❑
Do you have support for making this change from friends, family, and loved ones?	❑	❑
Besides health reasons, do you have other reasons for wanting to change this behavior?	❑	❑
Are you prepared to be patient with yourself if you encounter obstacles, barriers, and/or setbacks?	❑	❑

After confirming that Rick is in the preparation stage, the health coach clarifies Rick's goals and explores options available to him for change. Further, having Rick explain what has been successful for him in changing and achieving these or similar goals in the past and understanding Rick's perceived barriers for change are appropriate actions to take at this time. The following statements are helpful in starting this conversation. "Here are some ideas others have found helpful. I wonder, what are your impressions of these interventions?" In addition, the health coach can use the DISC model to gain insight into Rick's behavioral style and preferences and get a sense of how best to structure communication with him (see Chapter 5).

The health coach may choose to do a systematic screening of Rick's disease history, risk factors, emotional issues, and family history. At the least, the PAR-Q would be an appropriate initial assessment (see Figure 10-3, page 272). Additional tools to consider using with Rick are the health-history checklist (see Figure 15-1, pages 412–414), the exercise history and attitude questionnaire (see Figure 10-5, page 276), a weight-loss readiness quiz (see Figure 10-6, page 278), and the sample medical release form (refer to the *ACE Personal Trainer Manual*). Given that Rick's physician referred him for coaching, communication between the health coach and his physician is an important part of the professional relationship on Rick's behalf. The health coach needs to understand Rick's goal weight and diabetes profile numbers. This can be discussed with his physician (with Rick's written permission) and shared with Rick.

Visit www.ACEfitness.org/HealthCoachResources to download a free PDF of the documents listed here, as well as other forms and assessment tools that you can use throughout your career as a health coach.

Assessments

Body-composition assessment that motivates clients and aims to help them develop realistic **SMART goals** is a standard part of the health coach's toolkit. In Rick's case, it is a fundamental part of the initial assessment. Because of Rick's excess weight, performing skinfold measurements or **bioelectrical impedance analysis** procedures would not result in an accurate assessment, so circumference measures would be more appropriate.

An assessment of Rick's functional mobility is also a primary element in the initial evaluation. Rick's posture, movement, and **range of motion (ROM)** are important early-phase assessments. Because he has been sedentary and is deconditioned, a cardiorespiratory endurance test will undoubtedly show this, so an assessment of Rick's aerobic endurance is not crucial at this time. Rick's assessment results are listed in Table 19-1.

Table 19-1

Rick: Assessment Results

Assessment	Results	Observations
Circumference measurements	Waist: 40 inches (101.6 cm) Hips: 36 inches (91.44 cm) Waist-to-hip ratio: 1.11	Both Rick's waist measurement and his waist-to-hip ratio place him in a high-risk category for cardiometabolic disease and show that he has android body-fat deposition.
Posture	Stands with slight kyphosis and lordosis posture	Rick needs to improve postural stability and mobility. Because of low-back pain, McGill's core function test battery was avoided.
Modified body-weight squat	5 repetitions with approximately 45 degrees of knee flexion	Rick's results were poor due to performing fewer than 6 repetitions and inability to squat below 45 degrees of knee flexion. He also reported that he "felt it in his lower back" during the test.
Overhead reach	Both hands were able to reach the floor; however, the back arched excessively off of the mat	Rick lacks appropriate shoulder mobility and core stability.

Exercise Program

The ACE IFT Model encompasses four phases and two training components (see Chapter 16). In Rick's case, given his goals of weight loss and dealing with lower-back discomfort, the first two phases of both the functional movement and resistance training component and the cardiorespiratory training component are important starting points.

The initial functional movement and resistance training element for Rick—stability and mobility training—is aimed at core and balance exercises to improve postural stability throughout the kinetic chain, without compromising mobility throughout the chain.

Low-intensity exercise is introduced to help Rick enhance muscular balance, endurance, core function, and **flexibility.** Postural exercises to improve **static** and **dynamic balance** are also featured in the early stages of work with Rick. Bending and lifting, single-leg movement, pushing, pulling, and rotational movements—all aspects of movement training—are designed to help Rick develop mobility in the kinetic chain without compromising stability. Table 19-2 lists an initial stability and mobility training program for Rick.

Table 19-2

Rick: Stability and Mobility Exercise

Exercise	Intensity	Repetitions	Rest Interval	Sets
Exercise progression for core activation	<50% MVC	1	10–15 seconds	1-2
Pelvic tilts, progress to bent-knee marches	Body weight	12-15	30–60 seconds	2-3
Reverse flys with supine 90–90	<50% MVC	2-4	10–15 seconds	2-3
Cat-camel	Body weight	10–12	30–60 seconds	2-3
Quadruped drawing in with extremity movement	Body weight	10–12	30–60 seconds	2-3
Anterior capsule (pectoralis) stretch	Body weight	1-2	10–15 seconds	2-4
Closed kinetic chain weight shifts for upper body	Body weight	2-4	10–15 seconds	1-2
Body-weight squats	Body weight	12-15	30–60 seconds	2-3

Note: See Chapter 17 and the ACE Exercise Library (www.ACEfitness.org/exerciselibrary) for instructional guidelines for the exercises listed.

Note: MVC = Maximal voluntary contraction

Rick's sedentary lifestyle is an issue that exercise, particularly cardiorespiratory training, will address. Based on his cardiorespiratory fitness assessment, cardiorespiratory training is chosen to accommodate his fitness and health status. The initial aerobic-base training focuses on establishing a baseline to serve as the foundation upon which aerobic-efficiency training will be built. Rick's **self-efficacy** will grow with the improvements he sees in his health, endurance, energy, mood, and caloric expenditure during aerobic-base training. In the second phase of cardiorespiratory training, aerobic-efficiency training, Rick will experience increased duration and frequency of cardiorespiratory sessions, as well as interval training. Table 19-3 lists an initial cardiorespiratory endurance training program for Rick.

Table 19-3

Rick: Cardiorespiratory Endurance Exercise

Warm-up	Workout	Cool-down
Walk for 5 minutes	Frequency: >3 days per week Intensity: Below the talk-test threshold, or at a perceived exertion that is "moderate" to "somewhat hard" (RPE = 3 to 4) Time: Work up to 30 minutes of continuous exercise Type: Walking	Walk for 5 minutes Static stretching of the anterior shoulder capsule, hip flexors, hip adductors, hamstrings, and calves

Note: RPE = Ratings of perceived exertion

Motivation and Adherence

Given Rick's age and retired status, he faces potential challenges in terms of motivation, including illness, erroneous beliefs, lack of peer-group support, a sense of disempowerment, fear of injury, and "too much time on his hands." Promoting goal-oriented, empowering, cost-effective, gradual activity progressions and accessible weight-management programming are appropriate steps for the health coach to provide.

Developing more specific goals with Rick is important when determining how to best move into the subsequent phases of the ACE IFT Model. The health coach uses coaching skills to help Rick move through what is assumed to be the preparation stage by helping him solidify his plan for change. Writing down a formal statement of his behavior-change commitments may be helpful at this stage. Doing so in SMART goal language is important (see Chapter 13). Working with Rick to develop short-term, achievable goals, and then posting them where Rick can readily see them is useful.

Some examples of poorly written goals include the following:

- "I'm going to do more cardio this week."
- "I'm going to shop for healthier foods."
- "I'm going to watch my sugar intake."

Better-written goals avoid vague alternatives, are quantifiable and action-oriented, start with moderately difficult but doable steps, have specific time limits, are recorded, and can be easily reset when necessary. Examples of well-written goals include:

- "I will walk on a treadmill at the gym for 15 minutes, four days this week, and keep a minimum heart rate of 65%."
- "I will use a shopping list I have made to purchase more fruits and vegetables, organic lean proteins, omega-3 fatty acids, and purified water."
- "I will cut my sugar intake by eating three meals and two snacks, or five small meals, each day; keep sugar out of reach; and be mindful of my emotions."

The health coach can encourage Rick to associate with others who have similar goals and enlist support from his family. Designing other forms of environmental support, such as weight-management groups and group exercise programs, is also relevant. Active hobbies and volunteer efforts will be of value to him, given his retirement. **Social support** is a robust correlate of physical-activity **adherence,** particularly when it comes from friends and family. Helping Rick modify his environment to reduce access to sedentary behaviors and promoting physical activity will be useful to him.

The health coach can teach Rick the triggers that may work to derail his healthy eating and exercise plan. These triggers, real or imagined, internal or external, may include:

- The opportunity to eat unhealthy foods
- Conditioned responses
- Unpleasant emotions and physical sensations
- Socializing

Helping Rick identify how he will deal with these triggers in advance is an important part of coaching for him. The health coach can "brainstorm" with Rick to help him identify small steps he can take that are action-oriented and realistic for him. Helping Rick explore potential difficulties is also an important step in moving him through this stage. Instead of telling Rick what to do, the health coach can help him develop strategies to cope with obstacles before they arise.

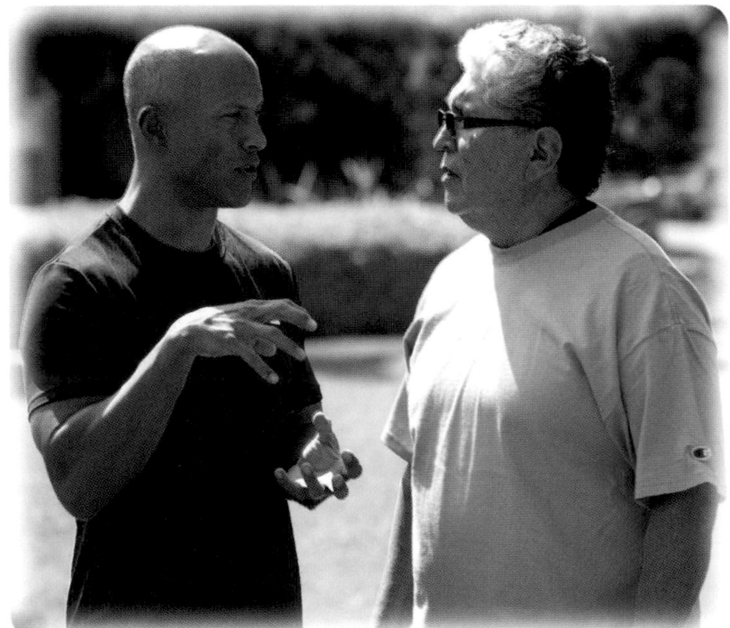

Lower adherence is often observed in exercise programs designed for overweight and obese populations, due, perhaps in part, to less pleasurable experiences during exercise. Thus, the health coach should pay close attention to Rick's appraisals of exercise, particularly negative ones, since these may become adherence issues later. The health coach should examine Rick's affective responses carefully, as this is essential in helping him change his thoughts, which are the foundation of his behaviors.

The health coach can explain to Rick that his behaviors are in large measure determined by what he thinks about the events in his life, more than the actual events. His thoughts create what he feels, and his feelings in turn fuel his behavior. The health coach can offer examples of how this can occur with respect to weight management and exercise adherence, and ask Rick for examples as well.

To deal with Rick's self-efficacy issues, the health coach can watch for inappropriate or unrealistic and misinformed thinking and goal-setting. The health coach should listen for self-talk that reflects cognitive distortions, such as:

- "I can't do this."
- "It's too hard."
- "I won't be able to… (enjoy life, eat with friends, or go to parties)."

Other cognitive distortions Rick may make include thinking in absolute, black-and-white terms, discounting anything positive, jumping to conclusions not warranted by facts, and criticizing, labeling, and blaming himself. The health coach can help Rick by asking him the following types of questions about his incorrect thinking:

- Is it true? What is the grain of untruth?
- Is this thought empowering or disempowering? What thought would be more empowering?
- How can you leverage this experience to become even better? What can you do to rework this to catapult you forward?
- What is one thing you could stop doing today that would have the most positive impact in your life? What could you start doing that would have a more positive impact on your life?
- What is it that you are not facing?

Rick may also write SMART goals for cognitive restructuring:

- "I will define my three to five top motivators and goals for this week."
- "I will bring in a list of pros and cons for calorie counting in my next visit."
- "I will keep a journal of my thoughts as I eat for one day and bring it to our next visit."
- "I will create five cards that I will carry with me that are 'rational response thoughts' to counter any erroneous thinking I have about exercise and diet."

Specific erroneous, incorrect, irrational thoughts may surround the urge to:

- Eat inappropriately
- Avoid the structured exercise plan
- Be more aggressive in either dieting or exercising

The health coach may help Rick cope with his urges by teaching him that when he gives in to an urge, the correct question to ask is, "How did I talk myself into it?" Rick will find more progress in that question than when asking, "What made me do that?" or "Why did I do that?" The health coach can teach Rick that the urge does not cause the relapse, as it is the client's beliefs that lead to the relapse. Four common beliefs that Rick may demonstrate include:

- "The urge is unbearable. I can't stand it."
- "The urge is so powerful, it makes me eat or avoid exercise."
- "The urge to eat or avoid exercise will not stop until I give in to it."
- "The urge is making me crazy."

These largely incorrect and inaccurate thoughts in turn lead to greater emotional upset and more urges. The health coach can coach Rick on how to dispute, debate, and challenge these irrational thoughts by asking, "Where is the evidence that your urge is unbearable and that you can't stand it? You appear to be tolerating it. Perhaps not well, but you are standing it." Rick will develop the rational response that there is evidence that bearing the urge is difficult, but not impossible. A rational response may be "I sure don't like it when I feel this urge, but I can stand it." Another may be, "I don't like feeling this way, but it's not killing me not to give in to the urge and I can keep on resisting it."

Next, Rick may tackle the "urge makes me" thought by asking, again, if there is any evidence for this belief. The answer, of course, is that there is no evidence that the urge *makes* Rick eat or avoid exercise. Instead, the health coach can teach Rick that while the urge to eat inappropriately or avoid exercise makes reaching goals difficult and generally makes life unpleasant, it does not force him to do anything. It is just a thought. The only thing that makes Rick do, or not do, anything is ultimately his own decision.

The thought that the urge will not disappear until the client gives into it is another false belief. Again, the client can be asked about the evidence for this thought and, again, there will be no evidence whatsoever that the urge remains until the client eats inappropriately or avoids exercise. It may take a while for the urge to evaporate, but urges (like all thoughts) are generally time-limited, and they go away, or stay, regardless of whether the client eats or does not eat, exercises or does not exercise.

Finally, the thought that the urge is driving the client crazy is another one that has no proof behind it. The client may drive him- or herself crazy about the urge and need to learn that he or she can *decide* to not to go crazy because of the thought (urge). The client may think instead, "I can remain calm and get through this urge."

Lastly, a client facing issues such as Rick faces may experience low frustration tolerance, self-doubt, and self-pity. The health coach may teach Rick that even though he may inaccurately believe that others are stronger than he is and that others can succeed and he cannot, the truth is that traits such as self-regulation are not something some people "have" while others, like Rick, do not have. These skills can be learned, and Rick can come to recognize that working with the health coach will give him the opportunity to practice and learn these skills. Rick needs to learn to believe that he can change his behaviors and will, with the structured set of interventions the health coach has developed with him. If Rick believes that "it is *too hard* to change," the health coach can help arm Rick with the healthier belief that it is hard but not "*too* hard." He also would do well to learn that not changing will eventually be more difficult for him.

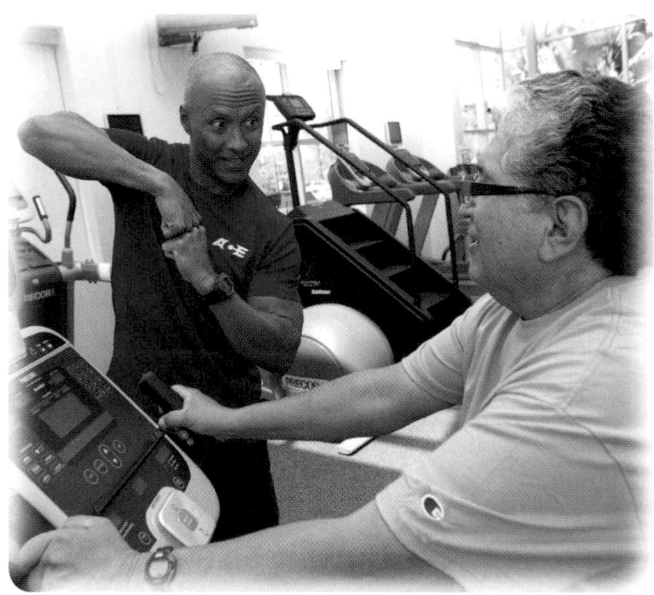

If in the course of active listening, the health coach picks up that Rick believes that "it *shouldn't be* this hard," or that "it *must* be easy," the health coach may help Rick identify this belief and help him replace it with the idea that there is no rule as to how difficult it "should be," and that although he would *prefer* it to be easier, that does not mean therefore it *must* be. Rick is not doing himself any good by this absolutistic demanding thinking.

If Rick demonstrates the belief, "*It's not fair* that I can't eat what I want and 'have to' exercise," the health coach can help him challenge this thought and replace it with the idea that many things in life may not be "fair." It is far healthier for Rick to accept that fact and move forward as he does with many events in his life that he has deemed "unfair" and succeeded in spite of this belief. Rick can learn that life is not fair, but rather it is a sequence of events, some of which are unpleasant and some of which are pleasurable.

The health coach may suggest that Rick ask, "What is the worst thing that can happen to me if what I want to happen, does not happen?" Or, "What is the worst thing that can happen to me if what I want not to happen, does?" Rick can learn that he might be inconvenienced, deprived of some pleasurable experiences, and feel stress and tension. Alternatively, Rick might learn to tolerate frustration better than he has in the past, improve his coping skills, and begin to recognize that he can accept and deal well with unpleasant situations as they occur.

Follow-up sessions may be introduced with questions such as, "What is the most positive thing that has happened since we last spoke?" Or, "What was the best thing that you experienced related to your goals since we last spoke?" Or, "What was the best thing you learned about your goals this past week?" The health coach should stay connected to Rick through email if he has access to an email account, or make a follow-up phone call to see how his adherence and commitment to his SMART goals is being maintained.

Shane: Sedentary Businessman With High Cholesterol

Shane is a 35-year-old public relations manager who works long hours and sometimes works two weeks straight without a day off. He has contacted a health coach in hopes of making lifestyle changes to improve his health status. Shane's **cholesterol** was elevated at his last doctor's visit, one month ago. His doctor has recommended that he consume a more balanced diet and increase his physical activity. His body weight is normal and he claims that he has always had a slender build, which is why he reports that he is confused by the diagnosis because he is not overweight. According to Shane, he is too busy to engage in a regular exercise program and is currently sedentary. Upon reviewing his **food diary,** the health coach observes that Shane eats a poor-quality diet consisting mainly of fast food.

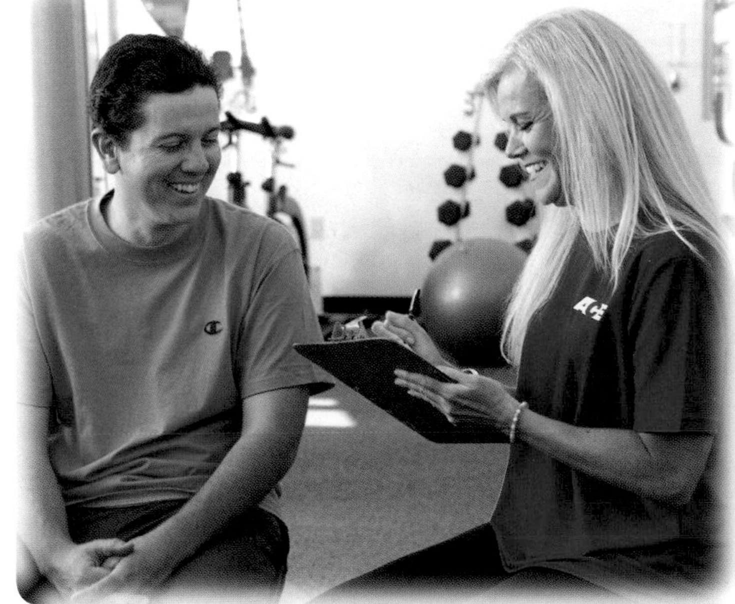

What do we know about Shane?

- He is 35 years old and works many hours, often without a break.
- He initiated contact with the health coach for lifestyle health changes.
- Health history includes:
  - ✓ Elevated cholesterol
  - ✓ Physician recommended a more balanced diet and physical activity
  - ✓ Normal body weight
  - ✓ Feels too busy to engage in regular exercise
  - ✓ Eats a poor-quality diet (fast food)
- His goal is to improve his cholesterol profile.

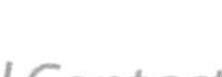

Initial Contact

As described in the previous case, the health coach should schedule the first appointment with Shane at the earliest convenient time. Similarly, it would be helpful for the health coach to spend a few minutes either in person or on the phone asking basic questions, getting to know Shane, and establishing the business side of the relationship. If the first appointment is set for more than a week away, a reminder call may be appropriate to confirm the meeting. However, in Shane's case, it might be prudent to ensure that the first meeting is scheduled for a day in the very near future because he appears to run a fast-paced schedule and might lose sight of the importance of starting his lifestyle change sooner rather than later.

Interview and Screening

Shane's goal, to improve his cholesterol profile, will be important in discussing many areas with the health coach. The initial screening will include the types of evaluations and related tools described for Rick, with greater focus on Shane's cholesterol levels, eating habits, work hours, time-management skills, and any negative thoughts about the time he has available for exercise. Shane's motivation for change will depend on a number of factors, including his **decisional balance** analysis, self-efficacy, the trust he has in the health coach, the support he feels, the degree to which he feels respected, and the clarity with which his goals are set.

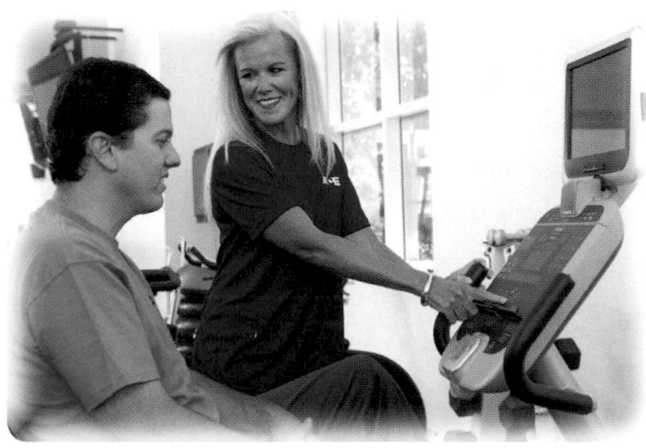

Communication with Shane's physician is necessary, with appropriate releases signed by Shane, to assure him that he has a team working together on his behalf. The assessment phase may be difficult given the limited time Shane has and the potential for unrealistic demands and expectations he may have on getting it done as quickly as possible. Still, the assessment phase is important to demonstrate the professionalism of the health coach, develop the unique program that will be drawn up for him, and make clear the level of individual care and attention he is getting. Assessments are an important part of the overall set of interventions the health coach will make and should not be cut short for any reason, regardless of Shane's "fast food" approach to life. The health coach needs to understand Shane's cholesterol levels to best understand the goals that Shane has set for himself.

Shane's *ideal* cholesterol profile will likely be as follows, but should be confirmed with his physician:

- Total cholesterol: less than 200 mg/dL
- **Low-density lipoprotein (LDL)**: less than 100 mg/dL
- **High-density lipoprotein (HDL)**: 60 mg/dL or higher
- **Triglycerides**: less than 150 mg/dL

As with Rick, it is likely that Shane is in the preparation stage of readiness to change, given that he has already contacted the health coach, and has agreed with his physician to get help for improving his cholesterol profile. Asking the same types of questions the health coach used with Rick may be of value (see Figure 19-1).

The health coach—after helping Shane identify his current behavior as it relates to his cholesterol profile, assessing his readiness to change, and gathering knowledge to help him make a commitment to change and create short- and long-term goals—can discuss anticipated obstacles, self-monitoring practices, methods to stay motivated, ways to cope with his potential ambivalences, and the continual reevaluation of his plan.

Assuming Shane's physician helped him understand the factors influencing his cholesterol levels, including age, body-fat deposition, gender, genetics, diseases, and lifestyle choices (e.g., diet, exercise, and stress management), the health coach can structure a set of interventions aimed at improving Shane's cholesterol profile. These interventions would focus on behavioral change in the following areas:

- Healthy eating
- Increased physical activity
- Stress reduction (particularly related to unusual work hours)

Regarding Shane's diet, the health coach may want to coach him on strategies for eating healthy before, during, and after his busy workday. Also, helping Shane progressively implement the following nutrition changes adapted from the U.S. Department of Agriculture's *2015-2020 Dietary Guidelines for Americans* (U.S. Department of Agriculture, 2015) would be appropriate:

- Eat less meat
- Add fish to the weekly diet
- Eat more fruits and vegetables
- Add more nuts daily
- Increase **complex carbohydrates** and **fiber**
- Choose low-fat dairy products
- Cut down on **saturated fat** in cooking
- Avoid palm and coconut oils
- Avoid or significantly reduce **trans fat**
- Reduce salt intake
- Avoid or significantly reduce highly processed, unhealthy snacks
- Drink alcohol in moderation
- Read labels carefully

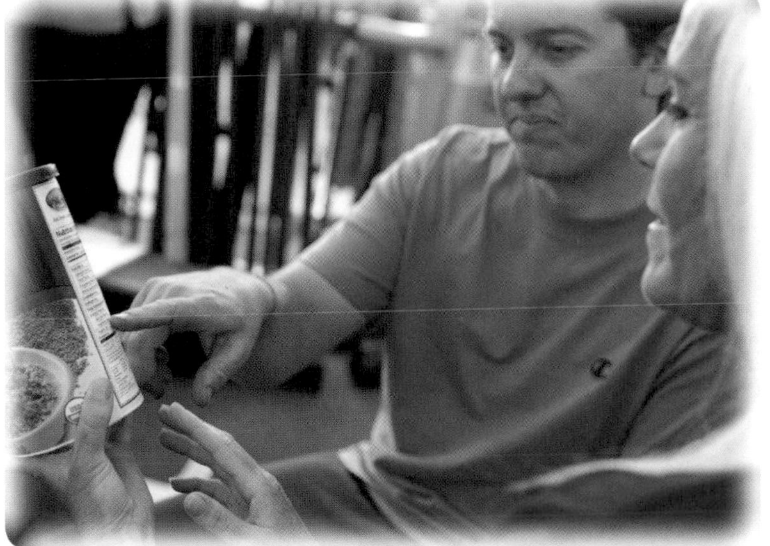

Assessments

Shane is of the mindset that he does not like to waste time. Thus, the health coach might consider conducting physical assessments with Shane as part of his first workout. That is, the health coach could explain to Shane that while the exercises he will be doing during his first meeting are also assessments, they will be challenging enough to "count" as a workout session. Postural and functional movement assessments are appropriate for Shane at this point. Before the physical assessments, however, the health coach would be wise to conduct a skinfold test on Shane and educate him about the differences between body weight and **body composition.** Table 19-4 lists Shane's assessment results.

Exercise Program

Shane will need to understand that exercise may improve his cholesterol profile (by increasing HDL and decreasing LDL levels), lower triglyceride levels and **blood pressure,** reduce excess weight, and improve his heart and lung function, while also helping him diminish or better manage his stress levels. As with Rick, Shane's self-efficacy and anticipated negative predictions about his inability to find time to exercise will need to be addressed using the methods outlined earlier for Rick.

Based on understanding Shane's DISC profile and level of behavioral readiness to change (the same strategies and techniques described earlier in the chapter for Rick),

Table 19-4		
Shane: Assessment Results		
Assessment	Results	Observations
Body composition: Skinfold measurements	25% body fat	Shane's body-fat percentage places him at the low end of the obese category for men.
Posture	Stands with slight flat-back posture	Flat-back posture appears to stem from posterior pelvic tilt
Modified body-weight squat	10 repetitions with approximately 90 degrees of knee flexion; noticeable varus knee movement at the lowest depth of squat	Shane's results reveal that he has good muscular endurance at 10 repetitions and the ability to tolerate a normal depth of squat. However, his knees bowed outward at the lowest point of the squat, indicating instability of the lower extremity.
Front plank	Held proper alignment for 20 seconds	Shane lacks appropriate stability and endurance in his core musculature.
Overhead reach	Both hands hovered approximately 2 inches (5.1 cm) above the floor	Shane lacks appropriate shoulder mobility.

Note: HR = Heart rate; VT1 = First ventilatory threshold

Shane can be helped to understand that a goal for exercise for cholesterol improvement includes an accumulated 150 minutes of moderate-intensity aerobic endurance activity each week in addition to resistance training. The health coach may choose to use a measure of effort with a 5 or 6 on a 10-point scale to properly define "moderate intensity" with Shane. Further, the health coach may assist Shane in understanding the value of wearing a pedometer to achieve a moderate pace of 100 steps per minute while walking. Tables 19-5 and 19-6 list Shane's initial stability and mobility training program and cardiorespiratory endurance program, respectively.

Table 19-5				
Shane: Stability and Mobility Exercise				
Exercise	Intensity	Repetitions	Rest Interval	Sets
Cat-camel	Body weight	10–12	30–60 seconds	2–3
Quadruped drawing in with extremity movement	Body weight	10–12	30–60 seconds	2–3
Front plank	Body weight	1 (15–30 second hold)	30–60 seconds	2–3
Side plank	Body weight	1 per side (10–20 second hold)	30–60 seconds	2–3
Thoracic matrix in neutral stance (seated or kneeling); progress to standing, staggered stance, and split stance	Body weight	15	30–60 seconds	2–3
Hip hinge progression	Body weight	5–10	30–60 seconds	1-2
Body-weight squats	Body weight	12-15	30–60 seconds	2-3

Note: See Chapter 17 and the ACE Exercise Library (www.ACEfitness.org/exerciselibrary) for instructional guidelines for the exercises listed.

Table 19-6		
Shane: Cardiorespiratory Endurance Exercise		
Warm-up	Workout	Cool-down
Fast walk or light cycling for 5 minutes	Frequency: >3 days per week Intensity: Below the talk-test threshold, or at a perceived exertion that is "moderate" to "somewhat hard" (RPE = 3 to 4) Time: Work up to 30 minutes of continuous exercise Type: A combination of walking and cycling	Walk for 5 minutes Static stretching of the entire shoulder capsule, hip flexors, hip adductors, hamstrings, and calves

Note: RPE = Ratings of perceived exertion

Since Shane spends so much time at work, the health coach may discuss the value of exercise at work, encourage him to join work- or community-wide events that promote physical activity, and suggest that he involve himself in any corporate wellness programs that may be available.

Motivation and Adherence

Stress reduction can be a powerful tool in creating enhanced motivation and adherence to a behavior-change program. Teaching Shane how he creates stress by the way in which he perceives and thinks about events in his life is based on cognitive behavioral coaching techniques.

For example, if Shane believes that it is *terrible* if he does not finish all the work on his desk, it is *awful* when people do not treat him as he demands they do in his business dealings, or it is *the end of the world* when life is not as fair as he insists it should be, he is creating a false sense of how bad life can be. Anticipating that things will be "horrible, awful, terrible, and catastrophic" if and when they do not turn out as Shane thinks they *should, must* and *ought to* be, will create mental and emotional stress. He would be far better off restructuring his thinking to reflect the following concepts: "It may be bad, but it is *not terrible* if I do not do as well as I would like to do," or "When people do not treat me well, it is *unfortunate* but not awful," or "If life is unfair, that is bad but it is *not the end of the world*." Teaching Shane that things could always be worse, that the event or situation is less than 100% bad, and that good can come from the event or situation would all be valuable in helping Shane reduce his stress.

Social support and a stimulating environment are also valuable to reduce stress and reduce cardiovascular risk. Talking with Shane about his social life, both in and out of work, may provide insight into the need for further coaching in this area.

Avoiding Relapse

Shane's ability to remain motivated and avoid relapse is an important element in the successful relationship the health coach creates with him. While relapse often occurs after a change has been implemented, it should be viewed as a time of increased vulnerability and *not* failure. Feelings of disappointment, failure, or frustration are common when a client has moved into relapse. The health coach will need to identify triggers that lead to relapse, recognize those barriers and obstacles that contribute to relapse, and take steps to overcome those obstacles.

Many experts believe that relapse is a part of the overall growth process. When relapse occurs, the health coach may need to help Shane re-enter an earlier stage of readiness for change such as **contemplation,** preparation, or **action.** Shane may need to reevaluate his goals and strategies. He needs to understand his own personal triggers and, with the help of the health coach, develop appropriate skills and strategies to cope with these triggers. When relapse occurs, peer support may be an additional tool for the health coach to bring into the overall intervention.

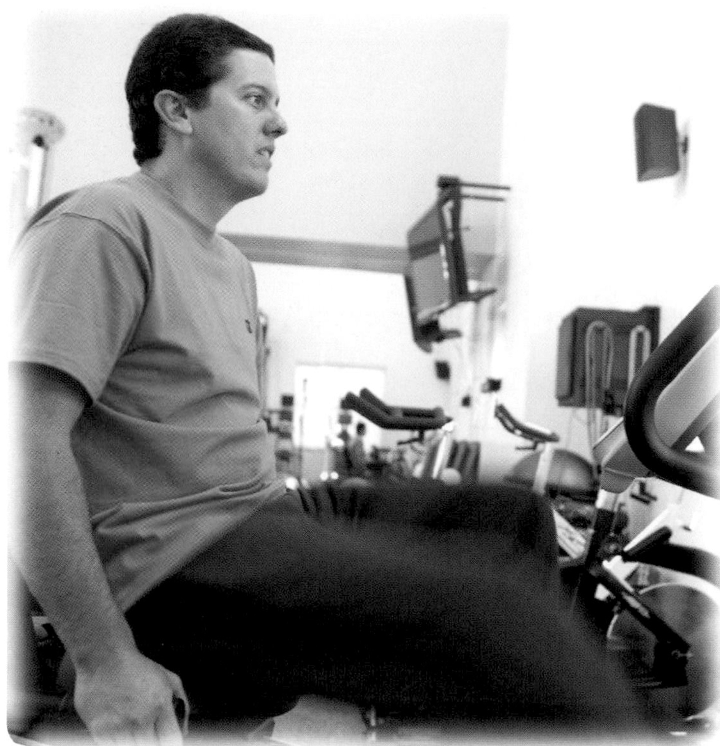

One area of potential relapse for Shane involves eating unhealthy foods. If he finds himself in a "high-risk" situation, such as being invited by his coworkers to go out to a fast-food restaurant for lunch, he can use a positive coping response such as, "I think I'll pass—I've decided to cut back on fast food and going to that restaurant probably wouldn't be good for me now." This will likely lead to increased self-efficacy and reduce the likelihood of relapse.

If Shane is not prepared with a positive coping response, his self-efficacy will be diminished, he will likely lapse, have a perceived loss of control, and increase the probability of relapse. He may say something like, "Even though I know it's not good for me, it's not fair that I can't go. I've had a lousy day and deserve a break." This might erroneously lead Shane to believe that he is weak and cannot resist temptation. It might also result in Shane believing that going with his coworkers will lift his spirits and make him feel better. He then goes out and eats unhealthy food, which strengthens the "giving-in" habit and enforces the "I'm hopeless, so why bother" belief, leading to more eating and increasing the likelihood of relapse.

By maintaining positive non-judgmental support, reframing the experience as a learning opportunity, identifying positive coping strategies, and developing a new plan, the health coach can help Shane try again, and again, until eventually he regains the commitment to healthy lifestyle change.

Andrea: Young and Overweight

Andrea is a 26-year-old retail clothing store manager who needs the guidance of a health coach to help her incorporate more exercise into her weekly schedule. Andrea is 15 pounds (6.8 kg) overweight and reports that the extra weight was gained during her last two years in college. She is frustrated because she claims that she is "constantly dieting and going hungry in order to not gain even more weight." Currently, Andrea takes two 10-minute walks per day (during her breaks) around the shopping mall where she works. While she is interested in exercising more and increasing the intensity of her exercise program, Andrea has dropped out of exercise

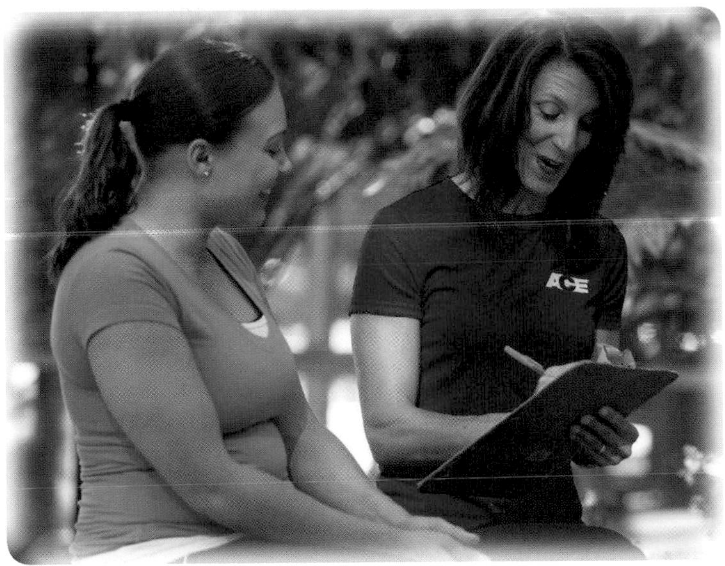

programs in the past due to a lack of time resulting from her often overwhelming time demands.

What do we know about Andrea?

- She is a 26-year-old, full-time employee.
- She is 15 pounds (6.8 kg) overweight.
- She gained this weight over the last two years in college.
- She reports that she has been dieting and "going hungry" to avoid more weight gain.
- She walks twice daily for 10 minutes each time while at work.
- She wants to adhere to an increasingly more intense exercise program.
- She has a history of dropping out of exercise due to "overwhelming time demands."
- Her goal is to lose weight and start a regular exercise program.

Initial Contact

As described in the previous cases, the health coach should schedule the first appointment with Andrea at the earliest convenient time. Similarly, it would be helpful for the health coach to spend a few minutes either in person or on the phone asking basic questions, getting to know Andrea, and establishing the business side of the relationship. If the first appointment is set for more than a week away, a reminder call may be appropriate to confirm the meeting.

Interview and Screening

Andrea presents with a common pattern that many health coaches may see in practice. Andrea has no apparent health problems other than being 15 pounds (6.8 kg) overweight. While a health-history review is still important to conduct in Andrea's case, the health coach will most likely not have to consider many (if any) health limitations for exercise testing or programming based on her age and current physical condition.

Andrea is young and has faced a frequent pattern of failed diet and exercise routines. It is likely that her self-efficacy is diminished, and while she did contact the health coach—suggesting that she might be in the preparation stage of readiness—it would be useful for the health coach to very carefully investigate Andrea's thoughts about her readiness and ability to change. Does Andrea believe *she* is the reason for her failure or does she believe she simply has not found the *right approach*? The answer to this key question will help the health coach best understand how to help Andrea move forward and where to begin with her.

The health coach may consider the following approaches, some of which were described with Rick and Shane earlier in the chapter:

- *Confidence booster:* Ask Andrea, on a scale of 1 to 10, the importance of change and then ask the reason that number was selected, followed by asking why a lower or higher number was not selected. Lastly, the health coach can ask what it would take for Andrea to move up one or two numbers.

- *Decisional balance:* Ask Andrea what she sees as the pros and cons of her changing her diet, exercise, and lifestyle habits. Then ask the pros and cons of not changing her behaviors. Additional information may be obtained by following up with, "What would you like to do with this information?" This technique is especially helpful in the **precontemplation** and contemplation stages.

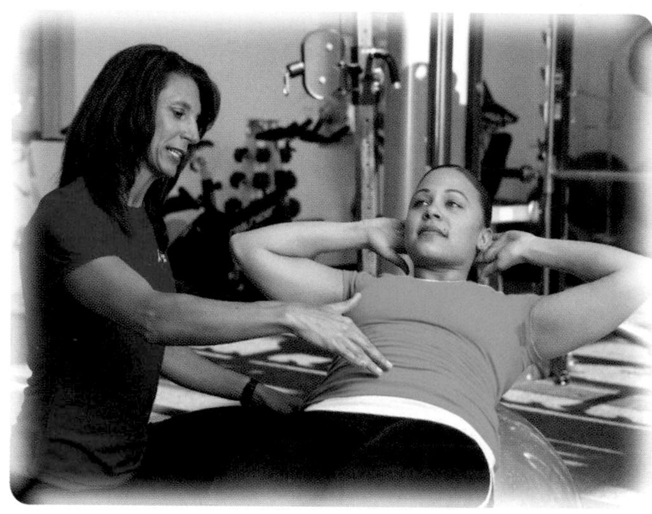

- *Goal-setting:* Behavioral goals are especially useful if Andrea is in the preparation stage. SMART goal language is most helpful. Similarly, when Andrea says she is going to attend the gym four days a week, the health coach can ask, "How important is that for you?" That question can be followed by a discussion of potential obstacles to her making it to the gym four days per week and how she may overcome them.
- *Positive history:* Asking Andrea what worked for her in the past and what strengths she believes she has will help reinforce her self-efficacy.

An empathetic and non-biased, thoughtful questioning approach will help elicit important information to determine an accurate nutritional and exercise understanding and intervention plan. The health coach needs to understand Andrea's desire to change ("I want to…"), ability to change ("I can…"), reasons for change ("I would look better…"), and need to change ("My doctor told me I have to…"). Asking the following questions can help the health coach gather this type of information:

- "What reasons do you have for wanting to exercise more regularly and lose 15 pounds?"
- "How important to you is that right now?"
- "Do you have any other reasons for wanting to lose weight and exercise more?"
- "I'd like to get to know the history of your eating patterns, the diet approaches you have used that have gone well, and a bit more about your exercise programs that have helped you in the past."

The OARS (open-ended question, affirm, reflectively listen, and summarize) model described in Chapter 5 is another valuable method that can be used to obtain information and understand Andrea's attitudes toward herself and changing her lifestyle. It is also a useful method to build a respectful connection, which is essential for any level of success.

- *Open-ended questions:* These questions encourage Andrea to do most of the talking.
  - ✓ "What made you decide now to do something about your weight and exercise?"
- *Affirm:* Affirming statements build Andrea's self-efficacy and validate her desire to change.
  - ✓ "I respect what you are saying and appreciate what you are telling me about how difficult it has been for you."
- *Reflectively listen*: The health coach should mirror what Andrea has said in a way that demonstrates that he or she has heard what Andrea said and meant.
  - ✓ "I hear that you are concerned about your weight and how frustrated and worried you are about not controlling it now."

- *Summarize:* Here, the health coach simply summarizes Andrea's key points.
  - ✓ "What I understand you've said is that you've been growing more worried and frustrated about gaining weight and the belief that you simply don't have the ability or time to cook for yourself, eat healthier, and exercise more regularly."

A proper fitness evaluation, connecting her to a healthy weight-loss regimen, discussing her schedule to help her see where she does have time for exercise, and using social support are foundational elements of Andrea's overall goal-setting.

Assessments

Because Andrea's primary goal is to lose body fat, it is prudent to assess her body composition at the beginning of, and at appropriate intervals during, her weight-management program. Furthermore, Andrea is interested in performing a variety of different types of exercises to keep her routine interesting. For example, she would like to engage in at least two different aerobic endurance modalities and several resistance-training modalities, including core training, circuit training, and traditional resistance training. Thus, considering her age and her physical-activity interests, conducting a full battery of assessments for Andrea is appropriate. Table 19-7 lists Andrea's assessment results.

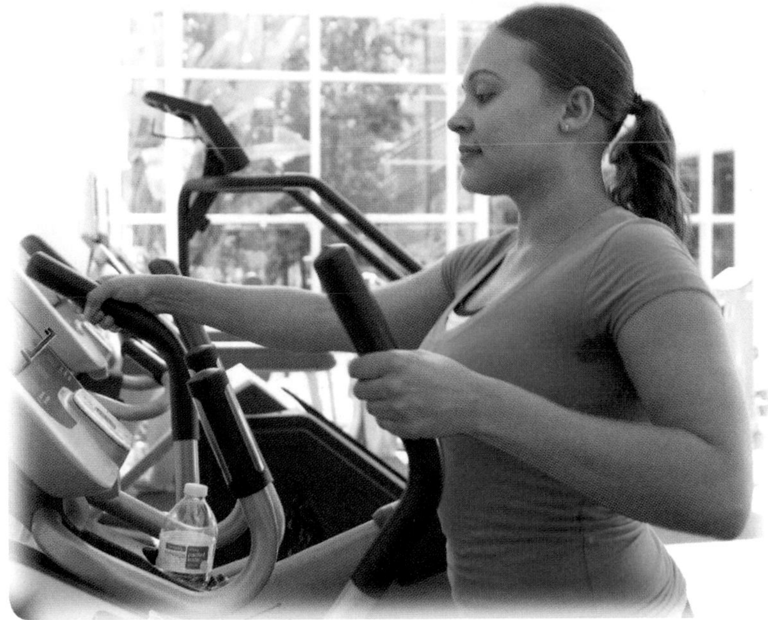

Exercise Program

Andrea appears motivated at this time to engage in a new exercise program. Because of her past failed attempts at sticking with an exercise program, the health coach should be sure to remain connected with Andrea in terms of her emotional responses to her current exercise program. Keeping the program varied, playful, and interesting (as perceived by Andrea) may help to increase her enjoyment and thus motivation to stick with it. Additionally, ensuring that Andrea is successful (and thus continually building self-efficacy during her workouts) will also go a long way toward facilitating motivation. Tables 19-8 and 19-9 list Andrea's initial stability and mobility training program and cardiorespiratory endurance program, respectively.

Adherence and Motivation

There are additional areas of behavioral change that Andrea may benefit from in understanding her failed diet and exercise pattern. These include a more "wellness" than "health" focus. The health coach may point out that exercise and nutrition emphasize the physical domain of life only. Helping Andrea see the value in stress management, positive relationships, emotional intelligence, humor, and "play," may also motivate her to seek overall "wellness," including a better work-life balance.

Through the initial interview process, the health coach learns that Andrea has tried everything from low- to no-carbohydrate meal plans, Jenny Craig®, South Beach®, Taking Off Pounds Sensibly® (TOPS), and every other diet available. She has also tried numerous exercise programs from popular magazines. She is now asking for lifestyle change coaching. The health coach may discuss the social value of commercial support programs with weekly support group meetings for weight loss, such as Weight Watchers®.

Table 19-7

Andrea: Assessment Results

Assessment	Results	Observations
Body composition: Skinfold measurements	28% body fat	Andrea's body-fat percentage places her in the "average" category for women. Recording and tracking this throughout her program will be useful in goal-setting and to measure progress.
Posture	Stands with lordosis posture	Lordosis appears to stem from anterior pelvic tilt
Core: Flexor endurance test	Maintained position for 60 seconds	See below.
Core: Back extensor test	Maintained position for 80 seconds	Flexion:extension ratio = 0.75 (60 sec/80 sec = 0.75); indicates an appropriate balance between core flexors and extensors
Core: Lateral endurance test—right side	Maintained right-side balance (RSB) for 50 seconds	See below.
Core: Lateral endurance test—left side	Maintained left-side balance (LSB) for 35 seconds	RSB:LSB ratio = 1.43 (50 sec/35 sec = 1.43), a differential score of 0.43 from 1.0; indicates a large discrepancy between the strength and endurance of the right and left sides of the core musculature, with the right side exhibiting more strength than the left side; also, Andrea reported shakiness and fatigue in her shoulders during both sides of the test, indicating weakness in her upper extremity.
Modified body-weight squat	10 repetitions with approximately 90 degrees of knee flexion	Andrea's results reveal that she has good muscular endurance at 10 repetitions and the ability to tolerate a normal depth of squat. Furthermore, she reports that she felt the squat mainly in her posterior hips and hamstrings, indicating that she practices a glute-dominant squat.
Front plank	Held proper alignment for 10 seconds	Andrea lacks appropriate stability in her core musculature. She also reports that she felt shaky and tired in her shoulders during the test, again indicating a lack of strength in her upper extremity.
Overhead reach	Both hands reached the floor, while her back remained in contact with the mat	Andrea possesses appropriate shoulder mobility.
Cardiorespiratory endurance: Rockport fitness walking test	13:00 minutes	Andrea scored in the average ranking for females between the ages of 18 and 30 years old.

Table 19-8

Andrea: Stability and Mobility Exercise

Exercise	Intensity	Repetitions	Rest Interval	Sets
Exercise progression for core activation	<50% MVC	1	10–15 seconds	1-2
Pelvic tilts, progress to bent-knee marches	Body weight	12-15	30–60 seconds	2-3
Front plank	Body weight	1 (15–30 second hold)	30–60 seconds	2-3
Side plank	Body weight	1 per side (10–20 second hold)	30–60 seconds	2-3
Supine arm lifts in various positions (I, Y, W, O): progress to standing and then stability ball (progress to prone)	Body weight	2–4 per position	30–60 seconds	2-3
Closed kinetic chain weight shifts for upper body	Body weight	2–4	10–15 seconds	1-2
Hip flexor mobility progression: half-kneeling triplanar stretch	Body weight	1 in each plane (hold >15 seconds each)	30–60 seconds	2-3
Body-weight squats	Bod yweight	12-15	30–60 seconds	2-3
Forward lunges, progress to include side, backward, and rotational lunges	Body weight	12-15	30–60 seconds	2-3

Note: See Chapter 17 and the ACE Exercise Library (www.ACEfitness.org/exerciselibrary) for instructional guidelines for the exercises listed.

Note: MVC = Maximal voluntary contraction

Table 19-9

Andrea: Cardiorespiratory Endurance Exercise

Warm-up	Workout	Cool-down
Fast walk for 5 minutes	Frequency: >3 days per week Intensity: Below the talk-test threshold, or at a perceived exertion that is "moderate" to "somewhat hard" (RPE = 3 to 4) Time: Work up to 30 minutes of continuous exercise Type: Walking (with jogging introduced as fitness improves) and a variety of group fitness classes	Walk for 5 minutes Static stretching of the entire shoulder capsule, hip flexors, hip adductors, hamstrings, and calves

Note: RPE = Ratings of perceived exertion

Summary

Rick, Shane, and Andrea are excellent examples of the types of clients that many health coaches work with on a daily basis. These case studies show different models of intervention that may be of use to health coaches in their practice of helping clients successfully achieve behavioral change that results in healthier lifestyles. Health coaches can build rapport during the initial interview, decide which assessments are appropriate, apply the ACE IFT Model, deal with relapse, and provide social and environmental support to clients. When the health coach meets his or her first real-life client, these basics will serve as a lens through which the myriad of human issues can be best understood.

Reference

U.S. Department of Agriculture (2015). *2015-2020 Dietary Guidelines for Americans* (8th ed.). www.health.gov/dietaryguidelines

Suggested Reading

American Council on Exercise (2014). *ACE Personal Trainer Manual* (5th ed.). San Diego, Calif.: American Council on Exercise.

SECTION VI

LEGAL, PROFESSIONAL, AND ETHICAL RESPONSIBILITIES

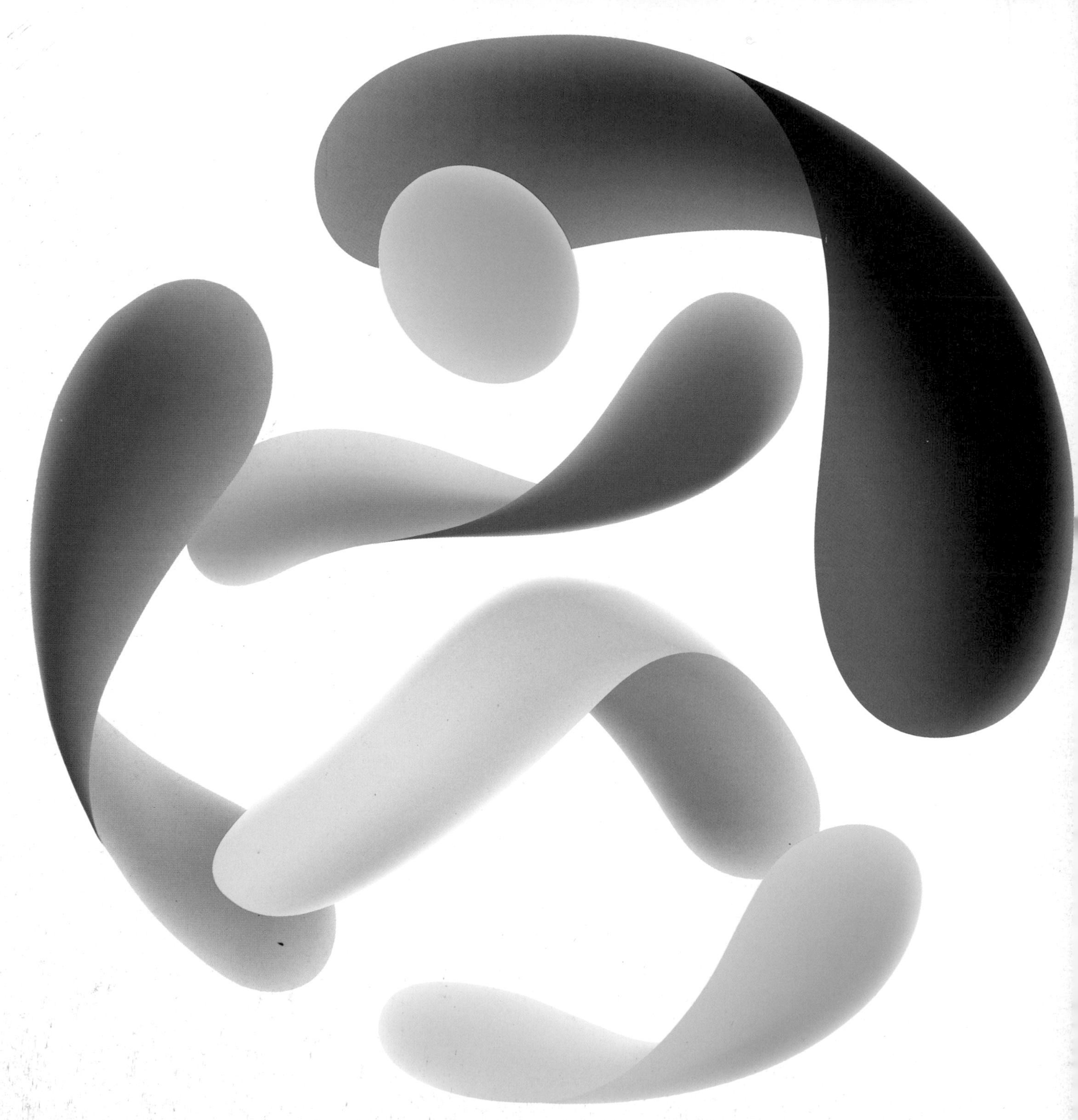

Chapter 20

Legal Guidelines and Professional Responsibilities

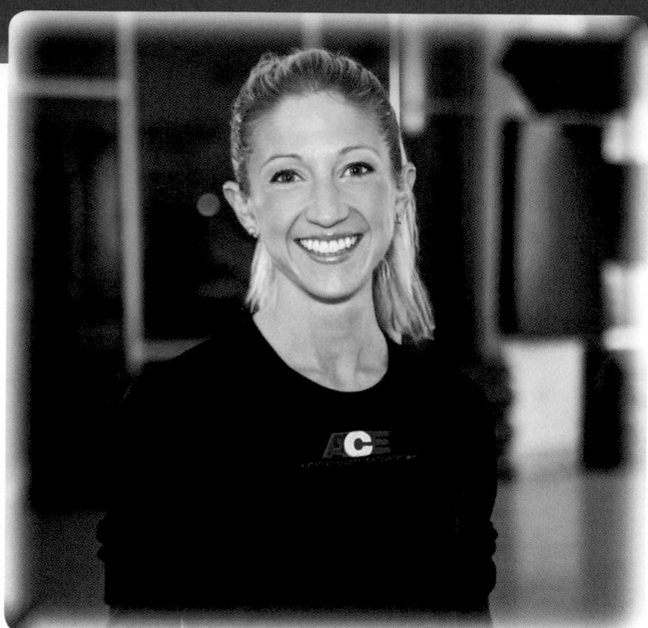

IN THIS CHAPTER:

20 Legal Guidelines and Professional Responsibilities

MARK S. NAGEL

Mark S. Nagel, Ed.D., teaches in the Sport and Entertainment Management Department at the University of South Carolina. Dr. Nagel has published extensively in a variety of areas of sport management, including law, finance, and marketing. Prior to becoming a professor, Dr. Nagel worked in campus recreation and intercollegiate athletics.

ACE-certified Health Coaches typically do not need to be reminded of the importance of studying the latest research related to weight management and nutrition. Most health coaches know that it is essential to spend considerable time and energy developing weight-management programs to help clients achieve their goals. However, the majority of health coaches often neglect the legal issues pertinent to operating a fitness business. Far too often, filed lawsuits are the first indication that a health coach has not adhered to established legal guidelines. In the vast majority of these cases, a simple understanding of the law and a coach's responsibilities can prevent a potential lawsuit, or reduce the financial damages if and when a lawsuit does occur.

This chapter addresses many of the standard legal and business concerns that health coaches may have regarding business structure, employment status, **contracts,** insurance, and **risk management.** It also describes the **scope of practice** in health coaching and summarizes legal responsibilities. The guidelines offered, while based on sport law and the experience of fitness professionals, are not intended as legal advice, but rather as guidance to help health coaches navigate the legal aspects of a career in the fitness industry. Every health coach should utilize these principles when consulting with attorneys who specialize in the appropriate areas. As a health coach's knowledge of the law increases, the ability to anticipate potential legal concerns is heightened, which not only helps to decrease potential litigation, but also provides a better environment for clients, vendors, and **employees.** Ideally, health coaches will regularly consult with an attorney who is aware of the unique laws governing the coach's city, county, and state to remain abreast of recent legal developments. In addition, health coaches should diligently read publications and attend conference presentations that address legal issues, as the **standards of care** and accepted business practices can change periodically as a result of legislation or case law.

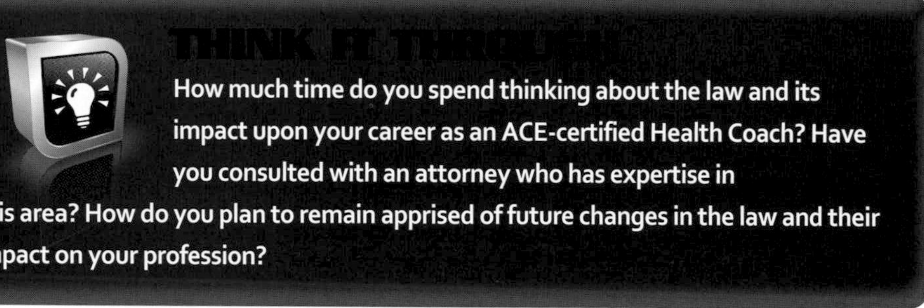

THINK IT THROUGH

How much time do you spend thinking about the law and its impact upon your career as an ACE-certified Health Coach? Have you consulted with an attorney who has expertise in this area? How do you plan to remain apprised of future changes in the law and their impact on your profession?

Business Structure

Much of the fitness industry is comprised of entrepreneurs—individuals who undertake new business ventures. Many fitness professionals start their careers as an offshoot of their own physical training. New personal trainers and health coaches often begin by working with close friends and family members before expanding their businesses to a greater assortment of clients. Most health coaches, like many entrepreneurs in other industries, do not realize that the moment they begin providing advice in exchange for financial compensation, they have created a business. Every business "owner," even one who is working part-time in a "hobby," should understand the ramifications of business structure.

Each health coach must decide the type of business structure under which he or she will operate. Each type retains certain legal and financial advantages and disadvantages. The size and scope of the business—both in the short- and long-term—will be important factors in the initial selection of the business entity. The business can be altered if conditions warrant, but health coaches must understand that legal issues that arise at a time when one structure was utilized cannot be mitigated by simply switching to a different business structure. The business entity employed at the time of an incident will usually be referenced by the courts in the event of a lawsuit. Typically, for-profit businesses* operate under one of the following three structures: **sole proprietorship, partnership,** or **corporation.** Refer to the *ACE Personal Trainer Manual* for more detail about each of the various business structures.

*Though this chapter primarily focuses on for-profit businesses, there are government-operated businesses as well as non-profit organizations that operate within different legal and financial constraints. Even though a health coach may be working with a client at a government-operated business (e.g., a community recreation center) or a nonprofit organization (e.g., a YMCA fitness center), the health coach may retain a different business structure for liability purposes. Health coaches should consult legal counsel prior to training or coaching any client.

Independent Contractors versus Employees

Once the appropriate business structure has been identified and implemented, health coaches need to address other legal concerns. Of particular note for the fitness industry is the definition of an employee versus an **independent contractor.** Employees "regularly" work for their employer, while independent contractors typically are hired on a short-term basis to perform a specific task or series of tasks. Once the specified tasks are complete, the independent contractor is compensated and then is no longer needed. A classic example of an independent contractor occurs when a homeowner has a leaking sink. The homeowner identifies the problem, hires a plumber, and pays the plumber once the leak is fixed. The plumber does not have an *expectation* of consistent work. Alternatively, an employer–employee relationship is created when a business hires a plumber full-time to address ongoing problems. In this case, the plumber would report to work daily, take direction from the employer regarding tasks, and be compensated on a regular basis (weekly, biweekly, monthly) rather than at the completion of each job.

The classification of a worker as an independent contractor versus an employee has numerous ramifications. In most cases, employers are responsible for training and supervising their employees and maintaining records regarding their employees' work performance. In addition, employers are generally required to withhold and match the employees' FICA (Federal Insurance Contributions Act) taxes for Social Security and Medicare. The employer usually offers and pays for unemployment coverage, workers' compensation coverage, and medical benefits. These requirements typically consume a tremendous amount of time and financial resources. In addition, employers generally must provide justification for firing an employee (unless they are employed in an "at-will" state where employers are not obligated to provide any justification for terminating an individual's employment). Conversely, someone hiring an independent contractor simply negotiates the job and the final compensation, and the independent contractor completes the work. If the independent contractor does not complete the work to the payer's satisfaction, the independent contractor will likely not be rehired in the future.

Certainly, most businesses would like to operate by limiting the number of employees and maximizing the number of independent contractors they retain. The time and expense necessary to adhere to laws regarding employer–employee relationships has caused some businesses to attempt to utilize *only* independent contractors. However, simply *designating* someone an independent contractor does not necessarily mean that an individual is *acting* as an independent contractor. Some companies have been penalized by the Internal Revenue Service (IRS) for improperly classifying an employee as an independent contractor to avoid their financial and administrative duties. Companies should ensure that they are properly classifying and utilizing independent contractors at all times if they choose to use this business model.

The main criteria the judicial system will utilize when addressing a potential complaint regarding independent contractor status is "control." In most cases, if the hiring authority maintains control over the worker, an employer–employee relationship has likely been established. Court cases have investigated control in the following areas:

- *Work details:* Creating schedules, requiring specific materials to be utilized, and overseeing procedures typically indicate an employment relationship.

- *Payment:* Regularly scheduled payments typically indicate employment, while payment by the "job" indicates an independent-contractor relationship.
- *Length of relationship:* People hired for short periods of time (a few weeks or less) are typically independent contractors.
- *Training and retraining:* An independent contractor will typically require no initial or ongoing training from the hiring agency.
- *Equipment:* Independent contractors typically provide their own equipment.
- *Number of clients:* Employees typically work for only one employer, whereas an independent contractor usually services multiple clients.
- *Nature of the work:* If the work provided is integral to the core function of the business, the person is more likely to be deemed an employee. In addition, if the work is *typically* performed by independent contractors, then the courts will usually utilize that in their determination.
- *Intention of the parties:* The intent of the parties is a factor, though certainly not the only or deciding factor, in the eventual classification.

It is important to note that each of these areas in and of itself will typically not be the sole criteria utilized by the courts when adjudicating a potential status dispute. The courts will examine the entire relationship and the extent to which the potential for employer "control" is present.

Both independent contractors and employees must be certain that every detail of their agreement is clear from the beginning of their professional relationship with a fitness facility or company. Often, the legal nature of the relationship is ambiguous, and fitness professionals have filed lawsuits attempting to collect worker's compensation or unemployment insurance from clubs that consider them independent contractors. Others who assumed that they were employees have been forced to pay back taxes once they were identified by the IRS as independent contractors. Ultimately, it is the responsibility of all parties to clearly define the work relationship and ensure that everyone's actions adhere to guidelines that govern the actions of independent contractors or employees.

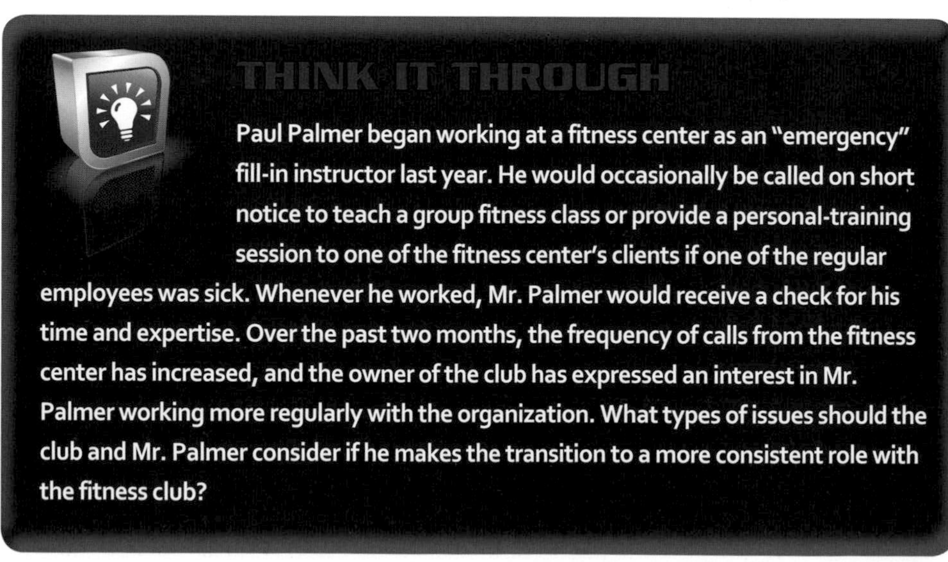

THINK IT THROUGH

Paul Palmer began working at a fitness center as an "emergency" fill-in instructor last year. He would occasionally be called on short notice to teach a group fitness class or provide a personal-training session to one of the fitness center's clients if one of the regular employees was sick. Whenever he worked, Mr. Palmer would receive a check for his time and expertise. Over the past two months, the frequency of calls from the fitness center has increased, and the owner of the club has expressed an interest in Mr. Palmer working more regularly with the organization. What types of issues should the club and Mr. Palmer consider if he makes the transition to a more consistent role with the fitness club?

Contracts

Contracts are the best method to ensure that all aspects of a relationship are properly established. Whether a health coach works as an independent contractor or an employee, the basic tenets of contract law should be understood. The following elements are necessary to create a binding contract:

- An offer and acceptance with a mutual agreement of terms
- Consideration (an exchange of valuable items, such as money for services)
- Legality (acceptable form under the law)
- Ability of the parties to enter into a contract with respect to legal age and mental capacity

For example, a health coach may talk to a prospective client and mention potential services, such as designing individualized exercise sessions or providing nutritional coaching. The health coach and client may agree on dates and times for specific workouts. This negotiation constitutes an offer and an acceptance. Stating a fee of $50 per hour for services establishes an exchange of consideration (i.e., coaching services for money). Once these negotiations are settled, the health coach should prepare a written contract by filling out a basic contract form or by having one specifically written for each agreement. Regardless of the type of form, legal counsel should be consulted to ensure that the written form is valid under contract law before it is utilized. This document becomes a valid contract when signed by both the health coach and the client, assuming both parties are of legal age to enter into contracts. Certainly, difficulty can arise if a minor seeks to retain a health coach's services. Since minors may not legally sign a contract, the health coach is retaining some risk in this situation. Having the parents sign the contract to perform services may mitigate, but not completely solve, this potential problem.

Some fitness professionals who are starting a business may feel that written contracts are unnecessary and that a brief chat and a handshake are sufficient when negotiating agreements. In the case of scheduling clients, that is often the standard practice. However, a potential miscommunication or misunderstanding may result in some difficulties, as any oral contract is subject to misinterpretation by the involved parties, and therefore is potentially dangerous. In the event of an oral contract dispute necessitating legal intervention, conflicting stories may be settled in a courtroom without sufficient evidence to support the health coach's account of what transpired.

In addition to scheduling, written contracts should be utilized to establish payment terms before any sessions occur. There should also be considerations for issues such as rescheduling, bounced checks, agreements to follow instructions and adhere to proper techniques, confidentiality, termination of the agreement, and other aspects critical to the client–health coach relationship. Typically, a **waiver** (Figure 20-1) will be signed as a component of the initial contract. Refer to "Vicarious Liability" on page 590 for more information on the purpose and proper use of waivers.

Health coaches should insist upon a written contract not only with clients, but also with fitness centers, vendors, and any other entities with which they conduct business. In any case in which the agreement involves real estate and/or goods or services worth $500 or more, or requires more than one year to complete, the **statute of frauds** requires that

I, ________________________________, through the purchase of personal training/coaching sessions, have agreed to voluntarily participate in an exercise program, including, but not limited to, strength training, flexibility development, and aerobic exercise, under the guidance of [name of health coach and/or business]. I hereby stipulate and agree that I am physically and mentally sound and currently have no physical conditions that would be aggravated by my involvement in an exercise program. I have provided verification from a licensed physician that I am able to undertake a general fitness-training program.

I understand and am aware that physical-fitness activities, including the use of equipment, are potentially hazardous activities. I am aware that participating in these types of activities, even when completed properly, can be dangerous. I agree to follow the verbal instructions issued by the health coach. I am aware that potential risks associated with these types of activities include, but are not limited to, the following: death; fainting; disorders in heartbeat; serious neck and spinal injuries that may result in complete or partial paralysis or brain damage; serious injury to virtually all bones, joints, ligaments, muscles, tendons, and other aspects of the musculoskeletal system; and serious injury or impairment to other aspects of my body, general health, and well-being.

I understand that I am responsible for my own medical insurance and will maintain that insurance throughout my entire period of participation with [name of health coach and/or business]. I will assume any additional expenses incurred that go beyond my health coverage. I will notify the [name of health coach and/or business] of any significant injury that requires medical attention (such as emergency care, hospitalization, etc.).

[name of health coach or business] or I will provide the equipment to be used in connection with workouts, including, but not limited to, benches, dumbbells, barbells, exercise bands, stability balls, and similar items. I represent and warrant any and all equipment I provide for training sessions is for personal use only. [name of health coach or business] has not inspected my equipment and has no knowledge of its condition. I understand that I take sole responsibility for my equipment. I acknowledge that although [name of health coach and/or business] takes precautions to maintain the equipment, any equipment may malfunction and/or cause potential injuries. I take sole responsibility to inspect any and all of my or the [name of health coach and/or business]'s equipment prior to use.

Although [name of health coach and/or business] will take precautions to ensure my safety, I expressly assume and accept sole responsibility for my safety and for any and all injuries that may occur during training sessions. In consideration of the acceptance of this entry, I, for myself and for my executors, administrators, and assigns, waive and release any and all claims against [name of health coach and/or business] and any of their staff, officers, officials, volunteers, sponsors, agents, representatives, successors, or assigns and agree to hold them harmless from any claims or losses, including but not limited to claims for negligence for any injuries or expenses that I may incur while exercising or while traveling to and from training sessions. These exculpatory clauses are intended to apply to any and all activities occurring during the time for which I have contracted with [name of health coach and/or company].

I represent and warrant I am signing this agreement freely and willfully and not under fraud or duress.

HAVING READ THE ABOVE TERMS AND INTENDING TO BE LEGALLY BOUND HEREBY AND UNDERSTANDING THIS DOCUMENT TO BE A COMPLETE WAIVER AND DISCLAIMER IN FAVOR OF [name of health coach and/or business], I HEREBY AFFIX MY SIGNATURE HERETO.

Client's name (please print clearly)____

Client's signature____ Date ____________

Client's address____

Parent/guardian signature (if applicable)________________________________ Date____________

Health coach's signature____ Date ____________

Figure 20-1
Sample waiver

Note: This document has been prepared to serve as a guide to improve understanding. Health coaches should not assume that this form will provide adequate protection in the event of a lawsuit. Please consult with an attorney before creating, distributing, and collecting any agreements to participate, informed consent forms, or waivers.

there be a written contract if the agreement is to be valid. The courts will not intervene in a potential oral contract dispute if the contract violates the statute of frauds—it will simply invalidate the agreement.

Using valid contracts can save businesses money and mitigate a tremendous amount of time and stress. Far too often, fitness professionals fail to understand the importance of operating with valid contracts. In addition, they often fail to thoroughly read and understand the contracts presented to them by fitness centers and other vendors. A visit to an attorney's office is advisable before signing any contract, but it is particularly important in cases where an employer–employee relationship is established or an ongoing time or financial commitment is created. Long-term contracts should be examined with particular scrutiny, since much can change over time.

Agreements to Participate, Informed Consent, and Waivers

There are a variety of potential contracts that health coaches may utilize in their day-to-day operations. Of particular importance are contracts detailing the relationship between the health coach and the client as they pertain to the potential injuries associated with physical activity. Health coaches should understand the concept and use of **agreements to participate, informed consent,** and waivers, as they can be important defenses to litigation for **negligence.** Ideally, each of these forms should be printed (avoid handwritten agreements) and signed by all clients *before* beginning the first exercise session.

> Before using any of these documents, it is critical that the health coach consult with an attorney who specializes in, or has experience with, the health and fitness industry.

Agreement to Participate

An agreement to participate is designed to protect the health coach from a client claiming to be unaware of the potential risks of physical activity (Figure 20-2). An agreement to participate is not typically considered a formal contract, but rather serves to demonstrate that the client was made aware of the "normal" outcomes of certain types of physical activity and willingly assumed the risks of participation. Typically, the agreement to participate is utilized for "class" settings (e.g., step training or aquatic exercise) rather than for individualized personal-training situations. The agreement to participate should detail the nature of the activity, the potential risks to be encountered, and the expected behaviors of the participant (Cotten & Cotten, 2009). This last consideration is important, as the participant recognizes that he or she may need to follow instructions while participating.

> Health coaches should have a process in place to formally warn their clients about the potential dangers of exercise.

Typically, agreements to participate are incorporated into other documents, such as informed consent forms and waivers. One potential consideration for each of these documents is a general request, or in some cases a requirement, that participants consult with a physician prior to beginning any exercise routine. Some attorneys may advise health coaches not to train anyone unless that person has verified that, at the very least, a basic health examination has been

I, _________, have enrolled in a program of physical activity including, but not limited to, traditional aerobics, weight training, stationary bicycling, and the use of various aerobic-conditioning machinery offered by [name of health coach and/or business]. I am aware that participating in these types of activities, even when completed properly, can be dangerous. I agree to follow the verbal instructions issued by the health coach. I am aware that potential risks associated with these types of activities include, but are not limited to, the following: death; serious neck and spinal injuries that may result in complete or partial paralysis or brain damage; serious injury to virtually all bones, joints, ligaments, muscles, tendons, and other aspects of the musculoskeletal system; and serious injury or impairment to other aspects of my body, general health, and well-being.

Because of the dangers of participating, I recognize the importance of following the health coach's instructions regarding proper techniques and training, as well as other organization rules.

I affirm that I am in good health and have provided verification from a licensed physician that I am able to participate in a general fitness-training program. I hereby consent to first aid, emergency medical care, and admission to an accredited hospital or an emergency care center when necessary for executing such care and for treatment of injuries that I may sustain while participating in a fitness-training program.

I understand that I am responsible for my own medical insurance and will maintain that insurance throughout my entire period of participation with [name of health coach and/or business]. I will assume any additional expenses incurred that go beyond my health coverage. I will notify [name of health coach and/or business] of any significant injury that requires medical attention (such as emergency care, hospitalization, etc.).

Signed ______________________________

Printed Name ______________________________

Phone Number ______________________________

Address ______________________________

Emergency Contact ______________________________

Contact Phone Number ______________________________

Insurance Company ______________________________

Policy #______________________ Effective Date ______________

Name of Policy Holder ______________________________

Figure 20-2
Sample agreement to participate

Note: This document has been prepared to serve as a guide to improve understanding. Health coaches should not assume that this form will provide adequate protection in the event of a lawsuit. Please consult with an attorney before creating, distributing, and collecting any agreements to participate, informed consent forms, or waivers.

performed by a medical professional within the past six months. Though most health coaches know to "start slowly" with new clients, fitness professionals cannot evaluate the overall health of a client in the same manner as a healthcare professional. Some agreements to participate also ask that health insurance information be provided. This not only lets the health coach know that the client has coverage, but also enables the health coach to provide that information if a client were in need of medical attention.

Informed Consent

An informed consent form can be utilized by a health coach to demonstrate that a client acknowledges that he or she has been specifically informed about the risks associated with the activity in which he or she is about to engage (Figure 20-3). Informed consent allows the client to have something done to him or her (e.g., strength test or flexibility assessment) by the health coach, and therefore can differ slightly from an agreement to participate. It is primarily intended to communicate the potential benefits and dangers

Informed Consent for Hydrostatic Measurement/Determination of Body Fat

Name____

1. Purpose and Explanation of Test

The purpose of hydrostatic weighing is to determine percent body fat from body density. Using this method of assessing body composition, my body density is determined through submerging myself underwater. Once my body density has been determined, my body composition can then be extrapolated. The results of this test are useful to warn me of a potential health risk associated with high body-fat percentages. Also, I can use this information as a comparison point for future body-composition assessments.

The hydrostatic weighing procedure will involve completely submerging my body underwater and holding my breath for approximately five to 10 seconds. I will be required to enter into the water slowly and position myself in front of the underwater weighing apparatus, which is suspended from a scale overhead. I will then be instructed to exhale as much air as possible above the water and then sit in the underwater weighing apparatus, thereby fully submerging myself. Once situated in the weighing apparatus, I will be required to stay as still as possible for approximately six seconds and then lift my head from the water to breathe. I understand that this procedure will be repeated several times to achieve reproducible results. It is also my understanding that while conducting the test, I will be required to wear a bathing suit to obtain the most accurate results. Once the test has been completed, I will be signaled to come to the surface of the pool and begin breathing normally again.

2. Risks

I hereby consent to voluntarily engage in the hydrostatic weighing procedure. I understand that there is a risk of adverse reactions to this test, which include dizziness, cramping, and, in rare cases, drowning. I understand and have been clearly advised that it is my right to request that the test be stopped at any time. I understand that I have the right to end the test at any point if I feel unusual discomfort or fatigue. I understand that I am responsible for monitoring my own condition throughout the test, and should any unusual symptoms occur, I will cease my participation and inform the fitness professional of these symptoms.

3. Confidentiality and Use of Information

I have been informed that the information obtained in this test will be treated as privileged and confidential and will be used only by the program staff to evaluate my body composition. The information will not be released or revealed to any person without my written consent or as required by law. I do, however, agree to the use of any information for research or statistical purposes so long as it does

Initial: _____

This figure uses the hydrostatic weighing test for illustrative purposes regarding the proper design and use of an informed consent form. The vast majority of health coaches will never administer such a test.

Figure 20-3
Sample informed consent form

Figure 20-3 Continued

Note: This document has been prepared to serve as a guide to improve understanding. Health coaches should not assume that this form will provide adequate protection in the event of a lawsuit. Please consult with an attorney before creating, distributing, and collecting any agreements to participate, informed consent forms, or waivers.

not provide facts that could lead to the identification of my person. Any other information obtained, however, will be used only by the facility staff to evaluate my exercise status or needs.

4. Inquiries and Freedom of Consent

I have been given an opportunity to ask questions about the procedure. Generally, these requests, which have been noted by the testing staff, and their responses are as follows:

____

____

____

I confirm that I have read this form in its entirety or that it has been read to me if I have been unable to read it, that I understand the description of the test, and that my questions regarding the test have been answered to my satisfaction. I consent to the conditions of all services and procedures as explained by all program personnel. I consent to the rendition of all services and procedures as explained herein by all facility personnel.

____

Date

____

Client's Signature

____

Witness' Signature

____

Test Supervisor's Signature

of the program or exercise testing procedures to the client. Informed consent forms should detail the possible discomforts involved and potential alternatives. Health coaches should remember that many potential clients will be unaccustomed to straining their bodies through physical exertion. The informed consent form, combined with oral communication, prepares the client for the positive and negative effects of certain types of exercise.

The documents presented in this chapter have been prepared to serve as a guide to improve understanding. Health coaches should not assume that they will provide adequate protection in the event of a lawsuit. Please consult with an attorney before creating, distributing, and collecting any agreements to participate, informed consent forms, or waivers.

Inherent Risks

Agreements to participate and informed consent forms, though potentially important in the defense against a lawsuit, primarily cover the **inherent risks** of participation in an activity. For example, even if proper stretching and lifting techniques are utilized, injuries can occur to ligaments, tendons, muscles, and other parts of the body. An agreement to participate and an informed consent form would help protect the health coach in the event that a lawsuit is filed by an injured client. However, it is often difficult to determine an inherent risk of participation and what might have been caused, in whole or in part, by the actions of the health coach. A client may claim that a health coach did not provide proper spotting during an exercise and that this action specifically caused an injury. The health coach might counter that an injury was unfortunate, but part of the normal, safe lifting process. This dispute would likely be settled in court. To potentially avoid this type of a scenario, health coaches should have all clients sign a waiver prior to beginning any exercise routine. The waiver (sometimes called a release) will typically incorporate similar language included in an agreement to participate and an informed consent form, but will also include an **exculpatory clause** that bars the clients from seeking damages for injuries caused by the inherent risk of activities and by the ordinary negligence of the health coach and his or her employees and agents (see Figure 20-1).

Procedures

Valid agreements to participate, informed consent forms, and waivers must be administered properly to clients. There should not be any underhanded attempt to hide the true nature of these agreements prior to a client signing the document. Though some states permit **group waivers** that have a list of spaces for multiple patrons to sign below the waiver, it is advisable to have a stand-alone document for each client. Often, health coaches properly insist that a new client sign a waiver prior to the first session, but then fail to allow sufficient time for the new client to read, understand, and ask questions about the document. Requiring a client to rush when reviewing a waiver can result in a court invalidating an otherwise properly crafted waiver. In addition, though courts have typically found that participants who cannot read English retain the responsibility to have someone translate the waiver prior to signing, it is a good practice to have someone available to assist with the translation if needed (Cotten & Cotten, 2009). If the document consists of multiple pages, a space for the client to initial the bottom of each page should be provided (see Figure 20-3 as an example).

Minors cannot legally sign a contract, so in most cases a waiver signed by a child will be invalidated by the courts. However, some states do allow parents to sign paperwork that may provide limited protection for the health coach. An attorney specializing in this area should be consulted if children will be utilizing a health coach's services. Health coaches should remember to have every member of a family sign an individual waiver. A waiver signed by one spouse may not cover the other spouse (Cotten, 2000a). Once agreements to participate, informed consent forms, and waivers have been signed, the health coach should retain the paperwork on file at least until the **statute of limitations**—the time allotted to sue for damages—has elapsed. Some attorneys even recommend retaining records past the statute of limitations to ensure that a sudden change in the law does not negatively impact the ability of the health coach to defend against potential litigation.

Ultimately, the goal of any fitness professional should be to prevent all client injuries. However, even in the safest conditions, physical activity may result in physical injury, even when proper care is provided. Health coaches should utilize paperwork to notify new clients of *all* risks and potential dangers associated with participating in physical activity. This creates a situation in which the client knows and assumes the risks of participation. Health coaches should also utilize waivers to protect against costly lawsuits that arise both from the normal physical injuries associated with physical activity and from mistakes that may occur during workout sessions.

Negligence

One of the most important aspects of health coaching is the adherence to established professional guidelines. Failing to perform as a reasonable and prudent person would under similar circumstances is considered negligence. In the case of health coaches, a reasonable and prudent person is someone who adheres to the established standard of care. Attainment of ACE **certification** indicates that the health coach has demonstrated an acceptable level of competence and understanding of the established standards. Since standards of care can and do change, it is critical that health coaches stay abreast of new guidelines. (*Note:* This is one of the many roles of continuing education.) A negligent act can occur if a health coach fails to act (**act of omission**) or acts inappropriately (**act of commission**). For example, a health coach could be successfully sued for neglecting to spot a client during a free-weight bench press (omission), or for programming straight-leg sit-ups for a client with known lower-back problems (commission). These actions would likely be found inappropriate as compared to what a reasonable and prudent professional would do in a similar situation.

To substantiate a charge of negligence in court, the plaintiff must establish four elements:

- The defendant had a duty to protect the plaintiff from injury.
- The defendant failed to uphold the standard of care necessary to perform that duty.
- Damage or injury to the plaintiff occurred.
- This damage or injury was caused by the defendant's breach of duty (proximate causation).

Negligence in a fitness facility could occur, for example, if a health coach agreed to provide instruction and supervision for a weightlifting regimen. The agreement between the health coach and the client establishes a legal duty that would not be present if both parties were simply working out at a fitness center at the same time. (Certainly there may be a moral duty to help a fellow patron in need, but there is not a legal duty to do so absent a special relationship such as parent–child.) If the health coach does not provide proper spotting during an exercise, the health coach has breached his or her duty to the client. If the client is injured as a direct result of the breach—which often happens when heavy weights are lifted without proper spotting—then the client will likely have a successful lawsuit for negligence against the health coach. The courts would examine the situation, the expected standard of care, the extent of the injury, and the result of the injury (e.g., medical bills or lost time at work) when assessing potential damages.

Vicarious Liability

Health coaches who hire employees need to understand the concept of **vicarious liability** (also known as **respondeat superior**). Employers are responsible for the employment-related actions of their employees. If an employee is negligent while working within the normal scope of employment, it is likely that the injured party will sue not only the employee who breached the duty to cause injury, but also the employer or employers. Since employees often do not have the financial resources of employers, courts have typically upheld the right of the injured party to seek damages from the employer's "deep pockets." In most cases, litigants name every possible entity linked to the employee when negligence occurs.

The use of waivers is critical in the fitness industry, as a properly worded exculpatory clause bars the injured from potential recovery (see Figure 20-1). There are some potential issues that every health coach must investigate with an attorney prior to crafting a waiver. Each state has slightly different rules regarding the validity of waivers, meaning that a waiver that is valid in one state may not be valid in another. In addition, confusion and litigation can arise when a fitness club or weight-loss facility utilizes health coaches who are not employees. Consider the following court case, which addressed a situation in which a member of a health club signed a supplemental contract for personal-training services in the club setting. When the client was injured in a session with the personal trainer, she contended that the waiver signed along with her membership contract did not extend and cover the services of the personal trainer. The court disagreed and ruled that the services of the personal trainer were part of the activities and benefits offered at the club and were therefore covered by the original waiver (Cotten, 2000b). Despite the outcome of this case, fitness professionals should utilize their own waivers in addition to the ones potentially already signed when the client joined the fitness center or club.

THINK IT THROUGH

Penelope Smith recently received a call from a potential client named Jennifer Burns. After discussing a variety of potential issues regarding weight-training options and prices, Ms. Smith met Ms. Burns at a fitness center. Before beginning her first session with a new client, Ms. Smith typically asks the client to complete a health-history form and sign a liability waiver. In this instance, Ms. Burns did not want to sign any paperwork before "trying out her first session" because she was "so excited to get started." What potential issues will arise if Ms. Smith does not require Ms. Burns to sign the waiver?

Waivers also must detail the types of activities and potential risks of injury that would be barred from recovery. A client must knowingly understand the nature of the activities and the potential risks before he or she can waive the right to potentially sue for injuries occurring during participation. Waivers also typically do not protect the health coach from injuries directly caused by **gross negligence**—an action that demonstrates recklessness or a willful disregard for the safety of others. As a general rule, gross negligence occurs when someone deliberately acts in a manner that extends beyond the scope of employment or fails to meet the accepted standard of care for his or her profession. For example, a correctly worded waiver would likely protect a health coach who did not properly spot a client completing a military press, as spotting would likely be considered part of the normal activities conducted during the course of training a client. In addition, it is expected that participating in vigorous activities such as the military press might lead to injury. However, if the health coach intentionally removed a safety screw from the seat prior to the client's arrival, the waiver would likely not apply, because removal of safety equipment is something that should *never* occur during the normal course of a health coach's activities. Ultimately, the use of proper waivers protects the health coach from lawsuits that arise not only from injuries that typically occur during exercises, but also from injuries that might occur due to mistakes the health coach may make while interacting with clients. Hopefully, mistakes are mitigated, injuries are limited, and potential lawsuits are completely avoided.

Even if a waiver is not utilized properly, a health coach may successfully defend against a negligence lawsuit in certain situations, even if he or she is partially at fault. In some cases, the client may have contributed to the potential injury. In certain states, **contributory negligence** laws prevent a plaintiff in a lawsuit who has played some role in the injury from receiving *any* monetary awards for damages. For example, if a client failed to notify the health coach that the soles of one of his shoes had been slipping, he would be partially to blame if his foot slipped while conducting a squat lift, even if the health coach did not properly spot the client. The clients' improper actions bar him from recovering any money, even though the health coach was partially at fault. Courts will typically examine every aspect of the scenario to determine potential responsibility.

The majority of states do not use the contributory negligence standard, instead utilizing **comparative negligence** when deciding negligence cases. When multiple parties may have caused injuries (e.g., the health coach and the client), the court will apportion guilt and any subsequent award for damages. For instance, in the earlier example the client may be deemed to be 40% at fault for the injury (for failing to inform the health coach of the issue with his shoes) and the health coach 60% at fault (for failing to spot the client during the lift). If the court were to normally award $100,000 in damages, the award would be lowered to $60,000 (i.e., 60% of the damages). There are a variety of state standards regarding comparative negligence and its potential impact on monetary awards.

Legal Responsibilities

The use of proper paperwork prior to working with clients can minimize the potential for litigation against the health coach. But even if clients waive their right to potentially sue, the health coach should still prepare for each training session with safety as the first priority. Not only is this a professional requirement, but it also provides a better experience for the client and increases the likelihood that the client will continue to utilize the health coach's services. One of the most important things a health coach can do is establish plans to regularly inspect facilities and equipment and review protocols regarding supervision and instruction.

Facilities

Health coaches have an obligation to ensure that the facilities where they work with clients are free from unreasonable hazards. At the very least, the physical environment should be inspected each day prior to beginning any training session, especially when the training area has been used by other patrons after the health coach was last present. Inspecting the facilities can be a problem if sessions are conducted outdoors or in a client's home. Health coaches should allocate sufficient time—which should *not* be charged to the client—to inspect the environment prior to the workout. In some cases, clients will recognize these inspections of the facility as a genuine concern for their well-being, which can have a positive impact on client retention and may generate new clients through referrals. The inspection should consider the following issues:

- Different floor surfaces are designed for different activities. Health coaches should ensure that floor surfaces will cushion the feet, knees, and legs from excessive stress.
- There should be sufficient free space available to protect the client from other patrons and from hurting him- or herself on equipment.
- Lighting must be sufficient for chosen exercises.
- There must be functioning heating and air conditioning systems.
- Proximity to drinking fountains and bathrooms is important for some clients.

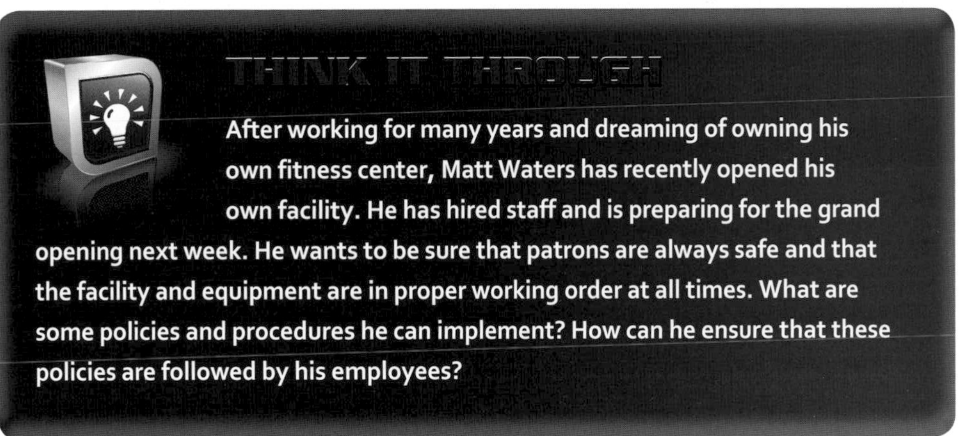

THINK IT THROUGH
After working for many years and dreaming of owning his own fitness center, Matt Waters has recently opened his own facility. He has hired staff and is preparing for the grand opening next week. He wants to be sure that patrons are always safe and that the facility and equipment are in proper working order at all times. What are some policies and procedures he can implement? How can he ensure that these policies are followed by his employees?

Because a health coach's primary responsibility is the client's safety, regular inspection using a safety checklist is recommended. If an unsafe condition is noticed, the health coach should notify the facility's management and avoid that area until it has been addressed. If a fitness club owner does not repair the problem and the client is injured, the health coach can still be held partially liable. Though juries have often looked favorably on independent contractors or employees who have tried unsuccessfully to persuade management to correct dangerous conditions, there is always a potential risk when training in an unsafe environment. For this reason, health coaches should develop relationships with reputable fitness centers that truly focus on safety. In addition, health coaches should develop contingency plans (outside of cancelling the session and losing potential revenue) for unsafe facilities.

Working with clients in their homes can pose potential safety challenges as well. Often, the client may be reluctant to alter the environment or change the overall décor. Though this type of situation may shift some or all of the responsibility for safety from the health coach to the client, an attorney should always be consulted in these circumstances.

Another consideration for training is the use of public spaces, especially the outdoors. For many health coaches and clients, it is much more enjoyable to run on a trail than on a treadmill in a fitness center. However, in some jurisdictions it is illegal to train clients on public beaches, parks, or trails. It is the health coach's responsibility to know the local laws prior to using these areas. Once a "legal" outdoor area has been identified and selected for a training session, the health coach should be sure to understand the potential dangers in the area before meeting the client. Outdoor areas pose specific risks. Running on a public street may involve evading oncoming vehicular traffic, while running on a mountain trail could involve dodging loose rocks or tree roots. Training outdoors certainly can be an enjoyable experience, but it is the health coach's responsibility to ensure that the activities will not pose a significant risk for clients.

While most courts recognize that outdoor activities pose certain risks that a typical person would assume (such as loose dirt or rocks on a hiking trail), the health coach should inspect the area to identify any particularly unusual dangers. In addition, certain aspects of the environment may impact the choice to utilize it for a training session. If a client has never run on a specific outdoor trail, it is advisable to walk the trail with the client the first time rather than expecting an all-out initial effort. The safety of outdoor activities is also impacted by the weather. The courts often will remove a person's potential **liability** for **acts of God** (e.g., earthquakes and mudslides), but if the weather forecast indicates heightened dangers, the health coach should not engage in the activity. For example, though earthquakes and lightning storms are both acts of God, in many cases a lightning storm can be predicted. Courts may be willing to absolve health coaches of potential liability from injuries caused by an earthquake, but they are less likely to rule in favor of a health coach if he or she knew, or should have known, that a lightning storm was in the area. In all outdoor training situations, extreme weather conditions such as freezing cold or excessive heat and humidity should be avoided. Acceptable exercise routines in 75° F (24° C) weather may not be acceptable in 95° F (35° C) or 35° F (2° C) weather conditions.

Some fitness professionals use fitness centers without informing the management that there will be a training session. This is certainly not an ethical business practice, and in many areas of the country is a violation of the law. In addition to adhering to the law and using good ethical behavior, developing a formal relationship with the fitness facility may eventually result in an expanded client base from fitness center referrals. An attorney should be consulted prior to establishing any formal relationship with a fitness center.

Equipment

Fitness programs may utilize a variety of equipment, and injuries from the use of exercise equipment are often a source of litigation in the fitness industry. All equipment should meet the highest safety and design standards and should be purchased from a reputable manufacturer. In most cases, the use of homemade equipment should be avoided, since designing and manufacturing are not considered part of the "normal" duties of a fitness professional. Equipment must be regularly inspected and properly maintained. Of particular concern is the protocol utilized when broken equipment is discovered. Once something is deemed unsafe, the health coach should immediately remove the equipment from the training area. If quick removal is not feasible, the equipment should be disabled to prevent further use until repaired. Unfortunately, broken equipment is often only marked with a sign that says "Do Not Use." Far too often, these signs easily fall off and unsuspecting patrons may be injured when trying to use the broken equipment. Manufacturers typically provide maintenance schedules for equipment that fitness professionals and club operators should follow. Regular maintenance should be logged and records retained for future referral in the event of a lawsuit.

The use of equipment owned by a client may create a conflict between professional practice and legal protection. A conservative legal stance would be to avoid any contact with the client's equipment, but most health coaches accept some liability by using their expertise to adjust a client's equipment or recommend maintenance. For example, a health coach may arrive at a client's home for an initial fitness session and find a leg extension machine with a frayed cable. The health coach should inform the client that the equipment needs to be repaired, suggest that he or she call the company to order a replacement part, and then conduct sessions without using this equipment until it has been repaired.

Health coaches should also understand the importance of non-exercise equipment when working with clients. Health coaches should require that proper clothing and shoes be worn by their clients during sessions. Failure to stop a client from exercising with improper shoes may be deemed an endorsement of a bad practice and be considered negligent. If the exercise sessions will be conducted outdoors, the health coach should provide a sufficient quantity of water for the time, intensity, temperature, and humidity during the workout.

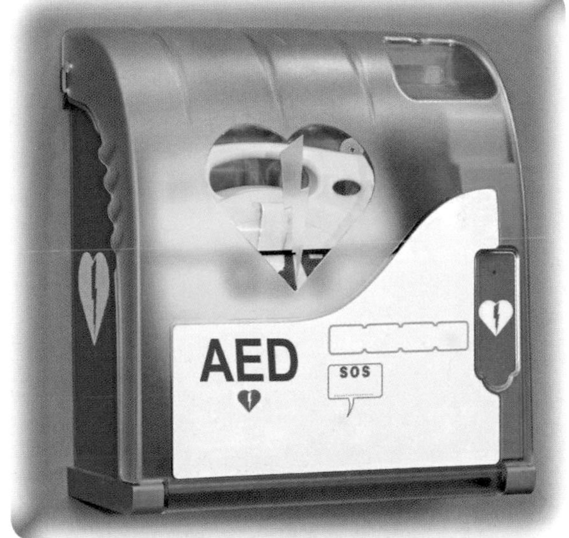

The use of safety equipment, such as **automated external defibrillators (AEDs),** has gained considerable attention in recent years. These devices can be found in a variety of public spaces (e.g., airports, shopping malls, and amusement parks) and are rapidly becoming standard emergency equipment in health and fitness facilities, not only because they can save lives, but also because they are legally *required* for fitness centers in many states (Agoglia, 2005). Even in states where AEDs are not required in fitness centers, courts can rule in favor of plaintiffs and change the standard of care (*Fowler v. Bally Total Fitness,* 2008).

Health coaches will familiarize themselves with AEDs through **cardiopulmonary resuscitation (CPR)** and first aid courses, which are required prior to certification, ACE-certified professionals in the United States and Canada are required to hold a current CPR with AED training certificate. Though usually not required, health coaches may want to consider purchasing an AED for use in their own studios or when working with clients in their homes. It is likely that future legislation will establish AEDs as a standard piece of equipment for fitness professionals working with clients in *all* settings (Wolohan, 2008). Every health coach should consult with his or her attorney to understand the local laws that may apply to a specific situation.

Supervision

General supervision involves overseeing a group of people, such as when a group fitness instructor leads a large class. **Specific supervision** occurs when an individual is supervised while performing a specific activity, such as what typically occurs during a personal-training session. When working with clients, health coaches need to remember that most personal-training activities require specific supervision for safety purposes. A health coach should never leave a client when there is a potential for injury (such as when a spotter is needed during a bench press). Health coaches who work with two or more clients during the same session should design the workouts to alternate between activities requiring general and specific supervision. For example, while the health coach provides specific supervision to one client (e.g., spotting), the other client should briefly rest or work on an activity that requires only general supervision (e.g., stretching or cardiovascular exercises). Health coaches should eliminate any time that a client is not in their direct view, as this is when injuries can quickly occur. In addition, a health coach should never leave a client during a session.

Before beginning any session, the health coach must adequately plan for any emergencies that may arise. A client's medical information should be immediately available in the event of an emergency or accident. This will eliminate the need to search for critical information about the client (such as emergency contact numbers) in the event of an emergency. If a workout is to occur in a remote area, cell phone coverage should be confirmed prior to the exercise session to ensure that 911 may be reached if necessary.

In addition to supervising their clients, health coaches need to be aware of the actions of their employees. This awareness includes properly screening potential employees prior to hiring them. It is the responsibility of an employer to determine if the potential employee would pose a specific danger to clients due to his or her personal history. Each employee should be trained regarding the unique aspects of the employer's operation and then supervised and retrained at regular intervals. Employers should conduct written performance evaluations with each of their employees and should keep those files even after an employee has stopped working at that particular facility.

Instruction

Health coaches should utilize instructional techniques that are consistent with current professional practices. If one fails to demonstrate a movement or give proper instructions regarding how to use a piece of equipment and the client is injured, the health coach may be found negligent. Legal standards require that clients be given "adequate and proper" instruction before and during an activity. In a courtroom, an expert witness could be asked to assess "proper" instruction. Adequate and proper instruction also means avoiding high-risk exercises, or those not recommended by professional peers. Advocating dangerous or controversial exercises puts the fitness professional at risk for a successful lawsuit if a client is injured. In one case (*Corrigan v. Musclemakers, Inc.*, 1999), a personal trainer put his client on a treadmill, but failed to appropriately adjust the speed for this first-time user or explain how to adjust the speed or stop the belt. The client could not keep pace, and she was catapulted backward and fractured her ankle in the ensuing fall.

Proper instruction also means individualizing workout routines for each client. An exercise may be appropriate for one client but completely inappropriate for another due to a variety of circumstances. In a reported case in the media, a personal trainer was sued for causing injuries to his client. The personal trainer, as is sometimes common, admitted to using the same workout routine with all of his clients. The injured woman was 42 years old and was not in proper physical condition to perform the same exercises as the trainer's other clients, who were much younger, healthier, and more advanced in their exercise training. After only two workouts, she was admitted to a hospital for nearly two weeks. Health coaches should insist on proper use of equipment and correct completion of activities at all times. Many fitness professionals remember to properly demonstrate how to operate equipment the first time a client uses it, but if the client becomes sloppy in the future, some professionals may become lax in terms of maintaining proper standards of performance. Health coaches should model proper instruction by always using good technique during their own workouts. If a client is not corrected when using bad form or sees a health coach "bending the rules," the client may be more likely to exercise improperly, which can increase the likelihood of injury.

A relatively new aspect of instructional liability concerns the physical touching of clients. Health coaches should avoid touching clients unless it is essential for proper instruction. Clients should be informed about the purpose of potential touching before it occurs. If a client objects, an alternative exercise should be utilized. Charges of sexual assault, even if groundless, can have disastrous consequences for a health coach's career.

Safety Guidelines

In reference to the above-mentioned areas of responsibility, health coaches should adhere to the following safety guidelines in the conduct of their activities:

- Be sure that all sessions are well-planned, appropriate, and documented.
- Communicate and enforce all safety rules for equipment use.
- Ensure that equipment meets or exceeds all industry standards.
- Inspect all equipment prior to use and document adherence to maintenance schedules.
- Never allow unsupervised activity by the client.
- Limit participation to those under contract (i.e., no friends or family members).
- Clearly warn clients about the specific risks of planned activities.
- Only select activities within the defined scope of practice and appropriate areas of expertise.
- Ensure that clients wear any necessary protective equipment (e.g., athletic supporter or sports bra).
- Review the emergency plan [access to a phone and 911 for emergency medical services (EMS)].
- Stay up-to-date with certifications and education in the field.

Scope of Practice

One of the biggest difficulties for a health coach—particularly one who constantly spends time seeking to learn new information—is to remember the extent of one's professional qualifications. While an ACE certification signifies the attainment of a specific level of competence and skill, it is narrowly focused in certain knowledge areas. Certainly, the more one learns, the greater the ability to help clients, but there is a danger that health coaches may extend their service offerings beyond their area of established expertise or scope of practice. Many states allow exercise "prescriptions" to be developed only by a licensed doctor. Therefore, it is important that health coaches provide exercise *programs,* not exercise *prescriptions.* Although the difference between these terms may sound like a technicality, it could become an important issue in a courtroom. Health coaches should attempt to develop a network of physicians and other healthcare professionals, such as **registered dietitians (R.D.s),** chiropractors, and physical therapists, who can provide meaningful information and services to their clients. Clients who need the specialized services of these healthcare professionals should be referred for treatment and counseling. In turn, these professionals may refer clients to the health coach.

In addition to having new clients undergo a physical exam from their primary care physician prior to beginning an exercise regimen with a health coach, it is also important for the health coach to have a completed health-history form on file. These documents should be utilized for the determination of an individual's existing health risk and level of fitness, rather than for the purpose of providing or recommending treatment for specific medical conditions.

Health coaches should use the health-history form to screen the client for appropriate placement in a fitness program. In cases where any significant risk factors are indicated, the client should be referred to his or her primary care physician for clearance before the fitness program begins. If health coaches were to use the health-history form to recommend treatment, they could be accused of practicing medicine without a license. Ideally, clients will have a physician sign a medical clearance form and produce a letter on the doctor's letterhead prior to beginning exercise. However, if a client forges a physician's signature to obtain acceptance to a fitness program, the health coach probably would not be held liable, unless the health coach had knowledge of the forgery prior to the client's participation.

Health coaches must understand how to use the information collected on the health-history form, asking only those questions that they can interpret and apply. Health coaches must read and fully understand the answers the client provides, as the forms are designed to alert the health coach to any potential problems that could occur. Therefore, health coaches should not just see the completed form as an item to "cross off the checklist." Instead, they should incorporate the information on the forms into the fitness programs they design for their clients.

Health coaches should know and follow the exercise program guidelines recommended by leading professional organizations such as the American Council on Exercise (ACE), the National Strength and Conditioning Association (NSCA), the American College of Obstetricians and Gynecologists (ACOG), the American College of Sports Medicine (ACSM), and the American Heart Association (AHA). Health coaches also should be familiar with the position statements for specific populations developed by these and other allied healthcare organizations. For example, the NSCA has produced a position statement on weight training for prepubescent youth; ACOG has produced resource material on pregnant women and exercise; and ACSM has published numerous position statements regarding various aspects of exercise, fitness, and health.

Most fitness professionals can easily recognize certain situations in which they do not have the necessary expertise. ACE has published established protocols for assessing posture, movement, flexibility, cardiorespiratory fitness, and muscular endurance, strength, and power (refer to the *ACE Personal Trainer Manual*). But there are instances where a client may ask for information that is not covered by ACE standards. For example, most health coaches would know immediately that a client who asked to have a sample of his or her blood drawn and analyzed would likely need to see a physician. However, in other situations, health coaches may not recognize that they are providing advice beyond their qualifications. The unique, close personal relationship that often develops between fitness professionals and their clients can cause potential areas of concern. Many clients view their health coach not only as their fitness advisor, but also as their physical therapist, registered dietitian, marriage counselor, or psychologist. When these types of perceived relationships develop, the health coach must pay particular attention to comments that may be construed by the client as qualified professional advice. It is important for health coaches to always stay within their scope of practice when providing professional advice, or a personal opinion that could be taken as professional advice. Though health coaches would never purposely hurt their clients, careless or misunderstood comments and actions can cause considerable pain, both physical and psychological.

When clients seek recommendations about exercise equipment, clothing, or shoes, it is important for health coaches to remain cautious when responding, particularly if they have a pre-existing endorsement arrangement with a service provider. Before giving advice, health coaches should become knowledgeable about the products and equipment available, as well as their advantages and disadvantages. Another option would be to limit potential liability by referring clients to their choice of retail sporting goods stores. Advice based solely on personal experience should be given with that express qualification.

Though the choice of shoes and other equipment is important, of far greater concern and consequence is the solicitation of advice regarding nutrition and supplements (refer to Appendix E for the ACE Position Statement on Nutrition Scope of Practice for Fitness Professionals). One of the most noteworthy cases in this area concerned a personal trainer who suggested dietary supplements for a client in writing (*Capati v. Crunch Fitness*, 2002). The client died from a brain hemorrhage due to complications from an adverse interaction between the supplements and other medication she was taking. Unless fitness professionals have received specific medical or nutritional training, and have earned appropriate professional licenses, credentials, or certifications (e.g., M.D. or R.D.), they should not provide advice in these areas. Most fitness professionals know and understand this potential area of concern, but they often unwittingly provide advice to their clients. For example, there is a distinct difference between telling a client that a certain food, beverage, or supplement contains a high amount of vitamins and minerals and specifically telling a client to eat more of a particular food, beverage, or supplement. When a client is told to do something, it creates a potential liability for the health coach.

Health coaches should also learn to recognize physical problems that their clients may be having. Unfortunately, impulsive behaviors regarding diet and exercise can lead some clients to engage in potentially destructive behaviors. It is important to learn to recognize eating disorders such as **anorexia, bulimia,** and **binge eating disorder.** In addition, despite various potential side effects, the use and overuse of supplements, anabolic steroids, and **growth hormone** has become more common. Health coaches should never state, or even imply, that they support their clients' use of these products. When health coaches recognize potential problems in their clients, they should have a plan to address the situation. Health coaches should seek the advice of experts in the field when developing these protocols and obtain legal counsel when necessary.

Though a health coach–client relationship does not legally require the same standards for confidentiality as a physician–patient or attorney–client relationship, health coaches should maintain that same level of professionalism. It is inappropriate for health coaches to discuss clients' workout regimens, strength and flexibility achievements, and weight loss with others. Violating a client's privacy is not only unethical, but can lead to significant negative repercussions (refer to Appendix A for the ACE Code of Ethics).

Liability Insurance

Even after taking precautions, health coaches must be aware of the importance of insurance. The recent increase in litigation throughout the healthcare and fitness industries has caused nearly every fitness professional to seek some sort of liability insurance. The need for insurance is always present, but as health coaches and their businesses become more financially successful, the importance of insurance becomes increasingly vital. Unfortunately, potential plaintiffs and their lawyers often "target" successful businesses, since there is a greater likelihood of "winning" a substantial financial reward. Though most trial attorneys will agree to work on a contingency fee basis (i.e., only receiving compensation if and when their client is awarded a judgment), some unscrupulous attorneys will take meritless cases simply with the hope that they will be "successful" in convincing a judge or jury that their client deserves compensation. Judgments for millions of dollars are not uncommon, and few individuals or businesses could survive such a substantial financial loss. Insurance protection provides some peace of mind, as health coaches can be secure in the knowledge that if someone were to be injured as a result of their actions or if a meritless lawsuit were to occur, insurance coverage would be adequate to cover such claims. There are a variety of important insurance aspects to understand.

Generally, an insurance policy is a contract designed to protect health coaches and their assets from litigation. There is, however, some truth to the saying that insurance companies are in the business of collecting premiums and denying claims. It is important to understand the basic components of insurance coverage before soliciting guidance from an insurance agent. Agents are in the business of selling policies, which means some agents will focus more on the potential sale than on providing accurate advice. Though it is important to never be "underinsured," health coaches can purchase too much insurance given their unique situation. Talking with established fitness professionals or seeking information from trusted industry organizations such as ACE can be a great way to be referred to a successful insurance agent who understands the unique aspects of the fitness industry. Not all insurance carriers are equal in their experience, acumen, and financial resources. The most reputable insurance carriers have a national affiliation, are licensed, have strong financial backing, have a reinsurer (a corporate policy to ensure that a policy holder's claims will be met even if his or her business collapses), and have not had any claims filed against them by the Better Business Bureau. It is the health coach's responsibility to carefully investigate insurance carriers and coverage options prior to beginning training sessions. In general, health coaches should not assume that any of their typically established personal insurance (e.g., auto and home) extends to their professional activities. For example, most homeowner's insurance has general liability to cover slips, trips, and falls that may occur while guests are visiting a person's home, but this type of coverage would likely not cover a client who fell while being trained, since the training would be considered a business activity.

Health coaches need to secure **professional liability insurance** that is specifically designed to cover the health and fitness industry. The selected liability insurance policy should cover personal injuries that can occur as a result of a training session. Injured clients may sue not only for medical expenses, but also for a variety of other compensation, such as lost wages from being unable to work, pain and suffering, and loss of consortium. ACE recommends retaining at least $1 million in professional liability coverage, as medical expenses can easily cost hundreds of thousands of dollars. In some instances, a higher liability coverage amount may be advisable.

> The American Council on Exercise has established relationships with reputable insurance carriers who specialize in the fitness industry. Visit www.ACEfitness.org/insurancecenter for more information.

Health coaches must understand the specific insurance needs that may arise given the location of the training activities. Home-based training has become popular, as many clients prefer to work with fitness professionals in their own residences. In addition, some health coaches would rather use their own homes for training activities than maintain a formal relationship with a fitness center. General liability policies may not cover a health coach who works with clients in a private residence. Health coaches who use their own home or a client's home should ensure that a specific insurance **rider**—a special addition to typical policy provisions—will cover those activities. In addition, specific language should provide liability protection for health coaches who utilize outdoor settings for their training activities. In cases where health coaches work outside of a fitness center, it is imperative that the insurance carrier is aware of the professional activities that will occur. In most cases, home-based or outdoor training will require insurance (typically at higher rates) that specifically covers the health coach for these locations. For health coaches who own their own businesses, insurance should be retained that covers potential problems with the facility as well as the instruction and supervision of the health coach.

Most insurance agents now recommend that all professionals purchase an **umbrella liability policy.** The umbrella policy provides added coverage for all of the other insurance (e.g., auto, home, and professional liability) that a person may have in place. For example, if a health coach was sued and the judgment exceeded his or her professional liability coverage, the umbrella policy would cover the insurance shortfall. When purchasing an umbrella policy, health coaches should be sure that it covers professional activities associated with health coaching. In addition, every liability policy should be examined to ensure that it covers the health coach while working in various locations (e.g., fitness center, personal home, clients' homes, and outdoors).

Health coaches who sell products may need to secure **product liability insurance** in the event a product fails to perform properly. This is particularly important for health coaches who own and operate their own businesses. Though the manufacturer of a product retains most of the liability for design flaws, manufacturing defects, and product malfunctions, there have been cases where the "middleman" was also successfully sued.

Health coaches who form partnerships or corporations may wish to investigate the purchase of **keyman insurance.** A keyman insurance policy is designed to compensate the business for the loss of a person who performs a unique and valuable function. If a business will experience significant financial trouble if one person experiences an extended illness or dies, keyman insurance should be purchased. Keyman insurance pays a specified amount to assist the business in its recovery from losing a critical human resource.

Employees and Independent Contractors

Many health and fitness industry employers now require their employees to demonstrate proof of liability insurance when they are hired, even though they will be potentially covered under the fitness center's insurance. Employers should ensure that employees renew and verify their liability insurance policies annually. Potential employees may wish to verify that the fitness center has adequate coverage and that the employer's insurance will assist them in defending against a potential lawsuit. It is *critical* that independent contractors working for fitness clubs or other facilities maintain adequate insurance, as the facility's legal representatives would likely seek to separate the facility itself from the actions of the fitness professional if a lawsuit occurs. The employment or independent contractor contract between the fitness center and the health coach should contain language detailing the insurance requirements and responsibilities of both parties.

One important aspect of insurance is to obligate the insurance carrier to pay in the event of a loss. The following statement, or some version of it, should be included in any basic agreement:

We agree to pay those sums that the insured becomes legally obligated to pay as damages because of bodily injury or property damage to which this insurance applies, and these will include damages arising out of any negligent act, error, or omission in rendering or failing to render professional services described in this policy.

One of the key provisions is that the insurance company will pay even if the health coach fails to provide a service. For example, if an injured person needed first-aid attention and the health coach did not provide it, the policy should still provide protection. If "failure to render" or "omission" is not specified, the policy covers the health coach only if the services provided were inadequate or improper.

A critical component of an insurance policy is related to coverage of legal fees, settlements, and defense charges. Health coaches should look for the following type of clause in their policy:

We will have the right and duty to defend any suit seeking damages under this policy, even if the allegations are groundless, false, or fraudulent and may, at our discretion, make such investigation and settlement of any claim or suit deemed expedient.

The best policies cover the cost of a legal defense *and* any claims awarded. Policies that only cover an amount equal to awarded damages are not recommended, as the health coach will be covered for the final judgment, but all of the legal expenses incurred will be the health coach's responsibility. One of the realities of insurance litigation is that the insurance company may make a strategic decision to settle rather than fight the case in court. It is important to have a policy that covers the cost of litigation, but the health coach should not necessarily be disappointed if the insurance company elects to settle a lawsuit out of court.

While it is important to identify and understand what is covered in the insurance policy, it is also critical to know what is not covered. Most policies delineate specific exclusions. The following liabilities are often excluded in fitness professional policies: abuse, molestation, cancer (resulting from tanning), libel, and slander. Health coaches should also inquire whether bodily insurance coverage will cover lawsuits alleging mental stress. Most policies differentiate between the two, and a standard bodily injury clause does not necessarily include mental injuries. A client filing a suit might claim that the health coach was overly critical and, as a result, mental injuries were suffered. Mental injuries are difficult to define and determine. The courts are split on the issue of inclusion and this is an evolving area of law.

Most policies exclude coverage for acts committed before the policy was purchased. Coverage also might be excluded for claims that occurred during the policy period but are filed after the coverage has been terminated. These issues are related to the "claims-made basis" of a policy. Though they can be expensive, health coaches can purchase "prior acts coverage" from most insurance carriers for an additional cost if they have already begun training without insurance coverage. An "extended reporting endorsement" will ensure that claims made in the future for injuries during the policy period will be covered even if the policy is cancelled. Ideally, insurance coverage should be maintained until after the statute of limitations has expired for anyone who has been a client of a health coach.

Understanding insurance policies initially can be difficult. Proper research of potential insurance agents is critical. Once an insurance carrier has been indentified, the health coach should maintain an open line of communication with his or her agent. Ultimately, the agent and the insurance company work for the health coach, but it is the health coach's responsibility to maintain open communication. Any changes in business activity should be immediately relayed to the insurance company so that appropriate changes in the policy can be made. Adequate levels of insurance can change as a health coach's client list, employees, and income increase.

Other Business Concerns With Legal Implications

In addition to the legal responsibilities in the areas of business structure, scope of practice, facilities, equipment, testing, instruction, and supervision, health coaches must be aware of the implications of certain other potential legal issues.

Marketing Activities

Identifying and procuring clients is the lifeblood of any business. Though most health coaches maintain high ethical standards, some health clubs and weight-loss centers have relatively little concern for ethical behavior. Unfortunately, it has become common for some fitness centers to utilize improper marketing tactics and long-term contracts that contain deceptive or misleading language to attract and retain clients. In some instances, "guaranteed weight loss" or other promises may violate consumer protection laws. In some extreme cases, fitness centers have even misused direct deposit agreements to commit fraud. Health coaches should understand the marketing and operating activities that their fitness centers may utilize. If a fitness center is behaving unethically or illegally, the health coach may be "associated" with those practices, even if he or she had no direct involvement in the improper behavior. The widespread use of the Internet has enabled customer complaints to be relayed to current and potential clients, as well as to the Better Business Bureau. Since a significant portion of a health coach's business is related to reputation, it is important to only associate with fitness facilities that maintain high legal and ethical standards.

Intellectual Property

Music recordings sold commercially are intended strictly for the private, noncommercial use of the purchaser. In addition, there are rules regarding the use of television programming as a key component of any non-food-or-beverage service business. This means that, in many cases, copyright violations occur when a fitness center utilizes music or television broadcasts as a key component of its business. Although two groups in America, the **American Society of Composers, Authors, and Publishers (ASCAP)** and **Broadcast Music, Inc. (BMI)**, as well as the **Society of European Stage Authors and Composers (SESAC),** will issue licenses for the commercial use of broadcasts and recordings, their fees may be prohibitive in many situations. A good option is to purchase recordings produced specifically for use in fitness facilities. When training clients in their homes, health coaches can have clients provide the music for each session. In effect, the clients are then using these recordings for their own private, non-commercial enjoyment during exercise.

Some health coaches may seek copyright or trademark protection for their own creative works. Health coaches who develop specific routines or who write books or other materials may wish to profit from their creativity. For example, a book or instruction manual can be copyrighted so that any future sales provide a **royalty** to the author. Health coaches who develop a company name or slogan may seek trademark protection so that other individuals or businesses cannot utilize that name or slogan without permission.

Proper Use of the ACE Name and Logo

The ACE-certified logo may be used by ACE-certified Professionals only and is a mark of excellence. ACE encourages its certified professionals to use this mark to promote themselves; however, it is important that ACE and its professionals work together to protect the American Council on Exercise name. The ACE logo and *ACE Logo Usage Guidelines* document are available for download by all ACE-certified Professionals at www.ACEfitness.org. This document provides complete details regarding proper and improper usage of both the ACE name and logo.

ACE-certified Professionals can use the ACE-certified logo mark to promote their credentials to current and prospective clients. Examples include business cards, stationery, advertisements, or brochures marketing any ACE certifications earned and actively maintained, as well as the fitness services provided to consumers. ACE-certified Professionals may also use the ACE-certified logo on their professional websites or apparel.

To ensure the ACE name and logo are protected, please also note where usage would violate the ACE Code of Ethics (see Appendix A) and trademark laws. ACE-certified Professionals must not use the American Council on Exercise name or ACE-certified logo on any materials that promote their services as a trainer or instructor of other fitness professionals, such as continuing education courses, seminars, or basic training, unless it is contained within their personal biographical material. In addition, ACE-certified Professionals must not use the American Council on Exercise name or ACE-certified logo in conjunction with any other product or merchandise that they sell, such as videos or clothing.

Transportation

In most cases, health coaches will meet their clients at a fitness center or some other location. However, there may be a situation where the health coach provides transportation for the client to or from a training or coaching session. Health coaches should be aware that many "standard" automobile insurance policies may not cover injuries sustained by clients riding in the health coach's vehicle. If the health coach is going to provide transportation for a client, the health coach should check with his or her auto insurance company to ensure that potential injuries from accidents are covered.

Financing

As health coaches create and expand their businesses, they may need to seek financing for certain activities. Regardless of the health coach's chosen business structure, banks and other lenders generally only loan money if it is personally guaranteed by an individual. Unfortunately, many companies have advertised "business loans" that are in fact personal loans. Health coaches who thought that only their businesses were liable for the financial obligation later learned that the lender was able to pursue the health coach for unpaid debts. Health coaches should read and understand the "fine print" of any loan (or, better yet, hire an attorney to review the documents) prior to signing.

Risk Management

One of the most important aspects of any business is risk management. There are risks to any activity, but exercise programs carry certain special risks due to the physical movement and exertion often required. Health coaches should constantly search for methods to make the environment safer for their clients. Periodically reviewing programs, facilities, and equipment to evaluate potential dangers allows the health coach to decide the best way to reduce potentially costly injuries in each situation.

Most authorities recommend a risk-management protocol that consists of the following five steps:

- *Risk identification:* This step involves the specification of all risks that may be encountered in the areas of instruction, supervision, facilities, equipment, contracts, and business structure.
- *Risk evaluation:* The health coach must review each risk, with consideration given to the probability that the risk could occur and, if so, what would be the conceivable severity. Table 20-1 can be used to assess the identified risks.
- *Selection of an approach for managing each risk:* Several approaches are available to the health coach for managing and reducing the identified risks:
  - ✓ *Avoidance:* Remove the possibility of danger and injury by eliminating the activity.
  - ✓ *Transfer:* Move the risk to others through waivers and insurance policies.
  - ✓ *Reduction:* Modify the risks by removing part of the activity.
  - ✓ *Retention:* Often there are risks that will be retained, especially if the removal of the risk would eliminate a potential benefit (e.g., no risks will occur if exercise is eliminated, but then no health benefits can be accrued).

  The recommended approach for extreme risks is to avoid the activity completely. Risks that fall into one of the high-risk categories can be managed either through insurance or specific actions that will reduce the likelihood of occurrence or the severity of

Table 20-1

Evaluating Risk Based on Frequency and Severity

	Frequency of Occurrence		
Severity of Injury or Financial Impact	High or often	Medium or infrequent	Low or seldom
High or vital	Avoid	Avoid or transfer	Transfer
Medium or significant	Avoid or transfer	Transfer, reduce, or retain	Transfer, reduce, or retain
Low or insignificant	Retain	Retain	Retain

outcome. Reduction is also the preferred method for addressing risks in the medium-risk category, while risks with low impact can be retained (see Table 20-1).

- *Implementation:* Execute the plan.
- *Evaluation:* Continually assess the outcome of risk-management endeavors. The standard of care regarding some risks may change over time. Therefore, risk-management approaches may need to be altered over time.

Health coaches can also manage risk by examining procedures and policies and developing conduct and safety guidelines for clients' use of equipment. Strict safety guidelines for each activity, accompanied by procedures for emergencies, are particularly important. Health coaches must not only develop these policies, but also become thoroughly familiar with them by mentally practicing emergency plans. Several lawsuits have resulted in substantial judgments against fitness professionals who failed to respond to the emergency medical needs of clients. In some cases, the initial injury was not a major concern, but the failure to adequately address the initial problem was the focus of the litigation. When an incident occurs, the health coach should first ensure the safety of all individuals involved. Once the immediate concern for safety has passed, the health coach should complete an incident report. The health coach should note any facts related to the incident and solicit information from any witnesses. When collecting information from witnesses, it is critical to get phone numbers, physical addresses, email addresses, and signatures for future verification and follow-up. This information should be retained in a secure location for future reference in a lawsuit or when reviewing past performance and emergency-management procedures.

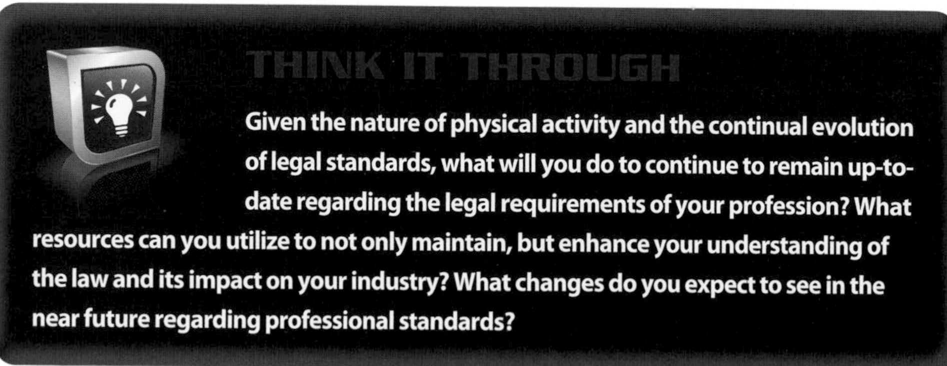

THINK IT THROUGH
Given the nature of physical activity and the continual evolution of legal standards, what will you do to continue to remain up-to-date regarding the legal requirements of your profession? What resources can you utilize to not only maintain, but enhance your understanding of the law and its impact on your industry? What changes do you expect to see in the near future regarding professional standards?

APPENDICES

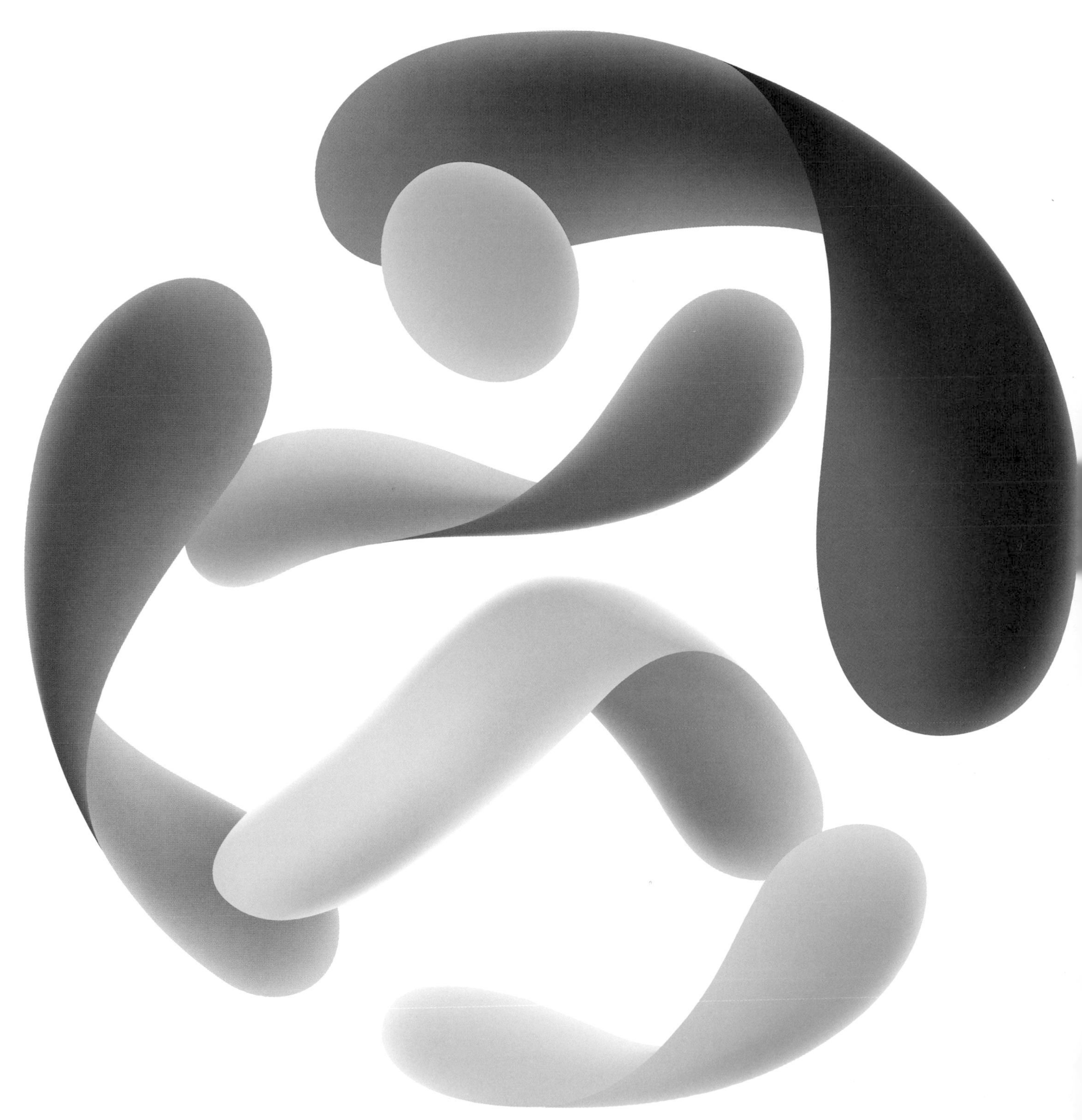

References

Agoglia, J. (2005). *The AED Agenda.* www.fitnessbusinesspro.com/mag/fitness_aed_agenda/

Capati v. Crunch Fitness International, Inc. et al. (N.Y. App. 2002). 295 A.D.2d 181.

Corrigan v. Musclemakers, Inc. (1999). 686 N.Y.S. 2d 143.

Cotten, D.J. (2000a). Non-signing spouses: Are they bound by a waiver signed by the other spouse? *Exercise Standards and Malpractice Reporter*, 14, 2, 18.

Cotten, D.J. (2000b). Carefully worded liability waiver protects Bally's from liability for personal trainer negligence. *Exercise Standards and Malpractice Reporter*, 14, 5, 65.

Cotten, D.J. & Cotten, M.B. (2009). *Waivers & Releases of Liability* (7th ed.). Statesboro, Ga.: Sport Risk Consulting.

Fowler v. Bally Total Fitness (2008). Maryland Case No. 07 L 12258.

Wolohan, J.T. (2008). Aftershocks. *Athletic Business.* www.athleticbusiness.com/articles/article.aspx?articleid=1758&zoneid=45

Suggested Reading

Broadcast Music, Inc. (2009). *Business Using Music: Fitness Clubs.* www.bmi.com/licensing/entry/C1299/pdf533620_1/

Herbert, D.L. & Herbert, W.G. (2002). *Legal Aspects of Preventive, Rehabilitative and Recreational Exercise Programs* (4th ed.). Canton, Ohio: PRC Publishing.

National Conference of State Legislatures (2008). *State Laws on Heart Attacks, Cardiac Arrest & Defibrillators.* www.ncsl.org/default.aspx?tabid=14506

Peragine, J.N. (2008). *How to Open and Operate a Financially Successful Personal Training Business.* Ocala, Fla.: Atlantic Publishing Group.

Reents, S. (2007). *Personal Trainers Should Not Offer Nutritional Advice.* www.athleteinme.com/ArticleView.aspx?id=264

Summary

Despite being commonly overlooked when considering the complexity of providing personalized fitness instruction and weight-management coaching, legal and business concerns are of paramount importance. Health coaches must always be aware of their scope of practice and the expected standard of care that should be provided. This chapter provides an introduction to the legal and professional responsibilities of health coaches. In every instance, health coaches should seek the guidance of qualified attorneys who specialize in the fitness industry. Health coaches should establish their business using the proper structure, understand and utilize contracts, know the changing nature of their legal responsibilities, secure proper insurance, and implement a comprehensive risk-management plan. Ultimately, it is the health coach's responsibility to not only continually educate him- or herself regarding the "science" of exercise, but also to thoroughly understand the legal guidelines that must be followed to create a safe and enjoyable environment for clients.

Appendix A
ACE Code of Ethics

Appendix B
Exam Content Outline

Appendix C
Frequently
Asked Questions

Appendix D
Effects of Medication
on Heart-rate Response

Appendix E
ACE Position Statement on
Nutrition Scope of Practice
for Fitness Professionals

Glossary

Index

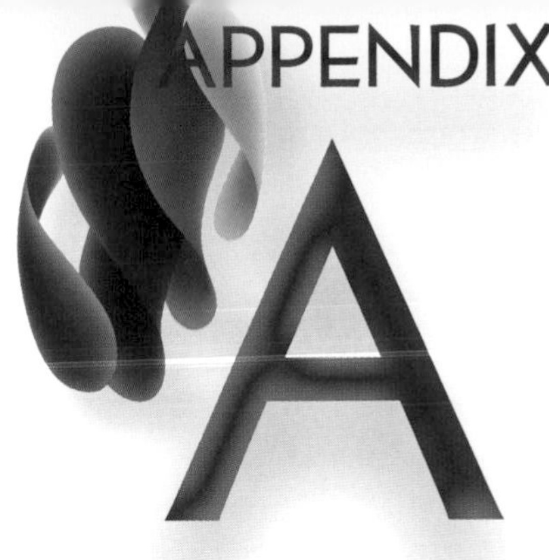

Code of Ethics

ACE-certified Professionals are guided by the following principles of conduct as they interact with clients/participants, the public, and other health and fitness professionals.

ACE-certified Professionals will endeavor to:

- Provide safe and effective instruction
- Provide equal and fair treatment to all clients/participants
- Stay up-to-date on the latest health and fitness research and understand its practical application
- Maintain current cardiopulmonary resuscitation (CPR) certification and knowledge of first-aid services
- Comply with all applicable business, employment, and intellectual property laws
- Maintain the confidentiality of all client information
- Refer clients to more qualified health or medical professionals when appropriate
- Uphold and enhance public appreciation and trust for the health and fitness industry
- Establish and maintain clear professional boundaries

Provide Safe and Effective Instruction

Providing safe and effective instruction involves a variety of responsibilities for ACE-certified Professionals. Safe means that the instruction will not result in physical, mental, or financial harm to the client/participant. Effective means that the instruction has a purposeful, intended, and desired effect toward the client's/participant's goal. Great effort and care must be taken in carrying out the responsibilities that are essential in creating a positive exercise experience for all clients/participants.

Screening

ACE-certified Professionals should have all potential clients/participants complete an industry-recognized health-screening tool to ensure safe exercise participation. If significant risk factors or signs and symptoms suggestive of chronic disease are identified, refer the client/participant to a physician or primary healthcare practitioner for medical clearance and guidance regarding which types of assessments, activities, or exercises are indicated, contraindicated, or deemed high risk. If an individual does not want to obtain medical clearance, have that individual sign a legally prepared document that releases you and the facility in which you work from any liability related to any injury that may result from exercise participation or assessment. Once the client has been cleared for exercise and you have a full understanding of the client's/participant's health status and medical history, including his or her current use of medications, a formal risk-management plan for potential emergencies must be prepared and reviewed periodically.

Assessment

The main objective of a health assessment is to establish the client's/participant's baseline fitness level in order to design an appropriate exercise program. Explain the risks and benefits of each assessment and provide the client/participant with any pertinent instructions. Prior to conducting any type of assessment, the client/participant must be given an opportunity to ask questions and read and sign an informed consent. The types and order of assessments are dictated by the client's/participant's health status, fitness level, symptoms, and/or use of medications. Remember that each assessment has specific protocols and only those within your scope of practice should be administered. Once the assessments are completed, evaluate and discuss the results objectively as they relate to the client's/participant's health condition and goals. Educate the client/participant and emphasize how an exercise program will benefit the client/participant.

Program Design

You must not prescribe exercise, diet, or treatment, as doing so is outside your scope of practice and implies ordering or advising a medicine or treatment. Instead, it is appropriate for you to design exercise programs that improve components of physical fitness and wellness while adhering to the limitations of a previous injury or condition as determined by a certified, registered, or licensed allied health professional. Because nutritional laws and the practice of dietetics vary in each state, province, and country, understand what type of basic nutritional information is appropriate and legal for you to disseminate to your client/participant. The client's/participant's preferences, and short- and long-term goals as well as current industry standards and guidelines must be taken into consideration as you develop a formal yet realistic exercise and weight-management program. Provide as much detail for all exercise parameters such as mode, intensity, type of exercise, duration, progression, and termination points.

Program Implementation

Do not underestimate your ability to influence the client/participant to become active for a lifetime. Be sure that each class or session is well-planned, sequential, and documented. Instruct the client/participant how to safely and properly perform the appropriate exercises and communicate this in a manner that the client/participant will understand and retain. Each client/participant has a different learning curve that will require different levels of attention, learning aids, and repetition. Supervise the client/participant closely, especially when spotting or cueing is needed. If supervising a group of two or more, ensure that you can supervise and provide the appropriate amount of attention to each individual at all times. Ideally, the group will have similar goals and will be performing similar exercises or activities. Position yourself so that you do not have to turn your back to any client/participant performing an exercise.

Facilities

Although the condition of a facility may not always be within your control, you are still obligated to ensure a hazard-free environment to maximize safety. If you notice potential hazards in the health club, communicate these hazards to the client and the facility management. For example, if you notice that the clamps that keep the weights on the barbells are getting rusty and loose, it would be prudent of you to remove them from the training area and alert the facility that immediate repair is required.

Equipment

Obtain equipment that meets or exceeds industry standards and utilize the equipment only for its intended use. Arrange exercise equipment and stations so that adequate space exists between equipment, participants, and foot traffic. Schedule regular maintenance and inspect equipment prior to use to ensure it is in proper working condition. Avoid the use of homemade equipment, as your liability is greater if it causes injury to a person exercising under your supervision.

Provide Equal and Fair Treatment to All Clients/Participants

ACE-certified Professionals are obligated to provide fair and equal treatment for each client/participant without bias, preference, or discrimination against gender, ethnic background, age, national origin, basis of religion, or physical disability.

The Americans with Disabilities Act protects individuals with disabilities against any type of unlawful discrimination. A disability can be either physical or mental, such as epilepsy, paralysis, HIV infection, AIDS, a significant hearing or visual impairment, mental retardation, or a specific learning disability. ACE-certified Professionals should, at a minimum, provide reasonable accommodations to each individual with a disability. Reasonable simply means that you are able to provide accommodations that do not cause you any undue hardship that requires additional or significant expense or difficulty. Making an existing facility accessible by modifying equipment or devices, assessments, or training materials are a few examples of providing reasonable accommodations. However, providing the use of personal items or providing items at your own expense may not be considered reasonable.

This ethical consideration of providing fair and equal treatment is not limited to behavioral interactions with clients, but also extends to exercise programming and other business-related services such as communication, scheduling, billing, cancellation policies, and dispute resolution.

Stay Up-to-Date on the Latest Health and Fitness Research and Understand Its Practical Application

Obtaining ACE-certification required you to have broad-based knowledge of many disciplines; however, this credential should not be viewed as the end of your professional development and education. Instead, it should be viewed as the beginning or foundation. The dynamic nature of the health and fitness industry requires you to maintain an understanding of the latest research and professional standards and guidelines and their impact on the design and implementation of exercise programming. To stay informed, make time to review a variety of industry resources such as professional journals, position statements, trade and lay periodicals, and correspondence courses, as well as to attend professional meetings, conferences, and educational workshops.

An additional benefit of staying up-to-date is that it also fulfills your certification renewal requirements for continuing education credit (CEC). To maintain your ACE-certification status, you must obtain an established amount of CECs every two years. CECs are granted for structured learning that takes place within the educational portion of a course related to the profession and presented by a qualified health and fitness professional.

Maintain Current CPR Certification and Knowledge of First-aid Services

ACE-certified Professionals must be prepared to recognize and respond to heart attacks and other life-threatening emergencies. Emergency response is enhanced by training and maintaining skills in CPR, first aid, and using automated external defibrillators (AEDs), which have become more widely available. An AED is a portable electronic device used to restore normal heart rhythm in a person experiencing a cardiac arrest and can reduce the time to defibrillation before EMS personnel arrive. For each minute that defibrillation is delayed, the victim's chance of survival is reduced by 7 to 10%. Thus, survival from cardiac arrest is improved dramatically when CPR and defibrillation are started early.

Comply With All Applicable Business, Employment, and Intellectual Property Laws

As an ACE-certified Professional, you are expected to maintain a high level of integrity by complying with all applicable business, employment, and copyright laws. Be truthful and forthcoming with communication to clients/participants, coworkers, and other health and fitness professionals in advertising, marketing, and business practices. Do not create false or misleading impressions of credentials, claims, or sponsorships, or perform services outside of your scope of practice that are illegal, deceptive, or fraudulent.

All information regarding your business must be clear, accurate, and easy to understand for all potential clients/participants. Provide disclosure about the name of your business, physical address, and contact information, and maintain a working phone number and email address.

So that clients/participants can make an informed choice about paying for your services, provide detailed information regarding schedules, prices, payment terms, time limits, and conditions. Cancellation, refund, and rescheduling information must also be clearly stated and easy to understand. Allow the client/participant an opportunity to ask questions and review this information before formally agreeing to your services and terms.

Because employment laws vary in each city, state, province, and country, familiarize yourself with the applicable employment regulations and standards to which your business must conform. Examples of this may include conforming to specific building codes and zoning ordinances or making sure that your place of business is accessible to individuals with a disability.

The understanding of intellectual property law and the proper use of copyrighted materials is an important legal issue for all ACE-certified Professionals. Intellectual property laws protect the creations of authors, artists, software programmers, and others with copyrighted materials. The most common infringement of intellectual property law in the fitness industry is the use of music in an exercise class. When commercial music is played in a for-profit exercise class, without a performance or blanket license, it is considered a public performance and a violation of intellectual property law. Therefore, make sure that any music, handouts, or educational materials are either exempt from intellectual property law or permissible under laws by reason of fair use, or obtain express written consent from the copyright holder for distribution, adaptation, or use. When in doubt, obtain permission first or consult with a qualified legal professional who has intellectual property law expertise.

Maintain the Confidentiality of All Client/Participant Information

Every client/participant has the right to expect that all personal data and discussions with an ACE-certified Professional will be safeguarded and not disclosed without the client's/participant's express written consent or acknowledgement. Therefore, protect the confidentiality of all client/participant information such as contact data, medical records, health history, progress notes, and meeting details. Even when confidentiality is not required by law, continue to preserve the confidentiality of such information.

Any breach of confidentiality, intentional or unintentional, potentially harms the productivity and trust of your client/participant and undermines your effectiveness as a fitness professional. This also puts you at risk for potential litigation and puts your client/participant at risk for public embarrassment and fraudulent activity such as identity theft.

Most breaches of confidentiality are unintentional and occur because of carelessness and lack of awareness. The most common breach of confidentiality is exposing or storing a client's personal data in a location that is not secure. This occurs when a client's/participant's file or information is left on a desk, or filed in a cabinet that has no lock or is accessible to others. Breaches of confidentiality may also occur when you have conversations regarding a client's/participant's performance or medical/health history with staff or others and the client's/participant's first name or other identifying details are used.

Post and adhere to a privacy policy that communicates how client/participant information will be used and secured and how a client's/participant's preference regarding unsolicited mail and email will be respected. When a client/participant provides you with any personal data, new or updated, make it a habit to immediately secure this information and ensure that only you and/or the appropriate individuals have access to it. Also, the client's/participant's files must only be accessed and used for purposes related to health and fitness services. If client/participant information is stored on a personal computer, restrict access by using a protected password. Should you receive any inquiries from family members or other individuals regarding the progress of a client/participant or other personal information, state that you cannot provide any information without the client's/participant's permission. If and when a client/participant permits you to release confidential information to an authorized individual or party, utilize secure methods of communication such as certified mail, sending and receiving information on a dedicated private fax line, or email with encryption.

Refer Clients/Participants to More Qualified Health or Medical Professionals When Appropriate

A fitness certification is not a professional license. Therefore, it is vitally important that ACE-certified Professionals who do not also have a professional license (e.g., physician, physical therapist, registered dietitian, psychologist, or attorney) refer their clients/participants to a more qualified professional when warranted. Doing so not only benefits your clients/participants by making sure that they receive the appropriate attention and care, but also enhances your credibility and reduces liability by defining your scope of practice and clarifying what services you can and cannot reasonably provide.

Knowing when to refer a client/participant is, however, as important as choosing to which professional to refer. For instance, when a client/participant complains of symptoms of muscle soreness or discomfort or exhibits signs of fatigue or lack of energy, it is not an absolute indication to refer your client/participant to a physician. Because continual referrals such as this are not practical, familiarize and educate yourself on expected signs and symptoms, taking into consideration the client's/participant's fitness level, health status, chronic disease, disability, and/or background as he or she is screened and as he or she begins and progresses with an exercise program. This helps you better discern between emergent and non-emergent situations and know when to refuse to offer your services, continue to monitor, and/or make an immediate referral.

It is important that you know the scope of practice for various health professionals and which types of referrals are appropriate. For example, some states require that a referring physician first approve visits to a physical therapist, while other states allow individuals to see a physical therapist directly. Only registered or licensed dietitians or physicians may provide specific dietary recommendations or diet plans; however, a client/participant who is suspected of an eating disorder should be referred to an eating disorders specialist. Refer clients/participants to a clinical psychologist if they wish to discuss family or marital problems or exhibit addictive behaviors such as substance abuse.

Network and develop rapport with potential allied health professionals in your area before you refer clients/participants to them. This demonstrates good will and respect for their expertise and will most likely result in reciprocal referrals for your services and fitness expertise.

Uphold and Enhance Public Appreciation and Trust for the Health and Fitness Industry

The best way for ACE-certified Professionals to uphold and enhance public appreciation and trust for the health and fitness industry is to represent themselves in a dignified and professional manner. As the public is inundated with misinformation and false claims about fitness products and services, your expertise must be utilized to dispel myths and half-truths about current trends and fads that are potentially harmful to the public.

When appropriate, mentor and dispense knowledge and training to less-experienced fitness professionals. Novice fitness professionals can benefit from your experience and skill as you assist them in establishing a foundation based on exercise science, from both theoretical and practical standpoints. Therefore, it is a disservice if you fail to provide helpful or corrective information—especially when an individual, the public, or other fitness professionals are at risk for injury or increased liability. For example, if you observe an individual using momentum to perform a strength-training exercise, the prudent course of action would be to suggest a modification. Likewise, if you observe a fitness professional in your workplace consistently failing to obtain informed consents before clients/participants undergo fitness testing or begin an exercise program, recommend that he or she consider implementing these forms to minimize liability.

Finally, do not represent yourself in an overly commercial or misleading manner. Consider the fitness professional who places an advertisement in a local newspaper stating: "Lose 10 pounds in 10 days or your money back!" It is inappropriate to lend credibility to or endorse a product, service, or program founded upon unsubstantiated or misleading claims; thus a solicitation such as this must be avoided, as it undermines the public's trust of health and fitness professionals.

Establish and Maintain Clear Professional Boundaries

Working in the fitness profession requires you to come in contact with many different people. It is imperative that a professional distance be maintained in relationships with all clients/participants. Fitness professionals are responsible for setting and monitoring the boundaries between a working relationship and friendship with their clients/participants. To that end, ACE-certified Professionals should:

- Never initiate or encourage discussion of a sexual nature
- Avoid touching clients/participants unless it is essential to instruction
- Inform clients/participants about the purpose of touching and find an alternative if the client/participant objects
- Discontinue all touching if it appears to make the client/participant uncomfortable
  - ✓Take all reasonable steps to ensure that any personal and social contacts between themselves and their clients/participant do not have an adverse impact on the trainer–client, coach–client, or instructor–participant relationship.

If you are unable to maintain appropriate professional boundaries with a client/participant (whether due to your attitudes and actions or those of the client/participant), the prudent course of action is to terminate the relationship and, perhaps, refer the client/participant to another professional. Keep in mind that charges of sexual harassment or assault, even if groundless, can have disastrous effects on your career.

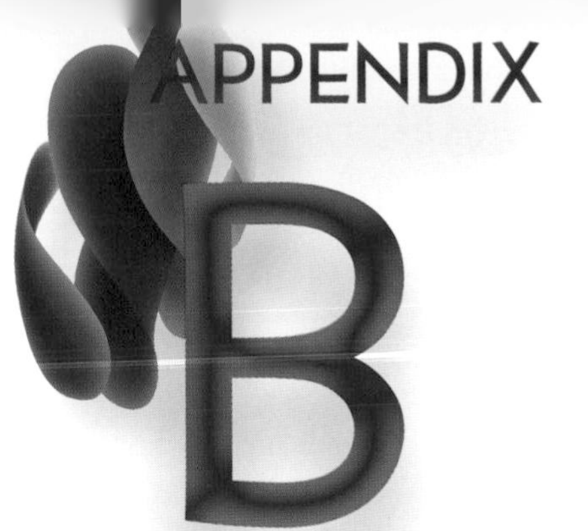

Appendix B Exam Content Outline

For the most up-to-date version of the Exam Content Outline, please go to www.ACEfitness.org/HealthCoachexamcontent and download a free PDF.

Attention Exam Candidates!

When preparing for an ACE certification exam, be aware that the material presented in this manual, or any text, may become outdated due to the evolving nature of the fitness industry, as well as new developments in current and ongoing research. These exams are based on an in-depth job analysis and an industry-wide validation survey.

By design, these exams assess a candidate's knowledge and application of the most current scientifically based professional standards and guidelines. *The dynamic nature of this field requires that ACE certification exams be regularly updated to ensure that they reflect the latest industry findings and research. Therefore, the knowledge and skills required to pass these exams are not solely represented in this or any industry text.* Go to www.ACEfitness.org/KeyIndustryUpdates for information. In addition to learning the material presented on our website and in this manual, ACE strongly encourages all exam candidates and fitness professionals to keep abreast of new developments, guidelines, and standards from a variety of valid industry sources.

Exam Content Outline

The Examination Content Outline is essentially a blueprint for the exam. As you prepare for the ACE Health Coach certification exam, it is important to remember that all exam questions are based on this outline.

Target Audience Statement

The certified Health Coach is an advanced fitness professional responsible for working independently and with other professionals to help a wide variety of individuals and groups adopt structured behavior-change programs that focus on lifestyle and weight management through physical activity, nutrition, and education necessary to improve and maintain health, fitness, weight, body composition, and metabolism. The following eligibility requirements have been established for individuals to sit for the ACE Health Coach certification examination:

- Must be at least 18 years of age
- Must hold a current adult CPR certificate and, if living in the U.S.A. or Canada, a current AED certificate
- Must hold one of the following:
  - ✓ A current NCCA-accredited certification in fitness, nutrition, healthcare, wellness, human resources, or a related field; OR
  - ✓ A minimum 2-year (Associate's) degree or comparable work experience in fitness, exercise science, nutrition, healthcare, wellness, human resources, or a related field

Exam candidates who do not hold an ACE certification must submit documentation to validate that they meet eligibility requirements. This can include a copy of their current NCCA-accredited certification, degree, transcripts ("unofficial"), or a letter from a supervisor who can confirm their comparable work experience. A listing of all NCCA-accredited certifications can be viewed at www.credentialingexcellence.org/NCCAAccreditation/AccreditedCertificationPrograms/tabid/120/Default.aspx.

Domains, Tasks, and Knowledge and Skill Statements

A Role Delineation Study, or job analysis, was conducted by the American Council on Exercise and Castle Worldwide, Inc., for the ACE Health Coach certification. The first step in this process was completed by a panel of subject matter experts in the various disciplines within the field of health coaching as an advanced specialization within fitness. The primary goal of the panel was to identify the primary tasks performed by Health Coaches in helping a wide variety of individuals and groups adopt structured behavior-change programs that focus on weight management. The panel first identified the major responsibilities performed by a professional health coach. These categories are defined as "Tasks" and it was determined that the profession of health coaching could be described in 14 task statements. These tasks were then grouped into four Performance Domains, or major areas of responsibility.

These Performance Domains are listed below with the percentage indicating the portion of the exam devoted to each Domain:

Domain I: Building Rapport and Facilitating Behavior Change – 26%
Domain II: Program Design and Implementation – 27%
Domain III: Program Progression and Adjustments – 32%
Domain IV: Professional Conduct and Competency – 15%

Each Domain is composed of Task Statements, which detail the job-related functions under that particular Domain. Each Task Statement is further divided into Knowledge and Skill Statements that detail the scope of information required to perform each Task and how that information is applied in a practical setting.

The Performance Domains, Task Statements, and Knowledge and Skill Statements identified by the panel of subject matter experts were then validated by a sample of currently practicing ACE-certified Health Coaches. This completed the Role Delineation Study, with the outcome of this study being the ACE Health Coach exam content outline detailed here. Please note that not all Knowledge and Skill Statements listed in the exam content outline will be addressed on each exam administration, as there are not enough questions on a certification exam to cover every knowledge and skill statement.

Throughout this exam content outline, the following definitions will be used:

Clients – Refers to individuals and groups with a variety of ages, fitness levels, etc.

Program – Refers to behavior-change programs that focus on lifestyle and weight management through physical activity, nutrition, and education necessary to improve and maintain health, fitness, weight, body composition, and metabolism.

DOMAIN I: Building Rapport and Facilitating Behavior Change 26%

Description: Use effective communication strategies to build and sustain relationships with individuals and groups by coaching behavioral change to improve and maintain health, fitness, weight, body composition, and metabolism.

Task 1

Use appropriate communication strategies to create and sustain rapport to establish and maintain credibility and trust with clients in order to recognize their current status (e.g., goals, barriers, progress, achievements, needs, expectations, and stage of change).

Knowledge of:

1. Special populations (including diseases and eating disorders) – include psychological and physiological populations
2. Communication, coaching, and teaching strategies (e.g., verbal, nonverbal, feedback, reinforcement, formal, informal, and nonjudgmental listening)
3. Goal-setting and motivational theories and strategies
4. Myths and misconceptions about fitness, health, nutrition, lifestyle, and metabolism
5. Theories of behavioral change
6. Importance and application of feedback, reinforcement, acknowledgement, and encouragement

Skill in:

1. Communicating results, program goals, expectations, and successes with diverse populations
2. Modifying interaction style and content appropriate to the client's personal characteristics
3. Establishing an effective climate for communication with diverse populations
4. Demonstrating empathy, nonjudgmental listening, and active listening
5. Educating the client on systems for self-reporting to the health coach
6. Successfully reframing client myths and misconceptions about fitness, health, nutrition, lifestyle, and metabolism

Task 2

Build client independence through teaching nutrition, exercise, and lifestyle-modification skills and by emphasizing the importance of a social-support network to enhance self-efficacy, motivation, program adherence, and behavioral change.

Knowledge of:

1. Nutrition, exercise, and lifestyle-modification strategies
2. Resources for community and personal support
3. Exercise physiology, anatomy, kinesiology, and nutrition
4. Communication, coaching, and teaching strategies (e.g., verbal, nonverbal, feedback, reinforcement, formal, informal, and nonjudgmental listening)
5. Motivational strategies, learning styles, and self-monitoring tools and techniques

Skill in:

1. Helping clients establish social-support networks
2. Empowering clients to become self-reliant
3. Preparing clients for lapses and plateaus and developing a plan of action to handle them
4. Explaining the effects of exercise and nutrition on health, fitness, and performance

Task 3

Educate and work with clients on key behavior-change strategies in order to impart the knowledge and skills necessary for program adoption and success.

Knowledge of:

1. Psychological factors that influence a client's self-image and their impact on the communication process
2. Behavior-change strategies
3. Communication, coaching, and teaching strategies (e.g., verbal, nonverbal, feedback, reinforcement, formal, informal, and nonjudgmental listening)
4. Motivational strategies that engage clients with various skills and limitations, preferences, and expectations
5. Learning styles
6. Factors that create positive experiences for clients
7. Personal issues and biases that may interfere with program effectiveness

Skill in:

1. Working with clients to establish attainable goals using appropriate goal-setting techniques
2. Selecting and using coaching strategies
3. Teaching clients how to manage lapses, barriers, and plateaus
4. Teaching clients about nutrition, healthful dietary intake, and strategies for weight management
5. Teaching clients about exercise and physical activity

DOMAIN II:
Program Design and Implementation 27%

Description: Create individual and group structured behavior-change programs that focus on lifestyle and weight management through physical activity, nutrition, and education necessary to improve and maintain health, fitness, weight, body composition, and metabolism.

Task 1

Identify potential areas for behavioral change and/or the need for referral by collecting

and assessing clients' current fitness, health, dietary, and lifestyle information using appropriate screening tools and techniques.

Knowledge of:

1. Screening tools and techniques (e.g., interviews, surveys, and questionnaires)
2. Theories and techniques of behavioral change, motivation, and social support
3. Scope of practice, indicators for referral, and referral sources
4. Fitness, health, nutrition, and lifestyle guidelines and standards
5. Special populations (including diseases and eating disorders) – include psychological and physiological populations
6. Communication, coaching, and teaching strategies (verbal, nonverbal)

Skill in:

1. Evaluating data from screening tools and techniques
2. Evaluating fitness, health, nutrition, and lifestyle information
3. Assessing physiological and psychological risk
4. Communicating with diverse populations
5. Assessing readiness to change
6. Referring clients to appropriate healthcare professionals as needed

Task 2

Select and conduct appropriate assessments based on clients' unique health, fitness, nutritional, and lifestyle data and goals to facilitate program design and implementation.

Knowledge of:

1. Fitness, health, nutrition, and lifestyle assessments, guidelines, and standards
2. Special populations (including diseases and eating disorders) – include psychological and physiological populations
3. Physiological responses to testing
4. Scope of practice
5. Contraindications for testing
6. Purpose and benefits for conducting assessments
7. Termination criteria for testing

Skill in:

1. Selecting and administering appropriate assessments for individuals and groups
2. Documentation of assessment data
3. Determining contraindications for fitness assessments
4. Evaluating fitness, health, nutrition, and lifestyle-assessment data
5. Identifying signs and symptoms that merit immediate termination of exercise

Task 3

Design and implement programs based on clients' interview, screening and assessment data, and goals to progress clients toward healthy lifestyle, weight management, and behavioral change.

Knowledge of:

1. Program-design guidelines for safe and effective nutrition, exercise, and behavioral change

2. Weight management, physiology of obesity, and metabolism
3. Communication, coaching, and teaching strategies (verbal, nonverbal)
4. Programming considerations for special populations
5. Physiological, psychological, and motivational adaptations and changes to program components (e.g., exercise and nutrition)
6. Theories and techniques of behavior change, motivation, and social support
7. Goal-setting theories and strategies

Skill in:

1. Program design and implementation based on evaluation of fitness, health, nutrition, and lifestyle-assessment data, guidelines, and standards
2. Communicating assessment results, program goals, and expectations with diverse populations
3. Creating positive program experiences
4. Collaborating with clients and other stakeholders on goal setting

DOMAIN III: Program Progression and Adjustments 32%

Description: Monitor, evaluate, and modify individual and group structured behavior-change programs designed to improve and maintain health, fitness, weight, body composition, and metabolism.

Task 1

Work with clients to facilitate progression toward established goals and self-efficacy using observed and self-reported data and appropriate communication strategies (e.g., feedback).

Knowledge of:

1. Goal-setting theories and strategies
2. Proper progression techniques
3. Communication, coaching, and teaching strategies (e.g., verbal, nonverbal, feedback, reinforcement, formal, informal, and nonjudgmental listening)
4. Obstacles and barriers to successful program adherence
5. Self-monitoring techniques
6. Subjective and objective observation techniques

Skill in:

1. Collaborating with clients and other stakeholders on goal-setting
2. Interpreting and evaluating observed and self-reported data
3. Interpreting and evaluating clients' progress toward goals
4. Helping clients develop coping and problem-solving strategies to overcome barriers to successful programs, including support systems
5. Facilitating behavior change
6. Building self-efficacy

Task 2

Evaluate program effectiveness by reassessing current fitness, health, dietary, and/or

lifestyle data and comparing with previous results in order to recognize successes, and determine and implement appropriate program adjustments and progressions.

Knowledge of:

1. Fitness, health, nutrition, and lifestyle assessments, guidelines, and standards
2. Special populations (including diseases and eating disorders) – include psychological and physiological populations
3. Physiological responses to testing
4. Scope of practice, indicators for referral, and referral sources
5. Proper progression techniques
6. Communication, coaching, and teaching strategies (e.g., verbal, nonverbal, feedback, reinforcement, formal, informal, and nonjudgmental listening)
7. Contraindications of testing
8. Goal-setting and motivational theories and strategies
9. Obstacles and barriers to successful program adherence
10. Program-design guidelines for safe and effective nutrition, exercise, and behavioral change

Skill in:

1. Interpreting, comparing, and evaluating fitness, health, nutrition, and lifestyle-assessment data to enable recognition of success
2. Communicating assessment results, program goals, and expectations with diverse populations
3. Determining contraindications for fitness assessments
4. Selecting and administering appropriate assessments for individuals and groups
5. Collaborating with clients and other stakeholders on goal-setting
6. Interpreting and evaluating client progress toward goals
7. Identifying signs and symptoms that merit immediate termination of exercise

Task 3

Monitor client attitudes (e.g., perceptions, experiences, and enjoyment) through continuous dialogue in order to make appropriate program adjustments.

Knowledge of:

1. Coaching procedures and techniques (e.g., motivational interviewing and nonjudgmental listening)
2. Subjective and objective attitude-assessment tools
3. Communication, coaching, and teaching strategies (e.g., verbal, nonverbal, feedback, reinforcement, formal, informal, and nonjudgmental listening)
4. Obstacles and barriers to healthy client attitudes
5. Learning styles
6. Cognitive, affective, and learning styles that influence progress and goal attainment (emotional states, self-motivation, self-perception, negative/positive self-talk, guilt)
7. Physical acceptance, competency, and self-efficacy

Skill in:

1. Selecting and applying appropriate coaching procedures and techniques (e.g., motivational interviewing)

2. Active listening and other communication skills
3. Selecting, interpreting, and evaluating subjective and objective attitude assessments
4. Helping clients develop coping and problem-solving strategies to overcome barriers to successful programs, including support systems
5. Identifying client cognitive and emotional patterns, including self-talk patterns such as guilt, self-verification
6. Building acceptance and self-efficacy

Task 4

Continuously revisit goals with clients and recognize achievements, challenges, and barriers in order to maintain and progress program participation, motivation, and success.

Knowledge of:

1. Theories of behavioral change
2. Goal-setting theories and strategies
3. Proper progression techniques
4. Communication, coaching, and teaching strategies (e.g., verbal, nonverbal, feedback, reinforcement, formal, informal, and nonjudgmental listening)
5. Obstacles and barriers to successful program adherence (perceived or real)
6. Reinforcement and motivation strategies
7. Behavior-maintenance strategies, maintaining lifestyle-change strategies

Skill in:

1. Interpreting and evaluating client progress toward goals
2. Helping clients develop coping and problem-solving strategies to overcome barriers to successful programs, including support systems
3. Communicating results, program goals, expectations, and successes with diverse populations
4. Collaborating with clients to modify goals
5. Facilitating change
6. Recognizing and preventing lapses

DOMAIN IV: Professional Conduct and Competency 15%

Description: Fulfill responsibilities through ongoing education, collaboration, and awareness of professional standards and practices necessary to protect clients, the profession, stakeholders, and yourself.

Task 1

Adhere to legal and ethical codes, scope of practice, and standards of care in order to protect the client, maintain professional standards, and manage risk.

Knowledge of:

1. Building and maintaining a collaborative referral network through various channels (e.g., community involvement and networking groups) in order to benefit clients and maintain professional standards

2. American Council on Exercise Code of Ethics
3. American Council on Exercise Professional Practices and Disciplinary Procedures
4. Scope of practice and accepted standards of care for fitness professionals
5. Liability issues associated with acting outside the standard of care, scope of practice, and ACE Code of Ethics
6. Standards, laws, and regulations governing confidentiality
7. Risk-management strategies
8. Various insurance policies and coverage (e.g., professional liability insurance, general liability insurance, workers' compensation insurance, and health and disability insurance) for fitness professionals working in a variety of settings (e.g., clubs, non-profit facilities, medical fitness facilities, community centers, homes, and outdoor settings)
9. Indicators for referral and referral sources
10. Intellectual property laws as they apply to video, DVD, written materials, Internet, music, copyright, and trademark

Skill in:

1. Assessing areas of risk (e.g., client, facilities, and use of technology)
2. Identifying professional boundaries based on scope of practice and professional and ethical obligations
3. Following industry guidelines to minimize risk for the health coach and clients
4. Determining appropriate insurance and levels of coverage necessary for the fitness professional based on the facility and client logistics
5. Referring clients to more qualified fitness, medical, or health professionals when appropriate

Task 2

Maintain and enhance competency by staying current on scientifically based research, theories, and best practices using credible resources such as continuing education, professional organizations, industry journals, and periodicals to provide safe and effective services and education.

Knowledge of:

1. Staying current with research for diverse populations
2. Reputable sources for product and service evaluation
3. Requirements for certification renewal
4. Available and credible continuing education providers and programs (e.g., conferences, workshops, college/university courses, online courses, and home study courses)
5. Appropriate agencies and organizations that establish and publish scientifically based lifestyle-modification standards and guidelines for the general public and special populations (e.g., USDA, ADA, ACSM, ACOG, NSCA, CDC, NIH, and OSHA)

Skill in:

1. Recognizing credible resources
2. Critically evaluating new products and services
3. Applying appropriate knowledge and skills gained through continuing education with clients

Task 3

Document client-related data, communications, and progress using a record-keeping system that is secure, confidential, accurate, current, and retrievable in order to manage risk.

Knowledge of:

1. Health, legal, and insurance obligations regarding confidentiality (privacy laws)
2. Terminology utilized in client-related data collection and communication (e.g., SOAP notes)
3. Effective and confidential record keeping and data security
4. Professional ethics regarding technology, communication, and protection of privacy
5. Importance of maintaining, and implications of breaching, client confidentiality
6. Paperwork and documentation related to client confidentiality and program participation (e.g., waivers, informed consent, medical history, health-risk appraisal, and client contracts)
7. Security laws, standards, and guidelines regarding client confidentially and storage of data

Skill in:

1. Appropriate use of social marketing tools
2. Maintaining confidentiality
3. Differentiating between confidential and non-confidential documents and information
4. Understanding the importance of confidentiality
5. Keeping professional records using healthcare technology and terminology (e.g., SOAP notes)

Task 4

Prepare for, practice, and respond to facility emergencies, acute medical conditions, and injuries by following established protocols and documentation requirements in order to maximize clients' safety and manage risk.

Knowledge of:

1. Components of a comprehensive risk-management program and worksite emergency plan
2. Credible resources for risk-management strategies (e.g., ACE, ACSM, IDEA, IHRSA, NSCA, and OSHA)
3. Cardiopulmonary resuscitation (CPR) and automated external defibrillator (AED) procedures
4. Appropriate emergency medical service (EMS) system activation
5. Basic first aid
6. Occupational Health and Safety Administration guidelines regarding bloodborne pathogens
7. Procedures for evaluating safety of equipment and the exercise environment
8. Industry standards for reducing risk of injury
9. Sources for, and limitations of, waivers and informed consent forms
10. How to communicate a sense of security and safety to clients

Skill in:

1. Identifying and responding to emergency situations

2. Identifying and responding to hazards in training situations
3. Implementing the emergency plan in a professional manner
4. Communicating the rationale for various techniques that limit the risk of injury
5. Using equipment properly and safely

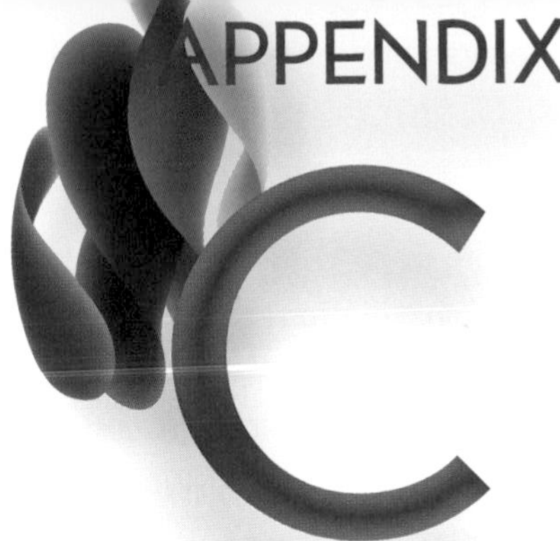

Appendix C Frequently Asked Questions

NATALIE DIGATE MUTH

Natalie Digate Muth, M.D., M.P.H., R.D., is a pediatrician, registered dietitian, Board-Certified Specialist in Sports Dietetics (CSSD), and Senior Consultant - Nutrition for the American Council on Exercise (ACE). She is also an ACE-certified Personal Trainer and Group Fitness Instructor, an American College of Sports Medicine Health and Fitness Instructor, and a National Strength and Conditioning Association Certified Strength and Conditioning Specialist. She is author of more than 50 articles, books, and book chapters, including the books "Eat Your Vegetables!" and Other Mistakes Parents Make: Redefining How to Raise Healthy Eaters *(Healthy Learning, 2012) and the upcoming textbook* Sports Nutrition for Allied Health Professionals *(F.A. Davis, in press).*

This appendix includes answers to some of the most common questions asked by both clients and ACE-certified Health Coaches themselves.

Frequently Asked Questions From Clients

Does exercise curb appetite?

Research suggests that appetite decreases for about the first hour after strenuous exercise and then normalizes. However, appetite regulation is a very complex process that relies on insulin, hormones, psychological factors, and blood sugar levels. This complexity makes it difficult to generalize the effects of exercise on appetite. Overall, people who participate in moderate exercise tend to eat about the same number of calories (or only slightly more) than they would if they did not exercise. Competitive athletes overall do consume a lot more food than usual after exercise, but they usually burn off much more than the excess calories they consumed (Lun, Erdman, & Reimer, 2009; Venkatraman & Pendergast, 2002; Blundell & King, 1999).

How long should I wait to exercise after eating?

It is generally recommended that exercisers wait about three hours after eating a full meal before engaging in a strenuous exercise program. That's about how long it takes for a balanced meal that includes some carbohydrate, protein, and fat to move from the stomach into the small intestines, where nutrients are absorbed and energy becomes available. Exercising before food has had time to empty from the stomach can cause cramps and abdominal discomfort. But people respond differently and there is no set amount of time to wait. If you exercise in the morning, a quick carbohydrate-dense snack might help to provide some energy during the workout without a lot of discomfort. Carbohydrates are generally digested in approximately an hour, while protein takes about two hours and fat about four hours. But remember, most foods are a combination of the three types of macronutrients.

What should I eat before my workouts?

In general, foods should be eaten about three hours before working out to give the body a chance to move the food out of the stomach and begin digestion and absorption. The food should be something that is relatively high in carbohydrate to maximize blood glucose availability, relatively low in fat and fiber to minimize gastrointestinal distress and facilitate gastric emptying, moderate in protein, and easy on the stomach. While the amount of food to eat varies from person to person, most people do well with approximately 2 grams (8 calories) of carbohydrate per pound of body weight. For morning workouts, eat a small amount of a rapidly digestible carbohydrate, such as a slice of bread or a banana, 30 to 60 minutes before exercise. If you exercise in the afternoon or evening, you may want to have a light snack right before a workout, especially if it's been more than three hours since your last meal.

What should I eat after a workout?

For optimal recovery after an endurance workout, it is important to eat carbohydrates to replace the stored energy (glycogen) that was utilized doing the workout. For best results, eat approximately 1.5 grams of carbohydrate per kilogram of body weight within 30 minutes of finishing the workout and then every two hours for four to six hours (American Dietetic Association, 2000). A little bit of protein will also help to repair muscles, which is especially important after a resistance-training workout. Of course, the amount of refueling needed depends on the intensity and duration of the workout.

Which is better for weight control: consuming three square meals or eating five to six small meals spread out over the day?

Weight control is achieved by balancing the number of calories consumed with the number of calories burned. Therefore, it doesn't matter if the calories come in the form of three larger meals or five to six smaller meals. However, some people find that they're better able to control their caloric intake in one way or the other. For instance, people who consume three or fewer meals per day may find that long periods between meals leave them feeling famished, which leads them to overeat to compensate. Eating smaller meals spaced throughout the day may help some individuals with calorie control. On the other hand, someone who eats five to six meals per day may forget to make them small meals and instead consume more calories than he or she would with three meals. In the end, it's a matter of preference. One strategy for effective meal planning is to determine the total number of calories (or, alternatively, the total number of servings from each of the food groups) and divide them somewhat equally throughout the day—whether that's three meals or six. It is important to note that people who have diabetes should consume five to six equally small-sized meals to maintain healthy blood sugar levels throughout the day.

How many calories should I eat and how often should I exercise for optimal weight loss?

Several formulas have been developed to estimate caloric needs for weight maintenance. One that is particularly useful is the Mifflin-St. Jeor equation:

For men: RMR = 9.99 x weight (kg) + 6.25 x height (cm) – 4.92 x age (years) + 5

For women: RMR = 9.99 x weight (kg) + 6.25 x height (cm) – 4.92 x age (years) – 161

Multiply the RMR value derived from the prediction equation by the appropriate activity correction factor:

1.200 = sedentary (little or no exercise)

1.375 = lightly active (light exercise/sports one to three days per week

1.550 = moderately active (moderate exercise/sports three to five days per week)

1.725 = very active (hard exercise/sports six to seven days per week)

1.900 = extra active (very hard exercise/sports and a physical job)

Moderately active people are generally advised to consume approximately 1.5 to 1.7 times the calculated resting metabolic rate (RMR). Convert pounds to kilograms by dividing by 2.2. Convert inches to centimeters by multiplying by 2.54.

The numerical caloric value derived from this formula represents how many calories an individual should eat to maintain his or her current weight. To lose 1 pound of fat, a 3,500-calorie deficit is required. This can come from decreasing caloric intake, increasing caloric expenditure or, ideally, both. But keep in mind that losing weight is not the hard part. The hard part is keeping the weight off. It is well-established that people who are most successful at maintaining weight loss are those who engage in regular physical activity.

The *2015-2020 Dietary Guidelines for Americans* suggest that adults seeking to maintain weight loss accumulate 60 to 90 minutes of moderate physical activity most days of the week (U.S. Department of Agriculture, 2015). This goal, which may seem overwhelming, can be reached gradually over time by starting with 15- to 30-minute bouts of enjoyable activity.

Is it true that food eaten late at night is more likely to turn into body fat?

Eating late at night does not necessarily lead to greater weight gain, which is dependent on caloric intake and caloric expenditure. If people eat more than they expend, then they will gain weight—regardless of whether the calories come from breakfast, dinner, or a late-night snack. However, in reality, people who eat a lot of food late at night tend to consume more calorie-dense foods and thus eat more calories, which can cause weight gain. Ultimately, it's not when you eat, but what and how much. For example, if you find yourself mindlessly eating chips at 10 o'clock at night while watching TV, then it might be helpful to reverse this fat-promoting behavior by making a behavioral plan that includes not eating after 8 o'clock p.m.

Do I have to stop eating all of the foods that I enjoy to lose weight?

The most successful approach to weight loss and weight-loss maintenance is to make permanent lifestyle changes that include a healthful eating plan and ample physical activity. A diet—which implies short-term and hard-to-adhere-to changes—is not the answer. Thus, while certain foods are prohibited by various diet plans, a healthy lifestyle allows for all foods in moderation. This means that less-healthy foods can be eaten, as long as they make up only a small portion of the total daily caloric intake. The government's

MyPlate plan (www.ChooseMyPlate.gov) calls these "discretionary calories."

Should I be taking a supplement to obtain adequate nutrition?

The science on multivitamins is inconclusive. In 2006, a National Institutes of Health (NIH) panel convened to evaluate all of the research on multivitamins and develop recommendations for the public. The panel concluded that insufficient high-quality research has been done to be able to assess whether vitamins help in chronic disease prevention (NIH, 2006). Two exceptions are the strong indications for folic-acid supplements for all women of child-bearing age to prevent neural tube defects in the developing baby, and fish oil/omega-3 fatty acid supplements for the prevention of heart disease in people who are at risk. In general, most dietitians recommend that people take a multivitamin as "insurance" and, more importantly, aim to get optimal nutrition, including vitamins and minerals, from whole foods such as fruits, vegetables, fish, and low- or nonfat dairy products.

I've tried many diets and have lost a lot of weight, only to regain more back. How much weight should I lose? And how do I keep it off?

The key to permanent weight-loss success is to make lifestyle changes that include a healthy eating plan and ample physical activity. The changes need to be doable enough that you can maintain them indefinitely and not feel deprived or unhappy.

A realistic goal for someone who is overweight or obese is to aim to lose 7 to 10% of starting weight over a six-month to one-year period and then to keep the weight off for at least six months before trying to lose more. This amount of weight loss will provide significant health benefits, including decreases in blood pressure, cholesterol, and the risk of developing diabetes.

Also, weight loss is more easily maintained when the weight is lost slowly (about 1 to 2 pounds per week).

I don't have a lot of time. How can I fit a healthy exercise and nutrition program into my busy schedule?

One could argue that the extra time invested each day to healthy meal planning and physical activity will, in the end, add years to one's life and, as such, is worth the effort. While this is true, in a practical sense it may not be enough to encourage someone to make the time for these changes—at least not right away. So it is also important to note that small changes that do not take much extra time, such as taking the stairs instead of the elevator and parking in one of the far away slots at the grocery store, can add up. Also, most fast-food and take-out restaurants now offer healthier choices, such as grilled chicken, salads, and kids meals (that adults can order, too) with fruit and milk. Visit www.smallstep.gov for numerous tips on how to incorporate healthy living into a jam-packed schedule.

Frequently Asked Questions From Health Coaches

Why do nutritional experts advise people not to skip breakfast if they are trying to lose weight?

Breakfast is considered the most important meal of the day for several reasons. From a weight-loss perspective, research demonstrates that people who eat breakfast weigh less than those who skip breakfast. In fact, one study showed that rates of obesity and metabolic syndrome were 35 to 50% lower among people who eat breakfast (Kircheimer, 2003). This may be because people who skip breakfast tend to overcompensate throughout the day by eating larger portions of food. Some experts suggest that hormonal, metabolic, and appetite factors may play a role. Or, it may be that people who eat breakfast tend to be healthier in general for a variety of other reasons. Regardless, breakfast provides a good opportunity to eat heart-healthy foods such as whole grains, fruits, vegetables, and dairy, which tend to be low-calorie but filling because of their high fiber content. Notably, other types of breakfast foods such as sausage and biscuits or sugary cereals do not provide the same benefits (Kircheimer, 2003).

Why do some people have a more difficult time losing weight than others?

Genetics clearly is a factor in how easily someone loses weight. Also, gender differences play a role in that when men lose weight they tend to lose abdominal fat first, while women generally have a more difficult time losing abdominal fat. However, there are additional, more controllable factors as well. First, the amount of muscle mass an individual has is directly proportional to his or her metabolism, and thus caloric expenditure. People who have a large muscle mass can more easily lose weight when they control caloric intake than someone who has a low muscle mass. Secondly, people who have more weight to lose are more successful in their weight-loss efforts when they decrease their caloric intake and increase physical activity, because their baseline is often a very high-calorie diet. For example, if a 250-pound man normally eats 3,000 calories per day and he cuts back to 2,000 calories per day and expends 200 more calories per day with exercise, he can easily lose more than 3 pounds in one week. On the other hand, if a 125-pound (57-kg) woman who normally eats 2,200 calories per day cuts back to 2,000 calories per day and expends 200 more calories per day with exercise she will lose less than 1 pound per week. Finally, behavioral factors cannot be ignored. Some people are more successful at weight loss because they are better able to adhere to a lower-calorie diet and regularly engage in physical activity.

Are carbohydrates bad? What proportion of carbohydrates, fats, and protein should people eat for optimal weight loss and health?

As far as weight loss goes, the proportion of macronutrients consumed is not as important as the total caloric intake versus caloric expenditure. However, foods rich in fiber and protein tend to be the most filling, which in theory would lead to a reduced intake of food and calories compared to high-fat foods and low-fiber carbohydrates. It is important to remember that people often eat for reasons other than hunger, which means that they will occasionally continue to eat even when they are full. An effective weight-loss program addresses both the recommended food intake as well as the behavioral factors that sometimes get in the way of successful weight loss. From a heart-health perspective, the healthiest overall meal plan appears to be a Mediterranean-type eating plan, which is rich in fruits, vegetables, whole grains, and omega-3 fatty acids from fish, and low in saturated fat, trans fat, sodium, and added sugars.

What are the glycemic index and glycemic load, and how are they related to weight control (if at all)?

Glycemic index is a measure of the amount of increase in blood glucose levels after consuming a particular food. Carbohydrates (CHO) with a high glycemic index value are rapidly broken down into glucose and released into the bloodstream, which causes a rapid peak blood glucose. Some examples of high-glycemic foods are baked potatoes, white rice, most cookies and cakes, bananas, and white bread. Low-glycemic foods are slowly digested and glucose is slowly released into the bloodstream, which leads to a much smaller peak. Milk, sweet potatoes, oatmeal, and apples are low-glycemic foods.

Glycemic load is a measure of the glycemic index multiplied by the number of carbohydrates consumed divided by 100:

$$\text{Glycemic load} = \text{Glycemic index} \times \text{CHO (g)}/100$$

The glycemic load is useful in that it represents how much a given amount of a food will affect blood sugar levels. The thinking behind glycemic index and glycemic load is that if blood sugar is rapidly increased, insulin levels will rise quickly and lead to increased fat deposition. To date, it is not clear if glycemic index influences weight loss.

What guidelines can I use to evaluate the quality of a diet?

When evaluating popular diets, ask the following questions:

- *How does the diet cut calories?* For any diet to work, calories consumed need to be less than calories expended. Recall that it takes a 3,500-calorie deficit to lose 1 pound of fat.
- *Is it healthy?* A healthy diet promotes a variety of foods and exercise to improve the six primary modifiable risk factors for cardiovascular disease: high cholesterol, elevated blood pressure, impaired fasting glucose, physical inactivity, obesity, and smoking.
- *What is the nutrient density of the diet?* The best diets advocate at least nine servings daily of a variety of fruits and vegetables, which are generally low-calorie foods that provide most of the body's needed vitamins and minerals, as well as phytochemicals that help ward off infection and disease. Fiber-containing whole grains and calcium-rich, low-fat dairy products should also be encouraged. If the diet relies primarily on a supplement to ensure adequate vitamins and minerals, it probably is not the healthiest choice.
- *Does the diet advocate exercise?* Nutrition is only one component in making a long-term lifestyle change. Exercise moderately accelerates weight loss by increasing caloric deficit and is essential in keeping the weight off.
- *Does it make sense?* To sell books and win over dieters who have "tried everything," diet plans tend to make unbelievable claims that may only be substantiated by dieters' personal testimonies. From promises to lose 8 to 13 pounds (3.6 to 5.9 kg) in the first two weeks of a diet to promotion of magic supplements, diets are marketed as so easy and effective that they may seem irresistible, at least at first. Fitness professionals play a critical role in helping clients to see through the hype and misinformation.
- *Where is the evidence?* Research studies can be a rich source of information on the

effectiveness and safety of different diets. When assessing research results, it is important to note both the study limitations as well as the results. For example, most diet research has focused on obese middle-aged men and women. Thus, the results may not apply to younger people or those who are only slightly overweight. Also, the duration of most diet studies is one year or less. Therefore, the differences between the diets or the apparent benefits may not hold true for the long term.

- *Does it meet the client's individual needs?* The most negligent diet is one that advocates the same plan to all people regardless of their health status and other individual factors. Clients, especially those with existing health problems such as diabetes or heart disease, should always be encouraged to obtain physician approval before starting a diet or exercise regimen.
- *How much does it cost?* While some people may be able to scrape together enough money to begin an expensive weight-loss program, they may not be able to sustain the cost for an extended period of time. A wiser approach is to plan ahead and assess the individual's readiness to change and commit to a program before making huge lifestyle adjustments and financial sacrifices.
- *What kind of social support does the individual have?* Social support is key to successful weight loss. If a diet requires that an individual eats different food than the rest of the family, he or she probably won't be successful on the diet. If the individual's family is not supportive, he or she may struggle to adhere to the lifestyle change.
- *How easy is it to adhere to the diet?* Long-term adherence to a program (i.e., lifestyle change) is the most important factor for lifelong weight-loss success. And the specific diet really doesn't matter. Dansinger and colleagues (2005) conducted a one-year randomized trial to assess the adherence rate and effectiveness of the Atkins,® Ornish,® WeightWatchers,® and Zone® diets. They found that all of the diets modestly reduced body weight and cardiovascular risk factors after the one-year trial. Furthermore, for each of the diets, people who adhered to the diet had greater weight loss and risk-factor reductions. Of course, most of the study participants struggled with adherence, which overall was poor for all of the diets. This once again drives home the point that permanent lifestyle change, not a quick-fix, time-bound diet, is essential for successful weight loss and sustainable health improvement.

What can or should I do to help an individual I believe may have an eating disorder?

If you suspect that someone has an eating disorder, consider using the "CONFRONT" approach advocated by the National Association of Anorexia Nervosa and Associated Disorders (ANAD) (www.anad.org):

C—Concern. Share that the reason you are approaching the individual is because you care about his or her mental, physical, and nutritional needs.

O—Organize. Prepare for the confrontation. Think about who will be involved, the best environment for the conversation to take place, why you are concerned, how you plan to talk to the person, and the most appropriate time.

N—Needs. What will the individual need after the confrontation? Have referrals to professional help and/or support groups available should the individual be ready to seek help.

F—Face the confrontation. Be empathetic but direct. Be persistent if the individual denies having a problem.

R—Respond by listening carefully.

O—Offer help and suggestions. Be available to talk and provide other assistance when needed.

N—Negotiate another time to talk and a timeframe in which to seek professional help, preferably from a physician or registered dietitian (R.D.) who specializes in eating disorders as well as an experienced psychologist.

T—Time. Remember that the individual will not be "fixed" overnight. Recovery takes time and patience.

A health coach can play an important role in helping to identify individuals who may be suffering from an eating disorder and referring them to the appropriate trained professional. As such, it is important to keep in mind that it is outside the scope of practice of a health coach to attempt to counsel and treat individuals with a suspected eating disorder.

What are the strengths and weaknesses of the following popular diets: South Beach,® Atkins, WeightWatchers, NutriSystem,® Jenny Craig,® Zone, and the Paleolithic diet?

Table 1

Strengths and Weaknesses of Popular Diets

DIET	STRENGTHS	WEAKNESSES
South Beach	Differentiates "good" and "bad" carbs and fats Generally considered healthy after the first phase	Restrictive first phase Encourages too much initial weight loss Studied inadequately
Atkins	Good short-term results Recipes simple to prepare	Nutritionally deficient (too much fat, not enough fiber and fruits) Poor long-term adherence
WeightWatchers	Good variety of foods Behavioral support Lots of education Not too restrictive	Appeals to a specific audience Too costly for some Counselors not health professionals
NutriSystem	Food preparation easy to follow Serving sizes prepackaged	Requires prepackaged foods Expensive Not conducive to long-term adherence Studied inadequately
Jenny Craig	Good nutrition Behavioral support	Expensive Dependence on prepackaged food Counselors not health professionals Studied inadequately
The Zone	Lower in fat than Atkins Recipes simple to prepare Good short-term results	Poor long-term adherence Restricts many nutrient-dense foods
Paleolithic diet ("Paleo diet" or "Caveman diet")	Promotes "whole" foods (fruits, vegetables, fish, grass-fed meats) Discourages processed foods Low sodium	Restricts some nutrient-dense foods like whole grains and low-fat dairy High meat intake may lead to health problems, if meats are not lean Too costly for some Studied inadequately

What are some general exercise and nutrition guidelines for clients with diabetes?

It is especially important for people with diabetes to balance nutrition intake (particularly carbohydrate intake) with exercise and insulin or other diabetic medications to maintain a regular blood sugar level throughout the day. Because most people with diabetes have type 2 diabetes, which is linked to an increased risk for cardiovascular disease, a heart-healthy eating plan including vegetables, fruits, and whole grains is key. While advocates of popular low-carbohydrate programs such as the South Beach, Atkins, and Zone diets claim that consuming a carbohydrate-restricted diet is better for people with diabetes, to date research has not supported any long-term cardiovascular benefit of low-carbohydrate diets versus a MyPlate-like, moderate- to high-carbohydrate diet. However, it is prudent to recommend that clients limit consumption of simple sugars and carbohydrates with little nutritional value (e.g., cakes, cookies, and candy bars), as these foods cause a spike in blood sugar. However, people with type 1 diabetes (insulin-deficient by definition) should carry hard candy or other sugary items to eat if their blood glucose drops too low.

Table 2
Exercise Precautions for Clients With Diabetes
• Metabolic control before exercise ✓ Avoid exercise if fasting glucose levels are ≥250 mg/dL and ketosis is present or if blood glucose levels are >300 mg/dL and no ketosis is present. ✓ Ingest additional carbohydrate if glucose levels are <100 mg/dL.
• Blood glucose monitoring before and after exercise ✓ Identify when changes in insulin or food intake are necessary. ✓ Be aware of the glycemic response to different exercise conditions.
• Food intake ✓ Consume additional carbohydrate as needed to avoid hypoglycemia. ✓ Carbohydrate-based foods should be readily available during exercise.
• Avoid injecting insulin into the primary muscle groups that will be used during exercise, because it will be absorbed more quickly, potentially resulting in hypoglycemia.
• Avoid exercise during periods of peak insulin activity.
• Exercise at the same time each day with a regular pattern of diet, medication, and duration/intensity.
• Exercise with a partner and wear a medical identification tag.
• Proper hydration is extremely important. Drink water before, during, and following exercise to prevent dehydration. Be especially cautious on hot days, as blood glucose can be impacted by dehydration.
• Focus on careful foot hygiene and proper footwear. Cotton socks and correctly fitting athletic shoes are important. Regularly check feet for sores, blisters, irritation, cuts, and other injuries.
• Do not ignore pain. Discontinue exercise that results in unexpected pain.

What are some general nutrition guidelines for clients with hypertension?

Research has demonstrated that the DASH (Dietary Approaches to Stop Hypertension) eating plan is effective for the treatment and prevention of hypertension. The DASH plan emphasizes a diet low in saturated fat, cholesterol, and total fat that consists largely of fruits, vegetables, and low-fat dairy products. Fish, poultry, nuts, and other unsaturated fats and whole grains are encouraged as heart-healthy foods, while red meat, sweets, sugar-containing beverages, and high-salt foods should be limited. Salt restriction is recommended for individuals who are salt-sensitive, typically—but not always—African Americans and older adults. Unfortunately, there is not a simple test to determine if an individual is salt-sensitive, so the best precaution for all Americans is to limit salt intake to no more than 2,400 mg per day. For more information about the DASH eating plan, refer to www.nhlbi.nih.gov/health/public/heart/hbp/dash/.

References

American Dietetic Association (2000). Position of the American Dietetic Association, Dietitians of Canada, and the American College of Sports Medicine: Nutrition and athletic performance. *Journal of the American Medical Association*, 100, 12, 1543–1556.

Blundell, J.E. & King, N.A. (1999). Physical activity and regulation of food intake: Current evidence. *Medicine & Science in Sports & Exercise*, 31, 11 Suppl., S573–S583.

Dansinger, M.L. et al. (2005). Comparison of the Atkins, Ornish, Weight Watchers, and Zone diets for weight loss and heart disease risk reduction: A randomized trial. *Journal of the American Medical Association*, 293, 1, 43–53.

Kircheimer, S. (2003). Breakfast reduces diabetes, heart disease. *WebMD Medical News*. www.webmd.com/content/Article/61/71457.htm.

Lun, V., Erdman, K.A., & Reimer, R. (2009). Evaluation of nutritional intake in Canadian high-performance athletes. *Clinical Journal of Sport Medicine*, 19, 405–411.

National Institutes of Health State-of-the-Science Panel (2006). National Institutes of Health state-of-the-science conference statement: Multivitamin/mineral supplements and chronic disease prevention. *Annals of Internal Medicine*, 145, 5, 364–371.

U.S. Department of Agriculture (2015). *2015-2020 Dietary Guidelines for Americans* (8th ed.). www.health.gov/dietaryguidelines

Venkatraman, J.T. & Pendergast, D.R. (2002). Effect of dietary intake on immune function in athletes. *Sports Medicine*, 32, 323–337.

APPENDIX D Effects of Medication on Heart-rate (HR) Response

Table 1

Effects of Medication on Heart-rate (HR) Response

Medications	Resting HR	Exercising HR	Maximal Exercising HR	Comments
Beta-adrenergic blocking agents	↓	↓	↓	Dose-related response
Diuretics	←→	←→	←→	
Other antihypertensives	↑, ←→, or ↓	↑, ←→, or ↓	Usually ←→	Many antihypertensive medications are used. Some may decrease, a few may increase, and others do not affect heart rates. Some exhibit dose-related responses.
Calcium-channel blockers	↑, ←→, or ↓	↑, ←→, or ↓	Usually ←→	Variable and dose-related responses
Antihistamines	←→	←→	←→	
Cold medications:				
without sympathomimetic activity (SA)	←→	←→	←→	
with SA	←→ or ↑	←→ or ↑	←→	
Tranquilizers	←→, or if anxiety reducing may ↓	←→	←→	
Antidepressants and some antipsychotic medications	←→ or ↑	←→	←→	
Alcohol	←→ or ↑	←→ or ↑	←→	Exercise prohibited while underthe influence; effects of alcohol on co-ordination increase possibility of injuries
Diet Pills:				Discourage as a poor approach to weight loss; acceptable only with physician's written approval
with SA	↑ or ←→	↑ or ←→	←→	
containing amphetamines	↑	↑	←→	
without SA or amphetamine	←→	←→	←→	
Caffeine	←→ or ↑	←→ or ↑	←→	
Nicotine	←→ or ↑	←→ or ↑	←→	Discourage smoking; suggest lower target heart rate and exercise intensity for smokers

↑ = increase ←→ = no significant change ↓ = decrease

Note: Many medications are prescribed for conditions that do not require clearance. Do not forget other indicators of exercise intensity (e.g., client's appearance and ratings of perceived exertion).

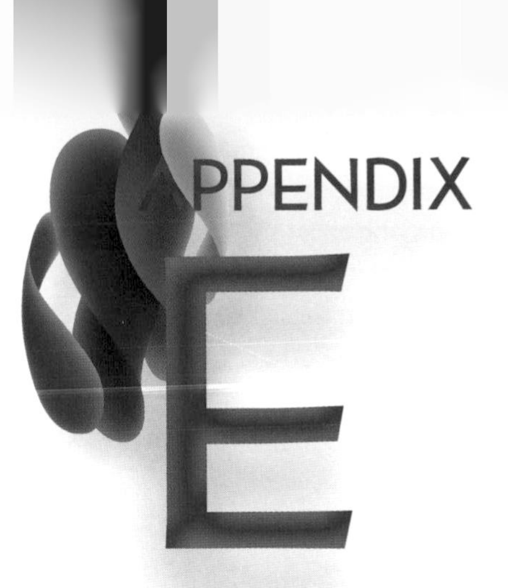

ACE Position Statement on Nutrition Scope of Practice for Fitness Professionals

It is the position of the American Council on Exercise (ACE) that fitness professionals not only can but should share general nonmedical nutrition information with their clients.

In the current climate of an epidemic of obesity, poor nutrition, and physical inactivity paired with a multibillion dollar diet industry and a strong interest among the general public in improving eating habits and increasing physical activity, fitness professionals are on the front lines in helping the public to achieve healthier lifestyles. Fitness professionals provide an essential service to their clients, the industry, and the community at large when they are able to offer credible, practical, and relevant nutrition information to clients while staying within their professional scope of practice.

Ultimately, an individual fitness professional's scope of practice as it relates to nutrition is determined by state policies and regulations, education and experience, and competencies and skills. While this implies that the nutrition-related scope of practice may vary among fitness professionals, there are certain actions that are within the scope of practice of all fitness professionals.

For example, it is within the scope of practice of all fitness professionals to share dietary advice endorsed or developed by the federal government, especially the *Dietary Guidelines for Americans* (www.health.gov/dietaryguidelines) and the MyPlate recommendations (www.ChooseMyPlate.gov).

Fitness professionals who have passed National Commission for Certifying Agencies (NCCA)– or American National Standards Institute (ANSI)–accredited certification programs that provide basic nutrition information, such as those provided by ACE, and those who have undertaken nutrition continuing education, should also be prepared to discuss:

- Principles of healthy nutrition and food preparation
- Food to be included in the balanced daily diet
- Essential nutrients needed by the body
- Actions of nutrients on the body
- Effects of deficiencies or excesses of nutrients
- How nutrient requirements vary through the lifecycle
- Information about nutrients contained in foods or supplements

Fitness professionals may share this information through a variety of venues, including cooking demonstrations, recipe exchanges, development of handouts and informational packets, individual or group classes and seminars, or one-on-one encounters.

Fitness professionals who do not feel comfortable sharing this information are strongly encouraged to undergo continuing education to further develop nutrition competency and skills and to develop relationships with registered dietitians or other qualified health professionals who can provide this information. It is within the fitness professional's scope of practice to distribute and disseminate information or programs that have been developed by a registered dietitian or medical doctor.

The actions that are outside the scope of practice of fitness professionals include, but may not be limited to, the following:

- Individualized nutrition recommendations or meal planning other than that which is available through government guidelines and recommendations, or has been developed and endorsed by a registered dietitian or physician
- Nutritional assessment to determine nutritional needs and nutritional status, and to recommend nutritional intake
- Specific recommendations or programming for nutrient or nutritional intake, caloric intake, or specialty diets
- Nutritional counseling, education, or advice aimed to prevent, treat, or cure a disease or condition, or other acts that may be perceived as medical nutrition therapy
- Development, administration, evaluation, and consultation regarding nutritional care standards or the nutrition care process
- Recommending, prescribing, selling, or supplying nutritional supplements to clients
- Promotion or identification of oneself as a "nutritionist" or "dietitian"

Engaging in these activities can place a client's health and safety at risk and possibly expose the fitness professional to disciplinary action and litigation. To ensure maximal client safety and compliance with state policies and laws, it is essential that the fitness professional recognize when it is appropriate to refer to a registered dietitian or physician. ACE recognizes that some fitness and health clubs encourage or require their employees to sell nutritional supplements. If this is a condition of employment, ACE suggests that fitness professionals:

- Obtain complete scientific understanding regarding the safety and efficacy of the supplement from qualified healthcare professionals and/or credible resources. Note: Generally, the Office of Dietary Supplements (ods.od.nih.gov), the National Center for Complementary and Alternative Medicine (nccam.nih.gov), and the Food and Drug Administration (FDA.gov) are reliable places to go to examine the validity of the claims as well as risks and benefits associated with taking a particular supplement. Since the sites are from trusted resources and in the public domain, fitness professionals can freely distribute and share the information contained on these sites.
- Stay up-to-date on the legal and/or regulatory issues related to the use of the supplement and its individual ingredients
- Obtain adequate insurance coverage should a problem arise

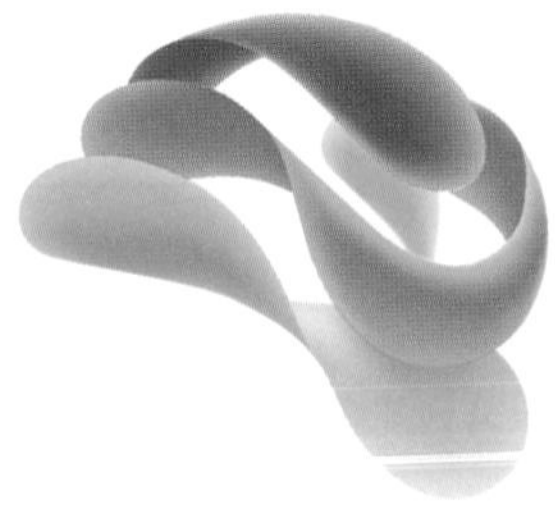

Glossary

Absorption The uptake of nutrients across a tissue or membrane by the gastrointestinal tract.

Abstinence violation effect The tendency to perceive lapses as indicators that one is no longer in a behavior-change program, and thus a rationalization for discontinuing one's behavior-change efforts.

Acceptable Macronutrient Distribution Range (AMDR) The range of intake for a particular energy source that is associated with reduced risk of chronic disease while providing intakes of essential nutrients.

Act of commission A form of negligence in which an individual acts inappropriately.

Act of God An unforeseeable and uncontrollable occurrence, such as an earthquake or flash flood, that may cause injury.

Act of omission A form of negligence in which an individual fails to act appropriately.

Action The stage of the transtheoretical model of behavioral change during which the individual started a new behavior less than six months ago.

Active isolated stretching (AIS) A stretching technique modeled after traditional strength-training workouts. Stretches are held very briefly in sets of a specified number of repetitions, with a goal of isolating an individual muscle in each set.

Active listening Mode of listening in which the listener is concerned about the content, intent, and feelings of the message.

Activities of daily living (ADL) Activities normally performed for hygiene, bathing, household chores, walking, shopping, and similar activities.

Acute Descriptive of a condition that usually has a rapid onset and a relatively short and severe course; opposite of chronic.

Adenosine trisphosphate (ATP) A high-energy phosphate molecule required to provide energy for cellular function. Produced both aerobically and anaerobically and stored in the body.

Adequate Intake (AI) A recommended nutrient intake level that, based on research, appears to be sufficient for good health.

Adherence The extent to which people follow their plans or treatment recommendations. Exercise adherence is the extent to which people follow an exercise program.

Adipocyte A fat cell.

Adipose Fat cells stored in fatty tissues in the body.

Adiposity The state of being fat; fatness; obesity.

Adulterated A supplement is considered adulterated if it, or one of its ingredients, presents a "significant or unreasonable risk of illness or injury" when used as directed, or under normal circumstances.

Aerobic In the presence of oxygen.

Agonist The muscle directly responsible for observed movement; also called the prime mover.

Agreement to participate Signed document that indicates that the client is aware of inherent risks and potential injuries that can occur from participation

Air displacement plethysmography (ADP) A body-composition assessment technique based on the same body volume measurement principle as hydrostatic weighing; uses air instead of water.

Allergen A substance that can cause an allergic reaction by stimulating type-1 hypersensitivity in atopic individuals.

Amenorrhea The absence of menstruation.

American Society of Composers, Authors and Publishers (ASCAP) One of two performing rights societies in the United States that represent music publishers in negotiating and collecting fees for the nondramatic performance of music.

Amino acids Nitrogen-containing compounds that are the building blocks of protein.

Anabolism A state in which the body produces more protein than it breaks down; occurs in times of growth such as childhood, pregnancy, recovery from illness, and in response to resistance training when overloading the muscles promotes protein synthesis.

Anaerobic Without the presence of oxygen.

Android obesity Adipose tissue or body fat distributed in the abdominal area (apple-shaped individuals).

Angina A common symptom of coronary artery disease characterized by chest pain, tightness, or radiating pain resulting from a lack of blood flow to the heart muscle.

Angina pectoris Chest pain caused by an inadequate supply of oxygen and decreased blood flow to the heart muscle; an early sign of coronary artery disease. Symptoms may include pain or discomfort, heaviness, tightness, pressure or burning, numbness, aching, and tingling in the chest, back, neck, throat, jaw, or arms; also called angina.

Anion Negative ion.

Anorexia *See* Anorexia nervosa.

Anorexia nervosa (AN) An eating disorder characterized by refusal to maintain body weight of at least 85% of expected weight; intense fear of gaining weight or becoming fat; body-image disturbances, including a disproportionate influence of body weight on self- evaluation; and, in women, the absence of at least three consecutive menstrual periods.

Antecedents Variables or factors that precede and influence a client's exercise participation, including the decision to not exercise as planned.

Anterior Anatomical term meaning toward the front. Same as ventral; opposite of posterior.

Antibody An immunoglobulin molecule produced by lymphocytes in response to an antigen and characterized by reacting specifically with the antigen.

Antioxidant A substance that prevents or repairs oxidative damage; includes vitamins C and E, some carotenoids, selenium, ubiquinones, and bioflavonoids.

Anxiety A state of uneasiness and apprehension; occurs in some mental disorders.

Arrhythmia A disturbance in the rate or rhythm of the heartbeat. Some can be symptoms of serious heart disease; may not be of medical significance until symptoms appear.

Ataxia Failure of muscular coordination; irregularity of muscular action.

Atherosclerosis A specific form of arteriosclerosis characterized by the accumulation of fatty material on the inner walls of the arteries, causing them to harden, thicken, and lose elasticity.

Atrophy A reduction in muscle size (muscle wasting) due to inactivity or immobilization.

Auscultation Listening to the internal sounds of the body (such as the heartbeat), usually using a stethoscope.

Autogenic inhibition An automatic reflex relaxation caused by stimulation of the Golgi tendon organ (GTO).

Automated external defibrillator (AED) A portable electronic device used to restore normal heart rhythms in victims of sudden cardiac arrest.

Autonomic nervous system The part of the nervous system that regulates involuntary body functions, including the activity of the cardiac muscle, smooth muscles, and glands. It has two divisions: the sympathetic nervous system and the parasympathetic nervous system.

Axial skeleton The bones of the head, neck, and trunk.

Balance The ability to maintain the body's position over its base of support within stability limits, both statically and dynamically.

Ballistic stretching Dynamic stretching characterized by rhythmic bobbing or bouncing motions representing relatively high-force, short-duration movements.

Basal energy expenditure (BEE) The calorie expenditure in a fasting state; also called basal metabolism.

Basal metabolic rate (BMR) The energy required to complete the sum total of life-sustaining processes, including ion transport (40% BMR), protein synthesis (20% BMR), and daily functioning such as breathing, circulation, and nutrient processing (40% BMR).

Base of support (BOS) The areas of contact between the feet and their supporting surface and the area between the feet.

Behavioral contract A tool used to establish an agreement to fulfill a specific set of behaviors within a specified timeframe.

Behavioral deficit Involves a desirable behavior that is not being performed often enough (e.g., physical activity).

Behavioral excess Involves an undesirable behavior that is being performed too often (e.g., unhealthy eating behaviors).

Beta blockers Medications that "block" or limit sympathetic nervous system stimulation. They act to slow the heart rate and decrease maximal heart rate and are used for cardiovascular and other medical conditions.

Beta cell Endocrine cells in the islets of Langerhans of the pancreas responsible for synthesizing and secreting the hormone insulin, which lowers the glucose levels in the blood.

Binge eating disorder (BED) An eating disorder characterized by frequent binge eating (without purging) and feelings of being out of control when eating.

Bioavailability The degree to which a substance can be absorbed and efficiently utilized by the body.

Bioelectrical impedance analysis (BIA) A body-composition assessment technique that measures the amount of impedance, or resistance, to electric current flow as it passes through the body. Impedance is greatest in fat tissue, while fat-free mass, which contains 70–75% water, allows the electrical current to pass much more easily.

Biomechanics The mechanics of biological and muscular activity.

Blood pressure (BP) The pressure exerted by the blood on the walls of the arteries; measured in millimeters of mercury (mmHg) with a sphygmomanometer.

Body composition The makeup of the body in terms of the relative percentage of fat-free mass and body fat.

Body density (BD) A measurement that expresses total body mass or weight relative to body volume or the amount of space or area that the body occupies.

Body fat A component of the body, the primary role of which is to store energy for later use.

Body mass (BM) The total weight of a person expressed in pounds or kilograms.

Body mass index (BMI) A relative measure of body height to body weight used to determine levels of weight, from underweight to extreme obesity.

Bolus A food and saliva digestive mix that is swallowed and then moved through the digestive tract.

Bone mineral density (BMD) A measure of the amount of minerals (mainly calcium) contained in a certain volume of bone.

Bradycardia Slowness of the heartbeat, as evidenced by a pulse rate of less than 60 beats per minute.

Broadcast Music Inc. (BMI) One of two performing rights societies in the U.S. that represent music publishers in negotiating and collecting fees for the nondramatic performance of music.

Brush border The site of nutrient absorption in the small intestines.

Bulimia *See* Bulimia nervosa (BN).

Bulimia nervosa (BN) An eating disorder characterized by recurrent episodes of uncontrolled binge eating; recurrent inappropriate compensatory behavior such as self-induced vomiting, laxative misuse, diuretics, or enemas (purging type), or fasting and/or excessive exercise (non-purging type); episodes of binge eating and compensatory behaviors occur at least twice per week for three months; self-evaluation that is heavily influenced by body shape and weight; and episodes that do not occur exclusively with episodes of anorexia.

Calorie A measurement of the amount of energy in a food available after digestion. The amount of energy needed to increase 1 kilogram of water by 1 degree Celsius. Also called a kilocalorie.

Capillaries The smallest blood vessels that supply blood to the tissues, and the site of all gas and nutrient exchange in the cardiovascular system. They connect the arterial and venous systems.

Carbohydrate The body's preferred energy source. Dietary sources include sugars (simple) and grains, rice, potatoes, and beans (complex). Carbohydrate is stored as glycogen in the muscles and liver and is transported in the blood as glucose.

Carbohydrate loading Up to a week-long regimen of manipulating intensity of training and carbohydrate intake to achieve maximal glycogen storage for an endurance event.

Cardiometabolic disease A condition that puts an individual at increased risk for heart disease and diabetes and includes the following factors: elevated blood pressure, triglycerides, fasting plasma glucose, and C-reactive protein, and decreased levels of high-density lipoprotein.

Cardiopulmonary resuscitation (CPR) A procedure to support and maintain breathing and circulation for a person who has stopped breathing (respiratory arrest) and/or whose heart has stopped (cardiac arrest).

Cardiorespiratory endurance The capacity of the heart, blood vessels, and lungs to deliver oxygen and nutrients to the working muscles and tissues during sustained exercise and to remove metabolic waste products that would result in fatigue.

Cardiorespiratory fitness (CRF) The ability to perform large muscle movement over a sustained period; related to the capacity of the heart-lung system to deliver oxygen for sustained energy production. Also called cardiorespiratory endurance or aerobic fitness.

Cardiovascular disease (CVD) A general term for any disease of the heart, blood vessels, or circulation.

Cardiovascular drift Changes in observed cardiovascular variables that occur during prolonged, submaximal exercise without a change in workload.

Cartilage A smooth, semi-opaque material that absorbs shock and reduces friction between the bones of a joint.

Casein The main protein found in milk and other dairy products.

Catabolism Metabolic pathways that break down molecules into smaller units and release energy.

Cation Positive ion.

Center of gravity (COG) *See* Center of mass (COM).

Center of mass (COM) The point around which all weight is evenly distributed; also called center of gravity.

Central nervous system (CNS) The brain and spinal cord.

Cerebral vascular disease A group of brain dysfunctions related to disease of the blood vessels supplying the brain.

Cerebrovascular accident (CVA) Damage to the brain, often resulting in a loss of function, from impaired blood supply to part of the brain; more commonly known as a stroke.

Certification A credential attesting that an individual or organization has met a specific set of standards.

Cholecystokinin A hormone released when fat is present in the small intestine; slows digestion and absorption.

Cholesterol A fatlike substance found in the blood and body tissues and in certain foods. Can accumulate in the arteries and lead to a narrowing of the vessels (atherosclerosis).

Chronic disease Any disease state that persists over an extended period of time.

Chylomicron A large lipoprotein particle that transfers fat from food from the small intestines to the liver and adipose tissue.

Chyme The semiliquid mass of partly digested food expelled by the stomach into the duodenum.

Claudication Cramplike pains in the calves caused by poor circulation of blood to the leg muscles; frequently associated with peripheral vascular disease.

Closed kinetic chain (exercises) Movements where the distal segment is more fixed; generally considered more functional, as they mimic daily activities closely.

Cofactor A substance that needs to be present along with an enzyme for a chemical reaction to occur.

Cognitive restructuring Intentionally changing the way one perceives or thinks about something.

Comparative negligence A system used in legal defenses to distribute fault between an injured party and any defendant.

Complete protein A food that contains all of the essential amino acids. Eggs, soy, and most meats and dairy products are considered complete proteins.

Complex carbohydrate A long chain of sugar that takes more time to digest than a simple carbohydrate.

Concentric A type of isotonic muscle contraction in which the muscle develops tension and shortens when stimulated.

Congestive heart failure Inability of the heart to pump blood at a sufficient rate to meet the metabolic demand or the ability to do so only when the cardiac filling pressures are abnormally high, frequently resulting in lung congestion.

Connective tissue The tissue that binds together and supports various structures of the body. Ligaments and tendons are connective tissues.

Consequences Variables that occur following a target behavior, such as exercise, that influence a person's future behavior-change decisions and efforts.

Contemplation The stage of the transtheoretical model during which the individual is weighing the pros and cons of behavior change.

Contract A binding agreement between two or more persons that is enforceable by law composed of an offer, acceptance, and consideration (or what each party puts forth to make the agreement worthwhile).

Contraindication Any condition that renders some particular movement, activity, or treatment improper or undesirable.

Contributory negligence A legal defense used in claims or suits when the plaintiff's negligence contributed to the act in dispute.

Core stability When the muscles of the trunk function in harmony to stabilize the spine and pelvis to provide a solid foundation for movement in the extremities. A key component necessary for successful performance of most gross motor activities.

Coronary artery disease (CAD) *See* Coronary heart disease (CHD).

Coronary heart disease (CHD) The major form of cardiovascular disease; results when the coronary arteries are narrowed or occluded, most commonly by atherosclerotic deposits of fibrous and fatty tissue; also called coronary artery disease (CAD).

Corporation A legal entity, independent of its owners and regulated by state laws; any number of people may own a corporation through shares issued by the business.

Correlates Variables associated with sustained physical activity and weight-loss behaviors; also called determinants.

C-reactive protein A pro-inflammatory substance that is elevated in the blood when there is inflammation present in the body.

Cultural competence The ability to communicate and work effectively with people from different cultures.

Cyanosis A bluish discoloration, especially of the skin and mucous membranes, due to reduced hemoglobin in the blood.

Cytokines Hormone-like low molecular weight proteins, secreted by many different cell types, which regulate the intensity and duration of immune responses and are involved in cell-to-cell communication.

DASH eating plan *See* Dietary Approaches to Stop Hypertension eating plan.

Deamination A process by which the liver removes nitrogen from an amino acid; essential before an amino acid can be used by the body.

Decisional balance One of the four components of the transtheoretical model; refers to the numbers of pros and cons an individual perceives regarding adopting and/or maintaining an activity program.

Degenerative disc disease (DDD) A condition of advancing age, and/or the result of the development of post-traumatic arthritis.

Dehydration The process of losing body water; when severe can cause serious, life-threatening consequences.

Denaturation A process by which a protein loses its unique shape; essential before it can be digested.

Deoxyribonucleic acid (DNA) A large, double-stranded, helical molecule that is the carrier of genetic information.

Depression 1. The action of lowering a muscle or bone or movement in an inferior or downward direction. 2. A condition of general emotional dejection and withdrawal; sadness greater and more prolonged than that warranted by any objective reason.

Diabetes *See* Diabetes mellitus.

Diabetes mellitus A disease of carbohydrate metabolism in which an absolute or relative deficiency of insulin results in an inability to metabolize carbohydrates normally.

Diastolic blood pressure (DBP) The pressure in the arteries during the relaxation phase (diastole) of the cardiac cycle; indicative of total peripheral resistance.

Dietary Approaches to Stop Hypertension (DASH) eating plan An eating plan designed to reduce blood pressure; also serves as an overall healthy way of eating that can be adopted by nearly anyone; may also lower risk of coronary heart disease.

Dietary fat Fats consumed through the diet.

Dietary fiber Fiber obtained naturally from plant foods.

Dietary Reference Intake (DRI) A generic term used to refer to three types of nutrient reference values: Recommended Dietary Allowance (RDA), Estimated Average Requirement (EAR), and Tolerable Upper Intake Level (UL).

Dietary supplement A product (other than tobacco) that functions to supplement the diet and contains one or more of the following ingredients: a vitamin, mineral, herb or other botanical, amino acid, dietary substance that increases total daily intake, metabolite, constituent, extract, or some combination of these ingredients.

Dietary Supplement and Health Education Act (DSHEA) A bill passed by Congress in 1994 that sets forth regulations and guidelines for dietary supplements.

Digestion The process of breaking down food into small enough units for absorption.

Digestive system The group of organs that break down food and absorb the nutrients used by the body for fuel.

Disaccharide Double sugar units called sucrose, lactose, and maltose.

Distal Farthest from the midline of the body, or from the point of origin of a muscle.

Diuresis An excessive loss of water from the body through urine.

Diuretic Medication that produces an increase in urine volume and sodium excretion.

Dorsiflexion Movement of the foot up toward the shin.

Dual-energy x-ray absorptiometry (DEXA) An imaging technique that uses a very low dose of radiation to measure bone density. Also can be used to measure overall body fat and regional differences in body fat.

Duodenum The top portion of the small intestine.

Dynamic balance The act of maintaining postural control while moving.

Dynamic stretching Type of stretching that involves taking the joints through their ranges of motion while continuously moving. Often beneficial in warming up for a particular sport or activity that involves the same joint movements.

Dyslipidemia A condition characterized by abnormal blood lipid profiles; may include elevated cholesterol, triglyceride, or low-density lipoprotein (LDL) levels and/or low high-density lipoprotein (HDL) levels.

Eccentric A type of isotonic muscle contraction in which the muscle lengthens against a resistance when it is stimulated; sometimes called "negative work" or "negative reps."

Electrocardiogram (ECG or EKG) A recording of the electrical activity of the heart.

Electrolyte A mineral that exists as a charged ion in the body and that is extremely important for normal cellular function.

Emotional eating Eating triggered by emotional states.

Emotional intelligence The ability to recognize one's own feelings, as well as the feelings of others.

Empathy Understanding what another person is experiencing from his or her perspective.

Employee A person who works for another person in exchange for financial compensation. An employee complies with the instructions and directions of his or her employer and reports to them on a regular basis.

Empty calories Calories that provide very little nutritional value; should be limited in the diet.

Emulsify Mix together two unmixable substances (such as water and fat).

Energy balance The balance between energy taken in, generally as food and drink, and energy expended through normal living and physical activity; when caloric intake equals caloric expenditure resulting in no change in body weight. A positive or negative energy balance will cause weight gain or weight loss, respectively.

Enzyme A protein that speeds up a specific chemical reaction.

Epilepsy A disorder that results from surges in electrical signals inside the brain, causing recurring seizures.

Esophagus The food pipe; the conduit from the mouth to the stomach.

Essential amino acids Eight to 10 of the 23 different amino acids needed to make proteins. Called essential because the body cannot manufacture them; they must be obtained from the diet.

Essential body fat Fat thought to be necessary for maintenance of life and reproductive function.

Essential fatty acids Fatty acids that the body needs but cannot synthesize; includes linolenic (omega-3) and linoleic (omega-6) fatty acids.

Estimated Average Requirement (EAR) An adequate intake in 50% of an age- and gender-specific group.

Estimated energy requirement The dietary reference intake for the daily requirement of energy; measured in calories.

Estrogen Generic term for estrus-producing steroid compounds produced primarily in the ovaries; the female sex hormones.

Etiology The cause of a medical condition.

Euhydration A state of "normal" body water content.

Eversion Rotation of the foot to direct the plantar surface outward.

Exculpatory clause A clause within a waiver that bars the potential plaintiff from recovery.

Express partnership A partnership created through formal paperwork

Extension The act of straightening or extending a joint, usually applied to the muscular movement of a limb.

External feedback Extrinsic reinforcement or encouragement.

Extinction The removal of a positive stimulus that has in the past followed a behavior.

Extrinsic motivation Motivation that comes from external (outside of the self) rewards, such as material or social rewards.

False-hope syndrome The tendency of people to set unrealistic goals.

Fascia Strong connective tissue that performs a number of functions, including developing and isolating the muscles of the body and providing structural support and protection. Plural = Fasciae.

Fat An essential nutrient that provides energy, energy storage, insulation, and contour to the body. 1 gram of fat equals 9 kcal.

Fat mass (FM) The actual amount of essential and non-essential fat in the body.

Fat-free mass (FFM) That part of the body composition that represents everything but fat—blood, bones, connective tissue, organs, and muscle; also called lean body mass.

Fat-soluble vitamin Vitamins that, when consumed, are stored in the body (particularly the liver and fat tissues); includes vitamins A, D, E, and K.

Fatty acids Long hydrocarbon chains with an even number of carbons and varying degrees of saturation with hydrogen.

Feedback An internal response within a learner; during information processing, it is the correctness or incorrectness of a response that is stored in memory to be used for future reference. Also, verbal or nonverbal information about current behavior that can be used to improve future performance.

Female athlete triad A condition consisting of a combination of disordered eating, menstrual irregularities, and decreased bone mass in athletic women.

Fiber Carbohydrate chains the body cannot break down for use and which pass through the body undigested.

First ventilatory threshold (VT1) Intensity of aerobic exercise at which ventilation starts to increase in a nonlinear fashion in response to an accumulation of metabolic by-products in the blood.

Flexibility The ability to move joints through their normal full ranges of motion.

Flexion The act of moving a joint so that the two bones forming it are brought closer together.

Food diary A tool used to track food consumption; involves having clients describe a "typical" eating day, including all foods and beverages.

Force-couple Muscles working as a group to provide opposing, directional, or contralateral pulls to achieve balanced movement.

Frontal plane A longitudinal section that runs at a right angle to the sagittal plane, dividing the body into anterior and posterior portions.

Fructooligosaccharide A category of oligosaccharides that are mostly indigestible, may help to relieve constipation, improve triglyceride levels, and decrease production of foul-smelling digestive by-products.

Fructose Fruit sugar; the sweetest of the monosaccharides; found in varying levels in different types of fruits.

Functional capacity The maximal physical performance represented by maximal oxygen uptake.

Functional fiber Fiber obtained in the diet from isolated fibers added to food products.

Functional food Any whole food or fortified, enriched, or enhanced food that has a potentially beneficial effect on human health beyond basic nutrition.

Galactose A monosaccharide; a component of lactose.

Gallbladder A pear-shaped organ located below the liver that stores the bile secreted by the liver.

Gastric emptying The process by which food is emptied from the stomach into the small intestines.

Gastric-inhibitor peptide A hormone that slows motility of the intestine to allow foods that require more time for digestion and absorption to be absorbed.

Gastric lipase An enzyme released by the stomach that aids in the digestion of fat.

Gastrin A hormone that maintains the pH of the stomach by signaling the cells that produce hydrochloric acid whenever food enters the stomach.

Gastroesophageal reflux disease (GERD) A chronic condition in which the lower esophageal sphincter allows gastric acids to reflux into the esophagus, causing heartburn, acid indigestion, and possible injury to the esophageal lining.

General supervision A method of supervision where the worker (or trainee) does not require the constant attendance of the supervisor (or trainer).

Ghrelin A hormone produced in the stomach that is responsible for stimulating appetite.

Glenohumeral joint The ball-and-socket joint composed of the glenoid fossa of the scapula and the humeral head.

Glucose A simple sugar; the form in which all carbohydrates are used as the body's principal energy source.

Glycemic index (GI) A ranking of carbohydrates on a scale from 0 to 100 according to the extent to which they raise blood sugar levels.

Glycemic load (GL) A measure of glycemic response to a food that takes into consideration serving size; GL = Glycemic index x Grams of carbohydrate/100.

Glycogen The chief carbohydrate storage material; formed by the liver and stored in the liver and muscle.

Glycogenolysis The breakdown of liver and muscle glycogen to yield blood glucose.

Golgi tendon organ (GTO) A sensory organ within a tendon that, when stimulated, causes an inhibition of the entire muscle group to protect against too much force.

Graded exercise test (GXT) A test that evaluates an individual's physiological response to exercise, the intensity of which is increased in stages.

Gross negligence A form of negligence that is worse than normal negligence. Generally, a waiver clause cannot prevent a suit for gross negligence or for wanton or recklessness or intentional misconduct in any state or jurisdiction.

Ground reaction forces The force exerted by the ground on a body in contact with it.

Group waiver Waiver that includes lines for multiple signatures.

Growth hormone A hormone secreted by the pituitary gland that facilitates protein synthesis in the body.

Gynoid obesity Adipose tissue or body fat distributed on the hips and in the lower body (pear-shaped individuals).

Habit strength The psychological and physiological factors involved in habitual behaviors; will change as one moves through the stages of the transtheoretical model of behavioral change.

Health belief model A model to explain health-related behaviors that suggests that an individual's decision to adopt healthy behaviors is based largely upon his or her perception of susceptibility to an illness and the probable severity of the illness. The person's view of the benefits and costs of the change also are considered.

Health psychology A field of psychology that examines the causes of illnesses and studies ways to promote and maintain health, prevent and treat illnesses, and improve the healthcare system.

Healthy Mediterranean-Style Eating Pattern One of three USDA Food Patterns featured in the *Dietary Guidelines for Americans;* modified from the Healthy U.S.-Style Eating Pattern to more closely reflect eating patterns that have been associated with positive health outcomes in studies of Mediterranean-style diets.

Healthy U.S.-Style Eating Pattern One of three USDA Food Patterns featured in the *Dietary Guidelines for Americans;* based on the types and proportions of foods Americans typically consume, but in nutrient-dense forms and appropriate amounts.

Healthy Vegetarian Eating Pattern One of three USDA Food Patterns featured in the *Dietary Guidelines for Americans;* modified from the Healthy U.S.-Style Eating Pattern to more closely reflect eating patterns reported by self-identified vegetarians.

Heart rate (HR) The number of heart beats per minute.

Heart-rate reserve (HRR) The reserve capacity of the heart; the difference between maximal heart rate and resting heart rate. It reflects the heart's ability to increase the rate of beating and cardiac output above resting level to maximal intensity.

Heat exhaustion The most common heat-related illness; usually the result of intense exercise in a hot, humid environment and characterized by profuse sweating, which results in fluid and electrolyte loss, a drop in blood pressure, lightheadedness, nausea, vomiting, decreased coordination, and often syncope (fainting).

Heat stroke A medical emergency that is the most serious form of heat illness due to heat overload and/or impairment of the body's ability to dissipate heat; characterized by high body temperature (>105° F or 40.5° C), dry, red skin, altered level of consciousness, seizures, coma, and possibly death.

Heterogenous Nonsimilar or nonuniform in nature, such as a group of lipids with differing basic structures.

High-density lipoprotein (HDL) A lipoprotein that carries excess cholesterol from the arteries to the liver.

High-viscosity fiber A type of fiber that forms gels in water; may help prevent heart disease and stroke by binding bile and cholesterol; diabetes by slowing glucose absorption; and constipation by holding moisture in stools and softening them.

Hormones A chemical substance produced and released by an endocrine gland and transported through the blood to a target organ.

Hydrostatic weighing Weighing a person fully submerged in water. The difference between the person's mass in air and in water is used to calculate body density, which can be used to estimate the proportion of fat in the body.

Hypercholesterolemia An excess of cholesterol in the blood.

Hyperglycemia An abnormally high content of glucose (sugar) in the blood (above 100 mg/dL).

Hyperplasia Increased cell production in normal tissue. An excess of normal tissue.

Hypersomnia A sleep disorder involving excessive sleep; a sign of depression.

Hypertension High blood pressure, or the elevation of resting blood pressure above 140/90 mmHg.

Hyperthyroidism A condition characterized by hyperactivity of the thyroid gland; the metabolic processes of the body are accelerated.

Hypertrophy An increase in the cross-sectional size of a muscle in response to progressive resistance training.

Hypoglycemia A deficiency of glucose in the blood commonly caused by too much insulin, too little glucose, or too much exercise. Most commonly found in the insulin-dependent diabetic and characterized by symptoms such as fatigue, dizziness, confusion, headache, nausea, or anxiety.

Hypokalemia A deficiency of potassium in the blood.

Hypokinetic disease Conditions associated with too little exercise or physical activity (e.g., cardiovascular disease, obesity, and diabetes).

Hyponatremia Abnormally low levels of sodium ions circulating in the blood; severe hyponatremia can lead to brain swelling and death.

Hypotension Low blood pressure.

Hypothyroidism Underactivity of the thyroid gland, leading to reduced secretion of thyroid hormones and a reduction in resting metabolic rate.

Ideal body weight A term used to describe the weight that people are expected to weigh for good health, based on age, sex, and height. Also called ideal weight or desirable body weight.

Ileum One of three sections of the small intestine.

Incomplete protein A protein that does not contain all of the essential amino acids.

Independent contractor A person who conducts business on his or her own on a contract basis and is not an employee of an organization.

Indirect calorimetry A method used to predict resting metabolic rate. Since oxygen is used in the metabolic process to create energy, a person's metabolic rate can be determined by measuring how much oxygen he or she consumes when breathing.

Inferior Located below.

Informed consent A written statement signed by a client prior to testing that informs him or her of testing purposes, processes, and all potential risks and discomforts.

Inherent risk Risks that can occur through normal participation in the stated activity. Inherent risks can only be avoided by declining to participate.

Insoluble fiber *See* Low-viscosity fiber.

Insomnia Inability to sleep; abnormal wakefulness.

Insulin A hormone released from the pancreas that allows cells to take up glucose.

Insulin resistance An inability of muscle tissue to effectively use insulin, where the action of insulin is "resisted" by insulin-sensitive tissues.

Interleukin-6 A pro-inflammatory substance associated with an increase in cortisol levels.

Interval training Short, high-intensity exercise periods alternated with periods of rest (e.g., 100-yard run, one-minute rest, repeated eight times).

Intrinsic feedback Feedback provided by the clients themselves; the most important type of feedback for long-term program adherence.

Intrinsic motivation Motivation that comes from internal states, such as enjoyment or personal satisfaction.

Inversion Rotation of the foot to direct the plantar surface inward.

Isometric A type of muscular contraction in which the muscle is stimulated to generate tension but little or no joint movement occurs.

Jejunum One of three segments of the small intestine.

Ketogenic Related to the accumulation of excessive amounts of ketone bodies in the body tissues and fluids as a result of fatty acid breakdown.

Keyman insurance Insurance that compensates a company for the loss of a representative of the company who was performing unique and valuable functions.

Knockouts Genetically manipulated animals that are made to lack specific genes and used to study the mechanisms of disease.

Korotkoff sounds Five different sounds created by the pulsing of the blood through the brachial artery; proper distinction of the sounds is necessary to determine blood pressure.

Kyphosis Excessive posterior curvature of the spine, typically seen in the thoracic region.

Lactase An enzyme that is needed to break the bond between the glucose and galactose molecules in lactose so that they can be digested; a deficiency of this enzyme leads to lactose intolerance.

Lactate A chemical derivative of lactic acid, which is formed when sugars are broken down for energy without the presence of oxygen.

Lactic acid A metabolic by-product of anaerobic glycolysis; when it accumulates it decreases blood pH, which slows down enzyme activity and ultimately causes fatigue.

Lacto-ovo-vegetarian A vegetarian that does not eat meat, fish, or poultry.

Lactose A disaccharide; the principal sugar found in milk.

Lactose intolerance A condition that results from a deficiency in the enzyme lactase, which is required to digest lactose; symptoms include cramps, bloating, diarrhea, and flatulence.

Lacto-vegetarian A vegetarian that does not eat eggs, meat, fish, or poultry.

Large intestine A component of the digestive system where certain minerals and a large amount of water are reabsorbed into the blood.

Lateral Away from the midline of the body, or the outside.

Lean body mass (LBM) The components of the body (apart from fat), including muscles, bones, nervous tissue, skin, blood, and organs.

Leptin A hormone released from fat cells that acts on the hypothalamus to regulate energy intake. Low leptin levels stimulate hunger and subsequent fat consumption.

Lever A rigid bar that rotates around a fixed support (fulcrum) in response to an applied force.

Liability Legal responsibility.

Lingual lipase An enzyme released in the mouth that marks the beginning of digestion; cleaves short- and medium-chain fatty acids.

Linoleic acid *See* Omega-6 fatty acid.

Linolenic acid *See* Omega-3 fatty acid.

Lipid The name for fats used in the body and bloodstream.

Lipoprotein lipase An enzyme in working cells that cleaves fatty acids so they can be used to produce energy.

Locus of control The degree to which people attribute outcomes to internal factors, such as effort and ability, as opposed to external factors, such as luck or the actions of others. People who tend to attribute events and outcomes to internal factors are said to have an internal locus of control, while those who generally attribute outcomes to external factors are said to have an external locus of control.

Lordosis Excessive anterior curvature of the spine that typically occurs at the low back (may also occur at the neck).

Low-density lipoprotein (LDL) A lipoprotein that transports cholesterol and triglycerides from the liver and small intestine to cells and tissues; high levels may cause atherosclerosis.

Low-viscosity fiber The structural part of the plant that does not form a gel in water; it reduces constipation and lowers risk of hemorrhoids and diverticulosis by adding bulk to the feces and reducing transit time in the colon. Also called insoluble fiber.

Lymphatic system A network of lymphoid organs, lymph nodes, lymph ducts, lymphatic tissues, lymph capillaries, and lymph vessels that produces and transports lymph fluid from tissues to the circulatory system.

Macronutrient A nutrient that is needed in large quantities for normal growth and development.

Maintenance The stage of the transtheoretical model of behavioral change during which the individual is incorporating the new behavior into his or her lifestyle.

Maltose Two glucose molecules bound together; used to make beer.

Maximal heart rate (MHR) The highest heart rate a person can attain. Sometimes abbreviated as HRmax.

Maximal oxygen uptake ($\dot{V}O_2$max) The maximal capacity for the body to take in, transport, and use oxygen during exercise; a common indicator of physical fitness.

Maximal voluntary contraction (MVC) The maximal effort of a muscle or muscle group during a muscular contraction.

Metabolic equivalent (MET) A simplified system for classifying physical activities where one MET is equal to the resting oxygen uptake, which is approximately 3.5 milliliters of oxygen per kilogram of body weight per minute (3.5 mL/kg/min).

Metabolic syndrome (MetS) A cluster of factors associated with increased risk for coronary heart disease and diabetes—abdominal obesity indicated by a waist circumference ≥40 inches (102 cm) in men and ≥35 inches (88 cm) in women; levels of triglyceride ≥150 mg/dL (1.7 mmol/L); HDL levels <40 and 50 mg/dL (1.0 and 1.3 mmol/L) in men and women, respectively; blood-pressure levels ≥130/85 mmHg; and fasting blood glucose levels ≥110 mg/dL (6.1 mmol/L).

Micelles Aggregates of lipid- and water-soluble compounds in which the hydrophobic portions are oriented toward the center and the hydrophilic portions are oriented outwardly.

Micronutrient A nutrient that is needed in small quantities for normal growth and development.

Mineral Inorganic substances needed in the diet in small amounts to help regulate bodily functions.

Minority partner A partner holding less than 50% of the company's ownership shares.

Mitochondria The "power plant" of the cells where aerobic metabolism occurs.

Mobility The degree to which an articulation is allowed to move before being restricted by surrounding tissues.

Monosaccharide The simplest form of sugar; it cannot be broken down any further.

Monounsaturated fat *See* Monounsaturated fatty acid.

Monounsaturated fatty acid A type of unsaturated fat (liquid at room temperature) that has one open spot on the fatty acid for the addition of a hydrogen atom (e.g., oleic acid in olive oil).

Morbidity The disease rate; the ratio of sick to well persons in a community.

Mortality The death rate; the ratio of deaths that take place to expected deaths.

Motivation The psychological drive that gives purpose and direction to behavior.

Motivational interviewing (MI) A method of questioning clients in a way that encourages them to honestly examine their beliefs and behaviors, and that motivates clients to make a decision to change a particular behavior.

Muscular endurance The ability of a muscle or muscle group to exert force against a resistance over a sustained period of time.

Muscular power The product of muscular force and speed of movement.

Muscular strength The maximal force a muscle or muscle group can exert during contraction.

Myocardial infarction (MI) An episode in which some of the heart's blood supply is severely cut off or restricted, causing the heart muscle to suffer and die from lack of oxygen. Commonly known as a heart attack.

Myofascial release A manual massage technique used to eliminate general fascial restrictions; typically performed with a device such as a foam roller.

Near infrared interactance (NIR) Body-composition assessment method that involves the use of light absorption and reflection to estimate percent fat and percent fat-free mass. It is based on the principle that body fat absorbs light while lean body mass reflects light.

Negative energy balance A state in which the number of calories expended is greater than what is taken in, thereby contributing to weight loss.

Negative reinforcement The removal or absence of aversive stimuli following a desired behavior. This increases the likelihood that the behavior will occur again.

Negligence Failure of a person to perform as a reasonable and prudent professional would perform under similar circumstances.

Neuro-linguistic programming (NLP) A coaching technique anchored in cognitive-behavioral psychology; employs techniques such as visualization and hypnosis to augment its effects.

Neuropeptide Y (NPY) An appetite-stimulating neuron.

Neurotransmitter A chemical substance such as acetylcholine or dopamine that transmits nerve impulses across synapses.

Nitrogen balance A measure of nitrogen consumed (from dietary intake protein) and nitrogen excreted (from protein breakdown). In a healthy body, the amount of protein taken in is exactly matched by the amount of protein lost in feces, urine, and sweat.

Nonessential amino acid Amino acids that can be made by the body.

Non-exercise activity thermogenesis (NEAT) Physiological processes that produce heat; a relative newly discovered component of energy expenditure.

Norepinephrine A hormone released as part of the sympathetic response to exercise.

Nutrient Components of food needed by the body. There are six classes of nutrients: water, minerals, vitamins, fats, carbohydrates, and protein.

Obesity An excessive accumulation of body fat. Usually defined as more than 20% above ideal weight, or over 25% body fat for men and over 32% body fat for women; also can be defined as a body mass index of >30 kg/m^2 or a waist girth of $\geq$40 inches (102 cm) in men and $\geq$35 inches (89 cm) in women.

Obesogenic An environment that tends to generate or create a state of obesity.

Ocular system Nerves, muscles, and organs associated with the eye, including vision and balance components.

Oligosaccharide A chain of about three to 10 or fewer simple sugars.

Omega-3 fatty acid An essential fatty acid that promotes a healthy immune system and helps protect against heart disease and other diseases; found in egg yolk and cold water fish like tuna, salmon, mackerel, cod, crab, shrimp, and oyster. Also known as linolenic acid.

Omega-6 fatty acid An essential fatty acid found in flaxseed, canola, and soybean oils and green leaves. Also known as linoleic acid.

One-repetition maximum (1 RM) The amount of resistance that can be moved through the range of motion one time before the muscle is temporarily fatigued.

Open kinetic chain (exercises) Exercises in which a muscle or muscle group is isolated to function alone.

Operant conditioning A learning approach that considers the manner in which behaviors are influenced by their consequences.

Osteoarthritis A degenerative disease involving a wearing away of joint cartilage. This degenerative joint disease occurs chiefly in older persons.

Osteomalacia Softening of the bone.

Osteopenia Bone density that is below average, classified as 1.5 to 2.5 standard deviations below peak bone density.

Osteoporosis A disorder, primarily affecting postmenopausal women, in which bone density decreases and susceptibility to fractures increases.

Overtraining syndrome The result of constant intense training that does not provide adequate time for recovery; symptoms include increased resting heart rate, impaired physical performance, reduced enthusiasm and desire for training, increased incidence of injuries and illness, altered appetite, disturbed sleep patterns, and irritability.

Overweight A term to describe an excessive amount of weight for a given height, using height-to-weight ratios.

Ovo-vegetarian A vegetarian who eats eggs, but avoids dairy products, meat, fish, and poultry.

Oxidation Process of oxidizing, or the addition of oxygen to a compound with a resulting loss of electrons.

Oxygen uptake ($\dot{V}O_2$) The process by which oxygen is used to produce energy for cellular work; also called oxygen uptake.

Palpation The use of hands and/or fingers to detect anatomical structures or an arterial pulse (e.g., carotid pulse).

Parasympathetic nervous system A subdivision of the autonomic nervous system that is involved in regulating the routine functions of the body, such as heartbeat, digestion, and sleeping. Opposes the physiological effects of the sympathetic nervous system (e.g., stimulates digestive secretions, slows the heart, constricts the pupils, and dilates blood vessels).

Partnership A business entity in which two or more people agree to operate a business and share profits and losses.

Pepsin An enzyme that breaks the peptide bonds between amino acids to shorten long protein complexes into shorter polypeptide chains.

Peptide bond The chemical bond formed between neighboring amino acids, constituting the primary linkage of all protein structures.

Peptide YY A satiety hormone that is released from the intestines.

Percent body fat (%BF) The ratio of fat mass (FM) and fat-free mass (FFM) to total body mass (BM).

Percentage daily value (PDV) A replacement for the percent RDA on the newer food labels. Gives information on whether a food item has a significant amount of a particular nutrient based on a 2,000-calorie diet.

Peripheral vascular disease A painful and often debilitating condition, characterized by muscular pain caused by ischemia to the working muscles. The ischemic pain is usually due to atherosclerotic blockages or arterial spasms, referred to as claudication. Also called peripheral vascular occlusive disease (PVOD).

Peristalsis The wavelike muscular contractions of the alimentary canal or other tubular structures by which contents are forced onward.

Phosphagen High-energy phosphate compounds found in muscle tissue, including adenosine triphosphate (ATP) and creatine phosphate (CP), that can be broken down for immediate use by the cells.

Phospholipid Structurally similar to triglycerides, but the glycerol backbone is modified so that the molecule is water soluble at one end and water insoluble at the other end; helps maintain cell membrane structure and function.

Physical Activity Readiness Questionnaire (PAR-Q) A brief, self-administered medical questionnaire recognized as a safe pre-exercise screening measure for low-to-moderate (but not vigorous) exercise training.

Phytochemical A biologically active, nonnutrient component found in plants; includes antioxidants.

Placenta The vascular organ in mammals that unites the fetus to the maternal uterus and mediates its metabolic exchanges.

Planning fallacy The tendency of people to underestimate the resources needed, in terms of time, effort, money, and so forth, to accomplish a given task or reach a certain goal.

Plantar fasciitis Inflammation of the plantar fascia, a broad band of connective tissue running along the sole of the foot; caused by stretching or tearing the tissue, usually near the attachment at the heel.

Plantar flexion Distal movement of the plantar surface of the foot; opposite of dorsiflexion.

Plyometric exercise High-intensity movements, such as jumping, involving high-force loading of body weight during the landing phase of the movement.

Polymorphism The quality of existing in several different forms.

Polysaccharide A long chain of sugar molecules.

Polyunsaturated fat *See* Polyunsaturated fatty acid.

Polyunsaturated fatty acid A type of unsaturated fat (liquid at room temperature) that has two or more spots on the fatty acid available for hydrogen (e.g., corn, safflower, and soybean oils).

Portal circulation A circulatory system that takes nutrients directly from the stomach, small intestines, colon, and spleen to the liver.

Portion The amount of a food or beverage consumed by an individual in one sitting.

Positive energy balance A situation when the storage of energy exceeds the amount expended. This state may be achieved by either consuming too many calories or by not expending enough through physical activity.

Positive reinforcement The presentation of a positive stimulus following a desired behavior. This increases the likelihood that the behavior will occur again.

Posterior Toward the back or dorsal side.

Posture The arrangement of the body and its limbs.

Precontemplation The stage of the transtheoretical model of behavioral change during which the individual is not yet thinking about changing.

Prehypertension A systolic pressure of 120 to 139 mmHg and/or a diastolic pressure of 80 to 89 mmHg. Having this condition puts an individual at higher risk for developing hypertension.

Prehypertensive *See* Prehypertension.

Preparation The stage of the transtheoretical model during which the individual is getting ready to make a change.

Product liability insurance Insurance that covers damages occurring due to product failure .

Professional liability insurance Insurance to protect a trainer/instructor against professional negligence or failure to perform as a competent and prudent professional would under similar circumstances.

Progression The systematic process of applying overload. For example, in resistance training, more resistance is added to progress the training stimulus.

Pronation Internal rotation of the forearm causing the radius to cross diagonally over the ulna and the palm to face posteriorly.

Proopiomelanocortin (POMC) An appetite-inhibiting neuron.

Proprioception Sensation and awareness of body position and movements.

Proprioceptive neuromuscular facilitation (PNF) A method of promoting the response of neuromuscular mechanisms through the stimulation of proprioceptors in an attempt to gain more stretch in a muscle; often referred to as a contract/relax method of stretching.

Proprioceptive system A combination of the vestibular (eyes and inner ears), subcutaneous (beneath and within the skin), and kinesthetic (muscles and joints) sensors that enables an individual to determine body position and its movement in space.

Protein A compound composed of a combination 20 amino acids that is the major structural component of all body tissue.

Protraction Scapular abduction.

Provitamin Inactive vitamins; the human body contains enzymes to convert them into active vitamins.

Proximal Nearest to the midline of the body or point of origin of a muscle.

Psychotropic medication Drugs that affect the mental state; capable of modifying mental activity.

Punishment The presentation of aversive stimuli following an undesired behavior. Decreases the likelihood that the behavior will occur again.

Qualified health claims A claim authorized by the U.S. Food and Drug Administration (FDA) that must be supported by credible scientific evidence regarding a relationship between a specific food or food component and a disease or health-related condition.

Range of motion (ROM) The number of degrees that an articulation will allow one of its segments to move.

Rapport A relationship marked by mutual understanding and trust.

Ratings of perceived exertion (RPE) A scale, originally developed by noted Swedish psychologist Gunnar Borg, that provides a standard means for evaluating a participant's perception of exercise effort. The original scale ranged from 6 to 20; a revised category ratio scale ranges from 0 to 10.

Recommended Dietary Allowance (RDA) The levels of intake of essential nutrients that, on the basis of scientific knowledge, are judged by the Food and Nutrition Board to be adequate to meet the known needs of practically all healthy persons.

Registered dietitian (R.D.) A food and nutrition expert that has met the following criteria: completed a minimum of a bachelor's degree at a U.S. accredited university, or other college coursework approved by the Commission on Accreditation for Dietetics Education (CADE); completed a CADE-accredited supervised practice program; passed a national examination; and completed continuing education requirements to maintain registration.

Relapse In behavioral change, the return of an original problem after many lapses (i.e., slips or mistakes) have occurred.

Respondeat superior A legal doctrine wherein the actions of an employee can subject the employer to liability; Latin for "Let the master answer."

Resting heart rate (RHR) The number of heartbeats per minute when the body is at complete rest; usually counted first thing in the morning before any physical activity.

Resting metabolic rate (RMR) The number of calories expended per unit time at rest; measured early in the morning after an overnight fast and at least eight hours of sleep; approximated with various formulas.

Retraction Scapular adduction.

Rheumatoid arthritis An autoimmune disease that causes inflammation of connective tissues and joints.

Ribonucleic acid (RNA) A chemical cousin of deoxyribonucleic acid (DNA), RNA is responsible for translating the genetic code of DNA into proteins; found in the nucleus and cytoplasm of cells.

RICE An immediate treatment for injury: rest, ice, compression, and elevation.

Rider Specific additions to a standard insurance policy.

Risk factor A characteristic, inherited trait, or behavior related to the presence or development of a condition or disease.

Risk management Minimizing the risks of potential legal liability.

Rotation Movement in the transverse plane about a longitudinal axis; can be "internal" or "external."

Royalty A payment made to the owner of a copyright, patent, or trademark in exchange for use of the protected intellectual property; typically a percentage of each sale.

Sagittal plane The longitudinal plane that divides the body into right and left portions.

Satiety A feeling of fullness.

Saturated fat *See* Saturated fatty acid.

Saturated fatty acid A fatty acid that contains no double bonds between carbon atoms; typically solid at room temperature and very stable.

Scoliosis Excessive lateral curvature of the spine.

Scope of practice The range and limit of responsibilities normally associated with a specific job or profession.

Second ventilatory threshold (VT2) A metabolic marker that represents the point at which high-intensity exercise can no longer be sustained due to an accumulation of lactate.

Secretin A hormone that signals the pancreas to produce and secrete bicarbonate to neutralize the stomach acid.

Sedentary Doing or requiring much sitting; minimal activity.

Self-control The control people exert over their thoughts, feelings, and behaviors.

Self-determination theory (SDT) A psychological theory suggesting that people need to feel competent, autonomous, and connected to others in the many domains of life.

Self-efficacy One's perception of his or her ability to change or to perform specific behaviors (e.g., exercise).

Self-efficacy model An explanatory model for predicting initiation and maintenance of health behaviors. This model hypothesizes that all sustained changes in behaviors are mediated by the common mechanism of self-efficacy.

Self-regulation *See* Self-control.

Self-reliance The dependence on one's own powers, capabilities, and resources.

Serotonin A neurotransmitter; acts as a synaptic messenger in the brain and as an inhibitor of pain pathways; plays a role in mood and sleep.

Serving The amount of food used as a reference on the nutrition label of that food; the recommended portion of food to be eaten.

Shaping Designing a new behavior chain, including antecedents and rewards, to encourage a certain behavior, such as regular physical activity.

Shoulder girdle The articulation of the scapula with the thorax.

Simple carbohydrate Short chains of sugar that are rapidly digested.

Small intestine The part of the gastrointestinal system that is the site of the majority of food digestion and absorption.

SMART goals A properly designed goal; SMART stands for specific, measurable, attainable, relevant, and time-bound.

SOAP note A communication tool used among healthcare professionals; SOAP stands for subjective, objective, assessment, and plan.

Social support The perceived comfort, caring, esteem, or help an individual receives from other people.

Social-cognitive theory A behavior-change theory that posits that all health behaviors are goal-driven through anticipation of outcomes.

Society of European Stage Authors and Composers (SESAC) A performing rights organization designed to represent songwriters and publishers and their right to be compensated for having their music performed in public

Socio-ecological model (SEM) A tool that can be used to help the health coach better understand the health behaviors of their clients and more effectively structure behavior-change programs; examines interrelationships between individuals and the environments in which they live and work, as well as the many levels at which individuals are influenced, both in terms of support for healthy behaviors and barriers to improving health behavior.

Sole proprietorship A business owned and operated by one person.

Solid fats and added sugars (SoFAS) SoFAS are added to foods or beverages to make them more appealing, but they also can add a lot of calories. The foods and beverages with SoFAS provide the most empty calories for Americans.

Soluble fiber *See* High-viscosity fiber.

Specific supervision A method of supervision where the worker (or trainee) requires direct involvement of the supervisor (or trainer).

Stability Characteristic of the body's joints or posture that represents resistance to change of position.

Stages-of-change model A lifestyle-modification model that suggests that people go through distinct, predictable stages when making lifestyle changes: precontemplation, contemplation, preparation, action, and maintenance. The process is not always linear.

Standard of care Appropriateness of an exercise professional's actions in light of current professional standards and based on the age, condition, and knowledge of the participant.

Starch A plant carbohydrate found in grains and vegetables.

Static balance The ability to maintain the body's center of mass (COM) within its base of support (BOS).

Static stretch A low-force, long-duration stretch that holds the desired muscles at their greatest possible length for 15 to 30 seconds.

Statute of frauds A contract that must be in writing in order to be enforceable.

Statute of limitations A formal regulation limiting the period within which a specific legal action may be taken.

Steady state Constant submaximal exercise below the lactate threshold where the oxygen uptake is meeting the energy requirements of the activity.

Steady state heart rate (HRss) The point during aerobic endurance exercise where the heart rate will level off (and not continue to rise), assuming the work load remains constant or becomes only slightly more strenuous; the point at which the demands of the active tissues can be adequately met by the cardiovascular system.

Stepped-care model A model of treatment for obesity based on the premise that treatment can be cumulative or incremental.

Stimulant A substance that activates the central nervous system and sympathetic nervous system.

Stimulus control A means to break the connection between events or other stimuli and a behavior; in behavioral science, sometimes called "cue extinction."

Stroke A sudden and often severe attack due to blockage of an artery into the brain.

Stroke volume (SV) The amount of blood pumped from the left ventricle of the heart with each beat.

Sucrose Table sugar; a disaccharide formed by glucose and fructose linked together.

Superior Located above.

Supination External rotation of the forearm (radioulnar joint) that causes the palm to face anteriorly.

Supine Lying face up (on the back).

SWOT analysis Situation analysis in which internal strengths and weaknesses of an organization (such as a business) or individual, and external opportunities and threats are closely examined to chart a strategy.

Syndrome A collection of symptoms and signs indicating a particular disease or condition.

Systolic blood pressure (SBP) The pressure exerted by the blood on the vessel walls during ventricular contraction.

Talk test A method for measuring exercise intensity using observation of respiration effort and the ability to talk while exercising.

Telemetry The process by which measured quantities from a remote site are transmitted to a data collection point for recording and processing, such as what occurs during an electrocardiogram.

Testosterone In males, the steroid hormone produced in the testes; involved in growth and development of reproductive tissues, sperm, and secondary male sex characteristics.

Thermic effect of food (TEF) An increase in energy expenditure due to digestive processes (digestion, absorption, metabolism of food). Also called thermic effect of feeding.

Thermogenesis The process by which the body generates heat from energy production.

Tidal volume The volume of air inspired per breath.

Tolerable Upper Intake Level (UL) The maximal intake of a nutrient that is unlikely to pose risk of adverse health effects to almost all individuals in an age- and gender-specific group.

Total energy expenditure (TEE) Amount of energy expended in a 24-hour period, which includes basal metabolism, physical activity, and dietary-induced thermogenesis.

Trans fats *See* Trans fatty acid.

Trans fatty acid An unsaturated fatty acid that is converted into a saturated fat to increase the shelf life of some products.

Transamination The reversible exchange of amino groups between different amino acids.

Transtheoretical model of behavioral change (TTM) A theory of behavior that examines one's readiness to change and identifies five stages: precontemplation, contemplation, preparation, action, and maintenance. Also called the stages-of-change model.

Transverse plane Anatomical term for the imaginary line that divides the body, or any of its parts, into upper (superior) and lower (inferior) parts. Also called the horizontal plane.

Triacylglycerol Stored triglycerides.

Triadic reciprocal situation A social-cognitive theory that takes into consideration the client's cognitions and behaviors and the environment; posits that all health behaviors are goal-driven through anticipation of outcomes.

Trigger *See* Antecedent.

Triglyceride Three fatty acids joined to a glycerol (carbon and hydrogen structure) backbone; how fat is stored in the body.

Trypsin An enzyme responsible for breaking down proteins into single amino acids or amino acids joined in twos (dipeptides) or threes (tripeptides).

Tumor necrosis factor-alpha A pro-inflammatory protein involved in the acute phase of systemic inflammation.

Type 1 diabetes *See* Type 1 diabetes mellitus (T1DM).

Type 1 diabetes mellitus (T1DM) Form of diabetes caused by the destruction of the insulin-producing beta cells in the pancreas, which leads to little or no insulin secretion; generally develops in childhood and requires regular insulin injections; formerly known as insulin-dependent diabetes mellitus (IDDM) and childhood-onset diabetes.

Type 2 diabetes *See* Type 2 diabetes mellitus (T2DM).

Type 2 diabetes mellitus (T2DM) Most common form of diabetes; typically develops in adulthood and is characterized by a reduced sensitivity of the insulin target cells to available insulin; usually associated with obesity; formerly known as non-insulin-dependent diabetes mellitus (NIDDM) and adult-onset diabetes.

Type I muscle fibers A muscle fiber type designed for use of aerobic glycolysis and fatty acid oxidation, recruited for low-intensity, longer-duration activities such as walking and swimming.

Umbrella liability policy Insurance that provides additional coverage beyond other insurance such as professional liability, home, automobile, etc.

Unsaturated fatty acids Fatty acids that contain one or more double bonds between carbon atoms; typically liquid at room temperature and fairly unstable, making them susceptible to oxidative damage and a shortened shelf life.

Vagal afferent neuron A major nerve that transmits sensory information about the state of the body's organs (including the heart) to the central nervous system.

Valgus Characterized by an abnormal outward turning of a bone, especially of the hip, knee, or foot.

Varus Characterized by an abnormal inward turning of a bone, especially of the hip, knee, or foot.

Vegan A vegetarian that does not consume any animal products, including dairy products such as milk and cheese.

Vegetarian A person who does not eat meat, fish, poultry, or products containing these foods.

Very-low-calorie diet A weight-loss program that consists only of liquid meals, and a calorie content that usually ranges between 420 and 800 kcal/day. VLCDs should only be used when under the care and supervision of a physician.

Vestibular system Part of the central nervous system that coordinates reflexes of the eyes, neck, and body to maintain equilibrium in accordance with posture and movement of the head.

Vicarious liability Legal term meaning that employers are responsible for the workplace conduct of their employees.

Villi Finger-like projections from the folds of the small intestines.

Visceral adiposity *See* Visceral obesity.

Visceral fat *See* Visceral obesity.

Visceral obesity Excess fat located deep in the abdomen that surrounds the vital organs; closely related to abdominal girth. Its accumulation is associated with insulin resistance, glucose intolerance, dyslipidemia, hypertension, and coronary artery disease. Abdominal girth measured at the level of the umbilicus with values ≥40 inches (102 cm) in men and ≥35 inches (89 cm) in women are strong indicators of visceral obesity.

Vitamin An organic micronutrient that is essential for normal physiologic function.

$\dot{V}O_2$max Considered the best indicator of cardiovascular endurance, it is the maximal amount of oxygen (mL) that a person can use in one minute per kilogram of body weight. Also called maximal oxygen uptake and maximal aerobic power.

Waist circumference Abdominal girth measured at the level of the umbilicus; values ≥40 inches (102 cm) in men and ≥35 inches (89 cm) in women are strong indicators of abdominal obesity and associated with an increased health risk.

Waist-to-hip ratio (WHR) A useful measure for determining health risk due to the site of fat storage. Calculated by dividing the ratio of abdominal girth (waist measurement) by the hip measurement.

Waiver Voluntary abandonment of a right to file suit; not always legally binding.

Whey The liquid remaining after milk has been curdled and strained; high in protein and carbohydrates.

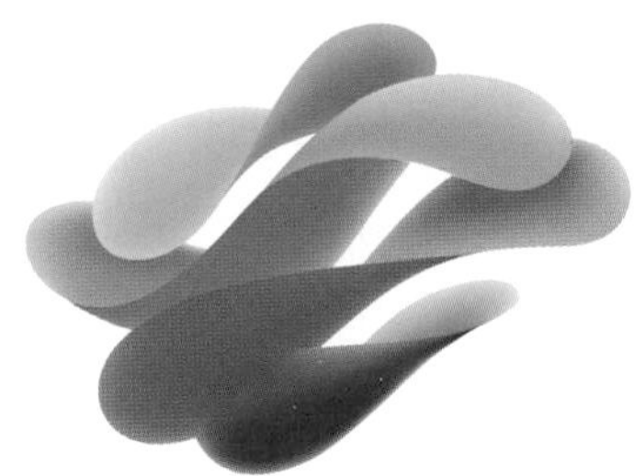

Index

A

B

F

H

I

M

O

P

U